# Advanced
# Pathophysiology

*Application to Clinical Practice*

# Advanced Pathophysiology

## Application to Clinical Practice

**MAUREEN WIMBERLY GROER, RN, MA, MSN, PHD, FAAN, EDITOR**

Associate Dean for Research and Evaluation
University of Tennessee, College of Nursing

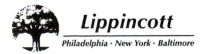

**Lippincott**

*Philadelphia · New York · Baltimore*

*Acquisitions Editor:* Lisa Stead
*Editorial Assistant:* Karin McAndrews
*Project Editor:* Debra Schiff
*Senior Production Manager:* Helen Ewan
*Senior Production Coordinator:* Nannette Winski
*Art Director:* Carolyn O'Brien
*Design:* BJ Crim
*Manufacturing Manager:* William Alberti
*Indexer:* Katherine Pitcoff

Library of Congress Cataloging-in-Publication Data

Advanced pathophysiology : application to clinical practice / [edited by] Maureen Wimberly Groer.
    p.  ; cm.
  Includes bibliographical references and index.
  ISBN 0-7817-2336-1 (alk. paper)
  1. Physiology, Pathological. I. Groer, Maureen Wimberly, 1944-
  [DNLM: 1. Pathology, Clinical—methods—Nurses' Instruction. 2. Primary Health Care—methods—Nurses' Instruction. QY 4 A244 2000]
  RB113 .A385 2000
  616.07—dc21
                                                              00-038467

Care has been taken to confirm the accuracy of the information presented and to describe generally accepted practices. However, the authors, editors, and publisher are not responsible for errors or omissions or for any consequences from application of the information in this book and make no warranty, express or implied, with respect to the content of the publication.

The authors, editors, and publisher have exerted every effort to ensure that drug selection and dosage set forth in this text are in accordance with the current recommendations and practice at the time of publication. However, in view of ongoing research, changes in government regulations, and the constant flow of information relating to drug therapy and drug reactions, the reader is urged to check the package insert for each drug for any change in indications and dosage and for added warnings and precautions. This is particularly important when the recommended agent is a new or infrequently employed drug.

Some drugs and medical devices presented in this publication have Food and Drug Administration (FDA) clearance for limited use in restricted research settings. It is the responsibility of the health care provider to ascertain the FDA status of each drug or device planned for use in his or her clinical practice.

# Dedication

*This book is dedicated to my parents,*

*Floyd and Dorothy Wimberly, who have, throughout my life,*

*inspired, encouraged, and motivated me to*

*question the obvious, search for the hidden, and*

*challenge the limits of my own possibilities.*

# Contributors

**Maria Cabrera,** MSN, RNCS
Family Nurse Practitioner
The Children's Heart Center
Atlanta, Georgia
CHAPTER 16 *Common Gastrointestinal Disorders*

**Laurie Elliot,** RN, MSN, FNPC
Staff Nurse
Ridgeview Psychiatric Hospital and Center
Oakridge, Tennessee
CHAPTER 5 *Behavioral Disorders*

**Ronda Hart,** MSN, RNCS
Family Nurse Practitioner
Morristown-Hamblen Healthcare System
Newport, Tennessee
CHAPTER 11 *Diabetes*

**Timothy L. Jones,** MSN, RNCS
Family Nurse Practitioner
Prompt Family Care
Morristown, Tennessee
CHAPTER 7 *Allergic Rhinitis*
CHAPTER 19 *Common Musculoskeletal Disorders*

**Leslie McQuay Klein,** MSN, RNCS
Family Nurse Practitioner
University Urology
Knoxville, Tennessee
CHAPTER 17 *Common Genitourinary Disorders*
CHAPTER 18 *Menstrual Cycle Disorders and Menopause*

**Marguerite L. Knox,** RN, MSN
Clinical Assistant Professor
University of South Carolina College of Nursing
Columbia, South Carolina
CHAPTER 21 *HIV Disease*

**Mary Kollar,** RNCS, PhD
Coordinator, FNP Concentration
University of Tennessee College of Nursing
Knoxville, Tennessee
CHAPTER 6 *Disorders of the Ear, Nose and Throat*

**Karen Lasater,** MSN, RNCS
University of Tennessee Medical Center
Knoxville, Tennessee
CHAPTER 4 *Dizziness and Headache*
CHAPTER 13 *Arthritis*

**Paula MacMorran,** RN, MSN, PhD
Psychologist/Clinical Specialist in Private Practice
Knoxville, Tennessee
CHAPTER 5 *Behavioral Disorders*

**Carolyn J. Moore,** MSN, RNCS
Nurse Practitioner
Knoxville, Tennessee
CHAPTER 18 *Menstrual Cycle Disorders and Menopause*

**Drema Phelps,** MSN, RNCS
Director of Nursing/FNP
Ironton City Health Department
Ironton, Ohio
CHAPTER 8 *Asthma and Allergies*

**Kenneth D. Phillips,** RN, PhD
Assistant Professor
University of South Carolina College of Nursing
Columbia, South Carolina
CHAPTER 21 *HIV Disease*

**Margaret Pierce,** MSN, MPH, RNCS, AOCN
Assistant Professor
University of Tennessee College of Nursing
Knoxville, Tennessee
CHAPTER 12 *Common Breast Disorders*

**Lisa Pullen,** RN, PhD
Knoxville, Tennessee
CASE STUDY FOR CHAPTER 5 *Behavioral Disorders*

**Penelope Perkey,** MSN, RNCS
Pediatric Nurse Practitioner
Allergy and Asthma Specialists
Knoxville, Tennessee
CHAPTER 5 *Behavioral Disorders*

**Ramona Scott,** MSN, RNCS
Women's Health Nurse Practitioner
Women's Care Group
Knoxville, Tennessee
**CHAPTER 17** *Common Genitourinary Disorders*

**Patricia Coulson Shivers,** PhD, HCLD
Assistant Professor
Pellissippi State Community College
Knoxville, Tennessee
**CHAPTER 10** *Thyroid and Endocrine Disorders*

# Reviewers

**Eileen M. Cerutchlow,** MSN, EdD, FNP, APRN
Associate Professor
Southern Connecticut State University
New Haven, Connecticut
Family Nurse Practitioner
Bridgeport Community Health Center
Bridgeport, Connecticut

**Peggy Ellis,** PhD, RNCS, FNP
Barnes College of Nursing
University of Missouri—St. Louis
St. Louis, Missouri

**Kathryn Fiandt,** ARNP, DNS
Assistant Professor and Coordinator
Family Nurse Practitioner Program
University of Nebraska Medical Center
Omaha, Nebraska

**Thomasine Guberski,** PhD
University of Maryland School of Nursing
Baltimore, Maryland

**Maureen Ryan,** RN, MSN, FNP
Grand Valley State University
Grand Rapids, Michigan

# Preface

This book was written in response to an obvious and significant gap in the educational resources available to teach pathophysiology to primary care health care provider students. The types of disorders seen in primary care patients tend to be vastly different than what is commonly covered in graduate pathophysiology textbooks. There is little available in these books on the pathophysiologic bases of common acute and chronic disorders such as is covered in this book. As a teacher of pathophysiology to graduate nurse practitioner students for nearly 25 years, this gap became more and more of a problem for me and the students. While it was essential that the student understand the health problems seen in primary care practice in much more depth, the books did not sufficiently cover the information, and many additional readings were required. The impetus for writing this book came from these experiences.

The aim of the book is to provide current, in-depth pathophysiology of common health problems. The approach is at genetic, molecular, cellular, tissue and organ levels. The major illnesses that primary care providers will treat are discussed as separate chapters in some cases, such as with diabetes, hypertension, or skin cancer. Other chapters describe common disorders within particular organ systems. The goal is not to be comprehensive, but to nevertheless be sufficiently broad enough to cover the usual, routine, common acute and chronic health problems that a provider would likely see on a regular basis in the office.

The book also seeks to provide a holistic perspective of the ill person. Illness is thus viewed in a multidimensional way, with attention paid to the impact of behavior, personality, stress, and coping on the etiology, progression, and outcome of various illnesses.

# Acknowledgments

The authors wish to acknowledge the many contributions of students at the University of Tennessee, who read versions of the manuscript, provided critiques, and helped with updating information in several areas of the book.

The help and support of Lisa Stead at Lippincott Williams & Wilkins is also acknowledged and much appreciated.

# Contents

## *C H A P T E R* 7

# Allergic Rhinitis 118

Timothy L. Jones

## *C H A P T E R* 8

# Asthma and Other Allergic Disorders 138

Drema Phelps

Maureen Groer

## *C H A P T E R* 9

# Common Respiratory Disorders 153

Maureen Groer

## *C H A P T E R* 10

# Thyroid and Endocrine Disorders 177

Patricia Coulson Shivers

*CHAPTER* **11**

## Diabetes   204

Ronda Hart

*CHAPTER* **12**

## Common Breast Disorders   231

Margaret Pierce

*CHAPTER* **13**

## Arthritis   245

Karen Lasater

Maureen Groer

## OSTEOARTHRITIS   245

*CHAPTER* **16**

## Gastrointestinal and Hepatic Disorders   308

Maria Cabrera

Maureen Groer

*CHAPTER* **17**

## Common Genitourinary Disorders   330

Leslie M. Klein

Ramona Scott

Maureen Groer

*CHAPTER* **18**

## Common Menstrual and Menopausal Disorders   363

Leslie M. Klein

Carolyn J. Moore

# CHAPTER 19

## Common Disorders of the Musculoskeletal System 385

Maureen Groer

Timothy L. Jones

# CHAPTER 20

## Common Hematologic Disorders 402

Maureen Groer

# CHAPTER 21

## HIV Disease 410

Kenneth D. Phillips

Marguerite L. Knox

# CHAPTER *22*

## Alzheimer's Disease   448

Maureen Groer

# Behavioral Processes in Human Illness States

## Maureen Groer

This chapter explores theories of health and illness and suggests approaches for viewing human illnesses and responses to illnesses through a holistic perspective. Primary care providers such as nurse practitioners have unique opportunities to interact with people throughout the life span and at many points along the health–illness continuum. The opportunity exists for providers to view their clients as biopsychosocial individuals interacting with the environment and endowed with unique and particular cultural, developmental, spiritual, social, biologic, and psychological attributes. This requires the provider to move away from a purely medical model of disease and to view illness as only one of many aspects of the person. It also changes the way that providers assess and evaluate the clients under their care. Such an approach requires a new paradigm for both diagnosis and treatment of the common illnesses than is commonly seen in primary care practices.

This text provides data supporting this perspective. While the focus here is on disease mechanisms, we will constantly try to understand the disease *within the human being*. This requires attention to many factors that might influence the occurrence of illness and the expression of disease symptoms. In particular, we examine pathophysiologic mechanisms through a holistic and biobehavioral perspective. Of importance to this approach is an understanding of how stress, mood, behavior, history, personality, and illness interrelate. A foundational area of interest in general pathophysiology is the emerging science of psychoneuroimmunology (PNI), which is described in this chapter and is integrated throughout other chapters as appropriate.

## THE HISTORIC PERSPECTIVE

The commonly accepted approach to patients throughout this century has been termed the *medical model*, and perhaps it has been unfairly castigated, without an appreciation for the origins and history of this approach. In its most negative connotation, the medical model is a paradigm in which patients' symptoms and their illnesses are the entire focus of care. The attention and treatment of the medical condition are the goals of medicine. The fact that the illness is occurring within an incredibly complex organism, the human being, is irrelevant because the goal is to eradicate a disease. Illness is viewed as an independent entity resulting from a single, identifiable cause, which, when discovered, can be treated pharmacologically or with surgery. Thus, in this view, health is the absence of disease. A medical failure occurs when the disease cannot be eliminated or when the patient deteriorates or dies.

The origins of such an approach can be appreciated only within the context of history and philosophy of science. The medical model approach has its origins in the ideas that occurred in the 17th century, which were the result of centuries of changing ideas, scientific discoveries, and historic, political, and religious influences.

Going back to the origins of modern thought, the influence of Aristotle, Plato, and other Greek philosophers remains important. Their fundamentally dualistic metaphysics remains an element of current science and philosophy. There was a physical reality and a separate, illusory, reality of the mind. Thus, for the Greeks, the mind and the body were two separate essences. This dualism continued through the centuries as a pervasive concept and was part of the metaphysical understanding of

Rene Descartes, the founder of modern science and, thus, of modern medicine.

## Cartesian Dualism

Descartes (1596 to 1650) developed a philosophy of science in the 1600s that remains influential. He was strongly influenced by Greek dualism, as well as by the Catholic Church's doctrine of the body as the repository of a spiritual and immortal soul. Descartes claimed that any problem could be broken down into basic elements, which could be isolated and explained by mathematical rules or rational first principles. Deduction was used as the rational approach, deducing all from the most perfect and rational of all—God. Deistic in its underpinnings, Cartesian philosophy assumed that properties of matter were endowed by God at the moment of creation and that the human mind was unable to fathom God's plan. Continuing the Aristotelian tradition, Descartes continued the belief in a fundamental difference in substance between mind and body. In this model, the workings of the mind are without substance, or at least of a different substance than that of inanimate matter: ephemeral, mysterious, and unmeasurable through normal science. However, the physical body was of substance and could be described in terms of rules that govern other inanimate matter in the universe. The material substance of the body was machinelike, composed of divisible parts that operated together and could be broken down into simpler and smaller units. There was no real mystery in the functioning of the body. Even the interaction of the mind and body was considered by Descartes, who proposed that the gateway to the mind was in the physical structure of the pineal gland in the brain. He acknowledged, as did many who followed him, that this mind stuff was able to influence the inanimate body stuff, and thus there had to be some seat of consciousness in the brain through which this interaction was possible. Descartes believed that matter was inert and had to be acted on by an outside influence to move and function. The fundamental problem with dualism is that it leaves the mind and consciousness outside of the realm of science as unknowable and, therefore, produces a dead end to possibilities for discovery about this mind (Dennett, 1991). Further, it does not provide any explanation of how the "ghost in the machine" could be of an unknowable and fundamentally different substance, yet still dramatically and constantly influence the material of the human body.

An outgrowth of Cartesian philosophy is materialism. In this view, the mind and the body are of the same material substance, which fundamentally is made of chemical compounds that behave according to immutable laws of physics. That is, the mind is the brain. Claude Bernard, the father of modern medicine and physiology, used this approach. Bernard legitimized the study of both body and brain but refuted the existence of a mysterious vital force that was independent of the brain.

Materialism, however, does not explain consciousness, which is a fundamental problem. Materialism led medicine to deal only with the aspects of human beings that it could understand and quantify. The mental processes occurring as a consequence of the functioning of the physical substance of the brain were separate phenomena that still retained a mystery. Thus, medicine developed its own type of dualism in which the physical body was understandable in terms of the growing body of knowledge in chemistry and physics; this concept became the focus of medicine. The mind, on the other hand, became the province of psychology, and it too was treated as independent. The mind and the body continued to be considered as separate entities. The problem of the spirit also challenged philosophers and presented a problem for the modern medical model of care. Was there a spirit independent of the physicality of the human mind, or was spirit essentially consciousness and thus dependent on the mind? How could spirit influence the physical body? This problem was even greater than the dilemma of the mind's influence on the body (or vice versa).

## The Medical Model

Materialism led to a reductionist approach to understanding both mind and body, which was useful for the development of medical science. The incredible accumulation of knowledge in the 20th century resulted in a need for medicine to organize, categorize, and reduce information so that it could be manipulated and applied practically. Another important factor was that most of the conditions treated by physicians through nearly the middle of this century were infectious. When it became clear that microbes caused infections, the goal of medical therapy became to discover the cause of the infection and eradicate the microorganisms, thus eliminating the disease and curing the patient. As antibiotics became increasingly available and tailored to be "magic bullets," the reductionist medical model approach was observed to be extremely effective.

In the matter of the mind, modern medicine developed the specialty of psychiatry to deal with mental illness. Freudian and psychoanalytic theories reduced these illnesses to germ theory–like etiologies. The physical health consequences of mental illness or the mental health consequences of physical illness generally were not recognized or treated.

## Modern Diseases

The medical model was successful in the early and middle 20th century. Its problems became more apparent when the nature of the common human illnesses began to change from acute life-threatening infections that killed both young and old to the more chronic, lifestyle-related diseases of the late 20th century. Table 1-1 depicts data on the causes of mortality for adults in the United States. Infectious diseases (pneumonia and influenza) appear on the list, but when the statistics are examined, it becomes apparent that primarily the elderly die of these infections now because they have been compromised by other health problems. The addition of HIV/AIDS to the list of the top 10 leading causes of death in recent years is a cause for concern not only because it is killing young people, but because it represents a new type of infectious illness. HIV is resistant to traditional antimicrobial therapy, is capable of evading the immune system through mutation, and infects macrophages and lymphocytes, destroying the immune system itself.

The diseases that currently are the common causes of mortality are largely multifactorial. Unlike infectious illnesses, a single etiology does not explain these often chronic conditions. Rather, the causes are multiple and interactive, not purely biologic. These diseases are associated with human behavior and habits, social setting, culture, diet, lifestyle, and biology. Therefore, a purely medical model may diagnose and treat symptoms but usually is not effective in reducing incidence, complications, progression, and morbidity. An example of this is atherosclerotic cardiovascular disease (CVD), which results in occlusion of coronary arteries. The medical model approach to a person with angina or a myocardial infarction would be to alleviate the occlusion and increase the perfusion to the myocardium so that the heart functions well. Unfortunately, this approach may produce only short-term positive results if the afflicted person is obese, highly stressed, sedentary, hypertensive, hypercholesterolemic, eats a high-fat diet, or smokes. Primary care providers continually interact with these individuals, often finding themselves frustrated. There seems to be so much that needs to be addressed, time is limited, reimbursement is restricted, the patient is resistant, and the medical model approach will produce a result, even if it is only short term. The other interactive factors must be acknowledged by the patient and require a long-term commitment from both the patient and provider for the necessary, significant behavioral changes, which never are accomplished easily, to take place. In reality, with a purely medical model approach, many of these interacting risks might never even be discovered, particularly if they are behavioral or psychosocial, and almost never if they are related to

---

**TABLE 1.1**

### Ten Leading Causes of Death in 1996

| Rank | Disease | Number of Deaths Annually |
|------|---------|---------------------------|
| 1 | Heart disease | 733,361 |
| 2 | Cancer | 539,533 |
| 3 | Stroke | 160,431 |
| 4 | Chronic obstructive pulmonary disease | 106,027 |
| 5 | Accidents | 94,948 |
| 6 | Pneumonia/influenza | 83,727 |
| 7 | Diabetes | 61,767 |
| 8 | HIV/AIDS | 31,130 |
| 9 | Suicide | 30,903 |
| 10 | Chronic liver disease and cirrhosis | 25,047 |

AIDS, acquired immunodeficiency syndrome; HIV, human immunodeficiency virus.
(From *National vital statistics reports* [1996], Vol. 47, No. 9. Atlanta: Centers for Disease Control. [www.cdc.gov/nchswww/fastats/deaths/htm]).

spiritual distress. The assessment of these nonbiologic factors can be lengthy and tedious; therefore, these factors often are ignored or incompletely addressed in primary care practices.

## HOLISM

A modern philosophic perspective is holism, which in popular parlance means that the whole is believed to be more than the sum of the parts, or that the whole emerges from the interactions of the parts. This also means that the whole cannot be accurately predicted by knowledge of the separate parts. In philosophic terms, it is the view that the parts of a system do not have significance as separate entities but mostly because of their interrelationship with other parts of the system. Another philosophical interpretation is that every person's experience is so unique that no generalizations across people can be made about a particular person's experience. Each person essentially is the center of the universe in that the center of the universe exists simultaneously everywhere. These concepts are applied to every system in existence. In terms of health care, this view is radically different from the medical model. Healing can occur only if the whole is addressed. Further, healing requires that the individual alone define and experience it, not an outsider such as a health care provider. Holism also implies that there is a resonance, or harmony, between the parts that contributes to health and wellness. For humans, the essences that make up the whole usually are considered to be the body, mind, and spirit, which produce the whole through their harmonic interaction. This whole, in a sense, is an indivisible entity because the whole emerges from the parts and never can be fully explained by the sum of the parts.

The implications for the primary care provider are obvious and profound if one ascribes to a holistic perspective. Patients' illnesses are but one expression of the interaction between body, mind, and spirit. Therefore, the provider cannot neglect the whole, even if a biologic disorder is present in the patient. Furthermore, the patient's experience of illness is so unique that generalizations become tentative and even dangerous. Such a model of health requires a different assessment, diagnostic, and treatment paradigm. The popularity of holistic health centers and holistic practitioners of every ilk makes it clear that people crave a holistic approach and often are willing to pay for it out of pocket. Yet, modern medicine tends to disdain holistic health approaches, and clearly the field of holistic health is ridden with charlatanism. Claims that any nontraditional and often untested approach is "holistic" have given the term a negative connotation. True adherence to the philosophical precepts of holism by professionally trained, credible providers would represent a new paradigm of caring and would be a revolution in modern health care.

For some providers, absolute adherence to holism is difficult. One problem is that the time commitment to the patient would increase because of the increased complexity of the assessment and diagnostic processes. At the very least, health care providers would need to pay more attention to the biopsychosocial perspective in dealing with patients. Numerous research studies support the fundamental interconnectedness of biology, behavior, and the social milieu. Understanding the relationship between stress and illness is critical when adopting a more holistic approach to patients and their illnesses. One developing science is the field of PNI. This new interdisciplinary science explains, at least in part, the stress–illness linkage. For years, stress has been implicated as a major risk factor in many human illnesses. PNI provides an explanatory model for how these effects could occur.

## THE STRESS–ILLNESS CONNECTION

The term *stress* has been used in so many ways that it often is difficult to ascertain what is being considered. Physics considers stress to be a demand or strain on the system, and it is reasonable to view human stress in the same conceptual way. In this section, stress is considered to be a psychophysiologic state that results when an individual perceives and reacts to stressors. Stressors, according to the concepts of Lazarus and Folkman (1984), are individualistic and unique. Persons appraise and evaluate stressors as either threats or challenges and then attempt to react appropriately to defend themselves.

In early studies, stress was conceptualized as a nonspecific response to any number and variety of stressors. This view was derived from the ideas of the "father of stress physiology," Dr. Hans Selye. Selye defined *eustress* and *distress*, the former being the normal and necessary challenges that make life interesting, and the latter being the negative, noxious events that provoke a physiologic defense response. He suggests that the stress (distress) response occurs in response to noxious stressors of all types (eg, cold, surgery, anesthesia, exercise) and, once evoked, follows a stereotypic pattern of arousal, resistance, and exhaustion. He also developed the concept of stress-related diseases, postulating that the demands of stress eventually break down the individual's resistance, leading to disease such as heart disease, diabetes, arthritis, and peptic ulcer disease. All of these can be provoked in animals by subjecting them to chronic stressors.

Whereas Selyes' work was foundational to stress research, many of his ideas are incomplete and are being challenged regarding their application to humans. The role of appraisal and coping is now considered important in stress physiology. A person's appraisal of a stressor is dependent on factors such as genetics, social factors, behavioral and personality influences, prior experience, and age. Furthermore, it is becoming clear that an organism responds to different types of stressors in specific ways, and a generalized, stereotypic, nonspecific stress response is not always found.

The physiologic and psychological response to stress generally is considered to be defensive and protective. Acute stressors are sensed through sensory data that are constantly being fed into the brain. This could be information from the special senses such as smell, sound, or vision. It is now known that immunologically processed information (such as neoantigens or microbial antigens) also is stressor information to the hypothalamus. When an event is perceived by the brain to be a stressor, requiring a stress response, an alerting and arousal response that is governed largely by activating the sympathetic nervous system (SNS) occurs (Fig. 1-1). This produces the release of norepinephrine and epinephrine from the adrenal medulla. These catecholamines pour into the body fluids and react with adrenergic receptors on many types of cells (eg, glandular, myocardial, vascular smooth muscle, and immune cells). The effect is to produce the classic "fight or flight" reaction. The heart rate increases, blood pressure rises, pupils dilate, respiratory rate increases, and blood is shunted to the heart, brain, and muscles. Metabolic fuel is made available to provide energy for the stress response. This reaction is almost simultaneous with the application of the stressor, and once the stressor is removed, the individual returns to a baseline state.

Human beings are unique in that they are able to imagine and recall stress states, thereby refueling the stress response, even in the absence of the stressor. The physiologic state that is produced through memory or imagination essentially is the same as the stress response to a real threat.

Hormones that are released during stress states (ie, catecholamines, glucocorticoids, vasopressin, prolactin) are defensive factors that allow the

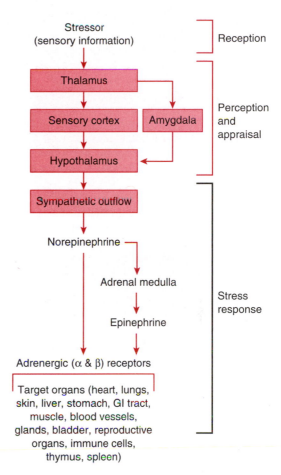

**FIGURE 1.1** ● The acute stress response.

organisms to respond physiologically or psychologically to the perceived stressor. Most stress responses that people elaborate are appropriate, and the physiologic changes they provoke probably are not major factors in human illness. For example, the acute arousal response that occurs when a person is suddenly threatened—as might occur when driving along the highway and another automobile suddenly maneuvers in a way to increase the driver's sense of danger—is a helpful reaction. People see, think, and act quickly and efficiently in responding to the threat, and once the threat is over, a baseline condition is resumed. It is inappropriate stress responsiveness, hypervigilant states, or chronic distress states that seem to be etiologic factors in disease.

*Stress reactivity* is a term used to define an individual who overreacts to stressors, who reacts excessively to perceived or imagined threat, or who is hypervigilant, producing greater sympathetic outflow than what might be ordinarily be expected for an appropriate response. Hypervigilance is a state characterized by chronically elevated levels of catecholamines, often associated with behavioral states of anxiety, anger, and hostility. This type of overactive sympathetic neural reactivity could lead to disease in several ways. It could produce pathophysiologic changes by exposing the organs and vasculature to repeated bursts of stress hormones; by resetting normal set points for physiologic regulators such as baroreceptors; by altering blood lipids, energy stores, and fat distribution; and by changing endocrine receptor responsiveness.

Chronic stress seems to be important in several disease mechanisms, and human beings experience chronic distress in numerous ways. Caring for an elderly, handicapped, or demented loved one is a major chronic human stressor. Poverty, prejudice, injustice, unfulfilling work, marital unhappiness, oppression, chronic illness, and any experience that is marked by feelings of helplessness and hopelessness can lead to chronic distress. Daily irritations and annoyances can become hassles that accumulate and lead to chronic stress. Ultimately, chronic stress is a burden that produces enormous physiologic and psychological costs. The hypothalamic-pituitary-adrenal (HPA) axis is chronically activated in this type of stress state, and the high levels of adrenocorticotropic hormone (ACTH), corticotropin releasing hormone (CRH), and glucocorticoids may produce pathophysiologic damage. Additionally, the immune system can become seriously suppressed, resulting in infections, cancer, atopy, and autoimmune diseases.

## History of Stress Research

The historic background to understanding the stress–illness link comes from a variety of studies. The predictive value of life events requiring social readjustment and morbidity and mortality were described in 1975 (Rahe, 1975), and, for many years, much of the stress–illness research focused on accumulated stressors, such as life events, causing illness and death. However, the strength of the relationship between life events and death was small, and much of the variance could be attributed to other factors such as age, socioeconomic status, and illness (Schlesinger & Yodfat, 1996). Personality began to be viewed as a moderating variable. Kobasa, Maddi, and Kahn (1982) introduced the concept of hardiness after studying stress and work, suggesting that people who view their work as challenging, experience control over their lives, and feel a sense of commitment to their work are stress hardy and therefore are able to

resist the effects of stressors in their lives. Other personality factors began to be discovered as risk factors for CVD and cancer. Lazarus and Folkman (1984) introduced a critical mediator between stress and illness—coping. Their ideas continue to be important: that stressors are perceived and appraised before the organism "decides" whether to produce a stress response. The moderating variables in coping efficacy include social support, life experience, and age. Social support has been found in many studies to be an important buffer between stress and illness.

Thus, the relationship between stress and illness is extraordinarily complex, even more complex in the human being compared with the laboratory rat.

Table 1-2 depicts possible stress-associated diseases based on several epidemiologic and experimental studies.

## Individual Differences

This chapter has alluded to the fact that people are unique in their assessment and responsiveness to stressors. These individual differences arise because each person's unique biologic, psychological, sociologic, and spiritual natures are translated into neuroendocrine and neurochemical differences that interplay with the environment in causing disease. Personality consists of fairly stable traits across a person's life span and is known to play a role in disease mechanisms. Anger and hostility are examples of personality traits that are influential in the etiology of CVD. The relationship between the type A personality pattern and CVD is known to be largely related to the *hostility* aspect of type A pattern. In particular, high scores on *cynical hostility* are associated with increased CVD mortality (Almada et al., 1991).

A distinction is made in *defense* versus *defeat* reactions to stress in the personality factors that play an important role in disease etiology (Ely, 1995). A defense reaction is an active response that might be pathophysiologic in that it could be associated with intense and excessive hostile mood states, which could increase the activity of the SNS. Highly hostile individuals view events through a lens of distrust and cynicism and react to environmental perturbations as if they were major threats.

Defeat reactions are passive responses characterized, at least in animal studies, by hopelessness and helplessness in the face of stressor application. When laboratory animals are subjected to experiments in which they always experience defeat, such as through inescapable shocks, they develop

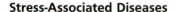

## TABLE 1.2

### Stress-Associated Diseases

| Disease/System | Mechanism |
| --- | --- |
| Cardiovascular disease | |
|    Myocardial infarction | Can be precipitated by acute stressor |
|    Coronary artery disease | Associated with hostility/anger; stress can accelerate atherosclerosis through effects on lipids, platelets |
|    Hypertension | Sympathetic hyperreactivity may lead to vascular and baroreceptor changes |
| Malignancy | Emotional suppression (especially anger) may play a role |
| | Chronic stress may increase risk of malignancy through immunosuppressive effects |
| Gastrointestinal disease | |
|    Gastritis and peptic ulcer disease | Associated with acute stress in animals; association with human stress made famous by the "executive monkey" experiments |
|    Inflammatory bowel disease | Major life events associated with exacerbation; ulcerative colitis associated with personality factors such as helplessness |
| Allergy/asthma/autoimmunity | Acute stress exacerbates asthma, eczema |
| | Relationship of life stress with symptoms of rheumatoid arthritis |
| Reproductive system | Amenorrhea common in stress |
| Musculoskeletal system | Tension headaches |
| | Low back pain |
| Viral infections | Relationship between stress and reactivation of latent viruses such as herpes |
| | Increased incidence of colds in stress |

"learned helplessness"; they come to expect constant defeat. Learned helplessness behaviors in laboratory rats resemble the symptoms found in human depression. Helplessness and hopelessness are factors in morbidity. In a study of 2428 men, those who had high hopelessness scores compared with men with low hopelessness scores were at three times the risk for violent death and had an increased risk for myocardial infarction and cancer (Everson et al., 1996).

Pessimism, fatalism, and depression are related dispositional states that also may influence morbidity. High levels of fatalism were associated with decreased survival in AIDS patients (Reed et al., 1994).

Another personality trait is that of emotional suppression, in which people do not express emotions or often do not recognize the experience of the emotion. Anger suppression, in particular, has been studied in relationship to cancer. A personality subtype has been identified, the type C personality, characterized by extreme emotional suppres-

sion and an unfailingly "pleasant" but ultimately pathologic niceness. Several studies show a high occurrence of these personality characteristics, particularly anger suppression, in patients with breast cancer.

These individual differences in stress response and disease morbidity risk can be explained partly through the influence of the immune system.

## PSYCHONEUROIMMUNOLOGY

A large and growing body of research suggests that there is a strong association between stress and altered immune function. The field of research identified with this association is termed *psychoneuroimmunology*. PNI is a new field of inquiry. The recognition that the immune system is not autonomous and is connected to other systems has been recent. In the beginning, when data were scant, this idea was met with skepticism by most of modern medicine. However, accumulated data over the last 20 years support the concepts of PNI at the molecular level and are convincing. Mood, behaviors, personality, stress, and coping ultimately are understood in biochemical changes that impact the integrated organism.

There appears to be a relationship between stress and immunity that differs, depending on the type and nature of the stressor, as well as which of the various cells and molecules comprising the immune system are studied. Evidence suggests that certain arms of the immune system are upregulated during acute stress, but chronic stress is most detrimental to immune function, particularly cellular immune and natural killer (NK) cell function. This makes teleologic sense in that the immune response thus would be activated to deal with the potential for injuries and wounding that might occur as a consequence of an acute threat situation with an aggressor. Chronic stress, on the other hand, does not result in helpful, adaptive responses and clearly is a threat to the survival of the organism (Fig. 1-2).

There are several multidirectional pathways through which the nervous, endocrine, and immune systems communicate with each other. The immune organs (lymph nodes, spleen, thymus and liver) are innervated by the SNS, and immune cells have receptors for neurotransmitters on their cell membranes. In some ways, the immune system acts like a giant neuroendocrine web that is able not only to receive neurologic and endocrine input, but also is able to elaborate cytokines and chemokines that can communicate with the nervous and endocrine systems. Cross-talk occurs between all of the systems in emotional states, during stress responses, and in the normal course of antigen recognition and response. The immune system, like the brain, is capable of memory, learning, and conditioning. Thus, stress may produce its immunologic effects through neurochemical and neuroendocrine pathways to the immune system. Once the immune system is compromised in any way, the risk for disease increases. The interactions between the nervous, immune, and endocrine systems are depicted in Figure 1-3.

Depressed immunity may increase risk for cancer, infectious illnesses, and atopic and autoimmune diseases. Stress, of course, also interferes with other systems, producing cardiovascular, neurologic, hormonal, and endocrine effects, which may contribute to disease risk. A meta-analysis of studies measuring stress and immune function found that 38 studies showed a decrease in mitogen responsiveness and NK cell activity with stress (Herbert & Cohen, 1993). CD4 and CD8 cells also generally decreased in number, and antibody titers to herpesviruses (indicating decreased suppression of antibody-secreting plasma cells and potential for latent virus reactivation) increased.

Chronic stress paradigms have been used in numerous animal studies, frequently producing immunosuppression. Stress may result in psychological depression, or depression itself, particu-

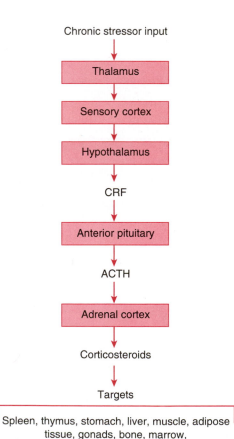

**FIGURE 1.2** ● The hypothalamic-hypophyseal-adrenocortical axis.

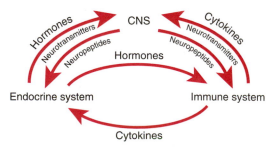

**FIGURE 1.3** ● Interactions among nervous, endocrine, and immune systems.

larly clinical depression, may act as a chronic stressor and be associated with activation of the HPA axis, causing increased secretion of CRH, ACTH, and glucocorticoids. There is evidence for chronic elevation of the stress hormones of the HPA axis in depression, anorexia nervosa, sexually abused women, alcoholics, drug and alcohol withdrawal, exercise, and malnutrition (Stratakis & Chrousos, 1995). The HPA axis likely is influential in producing the immune alterations that often are measured in depression: decreased cellular and humoral immunity, decreased response to mitogens, and decreased NK cell activity. Chronically stressed caregivers of patients with Alzheimer's disease have been studied and found to be immunosuppressed, with deficits such as higher antibody titers to latent herpes simplex and poorer specific T cell responses (Glaser & Kiecolt-Glaser, 1997). Kiecolt-Glaser, et al. (1996) discovered a poorer response to influenza vaccine in caregivers for patients with Alzheimer's disease than in controls. In another study (Pike et al., 1997), subjects reporting high levels of chronic stress were compared with controls reporting low levels and were found to differ in response to an acute laboratory stress challenge. Specifically, stressed subjects had higher epinephrine levels, a protracted decline in NK cell function, and a redistribution of NK cells.

Wound healing may be impaired by stress in both animals and humans. This has been measured in rodent models using restraint stress and in humans using wounds or punch biopsy. Generally, the time for tissue healing is lengthened in acute and chronic stress states.

The mechanisms through which stress impairs immune function are mediated particularly through the glucocorticoids. The cells most sensitive to glucocorticoids are a subpopulation of T

helper (Th) cells and the NK cells. The Th cell population normally differentiates from naive Th cells on antigen processing and presenting by antigen-presenting cells (APCs) such as macrophages and B cells. The direction of differentiation is in either the $T_H1$ or $T_H2$ cell direction, depending on the type of APC and the presence of various co-stimulatory molecules. The $T_H1$ population releases proinflammatory cytokines, such as interleukin-2(IL-2), interferon-gamma (IFN-$\gamma$), and IL-12. These cytokines generally increase cell-mediated or delayed hypersensitivity reactions, promoting the activation of CD8 (cytotoxic/suppressor cells). The $T_H2$ cells elaborate proimmune cytokines such as IL-4, IL-6, and IL-10, which increase the humoral immune response by stimulating B cell responses. In healthy, immunocompetent persons, a state of equilibrium or balance exists between the $T_H1$ and $T_H2$ cells and cytokines. In general, stress associated with elevated levels of glucocorticoids shifts the $T_H1$–$T_H2$ balance toward $T_H2$-dominant immune responsiveness by suppressing the $T_H1$ response. A change in the homeostatic balance between $T_H1$ and $T_H2$ immunity, therefore, could increase the risk for viral infection in particular, since cell-mediated cytotoxicity is mostly responsible for attacking and killing virally infected cells. It also would decrease the ability of cytotoxic cells to recognize and lyse cancer cells. These effects are illustrated in Figure 1-4.

An important observation is that the immune effects of stress are most pronounced in individuals who already are immunocompromised. This includes the elderly, who have diminished T cell responsiveness; children, who are still developing memory and expansion of immune clones; immunosuppressed persons, such as cancer or transplant patients; and immunodeficient persons, such as individuals with AIDS. Interventions to

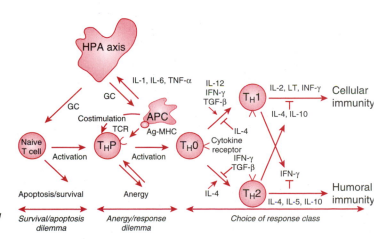

**FIGURE 1.4** ● T-helper cell differentiation. (From F. Hirsch and G. Kroemer [1998]. The immune system and immune modulation. In T. Kresina [Ed.], *Immune modulating agents.* New York: Marcel Dekker.)

reduce stress and improve coping, therefore, are more likely to improve immune function in these populations.

## CONCLUSION

This chapter provides historic background for the development of the medical model of illness care and advocates a newer approach, a holistic model of care. We have argued that human illnesses ordinarily encountered by primary care providers are multifactorial, encompassing biologic, psychological, social, and spiritual realms. We also provide evidence supporting a relationship between stress and illness that mandates providers to consider illness within a holistic paradigm. Finally, evidence is provided that PNI provides support for the more holistic concepts of illness and that the immune system may play a role in much of human disease. Throughout this book, these interactions and relationships are explored as the pathophysiologic mechanisms of the common illnesses generally diagnosed and managed by practitioners in primary care settings are described.

## REFERENCES

Almada, S., Zonderman, A., & Shekelle, R. (1991). Neuroticism and cynicism and risk of death in middle-aged men. *Psychosomatic Medicine 45*, 109–114.

Dannet, D.C. (1991). *Consciousness explained*. Boston: Little Brown & Co.

Ely, D.L. (1995). Organization of cardiovascular and neurohumoral responses to stress: Implications for health and disease. *Annals of the New York Academy of Sciences, 771*, 594–608.

Everson, S.A., Goldberg, D.E., Kaplan, G.A., Cohen, R.D., Pukkala, E., Tuomilehto, J., & Salonen, J.T. (1996). Hopelessness and risk of mortality and incidence of myocardial infarction and cancer. *Psychosomatic Medicine, 58*, 113–121.

Glaser, R. & Kiecolt-Glaser, J. (1997). Chronic stress modulates the virus-specific immune response to latent herpes simplex virus type 1. *Annals of Behavioral Medicine, 19*, 78–82.

Herbert, T.B. & Cohen, S. (1993). Stress and immunity in humans: A meta-anlytical review. *Psychosomatic Medicine, 55*, 364–379.

Hirsch, F. & Kroemer, G. (1998). The immune system and immune modulation. In T. Kresina (Ed.), *Immune modulating agents*. New York: Marcel Dekker.

Kiecolt-Glaser, J., Dura, J., Speicher, C., Trask, O., & Glaser, R. (1991). Spouse caregivers of dementia victims: Longitudinal changes in immunity and health. *Psychosomatic Medicine, 53*, 345–362.

Kiecolt-Glaser, J., Glaser, R., Gravenstein, S., Malarkey, W., & Sheridan, J. (1996). Chronic stress alters the immune response to influenza virus vaccine in older adults. *Proceedings of the National Academy of Science, 93*(7), 3043–3047.

Kobasa, S., Maddi, S., & Kahn, S. (1982). Hardiness and health: A prospective study. *Journal of Personality and Social Psychology, 24*, 168–177.

Lazarus, R.S. & Folkman, S. (1984). *Stress: Appraisal and coping*. New York: Springer.

McEwen, B. & Stellar, E. (1993). Stress and the individual. *Archives of Internal Medicine, 153*, 2093–2101.

Pike, J., Smith, T., Hauger, R., Nicassio, P., Patterson, T., McClintick, J., Costlow, C., & Irwin, M. (1997). Chronic life stress alters sympathetic, neuroendocrine, and immune responsivity to an acute psychological stressor in humans. *Psychosomatic Medicine, 59*, 447–457.

Rahe, R.H. (1975). Life events and near-future reports. In L. Levi (Ed.), *Emotions: Their parameters and measurement*. New York: Raven Press.

Reed, G.M., Kemeny, M., Taylor, S., et al. (1994). "Realistic acceptance" as a predictor of decreased survival time in gay men with AIDS. *Health Psychology, 13*, 299–307.

Scheier, M. & Bridges, M. (1995). Person variables and health: Personality predispositions and acute psychological states as shared determinants for disease. *Psychosomatic Medicine, 57*, 255–268.

Schlesinger, M. & Yodfat, Y. (1996). Psychoneuroimmunology, stress and disease. In H. Friedman, T. Klein, & A. Friedman (Eds.), *Psychoneuroimmunology, stress and infection*. Boca Raton, FL: CRC Press.

Stratakis, C. & Chrousos, G. (1995). Neuroendocrinology and pathophysiology of the stress system. *Annals of the New York Academy of Science, 771*, 118.

# Pathophysiologic Processes in Infectious Illnesses

## Maureen Groer

Infectious illnesses comprise most of patients' visits to primary care practitioners. Although antibiotics are readily available to treat bacterial infections, a surprising statistic is that worldwide mortality from infectious diseases increased by 58% from 1980 to 1992. Whereas most infections are self-limiting, more virulent infections occur and need to be recognized. The occurrence or reoccurrence in the 1980s of acquired immunodeficiency syndrome (AIDS) and tuberculosis reminds us to not be complacent about infectious disease. Additionally, novel influenza viruses pose threats to humans, as exemplified by an outbreak of avian influenza in Hong Kong in late 1997 by a strain (H5N1) not previously known to infect humans. The threat of emerging infectious illnesses is addressed by the Centers for Disease Control and can be read about at *http://www.cdc.gov/ncidod/ publications/eid_plan/about.htm.*

In aged, immunocompromised, or debilitated patients, even mild infections can become serious and possibly life threatening. Upper respiratory and gastrointestinal infections are the most common types in primary care practice, with skin and urinary tract infections also occurring frequently. An in-depth understanding of the pathophysiologic mechanisms underlying infection provides a solid basis for assessment, diagnosis, and management of patients with infections. This chapter covers the role of the nonspecific inflammatory mechanisms and immune defense processes that occur during acute and chronic infections and provides two case studies that illustrate aspects of these processes. Infection results when these normal nonspecific and specific defenses fail.

## MICROBIAL FACTORS

The infectiousness of a microorganism depends on both microbial and host factors. Whereas the remainder of this chapter focuses on the host response, the range of microbial factors that influence the inflammatory and immune responses of the host is discussed here. Microorganisms have varying *virulence* in the human host, with mild effects from organisms such as the common rhinovirus, or extreme effects caused by a virus from the same family, the poliovirus. Virulence is a characteristic of the microbe, but even a common cold in an immunocompromised host may lead to serious illness. Another variable is dosage, with virulent organisms often being dangerous in small quantities because of their extreme pathogenicity. However, in general, the higher the dosage of infective microorganism, the larger the host response. Portal of entry of the microorganisms also is a point to be considered. Another factor that determines host response is organ preference: some microbes have a natural predilection for certain types of tissues. Thus, mumps virus infects parotid gland and testicular epithelia, poliovirus infects the motor neuron cell bodies, and rhinoviruses infect nasal mucosa.

### Host Susceptibility

Numerous host factors influence susceptibility to infection, including age, immunity, genetics, nutrition, preexisting disease, health habits such as drug use or smoking, concomitant infections with other agents, and psychological factors (Kaslow & Evans, 1997). This chapter focuses on immune and inflammatory function in response to infectious agents, but the primary care provider must be aware of the multidimensional, cultural, and environmental influences on both risk and pathophysiologic mechanisms of infection.

## Mucocutaneous Barriers to Microorganisms

There are many ways that the body protects itself against the penetration of virulent pathogens and several ways that microorganisms are destroyed if they successfully overcome the barriers. The mucocutaneous linings that separate the internal from the external environments are obvious physical barriers but also act biochemically to destroy microorganisms. The secretions of oil glands inhibit microbial penetration, and the surface of the skin consists of five to seven layers of cells, with the top layer of squamous cells constantly being shed from the body's surface. The mucous membranes, which line orifices that are open to the environment, are part of a common mucosal immune system that acts specifically through secretion of secretory immunoglobulin A (IgA) into the mucosal fluids produced by these membranes. Mucus itself traps microorganisms, and there are many important, nonspecific molecules that are defensive and powerful bacteriostatic agents in mucus and liquid secretions such as saliva. Included in this group are lactoferrin, which binds iron and thus removes an important factor in some bacterial growth. Lysozyme also is present in mucosal secretions and acts in a bactericidal manner. Antiadhesive molecules prevent the attachment of microbes to the luminal epithelium of mucosal membranes. Molecules released by epithelial cells that have been damaged by infection initiate inflammatory responses that act to contain and resolve infections. Also, a *normal flora* in the gastrointestinal tract and vagina is protective against pathogenic invasions. The normal flora is physiologically part of the host but also colonizes the gut and vagina so as to compete with pathogens for nutrients, and usually the normal flora has a competitive advantage over pathogens. Pathophysiologic factors in these sites include eradication of the balance between normal flora and pathogens from antibiotic therapy. Then, superinfection with organisms normally held in check may occur.

Pathophysiologic factors that impair nonspecific defenses in the respiratory tract, a site of most human infections, include loss of ciliary activity, which may occur in viral infection or from irritating stimuli such as cigarette smoke, drugs, and airway obstruction.

These mechanisms are part of the nonspecific defenses and may destroy microbes even before a specific immune response is needed. However, as human defenses have evolved, microorganisms also have mutated and adapted to our defenses, and have many ways to thwart their destruction. They may elaborate coatings or capsules, release toxins that destroy defense molecules, evade attachment by inflammatory and immune cells, and develop latent or hidden states in which they are protected within the host's cells and cannot be recognized as dangerous.

## INFLAMMATORY MECHANISMS

Once microorganisms invade tissue, they act in different ways to cause infection. Viruses require living cells and invade cells for which they have a proclivity, using the nucleic acid of the cells to synthesize viral proteins and replicate themselves. Usually, unless the virus remains in a latent or chronic state, the virally infected cells are destroyed. Bacteria act differently to cause cell death by producing toxins that chemically destroy cells. In either case, when microbes kill cells, the result is cellular damage, debris, and necrosis. These are the most important signals, launching an acute inflammatory response. The goal of this response is to contain the infection, walling it off when possible, to dilute and destroy the offending microorganisms, to clean up and excavate the site of inflammation, and, ultimately, to produce healing. Usually, the nonspecific cellular response elements are the initial responders, followed by immune cellular elements.

## Exudate and Cellular Infiltration

Dead and dying cells activate inflammatory mechanisms. Many assaults on the body produce cell damage and death, some of which provoke immune and others, nonimmune, responses. Whereas inflammation is a normal and protective response, it can lead to morbidity and mortality. In some situations, the inflammation becomes a chronic state and ultimately harms the host. When acute, inflammation produces classic signs: rubor (redness), dolor (pain), calor (increased temperature), edema, and decreased function. These signs are produced by vascular and cellular events that typify the inflammatory response.

The initial signals of cell damage and death must take place in vascular tissue for an inflammatory response to occur. Vessels carry blood that supplies cells, important biochemical response molecules, and protein-rich fluid to the site of injury. In turn, inflamed cells secrete molecules that act on the supplying arterioles, capillaries, and venules. Vasodilatation, increased capillary permeability, development of an inflammatory exudate, and migration of leukocytes to the site of inflammation characterize the early stage of inflammation, as illustrated in Figure 2-1. Vasodilatation produces an increase in capillary hydrostatic pressure, which increases Starling forces, favoring net filtration out of the capillaries and into the interstitial fluid spaces. Capillary permeability is increased through the action of molecules released at the site of inflammation. Tissue cells that are damaged may leak mediators, and tissue macrophages and mast cells also are believed to be important early responders to damaged cells and debris produced by necrotic cells. The major vasodilator of inflammation is histamine, which is released by tissue mast cells in response to signals from the damaged cells. Histamine acts on $H_1$ receptors on the endothelium of postcapillary venules, causing the release of prostacyclin and nitric oxide. Histamine also acts on capillary endothelium to widen *gap junctions* between adjacent cells, thus markedly increasing the permeability of the capillary. These effects lead to exudate and tissue edema. An additional effect of histamine is the stimulation of P-selectin and platelet activating factor (PAF) on venule endothelium, a process that produces a stickiness on the endothelium, causing neutrophils to roll along the wall and ultimately to bind to endothelial cells. This is a necessary step before they can physically squeeze through the vessel lining into the tissues.

Mast cells are present throughout tissues, possibly arising from the basophils of the blood. They are essential components of other aspects of the inflammatory response. Granules containing a variety of inflammatory mediators are present within the mast cell's cytoplasm, and when appropriately stimulated, these cells release the granules' contents to the outside extracellular fluid, a process known as *degranulation*. Histamine is one of the many mediators contained within the granules of mast cells. Other mediators include leukotrienes, various chemotactic factors, and prostaglandins, which promote inflammation in a variety of ways. Prostaglandins and leukotrienes act on vascular endothelium, and chemotactic factors attract leukocytes from the blood into the inflamed tissue. Both prostaglandins and leukotrienes are produced from a common precursor, cell membrane lipid, which is acted on by the enzyme phospholipase $A_2$. Basophils and mast cells also are important in immune responsiveness because they have Ig receptors on their cell membranes, which allows them to physically transport Ig molecules through the blood and tissues.

Although the resident tissue macrophages and mast cells are important in the response to cell damage and death, these cells are down-regulated under normal circumstances. Resident cells become activated during the course of inflammation. In an inflammatory response, blood leukocytes migrate to the site, increasing in concentration and acting locally. This occurs by a process of *chemotaxis* in which proinflammatory chemoattractant chemicals released at the inflamed site cause migration of leukocytes into the tissue. In larger doses, these molecules also stimulate various aspects of leukocyte function such as bactericidal activity and production of the oxidative burst (see later section, "Neutrophils").

Generally, the cells observed emigrating into inflamed tissue are neutrophils and monocytes, some eosinophils and basophils, and occasional lymphocytes (these occur later in the course of inflammation and are associated more with chronic inflammation). Neutrophils enter the site early, digest microorganisms and cell debris, and die soon thereafter, sometimes within hours. The next cell type is the monocyte. Monocytes migrate from the blood, become activated as macrophages, and are phagocytic, ingesting neutrophils and other cells and debris, but typically they do not die and may even divide. Major chemotactic agents for neutrophils and macrophages, which are the usual cells that migrate into inflamed tissue, include bacterial formylpeptides, one of the complement cascade components (C5a), leukotriene

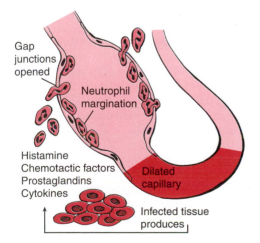

**FIGURE 2.1** ● Inflammation provokes vasodilatation, increased blood flow, increased exudate, and neutrophil emigration.

B4, PAF, and interleukin-8(IL-8) (Snyderman & Uhing, 1992). Low concentrations of these chemoattractants diffuse from the local site or are produced by endothelial cells and macrophages to act on leukocytes that have emigrated from the capillary blood. Chemoattractants act by increasing or mobilizing intracellular calcium ions, which then affect intercellular concentrations of other ions, intracellular pH, motility, superoxide production, degranulation, and aggregation.

For the neutrophils and monocytes to migrate from the blood into the tissue, several events occur within the capillary. First, because of histamine and other molecules that increase the permeability of the capillary endothelium, the enlarging gap junctions provide openings large enough for cells to emigrate from the blood vessels. Second, molecules that make the endothelium sticky and attract neutrophils to the luminal surface are expressed, causing *margination* of the leukocytes. These cells move to the outside of the column of blood through the capillary, change shape, and express *L-selectins*, which bind to endothelial cells and cause the neutrophils to stick to the walls, lying flat against the walls in a phenomenon known as *pavementing,* particularly against the side of the vessel closest to the site of inflammation. This step precedes the actual emigration of the cells into the extracellular tissue space. The increased vascular permeability allows more than cells to move out of the blood. Blood hydrostatic pressure is increased because of vasodilatation, and capillary permeability also is increased, so fluid and proteins exude through the capillary membrane into the tissue space along with the cellular emigration. This produces an inflammatory exudate rich in proteins and cells, which is the hallmark of an acute inflammatory locus, and which is responsible for edema occurring at the site.

## Neutrophils

The first cell type to be chemically attracted to an inflammatory site is the neutrophil (Fig. 2-2). Numerous neutrophils leave the blood and concentrate within inflamed tissue in the first hours after the tissue damage has occurred. Neutrophils are extremely phagocytic, nonspecific responders to the cellular damage that initiates the inflammatory response. Their only function is to be *professional phagocytes*, and they are efficient. On reaching the inflamed site, they become phagocytic and secretory. Their secretions are the products of phagolysosomal digestion.

Neutrophils have a short life span within inflamed tissue (about 48 hours), undergoing mor-

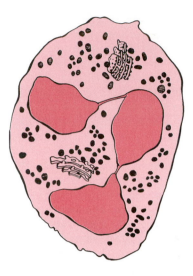

**FIGURE 2.2**   ●   The neutrophil.

phologic changes and, in severe inflammations, ultimately lysing and releasing their intracellular constituents. The death of the neutrophils also is related to the acid pH and higher temperature at the inflamed site. The emigration of neutrophils reaches its peak at 6 to 12 hours after inflammation has begun and then declines as the monocyte/macrophage becomes the dominant blood cell.

When neutrophils are actively phagocytic, a burst of metabolic activity accompanied by increased oxygen consumption, the *oxidative burst*, produces short-lived oxygen free radicals, which are capable of damaging biologic materials through oxidation or halogenation. Included in this group of oxygen metabolites are $OH-$, $H_2O_2$, and $HOCl$. Figure 2-3 illustrates the formation of these products in a phagocytic neutrophil and their effects on cells.

Damaging lysosomal enzymes are produced through non–oxygen-requiring metabolic pathways, and these also contribute to the breaking down of cells and biologic material at the inflamed site. Included are enzymes such as elastase and collagenase, which excavate damaged tissue in preparation for healing.

The monocyte, which becomes a macrophage when it migrates into tissue from the blood, begins to reach high concentration at the site as the neutrophil concentration declines by 24 hours. In fact, macrophages destroy old neutrophils at the site. The macrophage remains the major cell type during the second phase of inflammation. These cells reach their peak around 5 days after the initiation of inflammation. Macrophages are phagocytic, but also intensely secretory, and function as

## RESPIRATORY (OXIDATIVE) BURST

A

$$O_2 + e \xrightarrow{\text{NADPH oxidase}} O_2^{\bar{\cdot}} \longrightarrow \text{Toxic to biological molecules}$$

Oxygen accepts electron forming superoxide anion

B

$$O_2^{\bar{\cdot}} + O_2^{\bar{\cdot}} \xrightarrow{\text{superoxide dismutase}} O_2 + H_2O_2 \longrightarrow \text{Germicidal}$$

Two superoxide anions react to form hydrogen peroxide

C

$$Cl^- + H_2O_2 \xrightarrow{\text{myeloperoxidase}} HOCL + OH^- \longrightarrow \text{Germicidal}$$

Hydrogen peroxide reacts with chloride to form hypochloric acid

**FIGURE 2.3** ● Examples of highly reactive oxygen free radicals and $H_2O_2$ formation during the oxidative burst. These products are extremely toxic and damaging, and are released into the phagolysosome where phagocytosed.

the major surveillance cell that processes and presents antigen to the immune system.

## Phagocytosis

When tissue is invaded by microbial agents, professional phagocytes in tissue and from the blood are mobilized to actively destroy infected cells and microbes through phagocytosis. Phagocytosis is an active, energy-requiring mechanism in which cells first migrate toward the microbes through chemotaxis. It is facilitated by *opsonization* of the particles to be ingested, in which a coating of complement or antibody is layered onto the microorganisms, which makes them easier to be recognized; the microorganisms then are bound to cells and engulfed. Specific receptors on phagocytic cells bind the particles to the cell before it is internalized and digested. The cell then extends pseudopodia on either side of the particle, a process requiring actin, the same protein involved in muscle contraction. The pseudopodic cytoplasmic extensions completely surround the microbe and form a membrane-bound vacuole known as the *phagosome*. The internalized phagosome then binds with the intracellular cytoplasmic lysosomes, forming a *phagolysosome* (Fig. 2-4). Neutrophils and other phagocytic cells, including eosinophils, *degranulate* by releasing the contents of their lysosomes into the phagolysosome. They also degranulate several toxic substances from the intracellular granules into the intercellular space, which can destroy larger microbes, cancer cells, and normal tissue cells. In neutrophils, there is a release of highly reactive oxygen radicals and lysosomal enzymes. The oxygen free radicals can produce significant damage to biologic molecules in a short time.

## Complement

Phagocytosis is facilitated when the material to be ingested is "labeled" by complement so that it is

quickly identifiable to phagocytic cells as undesirable material. Complement is an enzymatically activated cascade of 20 factors that become sequentially activated. The initial stimulus to complement activation can be microbial cell wall polysaccharide or an antigen–antibody reaction. Figure 2-5 illustrates the complement cascade, showing that as complement factors are formed, they not only activate the next step in the sequence but also have important biologic activity on their own. Notice that C3b, when it is formed, binds in a covalent manner to microorganisms. This factor then binds to phagocytic cells, which actively remove the complement-labeled microorganism. The activation of C3b also causes the formation of C5b, which binds to microorganisms and induces the formation of the sequence of complement factors 6 to 9, which forms the *membrane attack complex* (MAC). The MAC drills holes in the membrane of some microbes, which causes osmotic lysis and destruction. (However, many Gram-positive organisms have such thick peptidoglycan layers that the MAC cannot penetrate

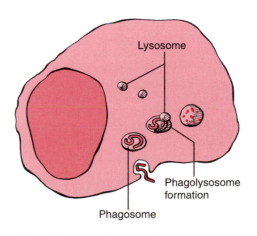

Lysosome

Phagolysosome formation

Phagosome

**FIGURE 2.4** ● Phagocytosis.

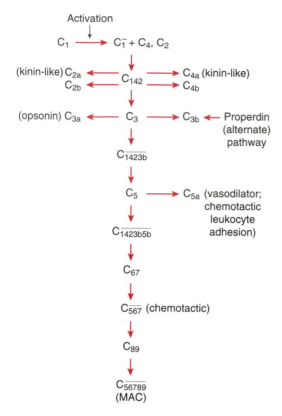

**FIGURE 2.5** ● Complement cascade.

through it to lyse the microbe.) Other components of complement act as opsonins, chemotactic factors, and mast cell degranulation stimulators.

## Macrophages

The macrophage is an essential cell, promoting inflammation and immune responses. It is phagocytic as well as secretory. Important products of activated macrophage secretions include complement factors, proinflammatory cytokines such as IL-1, IL-6, and tumor necrosis factor alpha (TNF-α), prostaglandins and leukotrienes, and protein-digesting enzymes (proteases). Macrophages are critical in the development of an immune response to a microorganism, which is discussed later in this chapter. Macrophages also participate in the regulation of hematopoietic responses to inflammation and infection, to connective tissue replacement, and phagocytic scavenging to prepare inflamed tissue for healing.

For macrophages to become activated, a membrane recognition event must occur between the macrophage and the microorganism. This involves receptor molecules on the macrophage surface. A respiratory burst, similar to that observed in neutrophils, may occur in the stimulated macrophage. Activation of the membrane enzyme phospholipase $A_2$ causes generation and release of prostaglandins and leukotrienes. Phagocytosis of the opsonized microorganism may occur, along with secretion of various mediator molecules of inflammation. Macrophages also are capable of binding to cancer cells and destroying them by releasing toxins into them.

During an acute inflammatory response to an infection, macrophages continue to emigrate into the tissue for about 5 days. Their phagocytic and immune functions usually are accomplished in this time, and the inflamed tissue is prepared for regeneration of new cells or replacement by connective tissue. During the inflammatory response, numerous neutrophils, followed by macrophages, emigrate from the blood into the tissue. This could cause these cells to become less available, but inflamed tissue responds to this threat by releasing specific hematopoietic substances that reach the bloodstream and directly stimulate stem cells in the bone marrow. The hematopoietic factors of importance are colony-stimulating factor–granulocyte macrophage (CSF-GM), CSF-G, and CSF-M. The term *colony-stimulating factor* comes from the ability of these substances to produce islands or colonies of growing, differentiating hematopoietic cells in organs such as the spleen or bone marrow.

Other substances produced at the inflamed site act at a distance to cause a variety of acute-phase effects. Because we have focused mostly on microbial infection as the initiator of inflammation in this chapter, it will be instructive to consider these systemic responses when the inflamogen is an infectious microorganism.

## SYSTEMIC RESPONSES TO INFECTION

### Hematopoietic Responses to Infection

A healthy host will launch a hematopoietic response to infectious disease. The signals for this response occur within the inflamed and infected tissue. Leukocytosis, or an increase in the total white blood cell count, is the general response in which leukopoietic molecules from inflamed tissue are carried to the bone marrow through the bloodstream, where they act on stem cells to increase proliferation of the leukocytes. Different types of leukocytes are differentially stimulated, depending on the type and stage of inflammation and the nature of the signal molecules from inflamed tissue. Clinically, it is wise in an acute infection to measure both total white blood cell count and to perform a differential count of the various subtypes of leukocytes.

## Neutrophilia

Neutrophilia is an increase in percentage of circulating neutrophils above the normal range of 50% to 80% of the total white blood cell count (Babior & Stossel, 1994). Infectious illness, particularly those that are pyogenic, localized, or caused by most cocci and some bacilli, produce a neutrophilic response. The degree of neutrophilia depends on the extent of the infection, the virulence of the microorganism, and general host defenses. The sources of the neutrophils that rise in the blood include both bone marrow stimulated cells and cells from the *marginal pool*. The latter are cells that are essentially sequestered from the circulation by adherence to vessel walls and are predominantly found in the lungs and spleen. However, they can be mobilized and thus can increase the total available circulating neutrophils. Physical stress, such as exercise and increased catecholamine levels, decreases the adherence of these cells and thus often cause a transient neutrophilia.

In early inflammation, when neutrophils marginate and emigrate from the circulation into the tissue spaces, neutropenia may occur. This is followed by a neutrophilia while the marrow releases stored neutrophils, cells from the marginal pool are made available, and bone marrow hematopoiesis is stimulated. If the infection continues and requires continuous emigration of neutrophils, the bone marrow eventually may not be able to keep up with the demands of the tissues.

## Neutropoiesis

The differentiation of neutrophils occurs within the red bone marrow and is stimulated by CSFs (see earlier section, "Macrophages"). Both granulocytes and macrophages arise from a common precursor stem cell, the colony-forming unit–granulocyte macrophage (CFU-GM). The CSF-GM stimulates this early cell to divide and produce phagocytic cells as the body needs them. There are about 100 billion neutrophils entering the circulation from the bone marrow every day (Bainton, 1992). Once the CFU-GM produces stem cells that are committed to the neutrophil lineage, the CFU-G, further differentiation produces the mature neutrophil. The stages of differentiation of neutrophils are illustrated in Figure 2-6.

The myeloblast is a large, undifferentiated, early progenitor cell that gives rise to promyelocytes and myelocytes. About 6 days into the development of the neutrophil, the metamyelocyte is formed. These cells rarely escape from the bone marrow into the peripheral blood, but the next cell type, the band, does appear. It may mature into a neutrophil in the blood, but only the mature form is a "professional phagocyte." The entire process of neutrophil development takes about 300 hours (Skubitz, 1999, p. 304). Neutrophils do not divide in the peripheral blood and have a life span of about 10 hours in the blood and only 1 to 2 days in the tissues.

When neutropoiesis is stimulated by the kinds of events described here, the marrow releases mature neutrophils from the large storage pool and begins to step up the production of neutrophils. A consequence of this may be release of neutrophils that are not yet fully mature from the marrow.

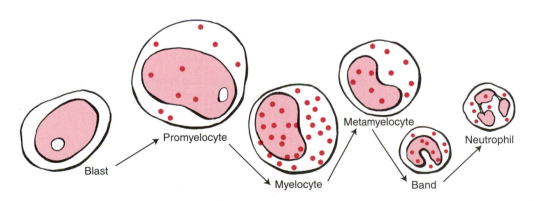

**FIGURE 2.6** ● Neutrophil differentiation.

*Band* cells, in particular, may become more numerous when stimulation of the bone marrow is markedly increased, but states of extreme stress can result in the myeloid precursor cells leaving the bone marrow. Additionally, the normally invisible granules inside neutrophils and neutrophil precursors change to blue-black, and their presence is termed *toxic granulation*. These granules are believed to be bits of partially digested material that has been incompletely phagocytosed, and their presence indicates poor phagocytic function of the cells. When there is a marked increase in bands and an associated toxic granulation, along with neutrophilia, the bone marrow is assumed to be under great demand to produce new cells. This is presumably because blood and marginal pool neutrophils are entering inflamed and infected tissue faster than they can be replaced. An ominous finding that can occur in Gram-negative septicemia is a *falling* white count associated with a marked shift toward neutrophil production, but with numerous band cells (> 25%) and toxic granulation. This indicates an inability of the bone marrow to respond any further to the signals from the periphery to produce fully functional neutrophils, and that remaining neutrophils are immature and have become sticky and poorly functioning.

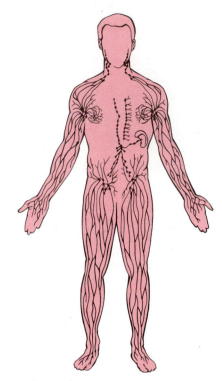

**FIGURE 2.7** ● Lymphatic channels and nodes.

## Monocytosis

The monocyte count rarely increases to the same degree as the neutrophils in acute infections. There is usually a mild stimulation to monocyte stores in the bone marrow, but a significant monocytosis usually is seen in chronic infectious diseases such as tuberculosis. Recall that the monocyte is the second cell to emigrate into inflamed tissue, and if it is unable to effectively clean and excavate the site, there will be continual inflammatory signals that promote local macrophage accumulation and an increase in the percentage of monocytes in the differential white blood cell count.

## Lymphadenopathy

Another generally healthy response to infection is enlargement of the lymphoid tissues that drain the sites of infection. These swollen lymph nodes are palpable, tender, movable masses of tissue in well-defined anatomic sites throughout the body. Figure 2-7 illustrates the major lymphatic channels and nodes. Recall that the inflammatory exudate, rich in proteins and cells, occurs in response to the acute phase of infection and inflammation. The fluid is reabsorbed through lymphatic channels draining the site. The lymph then is carried in ves-

sels that traverse lymph nodes, structures that are rich in macrophages and lymphocytes. Antigenic material can be identified and reacted to within the lymph nodes. The lymph nodes also are the site at which lymphocyte proliferation in an acute infection may occur, causing enlargement of these nodes. When infection is cleared, these nodes return to normal size in most cases but may be persistently enlarged in chronic infections and may sometimes become fibrotic and calcified after acute infection has passed. This is common in the pediatric population, particularly in the posterior occipital nodes.

## Acute Phase Reactants

When acute inflammatory reactions occur, a systemic effect in response to proinflammatory cytokines IL-1, TNF-α, and IL-6 is the release from the liver of several proteins, termed *acute phase reactants*. Included in this grouping are complement factors, serum C-reactive protein, fibrinogen, ferritin, haptoglobin, ceruloplasmin, alpha-1 antitrypsin, amyloid proteins, and alpha-1 acid glycoprotein.

The presence of these proteins in the blood changes the rate at which erythrocytes drop to the bottom of a tube of blood because of gravity. The proteins are thought to change the viscosity of the serum, making the sedimentation rate faster. The erythrocyte sedimentation rate (ESR) is a nonspecific indicator of an ongoing inflammatory process, but is not diagnostic of any specific infection. ESR is greatest during bacterial infections, but can still reach high levels in viral infections, and the use of ESR may help to monitor the course and response of an infection.

## Sickness Behavior

Behaviors associated with the phenomena of illness have long been recognized and generally are deemed to be of benefit to the host. This constellation of behaviors has been termed *sickness behavior* and in mammals consists of social and sexual withdrawal, lack of grooming behaviors, activation of the hypothalamic-hypophyseal-adrenocortical stress axis, sleep, anorexia, adipsia, and fever (Dantzer et al., 1998). These effects are illustrated in Figure 2-8. Administration of lipopolysaccharide, a component of bacterial cell walls that can act as an exogenous pyrogen, stimulates a large cytokine response both at the level of the immune cells and in the brain. In particular, the cytokines

IL-1, TNF-α, and IL-6 seem to be involved, but it also appears that different aspects of sickness behavior are produced by different combinations of cytokines.

Sleep is an essential aspect of sickness behavior. People with an acute infectious process sleep much more and have a different quality of sleep. TNF-α in particular causes an increase in non–rapid eye movement sleep (Krueger et al., 1998). An additional component of sickness behavior is anorexia, which is provoked particularly by IL-1α, which may reach the hypothalamic centers by crossing the blood-brain barrier or may be secreted into the brain by cells that have crossed over. IL-1α may act by binding to endothelial cells, which may be stimulated to produce vasoactive substances, such as nitric oxide, or could stimulate vagal afferent fibers, which then could affect hypothalamic function (Plata-Salaman, 1998). Generally, in chronic disease such as cancer or in chronic infections such as AIDS, cytokines are believed to contribute to the *anorexia-cachexia syndrome*. In this state, individuals have loss of appetite and extreme body wasting, probably in response to cytokines such as IL-1, TNF-α, IL-6, and interferon gamma (Plata-Salaman, 1998).

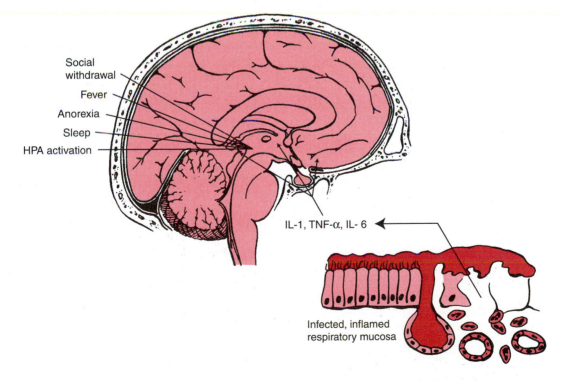

Social withdrawal
Fever
Anorexia
Sleep
HPA activation

IL-1, TNF-α, IL- 6

Infected, inflamed respiratory mucosa

**FIGURE 2.8** ● Inflamed tissue releases proinflammatory cytokines which act on the brain to produce classic signs of sickness behavior.

Activation of the stress response occurs along with sickness behavior and appears to be stimulated by the same proinflammatory cytokines. IL-1 provokes the release of corticotropin and also augments glucocorticoid release by the adrenal cortex. In turn, the glucocorticoids suppress the release of proinflammatory cytokines from T helper (Th) cells, acting in a feedback manner to down-regulate the inflammatory and immune processes.

Fever is a normal response to infection. It can be induced either by exogenous (eg, endotoxin) or endogenous pyrogens, which alter the hypothalamic set point for core body temperature. In most infectious illnesses, the febrile response is produced by the proinflammatory cytokines IL-1, IL-6, and TNF-α, which are released by stimulated monocytes/macrophages. These substances to-gether comprise endogenous pyrogen (EP). IL-1 appears to be a major pyrogen by its direct action on the preoptic area of the anterior hypothalamus. The action of IL-1 may be through the production of brain prostaglandin E. Fever is produced by hypothalamic-orchestrated heat gain mechanisms that regulate temperature around a new pyrogen-regulated set point. This set point is maintained only as long as there is a continuous supply of EP being produced in inflamed and infectious tissues. Only minute amounts are required for a febrile response to occur. Controversy exists over the potentially beneficial actions of fever. Evidence suggests that fever inhibits microbial growth in vivo, antibiotics are more effective in febrile states, immunologic defenses are more effective, and plasma iron levels are depressed and thus less available for iron-requiring microbial growth.

The physiologic and metabolic effects of fever are significant, and many of these effects are believed to be caused, at least in part, by the cytokines associated with EP. There is an increased metabolic rate associated with fever on the order of a 10% increase for every degree Celsius, which requires calories to meet this increased energy demand. In chronic febrile state, the metabolic demand associated with fever may waste body fats and proteins, leading to severe malnutrition. Part of this effect probably results from the anorexigenic effects of proinflammatory cytokines. There also is an increased insensible water loss on the order of 300 to 500 mL of water lost per meter squared per degree Celsius per day in fever. This may amount to water loss significant enough to cause dehydration. Other aspects of metabolism show increases, such as heart and respiratory rate.

The highest fevers in infectious diseases are associated with Gram-negative sepsis, bacterial meningitis, Legionnaire's disease, pyelonephritis, and viral encephalitis. Age is a factor affecting the ability to produce an EP-driven febrile response, with infants and elderly patients, malnourished patients, and patients receiving corticosteroids or nonsteroidal anti-inflammatory drugs sometimes unable to produce a significant fever, even in the presence of high levels of EP.

We have been describing a simple, acute inflammatory response to infectious microorganisms and the damage they produce, without examining how specific defenses of the body (ie, the immune system) might interact to protect the host. To understand this response, this chapter next describes the normal immunologic response of humans to infectious microorganisms.

## ANTIGENIC NATURE OF MICROORGANISMS

The immune system comprises the body's *specific* defense system. By recognizing foreign molecules such as viral proteins or bacterial cell wall polysaccharides, the immune system is able to marshal extraordinarily effective mechanisms for swift and complete destruction of most microbial invaders. The immune defenses, however, are not always successful. Microorganisms have evolved clever ways of surviving and multiplying even in the immunocompetent host. For example, some microbes are actually able to take up residence inside the macrophage itself, which attempts to destroy it through phagocytosis but is unable to do so. For example, *Mycobacterium tuberculosis* is taken up into phagosomes of macrophages but then secretes a substance that inhibits the acidification that is necessary for phagolysosomal enzymatic destruction (Kaufmann & Flesch, 1992). Thus, the organisms persist inside the cells. Some bacteria, such as staphylococcus, produce an outer capsule that is a difficult barrier for macrophages to penetrate. Other microbes secrete exotoxins that damage leukocytes. *Legionella* organisms inhibit the respiratory burst. Influenza viruses undergo regular antigenic drift in which mutations occur that alter the antigenicity of the virus, thus presenting novel viral epitopes to naive human immune systems. Multiple mechanisms have evolved by which microorganisms escape the normal specific and nonspecific host defenses.

## IMMUNE DESTRUCTION OF MICROORGANISMS

*Opsonization* greatly enhances the ability of the immune system to kill infectious microorganisms. This is a process by which complement and antibody coat the microbe, which increases the ability of phagocytic cells to bind them. Within the secretions of the mucosal systems of the body, the process of opsonization by secretory IgA is essential in preventing the adherence and penetration of microorganisms through the mucosa of the respiratory, gastrointestinal, and genitourinary tracts. Macrophages are not needed because the antigen–antibody complexes formed are removed and cannot harm the host.

## Components of the Immune System

The immune system consists of lymphocytes, accessory cells, and a wide array of molecules through which foreign material is rejected and destroyed in the human body. For the immune system to be effective, the microbial antigenic material must be identified by a group of cells known as the *antigen-presenting cells* (APCs). These cells are widely dispersed throughout the blood, lymphoid tissue, and extracellular spaces of the body. A major APC is the macrophage, which functions not only as an inflammatory cell, but also as the cell that introduces antigenic material to the immune system.

Macrophages are phagocytic and can ingest all sorts of foreign material. The foreign material goes through a sequence of events known as antigen *processing*. It is digested into smaller fragments and bound to peptides coded for by the major histocompatability (MHC) system. This is a multigenic complex of genes on chromosome 6 that is unique to each individual. It is essentially the same system of genes that is analyzed on lymphocytes (human lymphocyte antigens) for tissue typing. There are two major classes of MHC molecules: class I and class II. Class I molecules are on all nucleated human cells, whereas class II are on only immune cells and APCs. Digested antigenic material expressed in association with class I MHC peptides on the surface of cells is a signal to cytotoxic T cells, which are able to kill the presenting cell. This is a useful mechanism for killing virally infected cells and possibly malignant cells.

On immune cells and macrophages, the processed antigen is presented on the cell surface in association with MHC class II molecules. This antigen presentation then signals Th cells or B cells. Both Th and B cells have receptors for antigen on their cell surfaces. For the Th cells, a specific and unique T-cell receptor (TCR) is present. Through ontogeny of the immune system, over a million different TCRs develop on T cell surfaces, and on B cells, antigen receptors, which are Ig molecules, also display the same incredible diversity. Both Th and B cells have antigenic binding sites on their cell membranes that recognize the *epitope* region of the antigen. This is the part of the molecule that has a molecular configuration that allows it to fit into a lock-and-key reaction with TCRs, B-cell receptors, or Ig molecules. Before the cascade of immune responses can occur subsequent to macrophage processing and presenting, the antigen presented on the macrophage surface must bind to a specific TCR. The Th cells have many different cell surface receptors and markers along with their unique TCR. The CD4 and CD3 markers identify the cell as a Th cell, and Th cells sometimes are referred to as CD4 cells. CD markers are "cluster of differentiation" markers that occur on all lymphocytes as they mature in lymphoid tissue. Antigen binding with the TCR requires both CD3 and CD4 molecules to ensure the best fit of antigen and TCR. The CD4, therefore, is considered an adhesion molecule for MHC class II antigen binding. The binding of Th cells with macrophages is illustrated in Figure 2-9. Some bacterial antigens are considered "superantigens" in that they do not undergo antigen processing and presenting, but are able to elicit a Th cell–macrophage interaction that results in Th cell activation and cytokine release (see Fig. 2-10). Such superantigens are powerful mitogenic stimulators of the immune response.

Another marker of T cells is the CD8 marker that is found on cytotoxic and suppressor T cells. The CD8 marker is an adhesion molecule for MHC class I antigen binding. Another type of large granular lymphocyte also is involved in killing virally infected cells. The natural killer (NK) cell does not require MHC to recognize, bind, and attack virally infected cells. Thus, there is less specificity in the cell killing produced by NK cells.

## T Helper Cells

T helper cells help other lymphocytes function optimally. For example, Th cells preferentially activate cytotoxic/suppressor T cell populations or B lymphocytes. The populations of Th cells include $T_H0$ cells, $T_H1$, and $T_H2$ cells. Figure 2-10 illustrates the process by which the $T_H0$ cells differentiate into either $T_H1$ or $T_H2$ cells. The APCs and the mix of cytokine molecules regulate this process. Cytokines are important, hormonelike molecules that act both locally and at a distance to direct and amplify the immune response. Proinflammatory cytokines induce fever and produce sickness behavior. When stimulated by antigen, macrophages release the cytokines IL-1, IL-6, and TNF-α. IL-1 is a stimulatory molecule, acting on Th cells to activate them. These $T_H0$ cells then

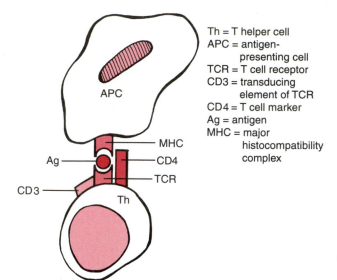

Th = T helper cell
APC = antigen-
          presenting cell
TCR = T cell receptor
CD3 = transducing
          element of TCR
CD4 = T cell marker
Ag = antigen
MHC = major
          histocompatibility
          complex

**FIGURE 2.9**  ●  Binding of presented antigen on an APC requires MHC molecules and CD3 and CD4 molecules on the Th cell.

"choose" to differentiate into the $T_H1$ direction, which helps cytotoxic reactions, or the $T_H2$ direction, which supports humoral immune responses. The direction is determined by costimulatory cytokines releases by the APCs involved in presenting the antigen. When stimulated, $T_H1$ cells release IL-2, IL-12, and interferon gamma, which are *proinflammatory* cytokines. These cytokines elicit a cellular immune response, producing localized inflammatory reactions. The $T_H2$ cells are stimulated to produce *proimmune* cytokines IL-4, IL-5, IL-6, and IL-10. These cytokines stimulate B cells and elicit a humoral immune response. The two types of Th cells mutually inhibit each other's functions and stimulate themselves in an autocrine manner through their cytokines and cell surface cytokine receptors. Depending on the nature of an infectious agent, its virulence, organ preference, and pathophysiologic mechanism of action, the Th cells direct either a stronger humoral or cellular immunity.

When CD8 cytotoxic T cells are stimulated by

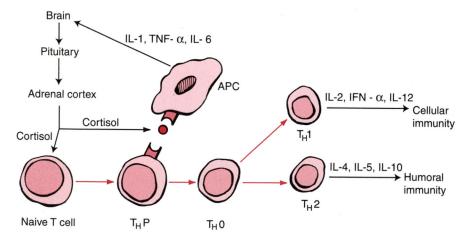

**FIGURE 2.10**  ●  Peripheral T cells are stimulated by APC-presented antigen. APCs secrete cytokines that act on the brain, producing an HPA axis arousal, which increases cortisol. Cortisol can suppress both T cells and APCs, thus down-regulating the immune response. $T_H0$ differentiates into either $T_H1$ or $T_H2$. The cytokines released by $T_H1$ are proinflammatory and promote cytotoxicity while those secreted by $T_H2$ are proimmune and stimulate B cells and humoral immunity. $T_H1$ and $T_H2$ cytokines mutually inhibit the opposing cells.

$T_H1$ cytokines, they kill cells that are displaying antigen. Often, these are class I MHC presenting cells, such as virally infected cells in which viral antigenic material is displayed with MHC on the cell surface. The CD8 cells bind to the target cell and synthesize a protein called *perforin*. Perforin produces circular membrane lesions, thus lysing the cell. This prevents virally infected cells from actively producing virions that could then infect other cells.

## B Cells

B cells are another type of lymphocyte with antigen receptor molecules and a variety of other markers and cytokine receptors, which identify them as B cells. When activated by antigen and $T_H2$ cell cytokines, B cells become *plasma cells*, which actively secrete Igs. These cells also divide when stimulated and form a clone of identical cells, all of which are capable of secreting the appropriate immunoglobulin that binds to the antigen. Immunoglobulins are classified according to shape and structure into five different types: IgG, which is the backbone of humoral immunity and sometimes is referred to as gamma globulin; IgM, the first immunoglobulin produced by stimulated plasma cells; IgA, the immunoglobulin found in mucosal secretions; IgE, the immunoglobulin associated with atopic disease; and IgD, whose functions are not understood well. Every Ig has two identical heavy and light chains, a constant region of amino acids, and a variable region containing the antigen-binding site called the *idiotype*. Every Ig has a unique idiotype that allows it to bind with unique antigen. Like T cells, B cells confer a specific immunity in that the Ig molecules produced by these cells bind only specific antigens. Immunoglobulins are important opsonins and provide antibody reactivity in the blood to circulating antigen material, combining with it and essentially removing it from circulation by aggregating, precipitating, or neutralizing it.

The clones of B cells that are produced by the first, or primary, immune response produce *memory*, sometimes lifelong, of the antigen. Then the clone of cells produced in the primary response is readily available to react with antigen if it should ever be reintroduced into the body. Furthermore, these cells secrete a low-level titer of measurable specific antibody in the blood, and when antigen is reintroduced, the secondary response is amplified, producing a larger titer of Igs than occurred in the primary response. The type of Ig also differs in the primary compared with the secondary response. The early responding plasma cells secrete IgM, but on later stimulation they undergo *isotype* switching, secreting IgG.

## Summary

The immune response to infection involves all components of the specific defense system. APCs recognize, process, and present microbial antigenic material, particularly if the microbe is opsonized with complement or antibody. Virally infected cells display viral antigens associated with MHC class I to CD8 cells that kill them. The killing done by NK cells also is directed at viral antigens on cell surfaces, without the need for MHC peptide association. CD4 positive cells interact with APCs to release cytokines, stimulating $T_H1$ or $T_H2$ cells, depending on whether a strong humoral or cellular immune response is needed. These immune reactions themselves may produce complement activation, and the products of infection also elicit an inflammatory reaction. Neutrophils emigrate into infected tissue en masse, and macrophages also enter from the blood. Neutrophilia is common in acute bacterial infections but also is seen in acute viral illness. Neutrophil phagocytosis, macrophage phagocytosis, antigen processing and presenting, and stimulation of Th cells to secrete cytokines together act on B cells or CD8 cells. These effects produce efferent responses of the immune system in which microbes, cells, and debris are removed from the host, and the host protects itself from further infection.

Patients frequently visit primary care providers because of upper respiratory infections, most of which are colds, although influenza, allergic rhinitis, and streptococcal pharyngitis must be routinely ruled out. There is little that can be done medically for patients with common colds other than symptomatic relief. It is conceivable that vaccines against cold viruses and viral therapy directed against the organisms causing the common cold may be available in the future. Nasal interferon decreases the severity of a cold but hardly warrants the expense. Whereas the symptoms of a cold are easily dismissed as insignificant, remember that colds predispose individuals to secondary infections that may produce significant morbidity. Studies using reverse transcriptase polymerase chain reaction to detect common cold viral genomes have established the importance of colds in predisposing to or causing otitis media, sinusitis, and exacerbations of asthma, as well as other lower respiratory tract disorders (Pitkaranta & Hayden, 1998). In debilitated or immunocompromised individuals, a cold can predispose to pneumonia. The following case is a typical presentation of an adult with a cold.

## Case Study 2.1

A 35-year-old white woman presents to the primary care provider with the following history and chief complaint. This previously well woman who is a 3rd grade school teacher began to get a "scratchy" throat 3 days ago, which progressed to nasal stuffiness, a low-grade fever of 99.6°F, and feelings of fatigue and malaise that were not, however, significant enough to interrupt her work or recreational activities. Yesterday, she began to have increasing amounts of clear nasal drainage, frequent sneezing, an irritating cough, and headache, and her ears felt "plugged up." She also stated that her chest felt "tight." She took over-the-counter cold medication, but it made her too sleepy, so she discontinued it. She is seeking antibiotics to treat her cold.

### History

#### Past Medical History

| | |
|---|---|
| Allergies | Seasonal; had asthma as child |
| Current medications | Low-dose oral birth control pills × 3 years |
| | Daily multivitamin |
| | No prescription medications |
| Surgeries | None |
| Injury/trauma | None |
| Childhood illness | Immunizations current. No hx influenza nor pneumonia, +hepatitis B vaccines |
| Pregnancy | G1P1A0 |

#### Social History

| | |
|---|---|
| Married | 6 years |
| Tobacco | Denies |
| Alcohol | Denies |
| Social drugs | Denies |
| Caffeine | Infrequent |
| Exercise | Walks in neighborhood nearly every day |
| | Works in yard when weather is good and allergies aren't bothering her |
| Employment | Full-time teacher |

#### Family History

| | |
|---|---|
| Mother | 54 years old, no current medical conditions |
| Father | 60 years old, diabetes |

### Review of Systems

| | |
|---|---|
| General | Has not slept well for last 3 nights because of nasal congestion |
| Skin | No problems; denies trouble with healing; no hx rash, pruritus, lesions |
| HEENT | Wears corrective lenses. Denies dizziness. Denies headache. Throat is sore, and she is experiencing mild pain on swallowing, slight hoarseness. Ears feel plugged up and she can't hear as well as usual |
| | No hx thyroid disease |
| Lungs | Denies SOB at rest or on exertion. No PND. No hx asthma, pneumonia, or bronchitis. Frequent colds. Chest feels tight today, as if she can't "draw a deep breath" |
| Cardiac | Denies chest pain or palpitations at rest or on exertion. No hx MRG. No prior ECG |
| GI | No nausea or vomiting. Complains of decreased hunger |
| GU | Denies dysuria, retention, hesitancy in starting a stream |

*(Case study continued on next page)*

| | |
|---|---|
| MS | Denies pain, tenderness, swelling of joints |
| Neurologic | Denies numbness, tingling, blackouts, seizures |

## Differential Diagnosis

1. Cold
2. Viral pharyngitis
3. Streptococcal pharyngitis
4. Allergic rhinitis

## Physical Examination

| System | Findings |
|---|---|
| Vital signs | T–99°F, P–74, R–18<br>BP–110/74 sitting, 106/68 standing<br>Height 5'4" Weight 134 lb |
| General | Alert and oriented, in no acute distress<br>Well-nourished woman in NAD |
| HEENT | Normocephalic. Vision 20/20 OU corrected<br>Cranial nerves intact. Funduscopic examination without hemorrhage or AV nicking. Optic disc margins well defined. Neck supple, no thyromegaly, no bruit, no palpable nodes. Turbinates enlarged, boggy, TMs dull with absent light reflex, pinkish gray, hearing normal at conversational levels. Throat erythematous without exudate, tonsils 2+. Sinus pain on palpation of maxillary sinuses |
| Lungs | Breath sounds equal. Occasional expiratory rhonchi heard over anterior chest, equal bilaterally |
| Cardiac | Heart rate regular. No MRG |
| Abdomen | Nontender. No masses. No HSM. BS × 4 quads |
| GU | Deferred |
| Extremities | Pulses 2+ bilateral lower and upper. No pedal edema. Skin warm, dry, and intact. Sensation intact |

## Laboratory Studies

| Test | Result |
|---|---|
| CBC | WNL |
| Streptococcus spot test | Negative |

## Impression

HRV infection
Serous otitis media, bilateral
Reactive airways with mild expiratory wheezing

## Physiologic Basis of Treatment Plan

Increase fluids to dilute organisms and hydrate the body
Prescribe antihistamines to decrease nasal mucosal swelling from inflammation and immune processes resulting in histamine release
Advise rest to increase immune and inflammatory efficacy
Follow up on wheezing and serous otitis media to determine if worsening of either condition occurs and to treat appropriately

AV, arteriovenous; BP, blood pressure; BS, bowel sounds; CBC, complete blood count; ECG, electrocardiogram; GI, gastrointestinal; GU, genitourinary; HEENT, head, eye, ear, nose, and throat; HSM, holosystolic murmur; HRV, human rhinovirus; hx, history; MRG, murmur, rub, or gallop; MS, musculoskeletal; NAD, not in distress; P, pulse; PND, paroxysmal nocturnal dyspnea; R, respiration; SOB, shortness of breath; T, temperature; TM, tympanic membrane; WBC, white blood count.

## PATHOPHYSIOLOGIC BASIS OF SYMPTOMS

Most colds in adults are caused by human rhinoviruses (HRVs), which are members of the picornavirus family (of which there are 89 types), and the occurrence of a cold every year caused by a different strain of HRV is thus a likely possibility for humans. Table 2-1 shows the etiologic factors important in causing both the common cold and viral pharyngitis. Most colds result from rhinoviruses that have been transmitted from another infected individual through hands or articles touched by the individual. Most are transmitted within the home.

When a particular rhinovirus infects an individual, an immune response occurs, leading to a measurable antibody titer to the specific HRV. However, lifelong immunity to that particular strain of HRV may not occur because minor antigenic changes in the virus may result in lack of antibody specificity over time. The peak antibody titers occur during early adulthood. In terms of epidemiology, the peak incidence of HRV infections occurs in September, with a rate of 1.28 per person-year (Gwaltney, 1997). School-aged children may have between three and eight colds each year. Many of the HRV serotypes have similar amino acid sequences (Skoner et al., 1995).

Figure 2-11 displays the steps in infection with HRV. Virus is carried through the lacrimal duct or by mucociliary activity to the nasopharynx, where it deposits and attaches to nasal epithelial cells, mostly using the intercellular adhesion molecule-1, with about 10% binding to the low density lipoprotein receptors, and a group of cells become infected. Surprisingly, few cells become infected in this process, and nearly no cell damage occurs, with most of the effects resulting from the cytokines being released in the mucosa after infection. Few cells show viral-induced cytopathic effects, even when the symptoms are severe. An inflammatory response occurs, which results in edema, engorgement of postcapillary venules,

## TABLE 2.1
● ● ●

### Viruses Associated With Respiratory Syndromes in Adults

| Virus | Common cold | Relative Importance for Indicated Syndrome | | | | |
|---|---|---|---|---|---|---|
| | | Pharyngitis | | Tracheobronchitis | Pneumonia | |
| | | Civilian | Military | | Civilian | Military |
| Rhinovirus, 89 types | 4+ | 2+ | + | + | + | + |
| Influenza virus type A | + | 2+ | + | 3+ | 2+ | 2+ |
| Influenza virus type B | + | 2+ | + | 2+ | + | + |
| Coronavirus | + | + | + | + | + | + |
| Adenovirus types 4 and 7 | + | + | 4+ | + | + | 4+ |
| Adenovirus types 1, 2, 3, and 5 | + | + | + | + | + | + |
| Herpes simplex virus | − | 2+ | + | + | − | − |
| Epstein-Barr virus | − | + | + | − | + | + |
| Respiratory syncytial virus | + | + | + | + | − | − |
| Parainfluenza virus types 1, 2, and 3 | + | 2+ | + | + | − | − |
| Group A coxsackievirus | + | + | + | + | + | + |
| Group B coxsackievirus | + | + | + | + | + | + |
| Echovirus | + | + | + | + | + | + |
| Poliovirus | + | + | + | + | − | − |

Symbols for relative frequency: +, occasional case; 2+, small proportion of cases; 3+, substantial proportion of cases; 4+, most cases; −, does not cause syndrome in immunocompetent host.
(From Douglas, R.G., Jr. [1984]. Respiratory diseases. In G.J. Galasso, T.C. Merigan, & R.A. Buchanan [Eds.], *Antiviral agents and viral diseases of man* [2nd ed.]. New York: Raven.)

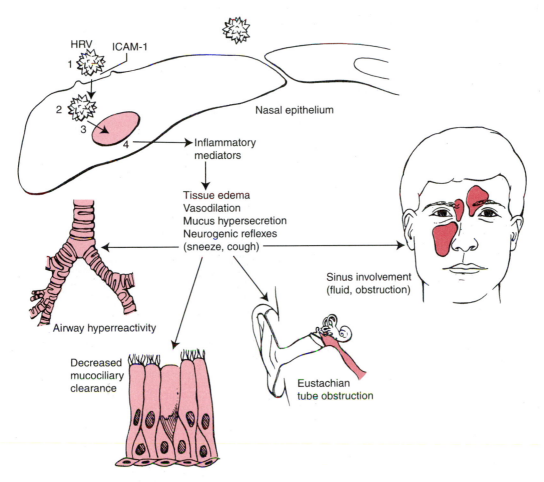

**FIGURE 2.11** ● Steps in infection with human rhinovirus.

mucus hypersecretion, and neurogenic responses such as sneezing and coughing (Pitkaranta & Hayden, 1998). Viral shedding occurs through nasal secretions in which the concentration is highest. Whereas HRVs can be recovered in saliva, the amount is small, and kissing usually is not an adequate mechanism for spreading infection (Gwaltney, 1997).

The common cold can be considered a cytokine-mediated pathophysiologic process. In vitro, HRV induces IL-6, IL-8, and CSF-GM from infected epithelial cells; in vivo, nasal washings of cold-infected people have high levels of IL-6 and IL-8. The effect of IL-8 may be to increase neutrophil and eosinophil emigration into the nasal mucosa. During the first and second day of illness, levels of both IL-1 and TNF-α are increased dramatically in the nasal mucus. The receptor for intercellular adhesion molecule-1 may be upregulated on epithelial cells either by the virus or

cytokines, making additional cells available for infection with HRV (Pitkaranta & Hayen, 1998). Cell-mediated immune activity is increased in response to HRV. Macrophages are competent in processing and presenting HRV antigen. The virus, however, does not replicate inside the macrophage. Macrophages respond to viral uptake by cytokine secretion.

Vasoactive peptides such as bradykinin, which increase IL-1 release, also increase in the nasal mucus of the patient with a cold. Bradykinin causes severe nasal stuffiness and rhinorrhea, probably related to its vasoactive effects.

There appears to be a relationship between stress and susceptibility to the common cold. Stone et al. (1992) found that susceptibility to the common cold was increased in subjects reporting more life events within the preceding year. Cohen, Tyrrell, and Smith (1993) exposed subjects to the common cold virus and then tested the relationship between appearance of cold symptoms and negative life events, negative affect, and perceived stress. They report that negative life events independently increased the risk of becoming infected. Cobb and Steptoe (1996) examined the relationship between incidence of upper respiratory tract illnesses in 107 adults over a 15-week study and again found that the risk of infection was increased in subjects reporting high levels of stressful life events and daily hassles.

Cohen and colleagues have studied the relationship between infectious illness and stress-immune processes using the cold virus inoculation technique, with subsequent follow-up for the appearance of symptoms, amount of mucous discharge, and ciliary clearance. This technique allows a more accurate assessment of infection compared with self-report data. Their landmark study in the *New England Journal of Medicine* in 1991 (Cohen et al., 1991) reports on the relationship between development of colds after cold virus nasal inoculation and psychological stress in 394 healthy adult subjects. Rates of clinical colds and respiratory infections increased in a dose-response pattern with level of psychological stress. In a recent report, they describe the influence of social ties on susceptibility to the common cold (Cohen et al., 1997). Risk and symptoms decreased as social ties and networks increased in subjects inoculated with the common cold virus.

There may be a differential effect of different types of stressors on susceptibility to the common cold. Stressors related to underemployment or unemployment and stress of an interpersonal

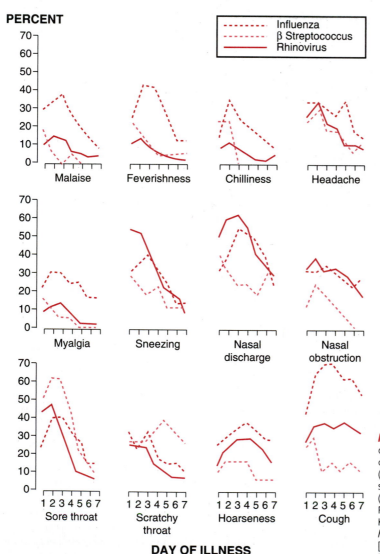

**FIGURE 2.12** ● Comparison of symptom profiles of rhinovirus colds (139) cases, type $A_2$ influenza (33 cases), and group A β-hemolytic streptococcal pharyngitis (17 cases). (Adapted from Gwaltney J. [1997]. Rhinoviruses. In A.S. Evans & R.S. Kaslow [Eds.]. *Viral infection in humans: Epidemiology and control.* [p. 829]. New York: Plenum Publishing.)

nature with families and friends were the types of stress most associated with susceptibility. The recent study of 276 volunteers subjected to the cold inoculation procedure shows that chronic stressors (greater than 1-month duration) were associated with a substantial risk of contracting a cold after cold virus inoculation (Cohen et al., 1998).

Clinical presentation of a cold mirrors the pathophysiologic mechanisms just described. The median time of infection is about 7 days, and people become most symptomatic on days 2 and 3. Figure 2-12 illustrates the type of symptoms; the patterns of occurrence; and the time course in HRV infections, streptococcal pharyngitis, and influenza. The latter is a major differential diagnostic feature that the primary care provider must consider when a patient presents with cold symptoms.

The HRV infection increases airway reactivity in the atopic host. HRV-activated cells secrete a factor that increases eosinophil activity within the mucosa. Infection with HRV-39 induced significant acute increases in serum IgE, leukocyte histamine release, and platelet aggregation, but only in patients with preexisting allergic rhinitis (Skoner et al., 1995), suggesting that allergic patients respond differently than nonallergic individuals to infection with HRV.

The patient described in Case Study 2-1 had a typical presentation, although two factors bear closer scrutiny. Her tympanic membranes were dull and had a diminished light reflex. This indicates fluid trapped in the middle ear caused by edema of the nasal and eustachian tube mucosa. Secondary infection is a threat in this patient. An additional concern is her feeling of "tightness" in her chest. This may indicate an early stage of exacerbation of asthmatic symptoms. A history of previous atopy is apparent, and a thorough respiratory system examination is essential to determine if there is bronchial tree involvement; these symptoms should be watched for worsening of her respiratory status. Her other symptoms resulted from cytokines released by epithelial and inflammatory cells in the nasal mucosa and should resolve with or without treatment. Her occupation predisposes her to exposure to strains of HRV, and she still is contagious. Exploration of stressful life events, lack of adequate sleep, or other psychosocial factors may be fruitful in preventing further frequent HRV infections. Her seeking antibiotics for relief of a common cold is a frequently seen fallacy in primary care practice. Antibiotics are necessary only if a secondary bacterial infection has occurred in the patient with HRV infection and should not be used to treat the common cold.

## REFERENCES

Babior, B. & Stossel, T. (1994). *Hematology: A pathophysiological approach* (3rd ed.). New York: Churchill Livingstone.

Bainton, D. (1992). Developmental biology of neutrophils and eosiniphils. In J. Gallin, I. Goldstein, & R. Snyderman (Eds.), *Inflammation: Basic principles and clinical correlates* (2nd ed.). New York: Raven Press.

Cobb, J. & Steptoe, A. (1996). Psychosocial stress and susceptibility to upper respiratory tract illness in an adult population sample. *Psychosomatic Medicine, 58*, 404–412.

Cohen, S., Frank, E., Doyle, W., Skoner, D., Rabin, B., & Gwaltney, J. (1998). Types of stressors that increase the susceptibility to the common cold in healthy adults. *Health Psychology, 17*, 214–223.

Cohen, S., Doyle, W., Skoner, D., Rabin, B., & Gwaltney, J. (1997). Social ties and susceptibility to the common cold. *Journal of the American Medical Association, 277*, 1940–1944.

Cohen, S., Tyrrell, D., & Smith, A. (1993). Negative life events, perceived stress, negative affect, and susceptibility to the common cold. *Journal of Perspectives in Social Psychology, 64*, 131–140.

Cohen, S., Tyrrell, D., & Smith, A. (1991). Psychological stress and susceptibility to the common cold. *New England Journal of Medicine, 325* (9), 606–612.

Dantzer, R., Bluthe, E., Gheusi, G., Cremona, S., Laye, S., Parnet, P., & Kelley, K. (1998). Molecular biology of sickness behavior. *Annals of the New York Academy of Sciences, 856*, 132–138.

Gwaltney, J. (1997). Human rhinovirus. In A. Evans & R. Kaslow (Eds.), *Viral infections of humans* (4th ed.). New York: Plenum Medical Book Co.

Horsnell, C., Gama, R.E., Hughes, P.J., & Stanway G. (1995). Molecular relationships between 21 human rhinovirus serotypes. *General Virology, 76* (Pt 10), 2549–2555.

Kaslow, R. & Evans, A. (1997). In A. Evans & R. Kaslow (Eds.), *Viral infections of humans* (4th ed.). New York: Plenum Medical Book Co.

Kaufmann, S. & Flesch, I. (1992). Life within phagocytic cells. In C. Hormaeche, C. Penn, & C. Smyth (Eds.), *Molecular biology of bacterial infection*. Cambridge: Cambridge University Press.

Krueger, J. M., Fang, J., Taishi, P., Chen, Z., Kushikata, T., & Gardi, J. (1998). Sleep: A physiological role for IL-1 and TNF-α. *Annals of the New York Academy of Sciences, 856*, 148–159.

Pitkäranta, A. & Hayden, F.G. (1998). Rhinoviruses: Important respiratory pathogens. *Annals of Medicine, 30* (6), 529–537.

Pitkäranta, A. & Hayden, F. (1998). What's new with the common cold: Pathogenesis and diagnosis. *Infections in Medicine 15* (1), 50–59.

Plata-Salaman, C. (1998). Cytokine-induced anorexia: Behavioral, cellular and molecular mechanisms. *Annals of the New York Academy of Sciences, 856*, 160–170.

Ransom, J. (1997). Sinusitis: Diagnosis and treatment. *Medscape Respiratory Care, 1* (8). [www.medscape.com].

Skoner, D.P., Doyle, W.J., Tanner, E.P., Kiss, J., & Fireman, P. (1995). Effect of rhinovirus 39 (RV39) infection on immune and inflammatory parameters in allergic and non-allergic subjects. *Clinical and Experimental Allergy, 25* (6), 561–567.

Skubitz, K. (1999). Neutrophilic leukocytes. In G. Lee, J Foerster, J. Lukens, F. Parakevas, & G. Rodgers (Eds.), *Wintrobe's Clinical Hematology* (10th ed.). Philadelphia: Lippincott Williams & Wilkins.

Snyderman, R. & Uhing, R. (1992). Chemoattractant stimulus–response coupling. In J. Gallin, I. Goldstein, & R. Snyderman (Eds.), *Inflammation: Basic principles and clinical correlates* (2nd ed.). New York: Raven Press.

Stone, A.A., Bovbjerg, D., Neale, J., Napoli, A., Valdimarsdottir, H., Cox, D., Hayden, F., & Gwaltney, J. (1992). Development of common cold symptoms following experimental rhinovirus infection is related to prior stressful life events. *Behavioral Medicine, 18,* 115–120.

# Skin Cancer

Maureen Groer

The pathophysiologic mechanisms of many common malignancies are described in appropriate chapters. This chapter provides an overview of current theories about how cancer develops in human cells and presents an example of this process, skin cancer, the most common malignancy. The pathophysiologic processes underlying carcinogenesis are being increasingly understood at the genetic and molecular mechanism. Understanding the stages of cancer development, including premalignant conditions, is an important tool for the primary care provider, who has many opportunities to screen for early signs of cancer and precancerous lesions. The skin, which is the largest organ of the body, is the most accessible organ for cancer screening, and skin cancers are the most common malignancy. This chapter begins with descriptions of general cellular responses to environmental influences and then discusses how malignant changes arise in cells. The chapter then moves to a discussion of the pathogenesis and pathophysiologic mechanisms of skin cancer.

## CELLULAR RESPONSES TO ENVIRONMENTAL INFLUENCES

Cells are extremely sensitive to environmental conditions and adapt in many ways to perturbations that threaten their survival. One way is through changes in their growth characteristics and morphology. These changes generally are reversible when they are adaptations to altered environmental conditions. Removing the stimulus causes the cells to revert to normal structure and function. However, in some cases, these alterations in cells can be premalignant, representing a significant change in cell function.

## Atrophy and Hypertrophy

When cells decrease in either number or size within a tissue or organ, there is an overall shrinkage of that structure, often accompanied by a decline in functional abilities. The loss of cell number may result from increased apoptosis (programmed cell suicide in which damaged cells are destroyed before they can proliferate) within a tissue, or it could result from necrotic events caused by decreased perfusion or innervation, physical compression, aging, or inflammatory changes. Atrophy of individual cells often results from lack of stimulation. For muscle cells, this is disuse atrophy. For endocrine cells, absence of trophic stimulation or negative feedback from exogenous administration of the hormone product of the gland causes cells to shrink markedly. Atrophy is not a premalignant change.

Hypertrophy occurs when cells increase in size within a tissue or organ, which may be significant enough to increase the size of that structure. Cellular synthetic pathways are involved in the production of increased intracellular constituents. Hypertrophy is seen when cells are subjected to increased workload. Muscle cell hypertrophy is a response to increased load. Cells that are called on to increase function as a compensatory response, such as the renal response that occurs when a kidney is removed, also undergo hypertrophy.

## Hyperplasia

Hyperplasia, in contrast, is when cells respond by increasing the rate of cell division, thus increasing the number of cells in a tissue. Inherent in hyperplasia, then, is cellular genetic processes that increase cell division as well as synthesis. Therefore, only dividing cells can become hyperplastic.

Hyperplasia may result from mitogenic or endocrine stimulation and may be a pathologic response. Excessive stimulation of the endometrial lining by estrogen–progesterone imbalance may lead to endometrial hyperplasia (Sirica, 1989). Hyperplasia may predispose a tissue to the development of malignancy.

## Metaplasia

Metaplasia is a response to stressful environmental perturbations that allow a particular cell type to adapt to the alteration. Chronic irritation is one such perturbation. The process again involves cellular DNA and differentiation of the cells. Metaplasia is the conversion of a population of cells from one type to another, either from altered stem cells within a dividing tissue compartment or from more mature cells. Chronic inflammation in a tendon leads to ossification and bony tissue formation. Cigarette smoke produces a change in bronchial epithelium so that the ciliated columnar epithelium converts to squamous epithelium. This type of tissue is more able to withstand the chronic irritation of cigarette smoke in the airways but also is more likely to undergo dysplastic changes over time.

## Dysplasia

Dysplasia is not adaptive and indicates that a disorderly proliferative process has occurred. The cells become atypical, with abnormal sizes, shapes, and orientations, a characteristic known as pleiomorphism. Dysplasia often is provoked by chronic irritation or inflammation and is found in a variety of epithelial and mesenchymal tissues such as the cervix, the bronchial epithelium, and the liver (Sirica, 1989). When cells display dysplasia, they often have an increased likelihood of converting to anaplasia, which is the term used to describe malignant cells.

## Anaplasia

The term *anaplasia* means "without form." Cancer cells display a loss of differentiation, thus losing the unique characteristics that mark differentiated cells. Anaplastic cells display striking pleiomorphism and an increased nuclear–cytoplasmic ratio and number of nucleoli. Bizarre and increased numbers of mitotic figures may be present, and there is an increased amount of DNA and chromosomes present within anaplastic cells. In contrast, the neoplastic growth seen in benign tumors is marked by growth of differentiated cells and little

mitosis. Anaplasia indicates that the cells have become more primitive, more proliferative, and less regulated. These cells also produce unusual, inappropriate, and sometimes primitive gene products, such as proteins normally produced only during embryonic life. Such a loss of differentiation also results in nonendocrine cancer cells occasionally synthesizing biologically active hormones such as parathyroid hormone.

Another important characteristic of anaplastic cells is that, in contrast to the cells of benign neoplasms, the cells are able to invade adjacent tissue and destroy normal cells. Malignant cells also release angioblastic factors that produce vascularization of the growing tumor mass. Other characteristics of malignant cells are that they are metabolically more efficient than normal cells, which must compete with them for nutrients. Anaplastic cells take up glucose and amino acids at a faster and more efficient rate than normal cells so that they are provided with fuel needed for their increased proliferative rate.

Anaplastic cells often are motile as well, and can break off either singly or in clumps from the primary site of tumor cell growth and spread to distant sites (metastasis). Benign tumors never spread from the local site of origin. Although certain skin cancers (basal cell carcinoma [BCC]) rarely metastasize, they are extremely invasive.

Cancer cells range in their degree of anaplasia, with the greatest degree of anaplasia indicating the most invasive and metastatic cell type. Therefore, biopsy specimens often are graded on the extent of loss of differentiation and degree of anaplasia. Figure 3-1 depicts the changes that occur in anaplasia.

## CARCINOGENESIS

### Initiation and Promotion

The process by which a normal cell is transformed into a malignant, anaplastic cell is *carcinogenesis.*

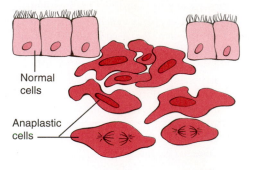

**FIGURE 3.1** ● Anaplasia.

Carcinogenesis is now thought to be a multistep, multistage process resulting from both genetic and environmental factors interacting in sequence in a susceptible host. Many chemicals cause cancer in laboratory animals and humans. Radiation exposure also has been shown to be carcinogenic. Viruses are important carcinogens in laboratory rodents, and a few human cancers are caused by viruses. All of these agents are external environmental influences that, when acting on normal or abnormal cells over time and in the appropriate sequence, may produce a malignant transformation. In chemical carcinogenesis, an agent that produces an irreversible genetic alteration in a cell *initiates* the cancer process. However, cancer does not occur unless a sequence of promoting events occurs (Fig. 3-2). Promotion is thought to result from changes that alter the growth characteristics of the cell. Most cancer is monoclonal; that is, arising from a single cell.

Although all body cells may be exposed at one time or another to chemical, radiation, or viral carcinogenic agents, cancer is a relatively rare event in which a single cell gives rise to a clone of malignantly transformed cells. The sequence and timing of the carcinogenic initiators and promoters are believed to be important. This also explains the long latency period occurring between exposure to the carcinogen and the development of cancer in an exposed individual. For example, the populations exposed to ionizing radiation in Japan during World War II developed thyroid malignancies 15 to 20 years after exposure. Presumably, the initiating

event, radiation, then was followed by many years in which some cells were exposed to promoters that ultimately resulted in the development of a cancer.

## The Cell Cycle

Cancer manifests itself as an abnormality of cellular proliferation, with the more aggressive tumors having increased proliferation rates. This rate is best characterized by *doubling time*, which is the time required for a population of cells to double in size. Doubling time can be increased by shortening of the length of the cell cycle, by decreasing apoptosis of cells within a population of cells, or by increasing the proportion of cells that are dividing with the population (Baserga et al., 1993). To understand the proliferative changes in cancer cells, it is helpful to review the normal regulatory controls on the cell cycle in dividing cells. The normal cell cycle is diagrammed in Figure 3-3. The mitotic period (M) is the shortest length of time, with cells in resting stages (G) most of the time. If the cell goes into G0, it rests until a stimulus causes it to enter G1. During G1 (Gap 1) the cells are synthesizing proteins and growing after just having gone through a cell division. When a cell becomes "ready" to divide, it leaves the G1 phase and goes into the synthesis phase (S). During the S phase, DNA is replicated, preparing the cell for a mitotic division. During G2, the cell again synthesizes protein and grows in preparation for the formation of two daughter cells and then enters mitosis (M). Several signals regulate the cell cycle and

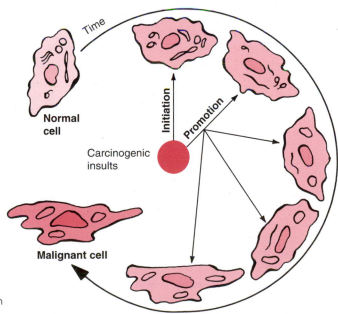

**FIGURE 3.2** ● Initiation and promotion in carginogenesis.

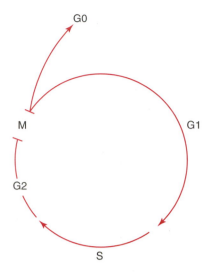

**FIGURE 3.3** ● The cell cycle.

control the rate at which cells divide. Primary to this is the effect of stimulatory growth factors such as insulin-like growth factors, platelet derived growth factor (PDGF), and epidermal growth factor (EGF), as well as inhibitory growth factors such as transforming growth factor-β, which activate or inhibit the cell in G1, stimulating it either to divide or delay division. One mechanism for these actions is through activation of cyclin-dependent kinases that bind to proteins (*cyclins*) that stimulate cell division. Notice that both stimulatory and inhibitory growth factors generally must bind to specific receptors on cells to function, and both the molecule and its receptor are needed to produce effects. In many cancers, there is evidence for either increased expression of stimulatory growth factors or their receptors, or inhibition of in-hibitory growth factors or their receptors, which then can induce excessive proliferation in the targeted cell population. The genes that code for these various growth factors are believed to be critical to the development of malignancy.

## Oncogenes and Tumor Suppressor Genes

Oncogenes are part of the normal genome, and they are genetic elements that generally code for growth factors or growth factor receptors. When these genes are part of the normal human genome, they are termed *proto-oncogenes*. When these same or closely homologous genetic sequences are found in viruses, they are termed *viral oncogenes*. Tumor suppressor genes are even more important in malignant transformation, and they code for

proteins that inhibit cellular proliferation. Notice that proto-oncogenes and tumor suppressor genes are a normal part of the genome and are appropriately regulated and activated in healthy cells. In the carcinogenic process, the essential difference seems to be the lack of regulation and inappropriate expression of proto-oncogenes resulting from mutations or deletions of these genes. Examples of known proto-oncogenes are the *sis* oncogene, which codes for platelet derived growth factor; the *erb B* oncogene, which results in alteration of the epidermal growth factor receptor; the *ras*, or *p21*, oncogene, which is a G protein binding guanine nucleotide and thus inhibiting receptor-mediated adenyl cyclase activation; *fos*, *jun*, and *myc* oncogenes, which code for proteins involved in regulating the cell cycle; and *bcl-2*, a mitochondrial oncogene, which, when activated, inhibits apoptosis. Then, instead of undergoing programmed cell suicide, the cells could enter the M phase of the cell cycle, and deleterious mutations could be carried on to daughter cells.

This interference with apoptosis is a major action of tumor suppressor genes. This second group of genes involved in human carcinogenesis seems to be more important than the proto-oncogenes. Tumor suppressor genes normally regulate the cell cycle by inhibiting cell division, and when they are mutated or absent, the cell cycle becomes dysregulated. Most tumor suppressor gene traits are recessive in that a person may inherit one copy of the normal allele and one copy of the abnormal. Only when both genes are abnormal does the trait manifest itself. So, for some cancers, an inherited predisposition may increase the risk of cancer, but exogenous carcinogens are required to mutate the normal tumor suppressor allele to cause a malignant transformation. For inherited types of cancer (eg, retinoblastoma, Wilms' tumor, BRCA mutations in breast cancer), the tumor suppressor genes are more involved in the carcinogenic process than the proto-oncogenes. Examples of tumor suppressor genes include *DPC-4*, which is involved in pancreatic cancer; *NF-2*, involved in several brain cancer types; *RB*, the gene involved in retinoblastoma; *WT1*, involved in Wilms' tumor; *BRCA1*, which is involved in breast cancer; *BRCA2*, which is involved in both breast and ovarian cancer; *p16* and *p53* (*http://www.cancergenetics.org/site-intro.htm*).

The *p53* tumor suppressor gene is a general model for how many tumor suppressor genes work. Mutations of the p53 gene are the most frequent abnormality identified in human tumors, with half of all human cancers showing a p53 mutation (Hussain & Harris, 1999). The function of p53 is described in Chapter 12, in which its role in breast cancer is discussed, and in Chapter 16, in which colorectal carcinogenesis is described. An important regulatory gene, p53 is located on chromosome 17 and is a major influence on gene transcription, DNA repair, stabilization of the genome, chromosome segregation, aging, and apoptosis (Soehgne, Ouhtit, & Ananthaswamy, 1997). This gene is stimulated by DNA damage or oncogene activity, and the p53 protein accumulates in cells thus damaged, inhibiting them from leaving the G1 phase of the cell cycle. The p53 protein can produce apoptosis by upregulating expression of certain proteins, and downregulating others. This shifts the balance toward apoptosis. A second effect is for the p53 proteins to bind to other proteins involved in DNA repair. Thus, damaged DNA can be efficiently repaired, or, if not repairable, the cell then can be stimulated to undergo apoptosis, thus eliminating any dangerous mutations from being inherited by daughter cells. These events are diagrammed in Figure 3-4. When there is a mutation in the p53 gene or if it is lost from the cell, this ability to repair damaged DNA and prevent damaged cells from replicating may become impaired.

## Interaction of Genetic Factors and Environmental Carcinogens

Cancer is viewed as a process in which carcinogenic insults act on genetically susceptible cells.

This interaction could take place by several possible mechanisms. The carcinogen could mutate proto-oncogenes or tumor suppressor genes. There could be an alteration in expression of these genes through mutation or changes in the regulatory genes that control the transcription of the proto-oncogenes or tumor suppressor genes. Viral carcinogenesis could result from the insertion of viral oncogenes into the human genome so that the expression of the oncogene and the production of its protein products (oncoproteins) are completely unregulated. Each of these mechanisms are explored in this chapter.

Carcinogenic chemicals are electrophilic compounds that usually are converted through enzymatic pathways into ultimate carcinogens, which then bind to DNA, forming DNA adducts. This binding permanently alters the DNA, causing mutations in the code, which are passed on to daughter cells. Some chemical carcinogens have been shown to mutate specific genes. For example, exposure to aflatoxin B, which is known to cause hepatocellular carcinoma, is related to a subsequent mutation in p53 in liver cells, so that a guanine–cytosine base pair is transversed to a thymine–adenine base pair at residue 249 (Hussain & Harris, 1999). This type of event is considered to be an initiation event, leading to an irreversible change in the DNA of the targeted cell. Promoting events then ensue in response to environmental exposure to mitogenic compounds, and a clone of potentially malignant cells then is produced.

All types of ionizing radiation cause cancer in tissues by forming highly reactive oxygen free radicals, which then damage DNA and other biologic molecules, or radiation can directly "hit" DNA bases, producing point mutations. This mechanism of damage is explored more fully when the carcinogenic processes involved in skin cancers are described later in this chapter.

Viruses appear to cause cancer by stimulating cell proliferation or incorporating viral sequences into the human genome. The viral oncogenes carried by some viruses are close to or identical with the human proto-oncogenes. The theory behind this fact is that these viruses have accumulated human DNA sequences while they infected human cells, and it is the presence of the human gene that confers the property of carcinogenicity on a particular virus. Only a few human cancers currently are known to be caused by viruses. One virus is the human papillomavirus, which causes cervical cancers by producing proteins that bind and inactivate p53. Another is the human T cell lymphotropic virus type I, a relative of HIV. However, several herpesviruses are suspected of being involved in

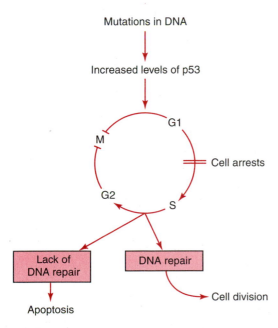

Mutations in DNA

Increased levels of p53

G1

M

Cell arrests

G2

S

Lack of DNA repair

DNA repair

Apoptosis

Cell division

**FIGURE 3.4** ● Action of p53.

some way with carcinogenesis, including both genital herpes, which is a factor in cervical cancer, and Epstein-Barr virus, which is involved in Burkitt's lymphoma.

## SKIN CANCERS

There are three common types of skin cancer: basal cell carcinoma (BCC), squamous cell carcinoma (SCC), and melanoma. Like other cancers, these malignancies undergo multistep carcinogenesis. Primary care providers should be familiar with the appearance of these lesions and should be able to identify premalignant changes in the skin.

The frequency of skin cancer is increasing, with half a million new cases diagnosed each year. Because of changes in the ozone layer, many authorities predict startling increases in the occurrence of skin cancer. All skin cancers are believed to be related to exposure to ultraviolet (UV) sunlight. The most frequent type of skin cancer is BCC (65% to 80%), with SCC second in incidence (10% to 25%), and melanoma the third most common type (Arndt, 1999).

### Basal Cell Carcinomas

Basal cell carcinomas arise in the basal layer of the epidermis (Fig. 3-5), with most occurring on the head or neck. They are slow growing and rarely metastasize, but they produce locally destructive, ulcerated lesions. Both SCCs and BCCs produce a variety of enzymes that degrade the basement membrane and extracellular matrix, allowing the tumor cells to invade underlying tissue. Slides of both BCCs and SCCs can be viewed at *http://tray.dermatology.uiowa.edu/ImageBase.html*. Another excellent dermatology atlas site is *http://dermis.net/bilddb/index_e.htm*.

Initially, BCCs appear as small, nonpainful, raised lesions that tend to bleed and do not heal.

### Squamous Cell Carcinomas

Also most frequently observed on the head and neck, SCCs are more likely to metastasize, particularly along nerves that supply the skin site. They arise from atypical keratinocytes (squamous cells) in the prickle cell layer of the epidermis (see Fig. 3-5), and they are most likely to arise from sun-damaged skin that has many actinic keratoses (Arndt, 1999). A gallery of photographs of SCCs in different areas of the body can be viewed at *http://matrix.ucdavis.edu/tumors/tradition/gallery-scc.html*. About 100,000 new cases of SCC are diagnosed each year, with a higher risk seen in people with blue, gray, or green eyes. They may arise in skin that has been damaged by chemicals, burns, or trauma, as well as in sun-damaged skin.

SCCs may be painful because of their rapid growth and inflammation around the lesion. Eventually, they may ulcerate and invade nerves.

### Malignant Melanoma

The most anaplastic, metastatic, and dangerous skin cancer is malignant melanoma. These lesions are the fastest growing cancer in the United States, with the incidence doubling every 10 years, so that it is predicted that 1 of 90 Americans will develop

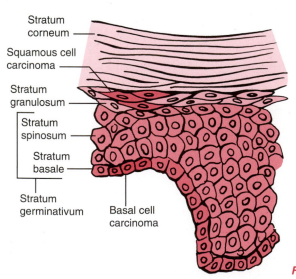

Stratum corneum

Squamous cell carcinoma

Stratum granulosum

Stratum spinosum

Stratum basale

Stratum germinativum

Basal cell carcinoma

**FIGURE 3.5** ● The epidermis.

a malignant melanoma in their lifetime (Arndt, 1999). Risk factors for melanoma include fair skin, significant sun exposure, the occurrence of a blistering sunburn before 15 years of age, family history positive for malignant melanoma, and the presence of either typical or atypical nevi on the skin. They are commonly located on the hands and feet, in the eyes, and on mucous membranes.

A melanoma arises from a change in a preexisting mole or presents as a new pigmented lesion. Occasionally, a lesion burns or itches, but most people with melanomas have no pain at the site.

## CARCINOGENESIS OF SKIN CANCER

### Basal and Squamous Cell Carcinomas

The major factor producing the transformation of normal skin keratinocytes to BCC or SCC is exposure to solar UV light. A premalignant lesion produced by this exposure is *solar keratosis,* which can convert to SCC. UV light consists of UVA, UVB, and UVC parts, which are of different wavelengths. UVC (wavelength of 200 to 290 nm) does not penetrate the stratospheric ozone layer, although concern over depletion of the ozone layer is justified because this UV light, with its short wavelength, is mutagenic. UVB (290 to 320 nm) and UVA (320 to 400 nm) do penetrate the skin, and both are carcinogenic to skin (Kanjilal & Ananthaswamy, 1996). UVB likely is responsible for initiation.

When UV light penetrates through the stratum corneum and reaches living epithelial cells, the genetic mutations that are produced are unique and are referred to as *signature* mutations. Pyrimidine dimers (covalently linked adjacent pyrimidines) are common effects of UV exposure. The sensitivity of the pyrimidine bases to photodamage is greater than the purine bases (Kanjilal & Ananthaswamy, 1996). Another type of mutation commonly produced is a *transition* mutation, in which a purine is converted to a purine or a pyrimidine is converted to a purine. The most common type of transition mutation is a conversion of cytosine to thymine. These molecular photolesions are produced either by direct hits of the DNA by UV light or chemicals in cells that have become irradiated and photoactivated, which then secondarily damage the DNA. DNA's chemical characteristics make it susceptible to UV light damage. The cell is able to repair photodamage in DNA efficiently in most cases; skin cancer requires multiple unre-

paired mutations to occur for the carcinogenic process to be complete.

Several repair mechanisms are involved in UV light-induced DNA damage. Cells that are damaged may be prevented from entering into cell division, with the delay allowing time either for DNA repair or apoptosis if the damage cannot be repaired. This prevents both the damaged DNA from being replicated and the new daughter cells containing the mutation from being produced. One important repair pathway is nucleotide excision repair (Sarasin, 1999). This pathway excises and repairs sections of light-induced DNA damage. An inherited autosomal recessive genetic disease in which this enzyme is missing is *xeroderma pigmentosum* (*XP*). Children with XP develop multiple freckles early in life, which then progress to multiple skin cancers. The continuous development of malignancies is correlated with amount of exposure to sunlight. The nucleotide excision repair pathway, depending on the circumstances, either is error free or error prone, the former resulting in complete repair of the DNA strand and the latter potentially resulting in a mutation.

The carcinogenic process in skin cancer involves unrepaired mutations in both proto-oncogenes and tumor suppressor genes, causing overexpression of growth-promoting genes or inactivation of tumor suppressor genes. As with other types of cancers, this is a multistep, multistage phenomenon, involving three to seven mutations in a cell occurring over an individual's lifetime. The probability of this happening is extremely small, especially when the cell compartment is one that is rapidly dividing and rapidly turning over, like the skin. Nevertheless, skin cancer is the most common type of human malignancy. The normal human being sheds 50,000 flakes of skin every minute, which translates into millions of cells being lost constantly. Yet, cancer does appear in the skin because of transforming events in keratinocytes (squamous cells) in the stratum corneum or in cells of the stratum germinativum. The mutational events that occur in SCCs and BCCs frequently involve the *ras* proto-oncogene and the p53 tumor suppressor gene.

### c-ras Proto-Oncogene Mutations

The c-*ras* proto-oncogene has been described previously as a gene that codes for a cell–membrane-bound protein that influences signal transduction through GTP binding. This allows c-*ras* protein to participate in regulating cell growth by being a mediator in hormonal or growth factor stimulation.

There is evidence that c-*ras* is mutated in some skin cancers, with XP patients having the most mutations. UV irradiation has been shown to produce c-*ras* mutations (Kanjilal & Ananthaswamy, 1996). However, tumor suppressor gene inactivation seems to be a major way that carcinogenesis proceeds in the skin.

## p53 Inactivation

Recall that p53 is a normal gene that codes for a necessary regulatory protein, which prevents mutational events from being carried forward in daughter cells. This is accomplished by delaying the entry of the cell into mitosis, which allows time for repair. If repair is not possible, then apoptosis is stimulated. Mutations in p53 that produce cancer thus inhibit repair mechanisms or promote DNA replication or synthesis when the DNA is damaged. Mutations in the p53 gene are numerous (5000 have been identified), and there are several types. The gene can be deleted partially or totally, which has been achieved by breeding p53 knock-out mice with a high incidence of cancer. Other mutations inhibit the ability of the p53 protein to bind to DNA. A third type of mutation produces a loss of tumor suppressor function (Soehnge et al., 1997). Inactivation of both alleles results in a loss of function, which contributes to the development of cancer.

In skin, p53 mutations are common and arise early in skin cells, in contrast to other types of cancer, such as colorectal cancer, in which the p53 mutation is a late event in carcinogenesis. p53 is upregulated by covalent dipyrimidine linkages that are produced by UV exposure in skin cells. The presence of this type of DNA damage blocks both RNA and DNA polymerase. This subsequently stimulates the expression of p53, which produces apoptosis in the damaged cell or allows the blocked polymerase in the transcribed strand of DNA to activate nucleotide excision repair mechanisms (McGregor, 1999). If p53 mutates, then this mechanism becomes impaired, and UV-damaged cells survive with unrepaired mutations and then divide to form a clone of potentially malignant cells.

Both BCCs and SCCs have been shown unequivocally to contain p53 mutations. The p53 mutations also are associated with increased cellular proliferation. Solar keratoses, which are the precursor lesions to SCCs, also have been shown to contain p53 mutations, in contrast to skin that has not been sun damaged (Shimuzu et al., 1999). There also is evidence that persons who use sunscreen are protected from p53 mutations (Rosen-

stein et al., 1999). Such pathophysiologic data provide the primary care provider with ample evidence supporting measures to protect patients from excessive sun exposure and to encourage sunscreen use beginning early in life.

## Malignant Melanoma

Melanomas arise from melanin-secreting epidermal cells called *melanocytes*. There is an epidemiologically higher risk in individuals with greater sun exposure. Fair-skinned individuals and people who have had a previous melanoma are at the highest risk.

Most melanomas are superficial spreading melanomas, which arise in the epidermal dermal junction and spread radially. They are only slightly elevated and usually are pigmented. The margins and colors are uneven. When melanomas are not pigmented, the degree of anaplasia is high, and the cells have lost their melanin-producing ability. Other less-common types of melanomas are nodular, lentiginous, and acrolentiginous. Examples of each of these types may be viewed at *http://matrix.ucdavis.edu/tumors/tradition/melanoma.html*. Melanomas are the most aggressive and metastatic forms of skin cancer with a 30% to 40% mortality rate, depending on the stage of disease when the lesion is diagnosed initially. Melanoma are staged according to the following criteria:

*Stage I*: Tumor cells are above basement membrane (in situ). The tumor is less than 1.5 mm ($^1/_{16}$ inch) thick.
*Stage II*: Tumor extends to dermis. The tumor is 1.5 to 4 mm.
*Stage III*: Tumor has spread below dermis and may have spread to other sites within 1 inch of the original tumor. The tumor is more than 4 mm and may have spread to adjacent lymph nodes.
*Stage IV*: Tumor has spread to distant sites.

Again, as in BCCs and SCCs, melanomas appear to arise from UV-induced mutations or deletions in a tumor suppressor gene. In melanoma, a suspect gene is CDKN2, a tumor suppressor gene located on chromosome 9. A hereditary risk for melanoma is associated with a mutation in the CDKN2 gene, which normally codes for p16 (Borg et al., 1996). In p16 knockout mice, the absence of the gene increases the risk for developing several types of cancer. Up to 10% of melanoma patients have relatives with melanoma, suggesting a possible shared genetic trait, with 25% of familial melanoma patients carrying the p16 mutation. Other potential melanoma genes also have been identified. Persons with dysplastic

---

### CLINICAL VIGNETTE 3.1

Mr. Joseph Cannon is a 75-year-old patient who comes complaining of a mole that bleeds and "looks funny." He has had several squamous cell cancers removed from his trunk in the last few years. He has had significant exposure to the sun during his life, having spent 40 years in Florida, never using sunscreen and enjoying being outside as much as possible. He is a former redhead with freckled, fair skin. He now has many actinic keratoses over all sun-exposed skin. There also are many large, dark moles, characteristic of dysplastic nevi syndrome, on his back.

The lesion of concern is on his left shoulder blade. It is raised and has black, reddish, and brown pigments, irregular borders, a slightly inflamed appearance, and measures approximately 1 cm. He has had this "mole" all his life, but in the last 2 months, its character has changed radically.

There are no palpable lymph nodes, and his general health otherwise is good. His medical history reveals a son who had a malignant melanoma diagnosed at the age of 35 years. Mr. Cannon is referred to a dermatologist. Biopsy reveals a grade II malignant melanoma. His familial history justifies genetic analyses of close relatives. His treatment includes excision and a trial of combined therapy, including interferon.

---

nevi are at higher risk for melanoma, and this trait is familial.

The cell cycle is regulated by tumor suppressor genes such as p23 or p16, as has been described previously. In the case of p16, the protein coded by the gene inactivates cyclin-dependent kinases. The cell cycle normally is regulated by proteins known as *cyclins* and cyclin-dependent kinases, which promote the cell moving from the G1 into the S phase. In the absence of normal amounts or function of p16, the mutated skin cell cycle is pushed into S and M phases.

Mutations in tumor suppressor genes provide one explanatory theory for the carcinogenic process in melanoma. As with BCC and SCC, the role of the primary care provider is in screening, early detection, and prevention of these skin cancers. Protective clothing, use of sunscreen, and avoidance of excessive exposure to UV light all are part of general health education for every patient.

### REFERENCES

Arndt, K. (1999). Manual of dermatological therapeutics. In *MAXX: Maximum Access to Diagnosis and Therapy, Version 2.0* (CD-ROM). Philadelphia: Lippincott Williams & Wilkins.

Baserga, R., Porcu, P., & Sell, C. (1993). Oncogenes, growth factors and control of the cell cycle. *Cancer Survey, 16*, 201–213.

Borg, A., Johannsson, U., Johannsson, O., Hakansson, S., Westerdahl, J., Masback, A., Olsson, H., & Ingvar, C. (1996). Novel germline p16 mutation in familial malignant melanoma in southern Sweden. *Cancer Research, 56,* (11), 2497–2500.

Hussain, S.P. & Harris, C.C. (1999). P53 mutation spectrum and load: The generation of hypotheses linking the exposure of endogenous or exogenous carcinogens to human cancer. *Mutation Research, 428* (1-2), 23–32.

Kanjilal, S. & Ananthaswamy, H. (1996). Molecular biology of skin carcinomas. In R. Weber, M. Miller, & H. Goepfert (Eds.). *Basal and squamous cell skin cancers of the head and neck*. Baltimore: Williams & Wilkins.

MacGregor, W.G. (1999). DNA repair, DNA replication, and UV mutagenesis. *Journal of Investigative Dermatology Symposium Proceedings, 4* (1), 1–5.

Rosenstein, B.S., Phelps, R. G., Weinstock, M. A., Bernstein, J.L., Gordon, M.L., Rudikoff, D., Kantor, I., Shelton, R., & Lebwohl, M.G. (1999). P53 mutations in basal cell carcinomas arising in routine users of sunscreen. *Photochemistry and Photobiology, 70* (5), 798–806.

Sarasin, A. (1999). The molecular pathways of ultraviolet-induced carcinogenesis. *Mutation Research, 428* (1-2), 5–10.

Shimuzu, T., Oga, A., Murakami, T., & Muto, M. (1999). Overexpression of p53 protein associated with proliferative activity and histological degree of malignancy in solar keratosis. *Dermatology, 199* (2), 113–118.

Soehnge, H., Ouhtit, A., & Ananthaswamy, H.N. (1997). Mechanisms of induction of skin cancer by UV radiation. *Frontiers in Bioscience, 2*, 538–551.

Sirica, A. (1989). *The pathobiology of neoplasia*. New York: Plenum Press.

# Headaches and Dizziness

Maureen Groer

Karen Lasater

Headaches and dizziness are nonspecific yet common symptoms confronted by primary care providers on a daily basis. The causes of these symptoms range from being completely innocuous to life threatening and deadly, and the list of diseases with headache or dizziness as a presenting syndrome is unbelievably long. Excellent diagnostic skills are needed to determine the differential diagnoses for both of these symptoms. The first section of this chapter covers the pathophysiologic basis for common types of headaches. The pathophysiologic mechanisms of common forms of dizziness are described in the second part of the chapter.

## HEADACHE

### CLINICAL PRESENTATIONS AND TYPES OF HEADACHES

Nearly every human being has experienced a headache, and most people have at least one a year. The International Headache Society (IHS) has published a comprehensive listing of diagnostic categories for headache, consisting of 129 types of headaches divided into primary and secondary types. Many of the secondary headache diagnoses are rare and are unlikely to be encountered in primary care practices. Ninety percent of the headaches managed by practitioners are primary headaches. Primary headaches are divided into the major subtypes: migraines, tension, cluster, rebound, and benign. Table 4-1 presents common primary headache diagnoses and the associated signs and symptoms for each.

### Tension-Type Headaches

Tension-type headaches arise from a culmination of factors influencing the muscles of the neck and cranium, leading to a headache. These headaches usually present bilaterally as a feeling of tight bands or viselike pressure on the occipital, frontal, or parietal regions of the head (Diamond, 1993a). The onset of tension-type headaches usually is concurrent with an emotional or physical strain (Graham, 1996). The psychological states of stress, anxiety, and depression are links to the development of this type of headache (Lance, 1997). Temporomandibular joint strain, eyestrain, and cervical spondylosis are physical conditions that exacerbate tension-type headaches. Many patients with chronic tension headache identify stress and worry, sleep deprivation or excessive sleep, and skipping meals as the most common headache precipitants. These patients are difficult to treat because they often overuse pain medication, may develop rebound headaches, or may have migraine headaches concurrent with chronic tension headache.

The IHS recognizes episodic and chronic tension-type headaches as separate entities, with episodic tension headaches being the most common headache. However, both anxiety and depression are factors relevant to both. Refer to Table 4-2 for the diagnostic criteria for differences. The primary care practitioner is most likely to see patients with chronic tension headaches (greater than 15 headaches per month, occurring for longer than 6 months).

To fully understand the pathogenesis of tension headache, the practitioner must be aware of the action of the central nervous system (CNS) on muscle tone and the contributing physiologic elements of emotional states. These are discussed

# TABLE 4.1

## Differentiating Common Primary Headaches

| Characteristic | Migraine Without Aura | Episodic Tension-type Headaches | Cluster |
|---|---|---|---|
| Location and radiation of pain | *(diagram)* Usually unilateral | *(diagram)* Bilateral | *(diagram)* Strictly unilateral |
| Quality and severity of pain | Achy to throbbing (50%), moderate to severe | Pressing or bandlike, mild to moderate | Boring, sharp, excruciatingly severe |
| Duration of pain | Usually 4 to 24 hours | Variable (30 minutes to 7 days) | Brief (30 to 90 minutes) |
| Frequency of attacks | Intermittent (usually two to five times per month) | Intermittent (< 15 per month) | Multiple (1 to 6) daily for several weeks to months |
| Time of occurrence | Anytime | Anytime | Frequently at night, same time each attack |
| Prodrome or aura | Often present | None | None |
| Associated symptoms | Photophobia, phonophobia, osmophobia, nausea, vomiting, anorexia, diarrhea, sensitivity to movement | Slight anorexia, photophobia or phonophobia, pericranial muscle tenderness, tooth grinding | Ipsilateral autonomic features (eg, nasal stuffiness, lacrimation) |
| Age at onset | Between 10 and 30 years | Any age | Adulthood |
| Gender predilection | Majority female | Majority female | Majority male |
| Family history | Often present | Present | None |
| Behavior during attack | Passive; rests in quiet, dark room | Variable | Active; pacing, head banging |
| Precipitating factors | Bright lights; fatigue; loss of sleep; hypoglycemia; stress; alcohol; menstruation; exercise; orgasm; certain drugs, foods, and food additives and allergies | Stress | Alcohol |
| Sleep pattern | ND | ND | Often awakens patient from sleep |
| Emotional status | ND | ND | ND |
| Allergy | Food allergies | ND | ND |

ND, Not different from nonheadache controls.
(From Smith R. [1997]. Diagnosing headache. *Hospital Medicine 33* [7], 26–42.)

## TABLE 4.2

### International Headache Society Criteria for Tension-Type Headache

Two of the following
- Nonpulsating, pressing, or tightening sensation
- Mild to moderate intensity
- Bilateral
- Not aggravated by walking stairs or physical activity

Both of the following
- No nausea or vomiting
- No photophobia or phonophobia

One of the following
- History and physical do not suggest organic or systemic disease
- Organic disease ruled out by testing
- Organic disorder present but does not appear related to headache

Episodic
- 10 previous headaches
- Less than 15 headaches per month
- Headache lasts for 30 minutes to 7 days

Chronic
- More than 15 headaches per month for longer than 6 months

next. A case study and treatment modalities also are included.

## Central Nervous System and Muscle Tone

Recall that the brain tissue and skull are not sensitive to pain, so the pain of headaches is derived from sensitive intracranial and extracranial structures. Intracranial structures that could be altered to cause headache include the fifth, ninth, and twelfth cranial nerves, the dural arteries, the arteries of the Circle of Willis, major venous sinuses, and the dura at the base of the skull. Extracranial structures usually implicated in primary headaches include the skin, fascia, muscles, blood vessels of the scalp, upper cervical root, and muscles of the neck.

In tension-type headache, the pain is thought to originate from muscle nociceptors and is caused by muscle contraction and spasm, muscle hypoxia, and, in chronic cases, tearing of tendons and ligaments from sustained, extreme muscle tension

(Jay, 1998). The pain is mild to moderate in intensity, causing a pressing or squeezing bilateral headache, often felt in the occipital region and neck, although the entire face and head can be involved. Muscle tension is believed to increase in the neck, shoulders, and lower back, and all contribute to the headache. Patients may develop a posture with their head held forward and the shoulders tensed to splint the pain of tension-type headache (Jay, 1998). The pain usually gets worse as the day progresses, and the headache can last from 30 minutes to 7 days.

Recall that muscle tone is maintained through a centrally organized multisynaptic reflex system consisting of gamma efferent neurons, alpha motor neurons, and the muscle spindle fibers. The CNS can produce an increase in muscle tone and a partially contracted tonic state through these reflex mechanisms. The gamma efferent neurons transmit information from the CNS toward an intended muscle group. Muscle contraction occurs when alpha motor neurons under control of the CNS stimulate the spindle fibers of the muscles. In tension-type headache, both cortical and subcortical signals to the muscles, as well as nociceptive signals from the muscle to the brain, may produce a pain-tension-pain cycle, which may lead to chronic contraction, spasm, and headache pain.

## Physiologic Basis for Relationship With Emotions

Because tension headaches are associated with emotionally distressful states, the stress-emotion-muscle contraction link is explored in this section. The response of the CNS to stressful stimuli is regulated partly by the limbic system, which receives sensory input from the frontal cortex, which has processed the sensory input. The amygdala, part of the limbic system, then interprets incoming sensory data and marshals appropriate autonomic and endocrine responses. Information from the amygdala goes either to the hypothalamus or multiple locations within the brainstem, such as brainstem aminergic nuclei (AMN) and nucleus paragigantocellularis (PGi). During a stressful situation, the hypothalamus coordinates the autonomic and endocrine responses, including release of cortisol by the adrenal cortex (Lovallo, 1997).

The AMN synthesizes neurotransmitters such as serotonin, noradrenaline, and dopamine. The hypothalamus and limbic system are innervated by the locus ceruleus and raphe nuclei (Lovallo, 1997). These two dense collections of neurons contain large amounts of noradrenaline and serotonin, respectively (Lance, 1993). These neurons and their neurotransmitters are believed to be involved in depression, anger, and aggression (Toates, 1995; Brown et al., 1986). Information from the amygdala also goes to the PGi, which has been linked to skeletal muscle reflexes. This link allows for the coordination of the autonomic nervous system and muscle reflexes through the amygdala (Lovallo, 1997).

### Pathogenesis of Episodic Tension-Type Headaches

The episodic tension-type headache is the result of an interaction between the CNS and the muscle reflex system (Solomon, 1998). Environmental stimuli, whether internal or external, may be precipitating factors for tension-type headaches. The triggering stimulus, traveling through the amygdala, initiates the multisynaptic reflex muscle contraction (Diamond, 1993a). This muscle contraction is further accentuated through a monosynaptic reflex between the afferent neurons and the motor neurons, which allows for a prolonged or continued muscle contraction to occur. The continued contracted state could result from repeated physical tasks such as looking over the shoulder or poor posture from sitting at a desk with an improperly placed computer monitor. A new form of tension-type headache results from ocular tendinitis related to computer screen fatigue. When these physical activities are combined with added psychological stress such as anxiety, the episodic tension-type headache occurs (Graham, 1996).

With continued muscular contraction, muscle lactic acid, serotonin, prostaglandin, and bradykinin levels rise, which are thought to activate the nociceptive relay system, evoking pain. Another pain-eliciting factor is the hypoxic state produced in the contracted muscles. Tense muscles compress small blood vessels, leading to a decrease in blood flow and thus hypoxia (Jay, 1993). In hypoxia, a buildup of byproducts or metabolites occurs, which further stimulates the nociceptive pathways (Jay, 1993). The episodic tension-type headache may be mainly a disorder of the nerves and muscles within the head and neck (Solomon, 1998). Recurrent episodes of these headaches may predispose a person to future attacks by changing the muscle tissue's threshold for contractions and decreasing the body's tolerance to pain.

### Pathogenesis of Chronic Tension-Type Headaches

The pathogenesis of chronic tension headaches still is undetermined. The role of serotonin has become the focus of recent study, since low levels of serotonin were found in persons with this headache (Solomon, 1998). Chronic tension-type headache may be the result of an alteration in the monoamine neurotransmitters, dopamine, noradrenaline, and serotonin, and in endogenous pain control (Diamond, 1993b). Depression and anxiety have been linked with these chronic headaches (Graham, 1996). Patients with chronic tension-type headache often report sleep disturbances (frequent awakening, decreased slow wave sleep), which may be related to serotonin dysregulation (Jay, 1998). Chronic tension-type headache also may be related to an abnormal endogenous pain control system.

### Anxiety and Depression

Most patients with depression experience chronic tension-type headaches (Diamond, 1993b). Although a complete understanding of this relationship is unknown, a biochemical etiology for depression could explain a connection between these two disorders. One biochemical theory suggests that decreased levels of the neurotransmitters noradrenaline and serotonin could lead to the development of depression (Ingram & Scher, 1998) (see Chapter 5). As previously mentioned, these neurotransmitters have been linked to chronic tension-type headache.

Persons who are chronically anxious are at risk for developing chronic tension-type headaches (Graham, 1996). These headaches may be caused by unconscious reactions toward life stressors. Suppressing anger or anxiety also leads to chronic tension-type headaches (Adler et al., 1987).

### Rebound Headache

Patients with tension-type headaches often begin a pattern of self-medication to relieve their pain, but this produces a vicious cycle. Medications containing caffeine or ergot most often are the cause of rebound headache. The pain is steady, dull, and perceived to be generalized to the entire head. The pattern that typifies this type of headache is one in which a person wakes up with this headache and takes medication for relief. The headache pain is relieved for a while but then returns. Treatment consists of discontinuing the medication until the headache subsides.

## PHYSIOLOGIC BASIS FOR TREATMENT OF TENSION-TYPE HEADACHE

Treatment for tension-type headaches focuses mainly on behavioral modification, including biofeedback, relaxation techniques, massage, acupuncture, and stress management. Biofeedback is a process in which a person learns to adjust muscle tension in response to an auditory or visual stimulus corresponding to their electromyographic levels. When combined with relaxation techniques, the patient can monitor decreases or increases in muscle contraction. Avoiding certain foods may be helpful for some patients with headache; milk products, chocolate, red wine, and foods containing monosodium glutamate are known to cause headache in some patients. Quality sleep also is important. Pharmacologic interventions for patients experiencing chronic tension headache include tricyclic antidepressants and monoamine oxidase inhibitors (MAOIs). Tricyclic antidepressants alter the reuptake of noradrenaline and serotonin, prolonging neural stimulation. MAOIs increase the levels of serotonin, dopamine, and noradrenaline within the CNS. These medications relieve depression and help patients to sleep. Muscle relaxants also are used occasionally. Over-the-counter analgesics, nonsteroidal anti-inflammatory depressants (NSAIDs), aspirin, and acetaminophen offer some relief. However, many of these medications contain caffeine, which can cause rebound headache. A possible new treatment is injecting botulinum toxin into the frontalis muscle in patients with tension headache, which produces muscle relaxation and relief for some.

A web site useful to primary care providers for information on common headaches and their treatment is *http://www.headachecare.com*.

### ● Case Study 4.1

A 35-year-old man presents to the office with episodic headaches for about a year. He describes the headaches as a band of pressure near his temples and at the base of his head. They occur mainly late in the afternoon when he is at work, although occasionally he has awakened with these headaches. The headaches have increased in intensity and frequency. He states that when the headaches are at their worst, his neck and shoulders ache and his scalp becomes tender. He feels that he is under a lot of stress at work because of the recent downsizing of his company. He states that an increase in workload has kept him from enjoying his hobbies of fishing and golfing. The headaches are interfering with concentration and relationships.

He has tried several OTC medications to alleviate the pain (acetaminophen 650 mg/q 4 h, ibuprofen 800 mg/qid, and aspirin 650 mg/q 4 h) but believes that none have been effective. He denies any aggravating factors and has not noticed changes in appetite or sleep patterns. He denies nausea, photophobia, auras or visual difficulties, phonophobia, recent head trauma, illness, fever, history of depression, neck stiffness, or vertigo.

No history of chronic illnesses or surgeries. Currently taking no medications. NKDA. Denies environmental or food allergies. No family history of headaches. Has worn glasses for reading for 10 years.

#### Differential Diagnoses

Episodic tension-type headache
Chronic tension-type headache
Depression
Hypertension
Cervical spondylosis
Migraine headache
Intracranial lesion
TMJ dysfunction

*(Case study continued on next page)*

### Physical Assessment

| | |
|---|---|
| Vital signs | T–98.5°F, P–90 beats/min, BP–145/88 |
| HEENT | Head: Normocephalic, no masses or lesions. Mild tenderness to palpation in the occipital region |
| | Eyes: Snellen 20/20 UO without glasses. Visual fields normal. EOM intact. Conjunctivae pink and sclera clear. PERRLA, red reflex and optic disc noted. No AV nicking or exudates noted |
| | Ears: Canal clear. TMs pearly gray and intact. Light reflex noted |
| Neck | Supple. Carotid pulse palpated at 88. No bruit auscultated |
| Musculoskeletal | Neck with full ROM. Tenderness and tightness noted in trapezius and occipitalis muscle groups. No TMJ clicking or tenderness. No weakness, contractures, or atrophy noted. Gait smooth |
| Neurologic | CN I–XII intact. Speech clear. Alert and oriented × 3. Recent and remote memories intact. DTRs 2+, no Babinski reflex noted, bilaterally strong, no weakness or atrophy noted. Negative for Romberg sign. Light touch, pin prick, position and vibration intact. |

### Diagnostic Tests

1. CT scan or MRI if assessment leads toward possible intracranial lesion or mass
2. CBC with differential if patient presents with symptoms of infection (chills, fever)
3. X-ray to rule out cervical spondylosis
4. Lumbar puncture to rule out infection/meningitis in febrile patient

AV, arteriovenous; BP, blood pressure; CBC, complete blood count; CN, cranial nerve; CT, computed tomography; DTRs, deep tendon reflexes; EOM, extraoccular muscles; HEENT, head, eye, ear, nose, and throat; MRI, magnetic resonance imaging; NKDA, no known drug allergies; OTC, over-the-counter; P, pulse; PERRLA, pupils equal, round, regular to light and accommodation; ROM, range of motion; T, temperature; TMs, tympanic membranes; TMJ, temporomandibular joint.

## MIGRAINE HEADACHES

Although not as common as tension headaches, migraine is a frequent diagnosis made by primary care providers. Twenty-five million Americans experience migraine headaches, with a female-to-male ratio of about 3:1. However, this may be an underestimate because not every person who has migraines seeks medical help for their headaches, and many persons with headache use over-the-counter medication.

Because of the throbbing nature and location of the pain, migraine headaches had been considered to have a vascular origin, with a period of vasoconstriction followed by a period of vasodilation. This theory is being challenged, with the predominant migraine theory being that the headache has a neurogenic origin with vascular sequelae.

Migraine headaches usually are unilateral, throbbing, and moderately to severely painful. There is a circadian pattern to migraine, with many headaches occurring between the hours of 6 AM and 10 AM. Sleep disturbances are common in migraineurs, and decreased melatonin may play a role in this rhythmic pattern (MacGregor, 1999). The pain lasts from 4 to 24 hours, and migraineurs report headaches as frequently as once a week or more. The two major types of migraine are migraine without aura (common) and migraine with aura (classic), the former being the most common type. The classic form of migraine has a prodromal period of symptoms that occurs 10 to 60 minutes before the headache and disappears with the onset of headache. This prodrome may include auras and paresthesia in the face, fingers, and arms. A migraine aura usually is unique to the migraineur and may include vertigo, scotoma (losses in the fields of vision), scintillations (light flashes), fortication (zigzag forms in the visual fields), one-sided weakness, and other neurologic symptoms. Visual symptoms are most frequent (99%), followed by sensory (31%), aphasic (18%), and motor (6%) symptoms (Russell & Oleson, 1996). A visual aura begins as a flickering, clear, zigzag line in the center of the visual field, which affects the central vision. It progresses toward the peripheral field and may be followed by a scotoma. A typical sensory aura is one sided, beginning in the hand, then moving toward the arm and finally to the face and tongue. A typical motor aura affects the hand and arm of one side (Russell & Oleson, 1996). Most migraineurs report subtle warning signs of a migraine in the 24 hours preceding the headache. They report changes in mood and appetite, food cravings, decreased activity, and repetitive yawning.

A migraine is a combination of neural, vascular, and gastrointestinal alterations. Therefore, symptoms include not only head pain, but also nausea and visual disturbances. The symptoms of a migraine attack are the culmination of an interaction between the nervous system and cranial circulation. This interaction produces different physiologic reactions including the premonitory symptoms, aura, and headache (usually unilateral). Symptoms associated with the headache phase are nausea, vomiting, photophobia, phonophobia, and vertigo (Diamond, 1993c). In the following sections, the pathogenesis of the migraine attack are discussed, along with current theories for the different physiologic reactions experienced during an attack.

## Pathophysiology of Migraine

Current evidence suggests that migraineurs are genetically and biochemical different from those who do not have migraine headaches. Migraines run in families, and a rare genetic form exists involving the calcium channel subunit gene CACNaIA. Familial and twin studies suggest that migraine with aura has a stronger genetic determination than migraine without aura, but the genes involved have not been identified. Persons with migraine have both altered biochemical and neurologic function in their normal, nonmigraine state. The general state of cerebrocortical excitability seems to be higher in migraine patients. This may

be related to neuronal calcium ion channels, decreased levels of intracellular magnesium (Mg), mitochondrial function, and increased levels of certain neurotoxic amino acids such as glutamate (Ferrari, 1998).

Whereas a nonmigraineur occasionally may experience a true migraine headache, the threshold for migraine headache seems to be lower in susceptible individuals who respond to sensory triggers within the environment. Factors known to trigger migraine include fatigue, sleep deficit, menstruation, hunger, stress, orgasm, bright lights, certain foods and drugs, and allergies (Smith, 1997).

## Sequence of Events in Migraine

The sequence of events in a migraine is indicated in Figure 4-1. When a migraine arises, the initial hyperexcitability usually occurs in the visual cortex. This is followed by the *cortical spreading depression* (CSD), a wave of depressed neuronal excitability. Next, a wave of cerebral hypoperfusion follows (oligemia). Then, the trigeminal vascular reflex is activated, which causes neuropeptides to be released. These chemicals then cause vasodilation and produce a neurogenic type of inflammation, which is thought to be the cause of migraine pain.

### Cortical Spreading Depression

The origin of migraine appears to be related to a lowered electrochemical threshold in the cerebral cortex, which can be triggered through internal and external environmental factors. When a

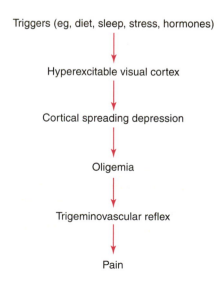

Triggers (eg, diet, sleep, stress, hormones)

↓

Hyperexcitable visual cortex

↓

Cortical spreading depression

↓

Oligemia

↓

Trigeminovascular reflex

↓

Pain

**FIGURE 4.1** ● Sequence of events in migraine.

migraine begins, it is characterized by CSD. This wave of electrical suppression begins with an initial period of neuronal hyperexcitability followed by electrical depression, which spreads throughout the brain surface, altering first brain and then vascular activity (Graham, 1996). It usually begins in the visual cortex, spreading across the cortex at a rate of 2 to 3 mm/minute. As it spreads, it produces marked depression of neuronal activity, which may last several minutes. This suppressed function is associated with efflux of excitatory amino acids (EAA) and alterations in cell membrane electrolyte fluxes (Ferrari, 1998). The aura also may be related to these electrical events, although research has not proven a link between these two events (Welch, 1997).

Hypoperfusion follows the CSD and spreads across the brain (Graham, 1996). The speed at which the oligemia spreads anteriorly from the occipital lobe has been recorded at 2 to 3 mm/minute, which is comparable to the rate of the CSD (Lance, 1997). The oligemia could be secondary to the CSD. However, a connection between the CSD and vascular changes has been confirmed only in patients with migraines with auras (Welch, 1997).

### Biochemical Events

The triggering mechanism for the initiation of the CSD is unknown, although several biochemical events are thought to be involved. A migraine threshold may exist that is sensitive to stimulation when the nervous system is influenced by certain biochemical agents, depending on the balance between excitation and inhibition of the nervous system (Lance, 1993). Potential agents include EAA, Mg, and serotonin.

Glutamate is one of the main neurotransmitters thought to be important in the development of CSD. It acts on the $N$-methyl-$D$-aspartate (NMDA) receptors, which are involved in neurotransmission (Chai et al., 1997). During a migraine, initial hypersecretion of EAA occurs, leading to a hyperexcited neural state. A subsequent efflux of EAA from the nerve cells follows, which could explain the initiation of the CSD.

Another agent implicated in altering the migraine threshold is Mg, which functions at the NMDA receptors by blocking ion fluxes across the nerve membrane (Farooqui & Horrocks, 1997). During a migraine, levels of Mg decrease (Ramadan et al., 1989).

### Vascular Effects

Decreasing concentrations of brain serotonin during a migraine may produce a vasodilatory response and contribute to the pain of migraine headache. Serotonin is a prominent neurotransmitter and potent vasoconstrictor. It can be found in large amounts throughout the body in the gastrointestinal tract, platelets, and brain. High concentrations are found in the neurons of the raphe dorsalis—located in the midbrain and forebrain—which projects into the hypothalamus and cerebral cortex. Projections from the raphe dorsalis also innervate the cerebral arteries (Raskin, 1998). There are also many serotonin receptors on the trigeminal nerve, and normally serotonin occupies these receptors and prevents pain. During a migraine, serotonin released from the raphe neurons is sporadic and decreased. The inadequate amounts of serotonin released can lead to an increase in spontaneous neural firing rate (Packard & Ham, 1997). Low levels of serotonin appear to cause activation of trigeminal nerve activity, leading to migraine pain. The increased blood flow found in the pons and midbrain during a migraine attack could result from this increased neural activity of the raphe dorsalis and another bundle of neurons, the locus ceruleus (Raskin, 1998).

Serotonin also is produced by aggregating platelets. Free serotonin from platelets, working in conjunction with peptides, could sensitize the cranial vessels to dilation, resulting in head pain (Lance, 1993).

The locus ceruleus, which contains numerous norepinephrine-containing neurons, also has been linked to vascular changes within the brain. The locus ceruleus is located in the pons near the fourth ventricle and contains many noradrenaline-containing neurons with connections to the hypothalamus, thalamus, trigeminal nerve, and spinal cord. Its neurons spread into the cerebral cortex, and its axons innervate the "intraparenchymal vessels" of the forebrain. When simulated, the locus ceruleus releases noradrenaline, which induces vasoconstriction though $\alpha$-receptors and vasodilation through $\beta$-receptors. Its also has been shown to play a role in regulating transmission of pain stimulus down the spinal cord (Lance, 1993).

### The Trigeminal Vascular Reflex

The pain of migraine is a result of the vascular changes as well as neural inflammation (Graham, 1996). The pathogenesis of migraine pain is based on an inflammatory response resulting from activation of the trigeminovascular reflex. This reflex is triggered by stimulation of the trigeminal (fifth cranial) nerve, which is the main sensory nerve in the head. Branches of this nerve dilate intracranial vessels and extracranial vessels though parasympathetic pathways. The trigeminal nerve has three major branches that innervate the ophthalmic, maxillary, and mandibular regions of the head. When afferent, nociceptive trigeminal nerve fibers are stimulated, they carry the pain message to the thalamus and cortex. This is followed by retrograde perivascular neuropeptide release at the synapses with blood vessels (Fig. 4-2). Some of the vasodilatory neuropeptides released in this manner include substance P, neurokinin A, vasoactive intestinal peptide, and calcitonin gene-related peptide. Along with the dilation, leakage of proteins from the cranial vessel walls and neurogenic inflammation occur (Gillies & Lance, 1993). This inflammation activates the pain receptors within the vessel walls, further evoking the transmission of pain stimuli through neuropeptide release (Raskin, 1998).

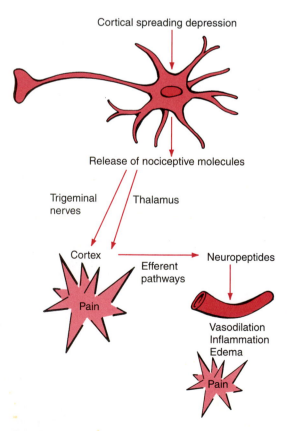

**FIGURE 4.2**  •  The pain of migraine.

## Symptoms Associated With Migraine Headache

Some of the main symptoms associated with a migraine are nausea and vomiting, anorexia, cold hands and feet, and pallor. These symptoms are thought to be a response of the secondary autonomic nervous system to the pain of migraine. This response could be caused by overactivation of the sympathetic nervous system (SNS) in response to the pain (Spierings, 1996). Most migraineurs also have sensory symptoms during the headache. These include blurring of vision and extreme sensitivity to light, noise, and smell.

## Pathophysiology of Premonitory Symptoms

Premonitory symptoms may arise days or hours before the head pain begins and continue throughout the migraine (Blau, 1986). Silberstein and Silberstein (1993) divided these symptoms into different categories: neurologic, mental, and general. These symptoms can be found in both types of migraines.

The pathophysiologic process of the premonitory symptoms still is undetermined. Symptoms such as hunger, thirst, drowsiness, and elation have been linked with a possible alteration in the hypothalamus (Lance, 1993). Dopamine and serotonin also have been suggested as possible contributors in the pathogenesis of these premonitory symptoms (Gillies & Lance, 1993).

## Pathophysiology of the Aura

The aura has been described as the hallmark trait for the migraine with aura. It usually begins about 20 minutes before the headache starts and subsides as the headache begins. There are different types of auras. The visual aura has been described as zigzag lines surrounded by darkened areas in which visual acuity is limited, whereas the motor and sensory auras are paresthesia and muscle weakness (Silberstein and Silberstein, 1993). Multiple research studies show an association between the aura and the decrease in blood flow observed during the initial stage of the migraine attack (Goadsby, 1997). Current research focuses on the concept that the CSD is responsible for the aura. Clinical studies and research have found that the rates of the CSD and the spreading oligemia are equal, suggesting this link (Appenzeller, 1997). The mechanism of initiation and propagation for the aura remains under investigation.

## Physiologic Basis of Treatment of Migraine Headache

The management of migraines involves lifestyle modifications and pharmacologic intervention. Lifestyle modifications include avoiding environmental agents that trigger migraine, making dietary changes, reducing stress, and establishing consistent sleep patterns (Diamond, 1993a). Pharmacologic treatment involves symptom-relieving drugs and prophylactic drug therapy.

## Avoidance of External, Physiologic, and Psychological Stimuli

Silberstein and Silberstein (1990) identified migraine patients as "hyperresponsive" to certain stimuli within their internal and external environment. The mechanism linking these stimuli with the initiation of the migraine is undetermined. Graham (1996) classifies these stimuli into three categories—external, physiologic and psychological—and lists some of the most commonly identified precipitating factors (see Table 4-1). Avoiding these stimuli has been effective in reducing migraine attacks (Diamond, 1993a). The triggering stimulants may depend on each other to initiate the migraine (Spierings, 1996). Decreasing the number of different stimuli in a person's lifestyle can reduce migraine frequency. However, Graham (1996) states that a person's susceptibility to migraine varies, most likely in relationship to life stress or the rhythmical cycle of the migraine itself.

## PHARMACOLOGIC THERAPIES

### Symptomatic Treatment

*Sumatriptan and dihydroergotamine*: Current research identifies several serotonin receptors playing a role in migraines. The 5-HT receptor has been divided into four families—1, 2, 3, and 4—with subdivisions (Raskin, 1998). Agonists of the receptors 5-HT$_{1D}$ and 5-HT$_{1A}$ offer relief during a migraine, whereas antagonists to the 5-HT$_2$ family are effective as prophylaxis. Sumatriptan activates the 5-HT$_1$ receptors (Ellsworth, 1998); however, it is most active toward the subdivision 5-HT$_{1D}$ (Raskin, 1998). Its mechanism of action involves activating these receptors, leading to the vasoconstriction of the cranial vessels. Dihydroergotamine works in the same manner, focusing on the 5-HT$_{1A}$ receptors (Raskin, 1998). The importance of the different subdivisions of the receptor families is their location within the brain.

*Ergotamine*: This drug is a potent vasoconstrictor known for its antimigraine properties. It works by constricting the cranial vessels, which branch from the external carotid (Diamond, 1993c). It also may reduce vascular inflammation and affect serotonin synthesis (Kunkel, 1993).

*NSAIDs*: The anti-inflammatory effects of NSAIDs make them useful in treating migraine pain. Their antiprostaglandin effect decreases the inflammation, and thus pain, by acting on cyclooxygenase, an enzyme necessary in the synthesis of prostaglandins (Diamond, 1993b). NSAIDs also have been found to be useful in prophylactic treatment (Diamond, 1993a).

### Prophylaxis Therapy

*Methysergide*: This drug is a serotonin antagonist, blocking the 5-HT$_2$ receptor site. A decrease in neurogenic inflammation can be seen with continued use of this drug.

*Tricyclic antidepressants*: The mechanism of action for tricyclic antidepressants involves the synthesis and metabolism of serotonin and norepinephrine.

*Nonselective beta blockers*: These medicines work by blocking the β$_1$- and β$_2$-receptor sites, thereby blocking the SNS from stimulating β-receptors. These blocking agents prevent dilation of the vascular smooth muscle.

*Calcium channel blockers*: This group of drugs is considered "vessels stabilizers." They inhibit the movement of calcium ions across the cell membrane, which decreases the number of calcium channels open for a membrane depolarization.

## CLUSTER HEADACHE

Cluster headaches sometimes are described as ice pick or suicide headaches because of the ferocity of the pain. The headache, more common in men than women, is characterized by excruciating, unilateral pain felt in the eye, the oculotemporal area, or the oculofrontal area. The incidence in men is between 0.4% and 1% (Jay, 1998). Like tension-type headache, it can be episodic or chronic. The term *cluster* headache refers to the fact that the headache often occurs in a series, sometimes for months, and then disappears for months to years before recurring.

Most patients have an accompanying ipsilateral tearing of the eye, nasal congestion or rhinorrhea, and conjunctivitis during the attack. The pain is so intense that afflicted individuals may become violently agitated. This is in contrast to the person with migraine who seeks a quiet, dark place.

### ● Case Study 4.2

A 26-year-old woman presents with a chief complaint of periodic headaches since early adolescence. She describes the headaches as pounding and sharp. The headaches usually are unilateral and are so severe that she has to lie down and go to sleep. She has at least one headache a week, usually lasting about 5 to 6 hours. She states, "Going to sleep for several hours helps a little." She has tried ibuprofen (400 mg) and acetaminophen (500 mg), but neither relieved the pain.

She has experienced nausea with some of the headaches and has visual disturbances ("tiny flashing lights") before the headache starts, which usually go away with the onset of the headache. She states that bright lights and loud noises aggravate the headache, and she has not noticed changes in moods or appetite. She has a positive family history of migraine headache; mother, maternal uncle, and grandfather. Denies vomiting, history of head trauma, fever, vertigo, difficulty sleeping, recent illness, or neck stiffness.

### Medical History

No previous diagnosis of headaches. Denies history of chronic medical conditions or diseases. No surgical history. Currently is taking no medications. NKDA. No environmental or food allergies

### Differential Diagnoses

Migraine with aura
Migraine without aura
Cluster headache
Tension-type headache
Cervical spondylosis
Depression
Intracranial mass/lesion
Posttraumatic headache

### Physical Assessment

| | |
|---|---|
| Vital signs | T–98.8°F, P–88 beats/min, BP–122/78 |
| General Appearance | Well-nourished 26-year-old woman. Neatly dressed. No distress noted |
| HEENT | Normocephalic, no masses or tenderness noted. Denies sinus pain |
| | Eyes: Snellen 20/20: OU, visual fields normal, conjunctivae pink, sclera clear, EOM intact, PERRLA, red reflex and optic disc noted, vessels without nicks or exudates |
| | Ears: Canals intact with small amount of soft brown cerumen. TMs pearly gray intact. Light reflex noted |
| Neck | Supple. Carotid pulse palpated at 84. No bruit auscultated |
| Musculoskeletal | Full ROM. Gait steady. Occipitalis, frontalis, temporalis, and trapezius muscles without tenderness or tightness |

*(Case study continued on next page)*

| Neurologic | Alert and oriented × 3. Speech clear. Recent and distant memory intact. CN I–XII intact. DTRs: 2+. No Babinski reflex noted. Bilaterally strong, no weakness or atrophy noted. Negative for Romberg sign. Light touch, pin prick, position and vibration intact. See Table 4-1 for the International Headache Society's Criteria for the Diagnosis of Migraines |

### Diagnostic Tests

1. CT scan or MRI if assessment leads toward possible lesion or mass
2. CBC with differential if patient presents with symptoms of infection (chills, fever)
3. X-ray to rule out cervical spondylosis
4. Lumbar puncture to rule out infection/meningitis if febrile

CBC, complete blood count; CN, cranial nerves; CT, computed tomography; DTRs, deep tendon reflexes; EOM, extraoccular muscles; MRI, magnetic resonance imaging; NKDA, no known drug allergies; PERRLA, pupils equal, round, regular to light and accommodation; ROM, range of motion; TMs, tympanic membranes.

The pain of cluster headache may arise in the cavernous sinus and may involve the trigemino-vascular reflex, as previously discussed. There is clearly an abnormality in the functioning of the autonomic nervous system in this type of headache. Problems in vasomotor regulation with hypoxia, vasodilation, and release of pain mediators such as bradykinin are thought to be involved. Abnormalities in rapid eye movement sleep also occur, which are characterized by decreased melatonin levels and sleep apnea. The occurrence of sleep apnea with its accompanying hypoxemia may "reset" chemoreceptors and increase the frequency of attacks.

# DIZZINESS

One of the most common reasons for patients to seek care in primary care practices is dizziness. What people consider to be dizziness ranges from feelings of faintness to vertigo to disequilibrium. Dizziness can be a difficult and frustrating symptom for the practitioner to work up and diagnose. The symptom is subjective, and a complete workup often reveals no known etiology. Yet, dizziness can be such an important symptom of underlying neurologic or otologic disease that it should never be ignored. In this section, the three major classifications of dizziness are described, and the pathophysiologic basis for each type is explored.

## CLASSIFICATION OF DIZZINESS

There are several ways to classify the symptom of dizziness. The approach used here is to view dizziness as *near syncope, vertigo*, and *nonsyncopal, nonvertigo* types. Table 4-3 shows the major pathophysiologic causes for each of these conditions. For each type of dizziness, the practitioner must take a complete medical history because events around the dizziness episodes may be important clues to the cause. Also, it is essential to completely account for all medications taken by the patient, since dizziness may be iatrogenic and related to drug toxicity.

A complete description of the dizziness episodes should be elicited because important clues may be found in the patient's accounting. The symptoms associated with dizziness provide important information for the diagnostic reasoning of the practitioner. For example, when questioned closely, a patient who complains of dizziness may describe a phobic fear of falling and associated panic disorder symptoms as dizziness. A cancer patient may describe fatigue and weakness as dizziness. A patient who is unsteady and afraid of falling because of cataracts may report feeling dizzy. On the other hand, terms like "wooziness" may be used when the patient has experienced profound vertigo. Several useful physical examination tools (see p. 54) and laboratory tests help the practitioner make the correct diagnosis in cases of dizziness.

## TABLE 4.3

● ● ●

### Causes of Dizziness

| Near Syncope | Vertigo | Nonsyncope, Nonvertigo Dizziness |
|---|---|---|
| Autonomic failure<br>  Autonomic neuropathy<br>  Medications<br>Cardiac<br>  Arrhythmia (supraventricular<br>    and ventricular tachycardias,<br>    bradyarrhythmias)<br>  Cardiac failure<br>  Ischemia<br>  Outflow obstruction<br>    (hypertrophic cardiomyopathy,<br>    myxoma)<br>  Valvular disorder<br>    (aortic stenosis, mitral<br>    regurgitation)<br>Hypovolemic<br>  Blood loss<br>  Dehydration<br>Reflexive<br>  Carotid sinus hypersensitivity<br>  Coughing<br>  Defecation<br>  Emotional distress<br>  Fainting<br>  Micturition<br>  Pain<br>  Swallowing<br>  Valsalva maneuver | Central pathways<br>  Ischemia<br>  Multiple sclerosis<br>  Tumor (astrocytoma)<br>Eighth nerve<br>  Ischemia<br>  Tumor (acoustic neuroma,<br>  meningioma, metastatic carcinoma)<br>  Vestibular neuritis<br>Medication<br>Physiologic (altitude, motion sickness)<br>Somatosensory dysfunction<br>Trauma (postconcussion syndrome)<br>Vestibular apparatus<br>  Endolymphatic fistula<br>  Ischemia<br>  Ménière's disease<br>  Paroxysmal positional vertigo<br>  Serous otitis media<br>  Tumor (cholesteatoma,<br>  glomus jugulare)<br>Visual dysfunction | Drop attacks<br>Hyperventilation<br>Hypoglycemia<br>Migraine<br>  Somatization disorder<br>Multiple sensory deficits<br>Seizures<br>Stroke |

(From Bowen, J. [1998] *Hospital Medicine 34*[1], 39–44.)

The causes of dizziness vary. The vestibular system often is a major contributor, but dizziness may result from hypoglycemia or cardiovascular, autonomic, psychological, or sensorimotor control problems (Baloh, 1998).

### Near Syncope

Dizziness associated with a feeling of faintness, or light-headedness, is described as *near syncope*. The patient may use a variety of terms to describe this symptom. An important distinguishing fact is that the patient does not describe the sensation of spinning in this type of dizziness. Rather, he or she speaks of light-headedness, which may resolve, or may progress to true syncope.

A common cause for near syncope, particularly in the elderly, is inadequate perfusion of the cerebral circulation. The perfusion pressure in the brain drops below the intraocular pressure, and the patient complains of "spots before their eyes," or "blacking out." Common causes for this type of near syncope include orthostatic hypotension and cardiac arrhythmias, especially atrial fibrillation. Orthostatic hypotension occurs when the patient quickly stands up from either a lying or sitting position, and the baroreceptor reflex is not able to adequately adjust blood pressure when the volume in the carotid artery drops. In the elderly, antihypertensive medication is a common cause for this phenomenon. Peripheral neuropathy also could lead to autonomic dysfunction, which impairs cardiovascular adaptation to gravitational changes. Other possible causes include true volume depletion from excessive perspiration and fluid volume loss through diuretics. Dizziness typically occurs when the blood pressure drops greater than 20 mm Hg when standing compared with lying down.

If the episodes of dizziness in an elderly patient are not related to posture, the cause might be cardiac arrhythmias or other cardiac problems such as pericarditis. A ventricular bradyarrhythmia may lead to inadequate cerebral perfusion pressure and volume. The pathophysiology of this response is related to a momentary drop in perfusion pressure of blood to the brain, causing cerebral hypoxia.

Another important mechanism in presyncope dizziness is vasovagal reflex activity. The pathophysiologic mechanism probably includes reflexive parasympathetic responses that are either hypersensitive or improperly regulated. The vagal response may occur when input reaches the brain from visceral sensations such as in hunger contractions, swallowing, coughing, a full bladder, or defecation. Other stimuli include heat exposure, stressful stimuli leading to profound fear responses, or acute pain. The parasympathetic output causes bradycardia and vasodilation, resulting in decreased cardiac output and cerebral perfusion. This mechanism is the most common cause of presyncope (Baloh, 1998), which often precedes fainting.

An often-misdiagnosed cause of dizziness is carotid artery disease, which results in dizziness when the head is turned in a certain direction. This symptom can be associated with carotid sinus hyperactivity or cerebrovascular insufficiency from atherosclerosis (Bowen, 1998).

The last cause of presyncope is psychogenic and may be related to hyperventilation. This should be considered in younger patients, particularly in anxious, stressed girls. The patient overbreathes, leading to a state of hypocapnia. The decreased $PCO_2$ leads to cerebral vasoconstriction and hypoxia. The patient also often experiences symptoms of hypocalcemia, since the respiratory alkalosis leads to increased binding of calcium to protein and a decrease in free calcium. In other cases of psychogenic dizziness, patients report that they are dizzy all day long. These patients may be highly anxious, phobic, or panicked.

The following clinical vignette illustrates a common occurrence in primary care—an elderly person with a head injury from a fall that occurred because of an episode of presyncope dizziness.

## Vertigo

Dizziness can be divided into vestibular and nonvestibular etiologies. When true vertigo is present, which is the sensation or hallucination of spinning motion, a vestibular imbalance is highly likely. Usually, the symptoms develop over a few seconds, and movements of the head make the sensation more pronounced. There may be pallor and nausea, or even vomiting, and people may develop an unsteady gait and loss of balance (Bowen, 1998). The causes of vertigo can be seen in Table 4-3.

Vertigo can occur in healthy individuals who are experiencing motion sickness or acclimating to high altitudes. Benign paroxysmal positional vertigo is common in elderly patients and may be caused by otolithiasis, which is the accumulation of

---

### CLINICAL VIGNETTE 4.1

Mr. Elwood is a 75-year-old African American man brought to the clinic with a laceration of the scalp caused by a fall in his home. He is known to the clinic as a compliant, hypertensive patient currently on a diuretic medication and a beta blocker. It is a hot summer day, and on questioning he reveals that his home is not air-conditioned. The patient is alert, oriented, cooperative, and jokes that he has come to the clinic to "cool off." His supine blood pressure is 126/84. Standing blood pressure is 96/60. Pulse is more rapid than usual at 90 beats per minute. He reports feeling "woozy" but can't remember the actual fall. He states that if he

gets up too fast, he sees spots before his eyes and feels a "little sick."

Because of the clear evidence of orthostatic hypotension, probably caused by his antihypertensive medication and possible heat-induced diaphoresis, which caused volume loss, this patient's dizziness does not need a full neurologic workup. His head injury needs a complete evaluation to rule out a concussion. His medications may need to be changed, and he should be advised about fluid replacement, not rising to a standing position too quickly, how to keep cool in the summer, and ways to prevent further falls in his home.

microscopic debris in the semicircular canals. These attacks typically last less than a minute and occur with positional changes. Most patients recover from this problem without treatment. Figure 4-3 illustrates how the presence of debris stimulates hair cells on the surface of the crista, or sensory epithelium in the semicircular canals. Cilia on the hair cells project into the gelatinous cupula and normally are influenced by position of the head in space. Debris can produce an abnormal stimulation of these cells as it moves within the canals, leading to a sensation of motion when none is present.

Whereas positional vertigo usually is benign, ruling out a brain lesion can be done through the Dix-Hallpike maneuver. The patient begins in a sitting position and is quickly shifted to a supine position, with the head tilted 45 degrees down and to the side. This position is kept for 60 seconds, then the head is tilted to the opposite side. When the maneuver reproduces the head position, the patient experiences positional vertigo (Bowen, 1998). This maneuver should not be performed in patients with atherosclerotic disease of the carotid or vertebral arteries or in elderly patients. The findings indicative of benign positional vertigo are the ability to reproduce the sensation of vertigo; nystagmus, in which the eyeball rotates in a clockwise or counterclockwise direction; a latent period of several seconds before the onset of nystagmus; and fatigue in response to repetition of the test (Browder, 1997). If the patient demonstrates benign positional vertigo, the Epley maneuvers can be done at the bedside. These are a series of positional changes to the head that change the position of debris in the semicircular canal, thus alleviating both vertigo and nystagmus (Bowen, 1998). The patient is instructed to sit upright for 48

hours and to wear a soft collar around the neck. The Epley maneuver may be accompanied by mastoid vibration. It usually is successful but should be performed by an otolaryngologist rather than a primary care provider (Wolf et al., 1999).

Nystagmus is an interesting and important finding in the assessment of vertigo. There are neurologic connections between the vestibular and ocular systems. Sensory nerves from the semicircular canals are associated with the motor neurons that supply the eye muscles, and stimulation of the sensory nerves supplying a canal causes eye movements in the same plane. So, if the left posterior canal were disturbed, then the left superior oblique and right lateral rectus muscles would be stimulated to contract. This relationship causes nystagmus (Baloh, 1998), which is rhythmic slow and fast movements of the eyeball in a particular direction. Nystagmus can be stimulated as described earlier in the Dix-Hallpike maneuver, or it can occur spontaneously. Damage to the labyrinth or vestibular nerve may cause spontaneous nystagmus, with the slow ocular movements moving toward the affected side. Horizontally beating nystagmus indicates unilateral vestibular disease, whereas vertical nystagmus suggests a brainstem lesion (Browder, 1997). Absence of nystagmus in a patient with acute, severe vertigo is so unusual that it indicates possible malingering.

### Neural Labyrinthitis

Neural labyrinthitis is a common type of vertigo thought to be related to a viral upper respiratory illness (URI); it has an increased incidence in the spring and summer. Attacks of vertigo follow the URI and may last for days. The vertigo usually is positional, and the patient may feel nauseous and unsteady. The vertigo may resolve spontaneously over several days to weeks, or it may reappear months afterward. The pathophysiologic mechanisms are unknown but may be related to inflammatory responses affecting inner ear balance mechanisms.

### Ménière's Disease

Ménière's disease is an important cause of vertigo during the third and fourth decade of life. It has an overall incidence of less than 0.5% in the general population and is characterized by a triad of symptoms: episodic vertigo, low-frequency hearing loss, and tinnitus. Patients also have a sensation of fullness in the affected ear. Although the cause is unknown, it can follow an ear infection or trauma. The most characteristic finding in Ménière's dis-

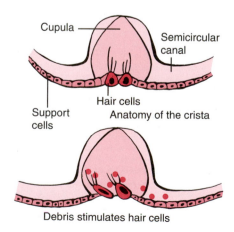

Cupula

Semicircular canal

Hair cells

Support cells

Anatomy of the crista

Debris stimulates hair cells

**FIGURE 4.3** ● Origin of vertigo in semicircular canals.

---

### CLINICAL VIGNETTE 4.2

Ms. Ellen Fulton is a 40-year-old school teacher who presents to the primary care clinic complaining of ringing and popping in the ears and dizziness. She first noted the symptoms while jogging the preceding week, and they have become more intense and frequent. She states that her hearing is good. She describes the dizziness as a tilting, spinning sensation. The tinnitus is worse at night when the ambient noises are reduced, but the episodes of dizziness are so severe and frequent that she has been unable to work.

Her history is unremarkable except for fairly frequent migraine headaches, for which she takes sumatriptan, and a recent upper respiratory infec-

tion, which she believed caused her ears to "become stuffed up." Results of a CT scan are normal. An audiogram of the patient indicates low-frequency, sensorineural hearing loss. Results of her otoscopic examination are normal, but during the examination she experiences an episode of vertigo in which horizontal nystagmus is noted.

The presence of the classic triad and the absence of findings suggestive of other neurologic or otologic disease indicate a probable diagnosis of Ménière's disease. She is begun on a sodium-restricted diet and started on furosemide (Lasix). She is cautioned about the danger of falls during the vertigo episodes and is referred to an otolaryngologist.

---

ease is an increased amount of endolymph in the inner ear. The cause of this abnormality is not known, although the entire endolymphatic system can become distended with fluid, giving rise to the term *endolymphatic hydrops*. The disorder may have a viral or an immunologic basis, since patients with Ménière's disease have antibodies against inner ear proteins. The current physiologic, nonsurgical treatment is diuretic therapy and sodium restriction to reduce endolymph. The disease can be extremely disabling, and patients often require psychological counseling. A web site for patients with Ménière's disease is *http://www. geocities.com/HotSprings/Spa/3143/info.htm*, which provides patients with information, chat rooms, and other supports.

### Nonsyncopal, Nonvertigo Dizziness

The third common type of dizziness, nonsyncopal, nonvertigo dizziness, sometimes is referred to as disequilibrium. It is not true dizziness, but rather a feeling of imbalance and a fear of falling. Causes are nonvestibular. Proprioceptive abnormalities may cause decreased sensations of joint positions, leading to unsteadiness. Hypoglycemia may lead to disequilibrium. Stroke, seizure, and mental confusion also are possible causes. Patients with neuropathies and visual defects also report this form of dizziness.

### REFERENCES

Adler, C., Adler, S., & Packard, R. (1987). *Psychiatric aspects of headache*. Baltimore: Williams & Wilkins.

Appenzeller, O. (1997). Headache. In R. Dulbecco (Ed.), *Encyclopedia of human biology* (2nd ed., pp. 413–422). San Diego: Academic Press.

Baloh, R. (1998). *Dizziness, tinnitus and hearing loss*. Philadelphia: F.A. Davis.

Blau, J. (1986). Clinical characteristics of premonitory symptoms in migraine. In W. Avery (Ed.), *The prelude to the migraine attack*. London: Baillière Tindall.

Bowen, J. (1998). Dizziness: A diagnostic puzzle. *Hospital Medicine, 34*(1), 39–44.

Browder, J. (1997). Dizziness. In L. Dornbrand, A. Hoole, & R. Fletcher (Eds.), *Manual of clinical problems in adult ambulatory care*. Philadelphia: Lippincott-Raven.

Brown, G., Goodwin, F., Ballenger, J., Goyer, P., & Major, L. (1986). Aggression in humans correlates with cerebrospinal fluid amine metabolites. *Annals of the New York Academy of Sciences, 487*, 176–188.

Chai, S., Aldred, G., & Mendelsohn, F. (1997). Neurotransmitter and neuropeptide receptors in the brain. In R. Dulbecco (Ed.), *Encyclopedia of human biology* (2nd ed., pp. 207–222). San Diego: Academic Press.

Diamond, S. (1993a). *A pain specialist's approach to the headache patient*. Madison, Connecticut: International Universities Press.

Diamond, S. (1993b). Tension-type headaches. In D. Dalessio & S. Silberstein (Eds.), *Wolff's headache and other head pain* (6th ed., pp. 233–261). New York: Oxford University Press.

Diamond, S. (1993c). Medical management of recurrent migraine. In C. Tollison & R. Kunkel (Eds.), *Headache: Diagnosis and treatment* (pp. 89–106). Baltimore: Williams & Wilkins.

Ellsworth, A. (1998). *1998 Medical drug reference*. St. Louis: Mosby.

Farooqui, A. & Horrocks, L. (1997). Excitatory neurotransmitters and their involvement in neurodegeneration. In R. Dulbecco (Ed.), *Encyclopedia of human biology* (2nd ed., pp. 845–851). San Diego: Academic Press.

Ferrari, M. (1998). Migraine. *The Lancet, 351* (April 4), 1043–1051.

Gillies, J. & Lance, J. (1993). Pathophysiology of migraine. In C. Tollison & R. Kunkel (Eds.), *Headache: Diagnosis and treatment* (pp. 77–84). Baltimore: Williams & Wilkins.

Goadsby, P. (1997). Bench to bedside: What have we learned about headache? *Current Opinions in Neurology, 10 (3),* 215–220.

Graham, J. (1996). Headaches. In J. Noble (Ed.) *Textbook of primary care medicine* (2nd ed., pp. 1283–1319). St. Louis: Mosby.

Ingram, R. & Scher, C. (1998). Depression. In H. Friedman (Ed.), *Encyclopedia of mental health* (Vol. 1, pp. 723–732). San Diego: Academic Press.

Jay, G. (1993). Pathophysiology of tension-type headache. In C. Tollison & R. Kunkel (Eds.), *Headache: Diagnosis and treatment.* Baltimore: Williams & Wilkins.

Jay, G. (1998). *The headache handbook.* New York: CRC Press.

Kunkel, R. (1993). Medical management of acute migraine episode. In C. Tollison & R. Kunkel (Eds.), *Headache: Diagnosis and treatment* (pp. 85–88). Baltimore: Williams & Wilkins.

Lance, J. (1993). The pathophysiology of migraine. In D. Dalessio & S. Silberstein (Eds.), *Wolff's headache and other head pain* (6th ed., pp 59–95). New York: Oxford University Press.

Lance, J. (1997). Approach to the patient with headache. In W. Kelley (Ed.), *Textbook of internal medicine* (3rd ed., pp. 206–212). Philadelphia: Lippincott-Raven.

Lovallo, W. (1997). *Stress & health: Biological and psychological interactions.* London: Sage Publications.

MacGregor, A. (1999). *Managing migraine in primary care.* Oxford: Blackwell Science.

Packard, R. & Ham, L. (1997). Pathogenesis of posttraumatic headache and migraine: A common headache pathway? *Headache, 37,* 142–152.

Ramadan, N., Halvorson, H., Vande-Linde, A., Levine, S., Helpern, J., & Welch, K. (1989). Low brain magnesium in migraine. *Headache, 29* (7), 416–419.

Raskin, N. (1998). Migraine and the cluster headache syndrome. In A. Fauci (Ed.), *Harrison's principles of internal medicine* (14th ed., pp. 2307–2310). New York: McGraw-Hill.

Russell, M.B. & Olesen, J.A. (1996). A nosographic analysis of the migraine aura in a general population. *Brain, 119* (Pt 2), 355–361.

Silberstein, S. & Saper, J. (1993). Migraine: Diagnosis and treatment. In D. Dalession & S. Silberstein (Eds.), *Wolff's headache and other head pain* (6th ed., pp. 97–170). New York: Oxford University Press.

Silberstein, S. & Silberstein, M. (1990). New concepts in the pathogenesis of headache. *Pain Management, 3,* 297–303, 334–342.

Silberstein, S. & Silberstein, M. (1993). Migraine: Clinical symptomatology and differential diagnosis of migraine. In C. Tollison & R. Kunkel (Eds.), *Headache: Diagnosis and treatment* (pp. 59–75). Baltimore: Williams & Wilkins.

Smith, R. (1997). Diagnosing headache. *Hospital Medicine, 33,* 26–42.

Solomon, G. (1998). Headache. In H. Friedman (Ed.), *Encyclopedia of mental health* (Vol. 2, pp. 337–349). San Diego: Academic Press.

Spierings, E. (1996). *Management of migraine.* Boston: Butterworth-Heinemann.

Toates, F. (1995). *Stress: Conceptual and biological aspects.* New York: John Wiley & Sons.

Welch, K. (1997). Pathogenesis of migraine. *Seminars in Neurology, 17* (4), 335–341.

Wolf, J.S., Boyev, K.P., Manokey, B.J., & Mattox, D.E. (1999). Success of the modified Epley maneuver in treating benign paroxysmal positional vertigo. *Laryngoscope 109* (6), 900–903.

# Behavioral Disorders

Laurie Elliott

Maureen Groer

Paula MacMorran

Penelope Perkey

Primary care providers must be constantly vigilant for underlying mood and behavior problems in their patients. Patients may come for care manifesting physical symptoms that ultimately have a psychiatric cause. Another common occurrence is for patients to present with a physical disorder needing treatment, and, in the course of a holistic assessment, a coexisting psychiatric condition is discovered. Many patients thus may be misdiagnosed or underdiagnosed. Attention to the person as a whole, rather than to just symptoms and disease, may illuminate other problems that the patient may be experiencing. One third of depressed patients, for example, are incorrectly diagnosed by their primary care provider (Davis, 1998). This chapter describes the most common behavioral disorders encountered by practitioners in primary care, including depression and anxiety, attention deficit/hyperactivity disorder (ADHD), and addictive disorders such as alcoholism. Clinical vignettes are presented throughout the chapter to illustrate pathophysiologic processes.

## DEPRESSION AND ANXIETY

Depression and anxiety are potentially serious, disabling, but treatable illnesses commonly seen by the primary care practitioner. They differ from other health problems, however, in that the patient rarely presents with the statement, "I have a problem with depression," or, "My anxiety is making me sick." Instead, the patient complains of insomnia, restlessness, lack of energy, weight gain or loss, or chronic or vague symptoms such as headache, backache, or stomach upset. These complaints are, after all, what most patients assume the clinician can treat. Patients also may hesitate to share emotional difficulties with a relative stranger. Alternatively, they may be unaware of the presence of a serious emotional problem or may be unwilling to admit it to themselves or anyone else. If the clinician has ruled out other serious, immediate medical problems, a careful assessment of the patient's emotional status is in order.

Assessment of anxiety or depression differs from other medical assessments in that few of the physical signs and symptoms are diagnostically specific. Instead, the practitioner's intuition, careful and directed questioning, and ability to listen are the critical skills needed for diagnosis. In this sense, the interview *is* the examination. The careful clinician can emphasize to the patient that although the problem is not "all in your head," the mind is nevertheless very powerful in affecting how we feel, and addressing mental status is a natural part of a complete health assessment.

Continuing to search for a physical source of the patient's complaints while assessing psychiatric status is an invaluable skill that will save time and resources for both practitioner and patient. Depression and anxiety can amplify the effects of pain, illness, and disability, making them harder to treat. A sensitive interviewer can reassure patients that help for their medical problems will be ongoing, but that understanding their emotional status is just as important in helping them to improve.

A useful web site for primary care providers to learn more about depressive illnesses, anxiety disorders, and other mental health problems is *http://www.nimh.nih.gov.*

## Anatomy and Physiology of Mood

Despite intense and ongoing investigation for the last several decades, no definitive anatomic, physiologic, or biochemical lesions exist that completely explain mood disorders. However, many lines of research are under way that should illuminate our understanding of the biology of mood and suggest future therapeutic interventions. Meanwhile, the practitioner will benefit from an understanding of the complex biologic interactions known to influence mood, mental status, and behavior.

### The Nerve Synapse

The neuronal synapse (Fig. 5-1) is the basic functional unit of the nervous system. Neurons transmit information in the form of waves of electrical depolarization, which must be transmitted from cell to cell. *Neurotransmitters* allow transmission of these impulses from one neuron to the next through the synaptic cleft. The axon terminal of the presynaptic neuron contains granules that store neurotransmitters in membrane-bound vesicles. When the neuron is stimulated, the storage vesicles migrate to join with the cell membrane and release neurotransmitter into the synaptic cleft. Neurotransmitters then attach to membrane-bound receptors on the postsynaptic cell, allowing neurotransmission to proceed. Because each receptor site has a specific function and is specific for a particular neurotransmitter, the quality and quantity of neurotransmission can be controlled precisely. Excess amounts of specific neurotransmitter may be reabsorbed back into the presynaptic neuron

(reuptake) or may attach to presynaptic autoreceptors. Reuptake allows "recycling" of excess neurotransmitters and saves the energy costs of added biosynthesis. Autoreceptors are thought to provide feedback, which aids in *up-* or *down-regulation* (increased or decreased sending potential) of the presynaptic cell.

Up-regulation and down-regulation occur at both presynaptic and postsynaptic sites and are critical to homeostasis. For example, a prolonged excess of a given neurotransmitter may result in up-regulation (increased number) of presynaptic inhibitory sites for that neurotransmitter or down-regulation (decreased number) of postsynaptic receptor sites. A decrease in neurotransmitter concentration at presynaptic sites may result in up-regulation (increased number or sensitivity) of postsynaptic sites. Prolonged treatment with drugs that block postsynaptic receptors may cause up-regulation—increased number or affinity—of these receptors. This ongoing responsiveness of receptor sites to physiologic changes has important implications in the pathophysiology of emotion. Although it makes understanding and treating mood disorders and anxiety more complex (and confusing), it also offers insights that may aid in the development of new drug treatments.

Receptor sites at the synapse do not communicate directly with a target site within the cell. Instead, information is transferred from the membrane-bound receptor to *G proteins,* or "coupling proteins," so named for their dependence on guanine (Fig. 5-2). G proteins travel into the neuron and transfer information to *second messengers* such as cyclic adenosine monophosphate (cAMP) and cyclic guanosine 3',5'-monophosphate (cGMP). Second messengers initiate a cascade of events, which results in changes in cell membrane shape and permeability and altered activity of potassium, sodium, calcium, and chloride ion channels. These in turn generate the following possible changes in neurotransmission:

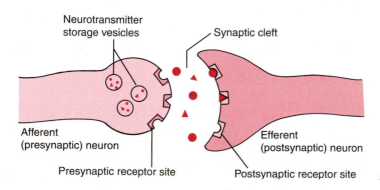

Neurotransmitter storage vesicles

Synaptic cleft

Afferent (presynaptic) neuron

Efferent (postsynaptic) neuron

Presynaptic receptor site

Postsynaptic receptor site

**FIGURE 5.1** ● Neuronal synapse.

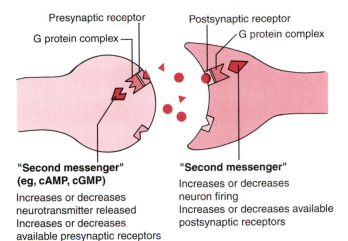

Presynaptic receptor

G protein complex

Postsynaptic receptor

G protein complex

**"Second messenger"
(eg, cAMP, cGMP)**

Increases or decreases
neurotransmitter released
Increases or decreases
available presynaptic receptors

**"Second messenger"**

Increases or decreases
neuron firing
Increases or decreases available
postsynaptic receptors

**FIGURE 5.2** ● Role of G proteins and second messengers.

1. Amount of presynaptic neurotransmitter released (up-regulation or down-regulation)
2. Firing rate of the postsynaptic cell
3. Number of presynaptic and postsynaptic receptors available for future neurotransmission

More information is sought on the exact role of G proteins. They are thought to be hormonally influenced, and with their role in second messenger activation, they are viewed as critical in regulation, amplification, and integration of nerve transmission and, therefore, of mood (Manji, 1992). Some medications such as lithium may exert their effects on G proteins, and a better understanding of these sites could lead to site-specific drug therapies.

## Neurotransmitters

Approximately 75 neurotransmitters have been identified, but some experts predict that the actual number is much greater. Not all neurotransmitters regulate mood, and those known to do so also have other roles in the body. For example, whereas the neurotransmitter serotonin is well known to modify mood, it also influences blood pressure, gastrointestinal (GI) activity, and uterine contraction. Such multiple effects create problems when pharmacologic interventions are being developed.

The transmitters most associated with emotional status are the monoamines; neural circuits carrying these substances project to many regions of the brain. Figure 5-3 depicts the major projections and centers involved in mood. *Norepinephrine* (NE), which is the primary postganglionic sympathetic neurotransmitter, increases the brain's sensitivity to external stimuli and is thought to play a significant role in the stress response (Schuyler, 1998). NE is associated with states of sadness, anxiety, agitation, and poor concentration and contributes to poor sleep and appetite. Low levels of NE are implicated in the lack of energy and pleasure (anhedonia) seen in depressive states. It also modifies the function of other neurotransmitters. Many antidepressants have marked effects on NE; thus, this has been the focus of most of the early research on mood in the United States.

Meanwhile in Europe, attention is centered on another monoamine, *serotonin* (5-HT). Generally inhibitory in its actions, this transmitter plays a critical role in dampening the function of other neurotransmitter systems and has widespread actions throughout the body. The cerebral cortex, basal ganglia, and limbic system all are heavily innervated by serotonergic tracts. There are at least seven subtypes of 5-HT receptors, which contribute to many diverse bodily functions. 5-HT is an important regulator of sleep cycles, appetite, and libido and is thought to modify the body's temperature and endocrine systems (Thase & Howland, 1995). It also is implicated in goal-directed motor behavior and inhibition of aggression. Significant reduction in 5-HT, therefore, is associated with disturbance of appetite, sleep, sexual function, and the increased impulsive thoughts and actions characteristic of violent aggression and suicide behavior.

A third monoamine, *dopamine* (DA), is a major component of psychotic disorders and possibly a factor in mania. Chemically similar to NE, DA is implicated in many of the same processes as NE. DA is thought to play a role in reward-motivated behavior (Fibiger, 1995). Its activity is intensified by drugs of abuse and known to be a key factor in the biology of addiction. Some researchers believe dopamine to be associated with the anhedonia that accompanies depression, and certain effective

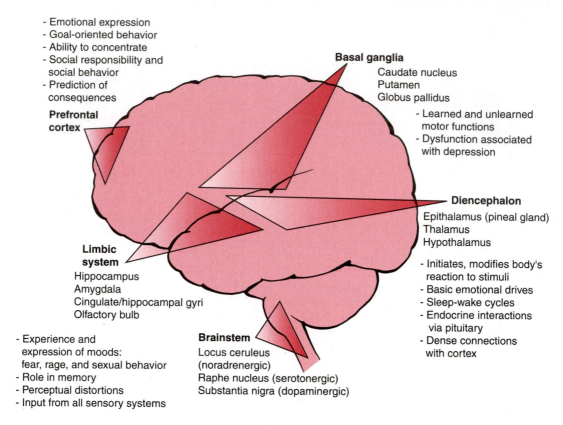

- Emotional expression
- Goal-oriented behavior
- Ability to concentrate
- Social responsibility and
  social behavior
- Prediction of
  consequences

**Prefrontal
cortex**

**Basal ganglia**
Caudate nucleus
Putamen
Globus pallidus

- Learned and unlearned
  motor functions
- Dysfunction associated
  with depression

**Diencephalon**
Epithalamus (pineal gland)
Thalamus
Hypothalamus

- Initiates, modifies body's
  reaction to stimuli
- Basic emotional drives
- Sleep-wake cycles
- Endocrine interactions
  via pituitary
- Dense connections
  with cortex

**Limbic
system**
Hippocampus
Amygdala
Cingulate/hippocampal gyri
Olfactory bulb

- Experience and
  expression of moods:
  fear, rage, and sexual behavior
- Role in memory
- Perceptual distortions
- Input from all sensory systems

**Brainstem**
Locus ceruleus
(noradrenergic)
Raphe nucleus (serotonergic)
Substantia nigra (dopaminergic)

**FIGURE 5.3** ● Brain structures associated with mood.

antidepressants are more active modifiers of DA. No firm evidence exists that DA abnormalities are central to depression, so it continues to be studied.

A critical point must be emphasized here. Because of the modulating effects of neurotransmitters on each other, attributing a given emotional presentation to a "pure" serotonergic or noradrenergic response most likely is erroneous. For example, levels of 5-HT and DA are correlated in the central nervous system (CNS), so that low levels of one are associated with low levels of the other. In contrast, 5-HT is thought to have an inhibiting, or at least modifying, effect on NE (Thase & Howland, 1995). This makes good evolutionary sense, since low 5-HT levels allow increases in NE as a compensatory mechanism in times of stress.

Another example of homeostatic interactions between neurotransmitters is the relationship between the monoamines and another transmitter, *acetylcholine* (ACh). The role of ACh in the chemistry of mood was recognized in the 1980s when it was found that increased cholinergic levels were associated with decreases in monoamines, and that, conversely, monoamine excess occurred with

decreased levels of ACh (Thase & Howland, 1995). Although it may function in a secondary role to the monoamines, ACh continues to be a subject of research interest. *Gamma-aminobutyric acid* (GABA) is another neurotransmitter long known as a major inhibitory neurotransmitter in the CNS. This amino acid also has been found to have an inverse relationship with NE levels (Roy, 1991) and may, therefore, affect mood and anxiety states. Several studies have found low levels of GABA in severely depressed patients, but the dynamics of GABA function in depression remain unclear. It is probably more important in anxiety states and is discussed later in this context.

Another neurotransmitter, the peptide *cholecystokinin*, is under investigation. This substance has a role in GI function, appetite, and, possibly, anxiety disorders and is discussed in a later section.

In summary, most dysfunctional emotional states are thought to be a particular and dynamic combination of neurotransmitter function and malfunction, and researchers are aware that reaching a complete understanding of psychopathophysiology is a distant goal.

## Brain Structures Associated With Mood

The brainstem, which represents the most primitive part of the brain, regulates basic body functions and as such does not participate directly in the creation and expression of complex subtleties of mood. It is, however, the site of several nuclei (clusters of cell bodies), which are responsible for the synthesis of specific neurotransmitters, which then send dense fiber networks upward to various sites in the forebrain. The *locus ceruleus*, *raphe nucleus*, and *substantia nigra* are major sources of noradrenergic, serotonergic, and dopaminergic neurons, respectively (see Fig. 5-3).

More complex emotions and behaviors are guided by higher, more recently evolved parts of the brain. The *diencephalon* forms the inner core of the cerebrum and is divided into areas that include the epithalamus, thalamus, and hypothalamus. The *epithalamus* (pineal gland), which forms the "roof" of the diencephalon, plays a role in some basic emotional drives. Pineal hormones affect reproductive function, and melatonin secretion is associated with circadian rhythms. The *thalamus* is the major relay station of information going to and from the cerebral cortex. It is responsible for the neural excitation essential for sleep-wake cycles, as well as awareness of general sensations such as pain, temperature, and touch. More pertinent to mood, it enables a person to experience emotional responses to these sensory stimuli. Lying beneath the thalamus, the *hypothalamus* regulates the coordination of behavioral patterns and emotional expression through dense connections with the autonomic nervous system. Among its other functions are influences on the endocrine system and hormone control through the pituitary gland.

Each of the preceding structures has extensive neural connections with a nearby surrounding area, the *limbic system*. Its principal structures include the amygdala, olfactory bulb, cingulate and hippocampal gyri, and the hippocampus. (Because of its close functional relationship with the thalamus and hypothalamus, some experts consider these to be limbic structures also.) In lower animals, the limbic system is involved primarily with the sense of smell. In humans, its principal effects are thought to be the experience and expression of mood, sleep, appetite, and (as in lower animals) sense of smell. The strong emotions of fear, rage, and sexual function are mediated here. Stimulation of specific areas of the limbic system can lead to feelings of dread, high anxiety, or intense pleasure, and can produce rage and violent behaviors. As is described later, emotional disorders such as depression and anxiety demonstrate many symptoms related to limbic dysfunction. Not surprisingly, the principal neurotransmitters here are monoamines (Schuyler, 1998).

Lying beneath the cerebral cortex are deep masses of gray matter, the *basal ganglia*. Whereas these nuclei are mostly associated with learned and unlearned motor functions, they also have been implicated in depression. Parkinson's disease and Huntington's chorea, two diseases affecting primarily the basal ganglia, often have been associated with a high incidence of depression.

Emotional expression and affect are largely a result of coordinated connections between the limbic system and the *prefrontal cortex*. This highest area of the brain is best associated with the personality, which arguably makes us unique as individuals and as a species. Prefrontal cortical function is responsible for goal-oriented behaviors, ability to concentrate, sense of social responsibility, and socially correct behavior. It governs creative thought, judgment, anticipation, and prediction of consequences of behavior. Many of these high cortical functions are impaired in serious depression or anxiety. Drugs of abuse such as alcohol also particularly depress this region of the brain.

Although assigning specific functions to specific localities in the brain is helpful, it is not scientifically accurate. In reality, many parts of the brain are involved with a given function, and much of brain function remains unclear. Another important concept of brain physiology is plasticity, the fact that brain structures are capable of change; for instance, with brain damage, certain functions can relocate elsewhere in the brain.

Initially, it had been hoped that depression and anxiety could be explained by simple models of disease, but this has not been true. Just as the brain's normal function mandates a complex interplay of many different nerve tracts and structures, depression and anxiety are increasingly seen as heterogeneous disorders with multiple etiologies. Each affected individual represents a particular combination of biochemical imbalances, genetic susceptibility, life experiences, social circumstances, and coping abilities. For the practitioner, such complexity may be frustrating, but it does explain why a treatment that works well for one patient may be ineffective for another. Although much remains unknown about the pathology of emotion, the practitioner should pursue assessment, treatment, and referral of depressed patients as vigorously as she or he would any other serious medical disease.

## Depressive Disorders

Our discussion of the pathophysiology of depressive disorders begins with an illustrative case (see Clinical Vignette 5-1, below).

### Clinical Presentation and Types of Depression

Depression is one of the most painful, distressing, and debilitating experiences that can afflict an individual. It commonly goes unrecognized and untreated in the primary care clinic and, as shown in the case just described, it also may go unrecognized by the patient. Depression may result from a traumatic life event or may have a gradual, insidious onset. Some patients describe "not feeling right," appear withdrawn, or have vague somatic complaints. Some individuals may perceive their problems as "just everyday life" and not be aware that their reaction has progressed past a temporary low mood. A certain cluster of symptoms is common, but these appear in different combinations in different people. Rarely will all be present and affect the patient to the same degree. Symptoms include the following:

- Feelings of sadness or despair
- Anhedonia (lack of interest or pleasure in most activities, diminished sex drive)
- Sleep disturbances (hypersomnia or insomnia, especially early morning wakening)
- Fatigue, loss of energy
- Psychomotor retardation or agitation
- Poor memory and concentration, difficulty making decisions
- Feelings of guilt or worthlessness, hopelessness
- Anorexia or overeating with concomitant weight change
- Regular thoughts of death, suicidal plans or actions

Types of depression most commonly seen in primary care are major depressive disorder (MDD), dysthymia, adjustment disorder with depressed mood, depression caused by a general medical condition, and bipolar disorder.

### *Major Depressive Disorder*

MDD is the most severe form of depression, with the greatest disability and the greatest risk of suicide. The diagnosis of MDD requires that at least five of the symptoms just described be present almost continuously for at least 2 weeks. One of the symptoms must be either depressed mood or anhedonia. Although less serious mood disturbances may respond well to care provided in the primary care setting, the practitioner who suspects MDD should refer the patient for psychiatric evaluation and treatment. This serious illness usually requires closely monitored drug therapy (with or without psychotherapy).

In some cases, the patient's thinking and perception of reality are grossly impaired. Hallucina-

---

## *CLINICAL VIGNETTE 5.1*

Mr. Roth is a 44-year-old who comes to the primary care provider requesting something to help him sleep. He is a neatly dressed, quiet man who is polite but avoids eye contact and seldom smiles. His insomnia has been a problem for at least a year. He states that he has no trouble falling asleep—indeed, he is tired all day and falls asleep on the couch at 9:00 PM nightly. He wakes again at about 4:00 AM, however, and is unable to get back to sleep. Lately, he has been getting up at 5:00 AM to exercise, "since I won't be able to sleep anyway." He says the exercise has not helped him sleep any better. His appetite is adequate and his weight has been stable for the last 5 years, but he no longer enjoys eating. When asked what he does enjoy, Mr. Roth is able to think only of things he used to like doing, but which no longer give him any pleasure. Asked to describe his usual day's activity, he says he spends most of his time at work, putting in 10- to 12-hour days, feeling a constant sense of pressure, and feeling as though he is never doing enough or doing well. He reports some stress at home, since his wife often is upset at his long work days and lack of involvement with her and the children. She accuses him of forgetting what she has told him, complains that he doesn't pay attention to her anymore, and is hurt that he is rarely interested in sex. Mr. Roth understands and accepts his wife's criticisms, but states that he loves his family and doesn't understand what has changed lately. He denies major stressful events at home or work that might have caused his current mood. When pressed to identify future goals or things he is looking forward to, he states sadly that he doesn't have much enthusiasm for life anymore and doesn't feel much hope that his life is likely to improve.

tions, paranoia, and other forms of disturbed thinking (*psychotic features*) accompany the major depression. These thoughts usually are consistent with low mood, following themes such as guilt, "deserved" punishment, somatic problems, and delusions of poverty. Psychotically depressed people are at greater risk for suicide, and require a more complex treatment than that of nonpsychotic depressive patients (Viguera & Rothschild, 1996). Such patients—as many as 30% of patients with major depression—require psychiatric referral. In the elderly, depression may cause a condition called "pseudodementia," which can be difficult to distinguish from other forms of dementia. These individuals also benefit from careful medical workup and referral to a gerontologic psychiatrist.

### Other Types of Depression

*Dysthmia* is a milder form of depression in which symptoms persist almost daily for at least 2 years; it also can result in significant disability. *Adjustment disorder with depressed mood* was formerly known as "exogenous depression," in that it is believed to result from an external event such as death or divorce. It is important to distinguish between a depressive disorder and the natural grieving process that follows a significant loss. The diagnosis is made when the patient experiences more impairment than normally would be expected. If depression lasts longer than 6 months and is not severe, the diagnosis changes to the catchall category, *depressive disorder not otherwise specified* (NOS). In any case, the treatment for depression remains the same, with antidepressant drugs and counseling being mainstays. A referral for psychiatric evaluation is needed for any mood disorder that persists despite several trials of antidepressants or counseling, or that poses a risk of harm to the patient or others. Again, the patient should be included in this decision-making process, since patients who do not understand or who reject the reason for the referral are much less likely to follow through with it.

*Depression caused by a general medical condition* (Table 5-1) is believed to be a direct result of physiologic changes ensuing from events such as stroke, thyroid disease, Parkinson's disease, or certain drug treatments (eg, reserpine). Every patient presenting with depression should be evaluated for other pertinent possibilities such as anemia or thyroid dysfunction. Whereas correcting the medical problem is the clinician's goal, the depression probably needs to be treated also. With incurable diseases or chronic pain syndromes, treatment of a coexisting depression may improve the patient's status by improving sleep, sense of energy, appetite, and coping abilities. Mental status is a powerful predictor of overall prognosis.

*Bipolar disorder* (formerly called manic depressive illness) and its milder form, *cyclothymia*, are not discussed in depth here, but merit a psychiatric referral if the clinician suspects more than a depressed mood. Bipolar disorders are marked by the presence of cyclic mood changes. Patients experience depression, as well as rare to frequent

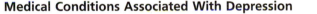

## TABLE 5.1

**Medical Conditions Associated With Depression**

| Type of Disease | Syndrome Associated With Depression |
| --- | --- |
| Cardiovascular disease | Cerebrovascular accident, myocardial infarction |
| Endocrine disorders | Diabetes, hypothyroidism, adrenal insufficiency |
| Cancer | All types |
| Neurologic disorders | Parkinson's disease, Alzheimer's disease, brain tumors, multiple sclerosis |
| Autoimmune disorders | Systemic lupus erythematosis, rheumatoid arthritis |
| Infectious diseases | HIV/AIDS, hepatitis, mononucleosis |
| Anemias | Blood loss; vitamin $B_{12}$, folate, or iron deficiency |
| Substance abuse | Alcohol, opiate, amphetamine, and cocaine abuse |
| Miscellaneous | Chronic pain, chronic fatigue syndrome, prolonged illness |
| Medications | Some antihypertensive drugs, anticonvulsants, hormones/oral contraceptives, steroids, antibiotics, antiparkinsonian agents, digitalis, antineoplastic agents, benzodiazepines |

episodes of manic or hypomanic thoughts and behaviors that contrast sharply with those seen in depression. Asking patients to describe themselves when *not* depressed may help in making a tentative distinction between unipolar and bipolar disorders.

Not all depressions are easy to treat; they may never resolve or may recur too frequently. However, most depressed patients (60% to 80%) improve with antidepressant medication (Dougherty & Rauch, 1997), and group or individual psychotherapy also may be beneficial. Many practitioners believe that a combination of medication and psychotherapy has the highest degree of success.

## Depression Throughout the Life Span

Mood disorders are common, affecting 5% to 10% of men and 10% to 20% of women. Despite much investigation, this large gender disparity is not fully explained by genetic and endocrine differences. It persists worldwide, through many cultures, and at all levels of income and education. Many researchers believe that sociocultural factors are more critical. These include gender differences, such as men not seeking help as often as women or men being more prone to blunting their depression with alcohol or overwork, and women more commonly exhibiting helpless or passive behaviors or reacting negatively to perceived power and control inequities with men. Women also may be more sensitive to personal relationships and therefore more vulnerable to loss. More study is needed to clarify these issues.

Depression has a high rate of comorbidity with other disorders. Individuals with another serious mental illness such as schizophrenia or anxiety are at increased risk for depression. Similarly, alcoholism and other forms of substance abuse (including cigarette smoking) frequently are associated with depression—although whether depression is a causative or secondary illness varies between individuals. Depression also may occur as a result of, or subsequent to, a medical condition such as cancer, coronary artery disease, or diabetes. Certain neurologic conditions (stroke, brain tumors, multiple sclerosis, Parkinson's disease, Alzheimer's disease) frequently present along with depression, although the extent to which this depression is caused by neurologic changes or ensues as a result of disease-induced disability is unclear and probably varies between patients.

The occurrence of depression in children and adolescents was questioned until a few decades ago. It was believed that dysfunctional behaviors such as delinquency represented a "masked depression," which would not manifest until adulthood (Birmaher et al., 1996). Recently, the prevalence of MDD in school-aged children has been acknowledged and is estimated to be approximately 3%, with rates being equal between between girls and boys; rates in preschoolers are undetermined. This changes in adolescence, with the overall prevalence of depression increasing—up to 8% in some studies—with girls affected twice as often as boys (Lewinsohn et al., 1994). This rate is similar to that observed in adults, and again, opinion is divided as to whether biologic, genetic, sociocultural forces, or a combination thereof, contribute to the gender difference.

Because adolescents frequently are in good health and often do not seek medical treatment, the clinician may have few opportunities to assess mood disorders in this group. However, suicide represents the second leading cause of death in 15 to 24 year olds, and homicide, the third. Clearly, an evaluation of a teenager's emotional status during routine examinations, such as sports physicals, is vital.

The prevalence of depression in the elderly is a source of debate. Some studies claim that rates equal those of younger adults, but others believe that symptoms are different in the elderly (more somatic complaints, higher risk of psychosis), and the diagnosis may be missed more often in elderly patients. A depression rating scale designed for younger populations may be invalid for elderly clients. Some studies (Georgotas, 1983; Raskin, 1979) report that the elderly are more likely to minimize feelings of sadness and deny their depression than younger patients. In any case, the elderly are seen to be at higher risk for depression because of their higher risk for major illness, greater use of medications that may cause depression, and the presence of stressors such as loss of role identity at work or home or death of significant others. Despite this, depression is *never* considered to be "normal" in the geriatric population.

Whether depression in older individuals results from illness or major loss or occurs without apparent cause, it may be assessed and treated successfully with the same modalities used for younger patients. Clients and their families should be taught that major depression reflects a true biochemical imbalance. Finally, the practitioner must be careful not to attribute vague somatic complaints to a depressed mood too quickly, since many symptoms of depression (fatigue, sleep disturbances, GI upset) also are seen in major illness. As in other age groups, the possibility of depression induced by medications must be considered (Clinical Vignette 5-2, page 65).

## Biologic Theories of Depression: Focuses of Research

Whereas certain areas of the brain are known to mediate and direct mood, and although it is assumed that dysfunction in these areas is partly or fully responsible for depression, the exact mechanisms remain obscure despite decades of research. Several lines of study are under way that approach the problem from several viewpoints; they are expected to yield important insights for diagnosis and treatment of depression.

The *monoamine hypothesis* of depression, which dominated the 1960s and 1970s, is based on the idea that depression results from a deficiency of NE (Schildkraut, 1965). This theory is attractive because most of the drugs that improve symptoms of depression act on monamines. At first, researchers thought NE to be the culprit, but 5-HT has been implicated recently. Many of the brain pathways involved in emotion also involve overlapping NE and 5-HT neurons, and another way of thinking about depression is that these neurotransmitter interact. Serotoninergic neurons are heavily concentrated in the raphe nuclei, which project to noradrenergic centers throughout the brain. This innervation thus may modulate neurotransmission of NE. Table 5-2 shows the major monoamine pathways, the enzymes that regulate them, and their relationships to depression.

The role of neuroendocrine abnormalities in depression is another area of intense interest. There is a close functional and spatial relationship between the limbic system, which controls mood, and the hypothalamus and pituitary gland, which govern endocrine function. Abnormal responses to several hypothalamic hormones have been well-documented in depression, especially those of the hypothalamic-pituitary-adrenal (HPA) axis. This system is of particular interest because of its primary role in the stress response. Depression is viewed by many as a stressor that generates a chronic stress response in the body, a view which is upheld by research. Elevated cortisol levels have been found in the cerebrospinal fluid (CSF) of approximately half of depressed patients, and these elevations remit with recovery from the depression (Schuyler, 1998). Similarly, hypersecretion of corticotropin-releasing factor (CRF) released from the hypothalamus and a blunted corticotropin (ACTH) (pituitary) response to CRF with hypercortisolemia have been observed. An abnormal result of a dexamethasone suppression test is diagnostic in some (but not all) cases of depression.

Whereas effects of HPA aberrations on the body are incompletely understood, they have practical significance for the clinician. Depressed individuals often complain of insomnia, particularly early morning wakening. This is attributed to cor-

---

### *CLINICAL VIGNETTE 5.2*

Mrs. Chase, 63 years of age, comes to the clinic with her husband who requests "something for her depression." The patient seems quiet and withdrawn, and her husband relates that about 6 months ago, she began to seem increasingly disinterested in her usual activities and resisted encouragement by her family to get out of the house and go places. No major changes have happened at home, and Mrs. Chase denies any knowledge of anything that would cause her change in mood. She has lost 5 lb and no longer enjoys cooking. Her husband also states that her former interest in sex has dwindled during the same time period and that they rarely have intercourse any more. As with the rest of her life, the patient complains that she "just doesn't have the energy for it." The couple has sought marriage counseling through their church and has been to a gyne-

cologist "to see if there's something wrong with her hormones." The gynecologist suggested that the patient seemed depressed and referred her to her primary care practitioner. On review of her medical history at this visit, it is noted that the patient was started on a beta blocker for mild hypertension at a clinic visit 9 months ago. After a physical examination, which reveals no new problems and a normal blood pressure, the practitioner decides to change to another antihypertensive class of medication and explains that the beta blocker may be causing the patient's problems. Mrs. Chase returns to the clinic in 6 weeks with a normal blood pressure, feeling much better, and reporting a noticeable improvement in her energy and interest levels. Her husband feels that "she's starting to seem like her old self again."

## TABLE 5.2

**Monoamines in Depression**

| Monoamine | Production | Enzymatic Breakdown | Potential Role in Depression |
|---|---|---|---|
| Norepinephrine | Tyrosine ▶ DOPA ▶ dopamine ▶ NE | Destroyed by MAO and COMT; also removed from synapse by presynaptic uptake transporter | Low levels at synapse; decreased concentration of NE metabolites in urine and CSF; NE and 5-HT interact throughout the brain: NE can increase ($\alpha_1$-receptors) or decrease ($\alpha_2$-receptors) 5-HT release |
| Dopamine | Tyrosine ▶ DOPA ▶ dopamine | Destroyed by MAO and COMT | Dopamine metabolites decreased in CSF |
| Serotonin (5-HT) | Tryptophan ▶ 5-hydroxytryptophan ▶ 5-HT | Destroyed by MAO and presynaptic uptake | 5-HT metabolites decreased in CSF; interacts with NE; decrease at synapse may decrease NE |

CSF, cerebrospinal fluid; COMT, catechol-*O*-methyltransferase; DOPA, dopamine; MAO, monoamine oxidase; NE, norepinephrine.

tisol secretion that persists into the evening and night rather than following normal diurnal variation. Treatment of the depression usually resolves or improves sleep problems.

Hypothyroidism often is associated with depression, and thyroid hormones can improve the course of some depressions and potentiate the action of antidepressants in others. A blunted response of pituitary thyrotropin to the hypothalamic hormone thyrotropin-releasing hormone has been noted in some depressed patients (Winokur, 1993), which may resolve with antidepressant treatment. Overall, the dysregulation of the hypothalamic-pituitary-thyroid axis, rather than hypofunction or hyperfunction of the thyroid gland itself, appears to underlie the thyroid anomalies associated with depression. The clinician should include thyroid function tests in early patient evaluation for depression.

A third endocrine system abnormality seen in depressed patients results in alterations in growth hormone (GH) secreted by the pituitary. Somatostatin secreted by the hypothalamus is decreased in the CSF of depressed patients, along with a blunted response of GH to several drug challenges.

In summary, evidence suggests hypothalamic-pituitary-endocrine dysfunction in depression. Furthermore, the clinical symptoms observed reflect alterations in food intake, libido, and circadian rhythms—all normally under hypothalamic control. Finally, the neurotransmitters that regulate communication between the hypothalamus and pituitary are the same as those implicated in depression: NE, serotonin, and DA (Schuyler, 1998). Further research is needed to illuminate this important relationship.

Sleep disturbances in depression are common and may manifest in a variety of forms. Early morning awakening, mentioned earlier, perhaps is the most common, but depressed individuals also complain of trouble getting to sleep (initial insomnia), multiple awakenings, or a sense of light sleep or poor sleep. Other patients experience hypersomnia—increased total sleep time. All of these alterations are reflected in electroencephalographic changes. Depression is associated with less time required to start rapid eye movement (REM) sleep and more REM sleep per REM period than normal. Whereas REM sleep is vital to normal nervous function, the excesses seen in depression reflect alterations that decrease the total time spent in the deep, slow-wave sleep (SWS), which also is essential. Serotonergic neurons normally are active during SWS and silent during REM periods, when ACh activity is greater (Thase & Howland, 1995). It is expected that changes in these and other neurotransmitters, as well as endocrine alterations, are responsible for the variety of sleep problems associated with depression.

A relatively new and exciting source of information comes from neuroimaging studies. Over the last 15 years, developments in the use of single-photon emission computed tomography, positron emission tomography (PET), and magnetic resonance imaging (MRI) offer new opportunities for the in vivo study of the brain's functional anatomy. Using isotope tracers, these techniques offer a visual display of both blood flow and regional metabolism of glucose in the brain. The most consistently identified finding has been left prefrontal cortical lobe dysfunction, as indicated by reduced cerebral blood flow (CBF) and glucose metabolism. Additional findings are less definitive but suggestive. Some neuroimages suggest atrophy of basal ganglia, whereas other results indicate abnormalities in specific limbic structures (Mayberg, 1997; Risch, 1997; Soares & Mann, 1997). The amygdala, a limbic structure that regulates memory for emotionally significant events, is more active than normal in both sadness and depression, and is believed by some to represent the primary functional abnormality (Dougherty & Rauch, 1997). But neuroimaging still is in its infancy, and much research is needed. Comparative studies analyze differences between affected and unaffected subjects, whereas dynamic studies are performed on subjects as they experience a variety of emotions. In the future, improved radiolabeling techniques should be able to perform a multitude of functions, including tracing the binding and behavior neurotransmitters in the body and brain.

Underlying much of the current work is an understanding of the importance of genetics in mood disorders. Studies of twins and adopted children demonstrate a hereditary vulnerability to depression, which is strongest in bipolar disorder. Through studies of specific bipolar family pedigrees, several genes that contribute to this illness have been identified. Unipolar depression shows a weaker genetic influence, and no genes have been directly associated with it. Given the neurologic complexity of human mood, it is reasonable to expect all mood disorders to be influenced by various combinations of genes, which differ in their effects, depending on the social and physical environment of the individual.

Another new focus of research is in the field of psychoneuroimmunology (see Chapter 1). First coined in 1981, this term refers to the discovery by scientists from several disciplines that a close connection exists between the CNS, the endocrine system, and the immune system, and that communication between the systems is multidirectional. Furthermore, as endocrine function is better understood, it is increasingly incorporated into the CNS/immune system dyad. Many believe that nervous, immune, and endocrine systems are so tightly linked that they represent a single rather than separate systems (Connor & Leonard, 1998). The associations between depression, the CNS, the endocrine system, and the stress response have been mentioned. It follows, then, that recent research has concentrated on the role of stress and immunity in mood disorders.

The effects of depression on the HPA axis result in hypersecretion of CRF from the hypothalamus. CRF in turn stimulates NE neurons in the locus ceruleus and promotes the release of ACTH and glucocorticoids, which eventually have immunosuppressive effects (Price & Rasmussen, 1997). Therefore, depression does affect the immune system. Can the opposite also be true? Research indicates that the immune system does affect mood through the action of *cytokines*, substances released by immune cells that normally play a major role in coordinating the immune response. Cytokines such as interleukin-1 (IL-1) have been shown to enhance the secretion of NE, serotonin, and DA in animal experiments. IL-1 reduces levels of ACh and has variable effects on GABA and other neurotransmitters (DeSimoni & Imeri, 1998; Muller & Ackenheil, 1998). More investigation is needed to identify other cytokines (eg, other interleukins, tumor necrosis factor) that may be active. There is an increasing consensus, however, that frequent and bidirectional interactions occur between immune cells and neurotransmitters in the CNS, and that the neurochemical changes induced by elevated cytokine levels play a role in the pathogenesis of depression (Connor & Leonard, 1998). Another interesting viewpoint regarding the HPA axis is the view that depression is an exaggerated and inappropriate form of sickness behavior (see Chapter 2). Proinflammatory cytokines released during antigenic threat and activation of macrophages normally cause brain release of cytokines that produce fever, lethargy, fatigue, anhedonia, and anorexia. This type of sickness behavior is appropriate and protective of the host, but in depression there may be inappropriate release of cytokines, producing HPA arousal and sickness-type behaviors characteristic of the depressed state.

## Physiology of Treatment: Matching the Patient With the Drug

Many mood-stabilizing drugs have been developed over the last 40 years, and despite the recent advent of important, new antidepressant drug classes, all of those currently marketed—new *and* old—have been proven equally effective in controlled tests. All exert their influence through one or more neurotransmitter systems. Therefore, it can be said that "each drug is a successful antidepressant treatment for some depressed persons, some of the time." A drug that has been effective for one individual may not work for another, and a prescription that worked well at first may lose its effect over time, requiring replacement or reevaluation.

### Pharmacology Update

There is no magic formula for predicting which drug will be most effective in a given patient, but knowledge of the major categories and their side effect profiles will help the primary care practitioner to make better educated guesses. As previously stated, the neurotransmitters affecting mood have other systemic effects. This fact helps to explain the various side effects of each drug class. The astute practitioner needs to use knowledge of side effects to tailor antidepressant drug choices to each patient's particular needs (Table 5-3).

The oldest class of antidepressants is the tricyclic antidepressants (TCAs), which work mainly by blocking reuptake of NE and serotonin and modifying the sensitivity of these receptors. Drugs in this class vary in the amount of noradrenergic and serotonergic effects produced and thus have individual differences. Their action is not immediate. The clinician must remind patients that these drugs may take up to a month to exhibit full antidepressant effects. TCAs have fallen out of favor recently, however, because of a several side effects. The most distressing to patients is the TCA effect on ACh. Anticholinergic effects include dry mouth, drowsiness, weight gain, constipation, dysuria, blurred vision, and dizziness. TCAs also have cardiovascular effects and should not be taken by anyone with heart disease, especially dysrhythmias. They are dangerous in overdose for this reason. A 2-week supply of medication taken at once may be fatal. No patient with any risk of suicide should be prescribed medication from this class. Despite their tarnished reputation, however, TCAs remain a valuable resource in the arsenal of available antidepressants (Clinical Vignette 5-3, page 71).

A second group of drugs, the monoamine oxidase inhibitors (MAOIs), blocks the action of monoamine oxidase, an enzyme that normally catalyzes monoamines. These generally are used as a last resort for patients who fail to respond to other drugs because they can cause a hypertensive crisis when taken with tyramine-containing foods (eg, chocolate, aged cheese or meat, red wine), and patient compliance is problematic.

Currently, the most popular drugs are selective serotonin reuptake inhibitors (SSRIs) such as fluoxetine (Prozac) and paroxetine (Paxil). These agents block the reuptake of serotonin in presynaptic neurons and allow higher concentrations of this neurotransmitter. They generally are safe to use, since overdose is unlikely to be fatal, and they have fewer side effects than TCAs. SSRIs are more expensive than older drugs, but the clinician may convince reluctant insurance companies of the need for coverage if the patient is obese, has significant medical problems (especially heart disease), is elderly, has failed previous TCA therapy, or poses a suicide risk (Clinical Vignette 5-4, page 72). Whereas the antidepressant effects of SSRIs may not be apparent for up to a month after initiating therapy, many patients report improvement sooner. Their most common side effects are insomnia, agitation, and altered sexual response (delayed orgasm). Drug–drug interactions can occur; SSRIs are metabolized through the P450 liver enzyme system and must be used with caution with other medications also metabolized this way. In addition, the combination of a SSRI with a MAOI can cause dangerously high blood pressure, tachyarrhythmia, and hyperthermia and should be avoided.

As pharmacologists gain a better understanding of neurotransmitter action and function, they will be able to design drugs with greater precision. Certain antidepressants, which act at specific points in noradrenergic and serotonergic pathways, are useful for specific purposes. Trazodone (Desyrel) has more sedating effects and is useful for insomnia. Bupropion (Wellbutrin, Zyban), primarily a DA blocker, affects the brain's reward pathway and has been approved for use in smoking cessation. Therefore, it might be an appropriate choice as an antidepressant for the patient who is trying to stop smoking. Bupropion also is one of several drugs (mirtazapine and nefazodone are others) that lack the sexual side effects of the SSRIs and might be used if the latter had been tried and rejected for this reason. The popular nonprescription herbal supplement St. John's wort contains a substance that is thought to have some degree of MAOI activity. It has been widely used in Europe and is believed to be fairly safe for individuals with mild depression. As with many other "natural" supplements, however, little is known about its biochemical makeup and long-term effects, and patients who are taking other medications or who have other health problems should avoid it.

## TABLE 5.3 ● ● ●

### Major Antidepressant Drug Classes

| Class | Example | Comments* |
|---|---|---|
| Tricyclics | Desipramine<br>Nortriptyline<br>Amitryptyline<br>Doxepin | Sedation, increased appetite, weight gain, dry mouth, dizziness, constipation, urinary retention, blurred vision. Contraindicated in cardiac conduction disorders, narrow-angle glaucoma, prostatic hypertrophy. Lethal in overdose<br>*Do not use in cases of potential suicide* |
| SSRIs | Fluoxetine (Prozac) | Agitation, insomnia, nausea, modest weight loss. Approved for anorexia treatment. Longest half-life. Try if patient lacks energy or is obese |
| | Paroxetine (Paxil) | Sedation, nausea, sweating, dizziness. Try in anxious, sleepless patients; may dose at HS. May cause weight gain |
| | Sertaline (Zoloft) | GI upset, nausea, diarrhea |
| | Citalopram (Celexa) | Respiratory: infection, flu Sx, sinus congestion, nausea, drowsiness<br>• Any SSRI may cause headache, nausea, insomnia. Sexual dysfunction common with all SSRIs<br>• Taper all drugs upward from lowest starting dose to minimize/monitor side effects<br>• SSRIs used for panic disorder, obsessive-compulsive disorder, sometimes used in anxiety. Also may be useful for social phobia (Paxil approved for this purpose)<br>*Caution: cytochrome P450 interactions* |
| Other heterocyclics | Trazadone (Desyrel) | Very sedating; used most often for sleep aid. (Therapeutic doses for depression seldom tolerated.) Anticholinergic, caution in elderly because of orthostatic effects |
| | Nefazodone (Serzone) | Sedating, orthostasis. Try in selected patients with anxiety, poor sleep. No sexual side effects |
| Miscellaneous newer agents | Venlafaxine (Effexor, Effexor XR) | Nausea, anorexia, constipation, sexual dysfunction. Side effects usually less with extended release. Monitor BP for dose-related effects. Higher doses associated with anxiety, may be effective for patients with low energy. No *CYP* interactions |

(continued)

**TABLE 5.3** (continued)

**Major Antidepressant Drug Classes**

| Class | Example | Comments* |
|---|---|---|
| | Bupropion (Wellbutrin, Zyban) | Dry mouth, constipation, sweating, nervousness, insomnia. May help depressed patient trying to quit smoking. Dose-dependent seizure risk; do not exceed recommended daily dosing. May help patients with low energy. No sexual dysfunction |
| | Mirtazapine (Remeron) | Sedation, appetite, and weight gain; dose at HS. Dizziness, dry mouth, constipation. No sexual dysfunction. Try in selected anorexic, anxious, sleepless patients. Paradoxical action: doses > 30 mg may reverse sedating effects |
| MAOIs | Phenelzine (Nardil) Tranylcypromine (Parnate) | Effective but rarely used because of safety and tolerability concerns. Interactions with tyramine-containing foods can cause hypertensive crisis; combining with other antidepressants can cause serotonin syndrome. Toxic in overdose |

BP, blood pressure; *CYP*, cytochrome P450; GI, gastrointestinal; HS, bedtime; MAOIs, monoamine oxidase inhibitors; SSRIs, selective serotonin reuptake inhibitors; Sx, symptoms.
*Side effects and precautions listed are not all-inclusive. Consult drug references for complete listing of side effects and precautions.

Patients may need to be reminded that just because a drug is advertised as "natural," it is not necessarily safe.

## GENERALIZED ANXIETY DISORDER

Anxiety is a protective and reasonable response to threat. It is a biologic mechanism for coping with danger. However, *generalized anxiety disorder* (GAD) represents much more than normal anxiety. It is chronic, exaggerated worry, although nothing in particular may be wrong. Individuals with GAD may consistently expect the worst and may be worried excessively about their health, money, family, or work. These fluctuating but persistent levels of worry are associated with symptoms of muscle tension and feeling irritable or "edgy," yet fatigued and drained. Unlike depressed patients who awaken in the early morning hours, individuals with GAD have trouble falling asleep (initial insomnia) and staying asleep. They complain of poor memory or concentration. They may startle easily or describe symptoms such as trembling, twitching, headaches, sweating, hot flashes, lightheadedness, breathlessness, nausea, a frequent urge to urinate, or a feeling of a lump in the throat (Table 5-4).

### Somatic Symptoms of Anxiety

Generalized anxiety disorder has a relatively slow onset and may not be recognized as a problem

**TABLE 5.4**

**Somatic Symptoms of Anxiety**

- Tremor
- Dyspnea
- Faintness
- Facial flushing
- Fatigue
- Nausea and vomiting
- Paresthesia
- Sweating
- Body aches, pain
- Dizziness
- Palpitations
- Insomnia
- Frequent urination
- Restlessness

---

### CLINICAL VIGNETTE 5.3

Mr. Williams, 38 years old, comes to the primary care provider asking for an antidepressant. He has had a myofascial pain syndrome (see Chapter 19) for 5 years, which has proven resistant to treatment, leaving him in chronic discomfort. Other than this, he is fairly healthy. The patient is exceedingly thin and clearly is tense because of discomfort with movement. He reports that he rarely sleeps more than 4 hours per night, has trouble falling asleep, and wakes by 5:00 AM daily. He cannot nap during the day and instead is always "on edge" and restless. He says he is always tired. Mr. Williams has no appetite and says he has to force himself to eat two meals daily. He has two small children and a supportive wife and says his family life is "pretty good, considering the shape I'm in." He denies suicidal thoughts or plans but reports that he struggles daily to keep his spirits up and frequently wonders if his life will ever be better. The patient had been prescribed fluoxetine (Prozac) a year ago but stopped taking it because, "It made me crazy and even more nervous. I felt a hundred times worse."

Mr. Williams is given a prescription for amitriptyline (Elavil) to be taken at bedtime on a gradually increasing dosage. He is an excellent candidate for tricyclic antidepressant (TCA) therapy because of his insomnia, anorexia, nervousness, and lack of suicidal ideation. The side effect profile of TCAs should prove beneficial. Because he had an adverse reaction to Prozac, another SSRI is ruled out at this point. He has no other known medical illnesses that would contraindicate a TCA. In addition, the drug may help with pain control, since TCAs such as amitriptyline have been shown to be effective in some chronic pain disorders.

Mr. Williams returns 1 month later feeling noticeably improved. He reports that the medication taken before bedtime helps him to get to sleep, and that he is sleeping 6 to 7 hours nightly and is feeling more energetic and relaxed during the day. His appetite has improved and he has gained 8 lb. He also says that his pain seems more tolerable lately and that he has started water exercises again. He now agrees with your suggestion of a referral to a local pain clinic.

---

immediately. Unlike patients with other anxiety disorders, those with GAD usually do not avoid certain situations or feel restricted in social settings or at work. But severe GAD can be debilitating, making it difficult to carry out even ordinary activities. To meet the *Diagnostic and Statistical Manual of Mental Disorders*, fourth edition, (DSM-IV) current criteria for the disorder, patients must have had some or all of these anxiety symptoms on more days than not for a minimum of 6 months. (Briefer episodes of generalized anxiety are placed in the residual category *anxiety disorder NOS*.)

How significant a problem is GAD? Anxiety disorders as a whole are the most common mental health disorders seen in the primary care clinic. GAD is one of the most common anxiety disorders, with a lifetime prevalence of 4% to 6%. For years it was considered to be a mild disorder, receiving attention only if it was accompanied by a more severe condition such as depression or panic. Currently, it is increasingly seen as a serious illness that often causes moderate impairment and often requires prolonged treatment. It may present during childhood but generally has its onset in the early 20s. It is more common in women and African Americans and more prominent in urban areas and lower income brackets, but thus far has shown no association with educational level. Opinions on the duration of GAD range from over 5 years to more than 20 years (Roy-Byrne & Katon, 1997). Remission may occur, but GAD has a high recurrence rate. It also is associated with a high rate of medical utilization. One study found GAD to occur at a rate of 22% in high users of medical health care (Katon, Von Korff, & Lin, 1990) (Clinical Vignette 5-5, page 73).

Whereas GAD is a common anxiety disorder, it is relatively rare in its "pure" form and usually coexists with other mental health disorders (Fig. 5-4). One study found only about 10% of GAD patients had GAD alone. The remainder had a comorbid condition such as phobia, panic disorder, major depression, or dysthymia (Roy-Byrne & Katon, 1997) (Fig. 5-4). Other comorbid anxiety disorders include obsessive-compulsive disorder and posttraumatic stress disorder. GAD also is accompanied by a higher than average incidence of substance abuse such as alcoholism, although less commonly so than in other anxiety disorders (Brawman-Mintzer & Lydiard, 1996). It may present with stress-related conditions such as headache, backache, or irritable bowel syndrome.

## CLINICAL VIGNETTE 5.4

Susan is a 15-year-old high school student who comes to the clinic requesting "diet medicine." She is clearly overweight at 220 lb and states she has put on 70 pounds in the last year and a half but says, "I just can't seem to stop eating!" On closer questioning, Susan tells you that her parents divorced in the last year, and she is still upset about it. She has several good friends and is doing fairly well at school but seldom leaves home otherwise. She is embarrassed about her weight and says she has no energy or motivation to diet or exercise. She naps in the afternoon, and falls asleep at 9:00 PM, only to find herself awake again at 3:00 AM, unable to get back to sleep. She has had more trouble concentrating at school this year and says her mother accuses her of being forgetful. She has crying spells at least every other day and feels overly sensitive about what people think of her. She eventually admits that she thinks she is depressed. She reports having wished she could "just drop off the face of the earth" many times but denies actual suicidal thoughts or plans.

After a complete physical examination and labwork reveal no medical problems, Susan (with her mother's support) agrees to a trial of antidepressants and several visits with a counselor. She agrees that her mood has a major effect on her living habits and that she is inter-ested in working toward a change. She is given a prescription for fluoxetine (Prozac) (any selective serotonin reuptake inhibitor [SSRI] would be an appropriate first choice) to be taken every morning and told to return in a month. SSRIs are antidepressants of choice here because of their effects on decreasing appetite and tendency to increase energy levels. They may worsen Susan's insomnia, but since she has no trouble getting to sleep, correction of the depression may allow her to sleep through the night. Finally, although Susan's suicide risk seems small, an SSRI is a safer choice for this patient.

Susan calls after 3 days and says that the medication is giving her a chronic headache. The prescription is changed to sertraline (Zoloft, another SSRI), also to be taken daily in the morning. Susan returns to the clinic in 1 month and reports that she is sleeping through the night and generally feeling much more energetic. She does not experience headache with the Zoloft. She feels the counseling sessions are helpful and plans to continue them for a while. She finds herself better able to concentrate at school and feels more motivated to participate in extracurricular activities. She and her mother have started on a diet together and she has lost 5 lb since her last visit. She also is thinking of starting an aerobics class soon.

---

Fortunately, GAD is relatively rare in the elderly. However, if an older person experiences severe anxiety, the patient may not see it as dysfunctional. Instead, the practitioner may be presented with a variety of physical symptoms or concerns about personal safety that may not be justified, but which may delay recognition of the real problem. Conversely, many physical illnesses may cause symptoms suggesting anxiety: dizziness, shortness of breath, and palpitations. The practitioner must never be too quick to assign a psychiatric diagnosis to what might be a significant organic problem or to underestimate the anxiety-inducing effects of medical illness. (Table 5-5).

The clinician treating GAD over a long time must be alert to emerging comorbid conditions that may require added evaluation and treatment. For example, most people with major depression also show symptoms of anxiety. A patient originally diagnosed with anxiety may later be rediagnosed

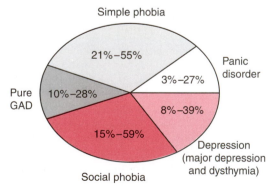

Current comorbid psychiatric diagnosis, except pure GAD (no other current or lifetime comorbid psychiatric diagnoses).

**FIGURE 5.4** ● Psychiatric comorbidity in generalized anxiety disorder. (Adapted from Brawman-Mintzer, O. & Lydiard, R.B. [1996]. Generalized anxiety disorder: Issues in epidemiology. *Journal of Clinical Psychiatry, 57*[Suppl 7], 3–8.)

### CLINICAL VIGNETTE 5.5

Mr. Jones is a 30-year-old who makes frequent visits to the clinic. He is here today requesting "something for my blood pressure," since he has been monitoring it at home four to six times daily and has noticed that it occasionally rises above 140/80. He also requests to have his cholesterol checked because he has been thinking about his diet lately and is wondering if he is eating too much fat. He denies a family history of hypercholesterolism or heart disease. A review of his records reveals that he has had regular physical examinations that reflected no major health problems. He does have ongoing bouts of low back discomfort that he treats with nonsteroidal anti-inflammatory drugs, recurring tension headaches for which he takes acetaminophen, and intermittent complaints of heartburn and stomach upset. He has been prescribed cortisone cream for intermittent skin rashes. Mr. Jones admits that he feels "edgy" most of the time, has trouble getting to sleep at night, and feels tired much of the day. He likes his job and enjoys his family but often feels tense just thinking about getting through the day. He feels guilty about his tendency to snap at the children and often finds himself worrying that something will happen to one of them. He gets little exercise and is at a loss when asked what he does to relax. Eventually, he says that two drinks after work each day help him unwind, and he reports that his alcohol use has increased in the last few years. He smokes two packs a day and feels this helps his nerves also. Mr. Jones admits that although eating also seems to help him calm down, he now is worried about becoming overweight.

as depressed. Panic disorder or phobia may be revealed (Table 5-6). Another pitfall arises from the natural human tendency to address the most prominent problem first then to underdiagnose or undertreat a less acute problem. Because GAD often falls into the latter category, the clinician must be careful not to put off addressing the real problems that it presents.

## TABLE 5.5

### Medical Conditions Associated With Anxiety

| | |
|---|---|
| *Drug reactions* | Neurologic conditions |
|   Stimulants |   Parkinson's disease |
|   Antidepressants |   Epilepsy |
|   Caffeine |   Dementia |
|   Tobacco | Infections |
|   Nonsteroidal anti-inflammatory agents |   Influenza |
|   Over-the-counter hypnotics |   Hepatitis |
|   Withdrawal of central nervous system |   Encephalitis |
|   depressants |   Pneumonia |
|     Alcohol | Cardiovascular disorders |
|     Barbiturates |   Congestive heart failure |
|   Benzodiazepines |   Myocardial infarction |
| *Physical illnesses* |   Pulmonary embolism |
|   Endocrinologic disorders | Metabolic disturbances |
|     Hyperthyroidism |   Dehydration |
|     Hyperparathyroidism |   Electrolyte imbalance |
|     Hypoglycemia | *Other conditions* |
|     Pheochromocytoma |   Constipation |
|   Cerebral infarction |   Pain |

(From Small, G.W. [1997]. Recognizing and treating anxiety in the elderly. *Journal of Clinical Psychiatry, 58,* [Suppl. 3], 41–47.)

## TABLE 5.6

### Other Anxiety Disorders

***Social phobia***
- Extreme, persistent fear of social situations
- Fear of humiliation or embarrassment
- Avoidance of situations
- Anxiety anticipating social situations
- Extreme anxiety in social situations
- Fears recognized as unreasonable or excessive

***Simple (isolated) phobia***
- Extreme, persistent fear of specific object or situation:
  - Objects include:
    - Animals (spiders, snakes)
    - Natural environment (heights, water, storms, dark)
    - Blood, injections, injury (may induce fainting)
  - Situations include:
    - Driving, flying, bridges, tunnels, elevators, enclosed spaces
- Avoidance of situation may produce severe limitations

***Panic attacks***
- Sense of escalating tension
- Chest pains, pounding heart, palpitations, tachycardia, sense of "heart attack"
- Sweating, chills, hot flashes
- Tremors
- Sense of choking, shortness of breath, smothering
- Nausea, other GI distress
- Dizziness, lightheadedness
- Weakness, numbness
- Sense of unreality
- Fear of dying, losing control

These symptoms develop quickly, reaching peak severity within 10 minutes. Duration of attack varies with nature of stressor, removal of subject from stressor, skill of subject in self-management of attacks.

***Panic disorder***
- Recurrent, unpredictable panic attacks (no specific stimulus)
- Fear of future panic attacks
- Change in behavior in response to attacks: isolation, avoidance. These may severely limit the individual's daily activities and affect job, school, and social performance

GI, gastrointestinal.

## Etiology of Generalized Anxiety Disorder

For a number of years, debate has persisted as to whether GAD existed as a distinct entity or whether it was a symptom of another diagnosis such as panic disorder or major depression. Perhaps for this reason, much less is known about its pathophysiology; research has been more sparse and has focused on comparisons with other diagnoses such as panic and depression. Areas of the brain thought to be involved with GAD are those also implicated in depressive disorders: thalamus, hypothalamus, the limbic system, basal ganglia, and parts of the cerebral cortex. There is debate about which regions are most critical, with different investigators favoring different limbic and cortical structures (Brawman-Mintzer & Lydiard, 1997; Soares & Mann 1997). As with the study of depression, the contemporary view is that the pathophysiology of anxiety is complex and does not represent a single pathologic state, but a disruption of multiple brain structures and neurotransmitter systems. Currently, investigators are interested in the specific factors that distinguish GAD from other emotional disorders, and more is being learned that reinforces the view of GAD being a distinct pathologic entity, different from other anxiety states.

*Neurotransmitter abnormalities* have long been suspected to exist in all of the anxiety disorders. Research on the biology of GAD generally has been based on the premise that prolonged anxiety creates a state in the body resembling a chronic stress response. Patients experiencing panic attacks show clear changes in NE levels, and early studies of GAD predicted similar, if less dramatic, alterations. Despite repeated testing, however, baseline NE levels in patients with GAD were found to be normal (Johnson & Lydiard, 1995; Pi et al., 1994). Recent work has refined this view, and GAD now is thought to be associated with subtle abnormalities in the nor-adrenergic system. One model of anxiety (Gray, 1988) proposes that whereas panic represents an activation of the sympathetic fight-or-flight response, GAD may reflect a state of "anticipatory anxiety" and be modulated through a different system or pathway. Further research is needed to validate and clarify this distinction.

The acknowledged role of serotonin in anxiety has been based largely on the observation that drugs affecting 5-HT activity have anxiolytic effects in GAD patients. The mode of action of these drugs varies, and their role in CNS function is poorly understood, but serotonergic drugs are increasingly becoming a mainstay of anxiety treatment. An important alternative to pharmacologic therapies used in the past, they are discussed in a later section.

In contrast to its more peripheral role in depression, GABA plays a critical role in anxiety disorders. In normal physiology, GABA-mediated hyperpolarization of neurons makes them less excitable. This is associated with alleviation of anxiety, particularly in specific modulating areas of the brain. There are two types of GABA receptors: GABA-A receptors, where benzodiazepine drugs enhance the binding of GABA; and GABA-B, where they do not. The former "benzodiazepine receptors" are found in large concen-

trations in the cerebral cortex, cerebellum, and amygdala of the limbic system (Pi et al., 1994) and are the focus of intense research interest. Unlike drugs that influence 5-HT levels, which may take weeks to relieve anxiety, benzodiazepines act rapidly after administration and are effective anxiolytics. Several lines of evidence suggest abnormalities in the GABA-benzodiazepine receptor complex in GAD. One study found patients with GAD to have abnormally low levels of *peripheral* lymphocyte benzodiazepine receptors, which normalized after treatment with benzodiazepines (Johnson & Lydiard, 1995). Other studies suggest that patients with GAD have alterations in the sensitivity of their *central* benzodiazepine receptors. Evidence is preliminary, however, and much remains unknown.

A recent focus of anxiety research concerns the role of cholecystokinin (CCK). This substance exists in several forms in mammals and is one of the most abundant peptide neurotransmitters in the human brain. CCK receptors are widely distributed through the CNS, with high densities in the hypothalamus, limbic system, basal ganglia, cortex, and brainstem. Experiments on patients with GAD and normal controls indicate that anxious patients are more likely to respond to a CCK challenge with panic and increased anxiety than are normal patients, and CCK is thought to be an important modulator of both normal and pathologic anxiety. Equally important are its interactions with other neurotransmitters implicated in anxiety. CCK increases the activity of NE neurons in the locus ceruleus and appears to antagonize the GABA and 5-HT systems. Certain subtypes of CCK increase secretion of ACTH and cortisol, and one study found CCK to inhibit thyroid and GH activity in the pituitary in rats (Brawman-Mintzer & Lydiard, 1997). More research will clarify the role of this lesser-known transmitter.

## Neuroendocrine Influences

Like depression, chronic anxiety is thought to represent a stressor that stimulates activation of the HPA axis, increasing the body's cortisol levels. No such elevated baseline levels have been demonstrated in GAD, however, and investigators believe that the HPA stress response is abnormally regulated, rather than elevated, in these patients (Brawman-Mintzer & Lydiard, 1997). Other researchers report abnormal GH responses in GAD (Abelson et al., 1991). No differences in thyroid function have been found, but the suspicion persists of hypothalamic dysfunction similar to that noted in depression.

Other subtle differences of body function have been identified in GAD. In drug challenges, GAD patients demonstrate more panic and anxiety symptoms than do normal controls when given sodium lactate infusion, although patients with panic disorder react even more strongly. GAD patients also have shown evidence of a weaker autonomic nervous system response to stress, as measured by respiration, blood pressure, and heart rate, when presented with a stress challenge. (Brawman-Mintzer & Lydiard, 1997).

*Neuroimaging studies* of patients with GAD have been limited. Work with normal subjects has shown increased total CBF with increased arousal and decreased CBF with reduced arousal. GAD patients show similar-to-normal patterns under resting conditions, but when they are exposed to stressful stimuli, CBF *decreases* (Brawman-Mintzer & Lydiard, 1997).

Differences also have been noted in the glucose metabolism of certain brain regions in GAD, with higher than normal metabolic rates in some areas and lower rates in others. Overall, imaging studies suggest potential brain changes in GAD, but more confirmation and clarification is required.

The degree to which *genetics* affects GAD has been studied, but debate over the diagnostic criteria for anxiety disorders has limited the validity of past research. This should improve now that distinctions between GAD, panic, and other anxiety states are more clearly defined. Several twin studies suggest a modest genetic effect in GAD, but less than that seen in major depression. No contributing genes have been identified.

## Physiologic Basis of Treatment

The clinician must approach the treatment of GAD with the realization that it is a chronic illness, so treatment needs to be chronic. This does not mean that patients will need to spend their lives on anxiolytic drugs; on the contrary, the goal is one of improvement to a maintenance state, with only intermittent use of medications if needed.

*Lifestyle changes* are a critical part of treatment. Caffeine use should be reviewed, since it worsens the condition of individuals with preexisting anxiety disorders, and abstinence has been shown to improve symptoms. Use of drugs, especially alcohol, to relieve anxiety symptoms should be evaluated, and dangers and disadvantages discussed with the patient. Regular exercise and adequate rest and relaxation time also should be encouraged. Psychotherapy and behavioral modification techniques also have been shown to be important. Behavioral therapy may include relax-

ation techniques such as deep-breathing exercises to counteract hyperventilation, which may occur with anxiety. Cognitive-behavioral therapy teaches patients to react differently to situations and body sensations that trigger their symptoms. They also learn how thinking patterns contribute to their anxiety response and how to change these patterns. Whereas extensive psychotherapy is beyond the scope of the primary care practitioner, brief counseling and structured problem-solving techniques are effective for many people and may be delivered in the family clinic (Clinical Vignette 5-6, page 77).

## Pharmacology Update

*Drug therapy* should be presented to patients with the attitude that some stress and tension are normal and probably unavoidable, but that the medication may help them to work through problems more constructively. Of the three major drug classes available, the *benzodiazepines* have been most extensively used and have the most rapid onset of action. They are effective for immediate relief of anxiety and are the most often requested by patients. For a chronic problem such as GAD, however, these medications pose a high potential for abuse and cause withdrawal symptoms after as little as 4 to 6 weeks' use (Schweizer & Rickels, 1997). Benzodiazepines are controlled substances, and state laws may require nurse practitioners to consult with a physician before prescribing them. For patients with panic or prominent adrenergic symptoms without panic, benefits of benzodiazepines may outweigh the risks. This is a difficult choice, however, and one referred by many primary care practitioners to a psychiatric specialist. Patients who have become accustomed to the rapid effects of benzodiazepines are difficult to manage without them, so the clinician should think carefully before introducing these drugs for the first time. It is best to choose those with a slower onset of action (oxazepam, clonazepam), which may cause less dependence and withdrawal symptoms than faster-acting drugs such as diazepam or lorazepam.

Benzodiazepines historically have been chosen to treat anxiety in the elderly, despite their added risks of dependence, excessive sedation, and increased potential for falls, depression, and confusion. Elderly clients also may be on a variety of other medications, increasing the likelihood of adverse drug interactions. If these drugs are chosen for use in an elderly client, remember that temazepam, oxazepam, and lorazepam are less likely to cause drug interactions.

A safer choice for most patients with GAD is an azaperone such as *buspirone* (Buspar). This rela-

## CLINICAL VIGNETTE 5.6

Mrs. Andrews is a 58-year-old who has just had a routine physical examination. She has been a patient at the prmary care clinic for years. She is widowed but has family in town and works full time at a job she generally enjoys. Her examination and laboratory results (including thyroid function tests) reveal that she is in fairly good health, but the patient admits that she experiences chronic worrying and an increasing inability to relax. She states that she has always been this way but has felt more anxious since her husband died a few years ago. About once a month, she says her tension at work and home increase to the degree that she finds herself unable to sleep for several nights in a row. She has spells of shaking and crying during these times but denies panic symptoms. She subsequently feels exhausted at work during the day and drinks six to eight cups of coffee per day to stay awake. Her memory and concentration have been poor lately, and despite a negative family history, she worries that she may be getting Alzheimer's disease. She is a nonsmoker, and denies a family or personal history of alcohol or drug use. She has tried over-the-counter Benadryl 50 mg for sleep without success. Mrs. Andrews says she has been thinking about exercising more but hasn't because her schedule is too busy. She also has been too busy to engage in craft projects that she used to find relaxing.

The primary care provider talks with Mrs. Andrews about her tension level, and she agrees that starting a regular exercise program is a high priority. Caffeine use is discussed, and Mrs. Andrews will switch to decaffeinated coffee and tea over the next week or two. A regular schedule of meals and sleeping is reviewed because the patient says she has been less regular about this since her husband died. The patient is taught basic deep-breathing exercises and told to do them several times daily. The patient returns to the clinic in 1 month, reporting some improvement in her symptoms but having had one 4-day period of sleeplessness and high anxiety. Based on your familiarity with the patient, her lack of substance abuse history, and the episodic nature of her anxiety symptoms, you decide to prescribe benzodiazepines in a limited dose. Mrs. Andrews is given a small supply of clonazepam in a low dose for use as needed only on the days when she cannot sleep or relax. She is told about the hazards of dependence and encouraged to try other methods of relaxing first. She returns in 1 month stating that she used three doses of the medication with good relief and a return to her normal state. She says she is nervous about overusing the medication but would like to keep the small supply she has for "emergencies." Future visits indicate that Mrs. Andrews is continuing her exercise program, has increased her recreational activities, reports better memory and concentration, is enjoying her life more, and is feeling less anxious. She reports using the clonazepam once or twice monthly.

---

tively new class of drug is a 5-HT receptor agonist and is thought to increase adrenergic activity of the locus ceruleus. Buspirone is the drug of choice in cases when:

- Impaired motor function, attention, vigilance, memory, or cognition is an issue (eg, the elderly, or patients who operate machinery or have dangerous job)
- There is concern about concomitant alcohol or drug use or abuse by the patient (especially if there is a personal or family history of drug or alcohol abuse)
- There is concern about the potentiated sedative effects of other medications taken by the patient
- The patient has problems with aggressivity or irritability; buspirone may decrease these symp-

toms, whereas benzodiazepines may decrease inhibitions and worsen symptoms.

Remember that buspirone is *not* effective for panic symptoms and should be avoided in those cases. Of greater importance is preparing the patient for what to expect from buspirone therapy. Many people expect relief of anxiety to be immediate, but like many antidepressants, buspirone exerts its effects more slowly and does not cause the muscle relaxation associated with benzodiazepine use. Relief of anxiety may be subtle and may not be noticed for 3 or 4 weeks. The clinician should start at low doses and increase gradually to avoid side effects such as dizziness, headaches, and nausea. These usually are signs that initial dosing has been too aggressive.

A third option for the patient with GAD is the use of *antidepressants*, especially the TCA imipramine. These have proven to be effective for some patients, alleviating anxiety as well as concomitant depression. As previously noted, TCAs have anticholinergic side effects that may be problematic. They may cause urinary retention and urinary tract infections, drowsiness, and postural hypotension and may be contraindicated in certain patients, especially the elderly. SSRI antidepressants are another possibility, especially if there are also signs of depression. Some patients may become more agitated on these medications, and some may do well. When using antidepressants for GAD, especially in the elderly, the clinician should start at low doses and gradually increase as tolerated by the patient to avoid problems. And as with buspirone, the patient should be counseled that effects might not be apparent for several weeks after beginning therapy.

Acute anxiety can be an extremely uncomfortable experience. There is a temptation to choose benzodiazepines for the patient on the basis of their rapid action and relief of anxiety symptoms. Patients also may press for these drugs based on their own experience or experience of others (Clinical Vignette 5-7, page 79). At this point, the clinician should know (and remind the patient) about several points of information. Studies show that the acute relief of symptoms achieved by benzodiazepines is not associated with long-term remission of anxiety. These drugs offer a "quick fix" but are not a good long-term solution for chronic anxiety. One study compares patient response to benzodiazepines versus the antidepressants imipramine and trazodone. After 1 week, benzodiazepines yielded the most rapid response; after 6 weeks, antidepressants had achieved comparable efficacy; and after 8 weeks, imipramine yielded the best results (Schweizer & Rickels, 1997). This study did not include a trial with buspirone, but with its slow onset of action, perhaps this drug would have performed similarly. Clinicians should encourage patients that they will do better to "invest" in a slower response and should support them in this decision. In this situation, a strong and trusting relationship between patient and clinician can make a substantial difference in the treatment outcome.

If patients already are taking benzodiazepines, it is possible (and probably preferable) to transfer them to buspirone or antidepressant therapy. As always, when starting the latter medications, the practitioner should remind the patient not to expect an immediate response to the new medica-

tion, and not to expect the muscle relaxation effects of benzodiazepines. Some clinicians suggest that buspirone or antidepressant therapy be started for 2 to 4 weeks before beginning a gradual withdrawal from benzodiazepines. Benzodiazepines need to be tapered at a rate of approximately 25% per week to avoid withdrawal symptoms (Schweizer & Rickels, 1997). The patient and clinician also should remember that if anxiety symptoms seem worse during this time, this is a result of the benzodiazepine tapering, rather than a failure of the new medication, and should improve with time. Patients may need ongoing support and reassurance during this period and should be congratulated for their efforts and willingness to work toward a change (Table 5-7).

## ATTENTION DEFICIT DISORDER

Attention deficit disorder has a high enough prevalence (3% to 5%) that primary care providers will have contact with patients with this disorder. Although the diagnosis requires testing not normally done in the primary care practice, the practitioner will suspect this problem and make proper referral if able to recognize the signs and symptoms. The pathophysiology of attention deficit disorders is just beginning to be understood, and pharmacologic treatment probably interrupts the biologic abnormalities that cause the disorder. Theories of etiology include preterm birth with lack of development of neurologic structures, genetic factors, and prenatal exposure to chemicals that affect the brain. The role of genetics is important, as there is a 25% concordance rate among first-degree relatives of a person with ADHD. Several studies indicate that the gene coding for the D4 dopamine receptor may be one of the inherited factors involved in ADHD.

ADHD clearly has been the "media pick" topic of the '90s. It would be difficult to find an adult who has not read something about ADHD in local newspapers or magazines or seen a discussion on popular television shows. One reason for the media's interest in ADHD is the controversy surrounding this disorder. Medical and psychological professionals often do not agree about whether an individual may or may not have ADHD. In 1989, the Church of Scientology picketed against the use of methylphenidate (Ritalin) to "control" children, and when CIBA-Geisy, the pharmaceutical company, ran out of Ritalin several years ago, many people felt that the shortage indicated that Ritalin was being overprescribed. The lack of consistency in assessment tools used by professionals to diag-

---

## CLINICAL VIGNETTE 5.7

Ms. Shea is a 28-year-old single mother of two small children who has just moved to town and is new to your clinic. Her physical examination reveals that she is generally healthy, but the patient requests "something for my nerves" several times during the examination. She describes her life as "really stressful," with working and raising her children taking most of her time. She reports daily tension, difficulty getting to sleep and staying asleep, and increasing irritability with her children. She gets no regular exercise outside of her daily work schedule, smokes one to two packs per day, and drinks "several beers" every evening to relax. She denies depression or suicidal thoughts. She states she was in a drug rehabilitation program 10 years ago for cocaine addiction but does not use recreational drugs now. The patient requests alprazolam (Xanax, a benzodiazepine), which she has used in the past, but states that she also has recently tried a friend's diazepam (Valium) with even better relief of anxiety. She assures the provider repeatedly that "I'm no drug addict. I don't want to get hooked on that stuff."

The practitioner discusses the problem of dependence with these drugs and the increased risk with this patient's history of drug addiction. She is reminded that self-medication with alcohol is a risk in people who are particularly anxious. Various behavioral techniques and lifestyle changes to promote relaxation are reviewed, and the patient is asked if she has ever talked with a counselor about her problems with anxiety. After being given the phone number for a community resource agency, the patient again asks for medication to control her anxiety. She is offered a prescription for imipramine on a gradually increasing dose, and it is explained that whereas it may not provide the immediate effects of a benzodiazepine, it will help to decrease her tension and help her cope with problems more easily. (Buspirone also would be a good choice for this patient, but her insurance will not pay for medications and her funds are limited. Because imipramine is much less expensive, it is a good initial choice here.) The patient seems dubious but takes the prescription and agrees to try it for the next month without expecting immediate results.

Ms. Shea returns in 6 weeks, stating that the medication does seem to be helping her to stay calmer and sleep more at night. She says the relaxation exercises "didn't work at all for me" and she stopped them after a few days. She plans to meet with a county agency to discuss financial assistance for child care and feels this will ease some of her concerns. The practitioner reviews lifestyle modifications, renews the prescription, and asks her to return in 3 months. Later, it is discovered through a pharmacist that Ms. Shea is buying Xanax prescribed by her previous provider in another town.

*Note:* It can be frustrating to work with individuals like Ms. Shea, but the practitioner can only work to promote a trusting and open relationship, educate the patient as much as possible, and support her efforts at self-improvement.

---

nose ADHD contributes to controversy. Many pediatricians believe that they can determine the presence or absence of ADHD during a single office visit based on the single criteria of hyperactivity. This approach is highly unreliable because people with ADHD often perform at their best in novel, one-on-one situations. Well-trained psychologists use a variety of well-validated behavioral scales designed to elicit information from parents and teachers. A thorough, structured interview and evaluation of academic records is included. One measure or test cannot reliably identify ADHD. This controversy makes "good copy" for the media.

Many people identify with the symptoms of ADHD and are quick to latch onto a label that explains some of their unsuccessful behavior patterns. These adults will present in the medical office with statements like, "I think I have ADHD, and I heard there was a pill I could take for it." These individuals may meet the DSM-IV criteria for ADHD, but they also may be seeking a source for the popular street drug, Ritalin. There also are many comorbid illnesses in ADHD. These included anxiety, bipolar disorder, oppositional or conduct disorders, hyperthyroidism, or sleep disorders. Symptoms of ADHD overlap with those of other disorders, and the symptoms for ADHD are present to some extent in many children and adults, but most children and adults do not meet the DSM-IV criteria for ADHD.

Debates exist about gender issues with ADHD. Clearly, more boys are referred for evaluation and treatment for ADHD. Some researchers believe

## TABLE 5.7

### Management of Generalized Anxiety Disorder

| Treatment | Comments |
| --- | --- |
| Benzodiazepines | Usually for short-term use; tolerance develops quickly |
| | Potential for addiction |
| | May cause depression |
| Antidepressants (tricyclics, SSRIs) | Not addictive, many side effects |
| | May increase anxiety initially |
| Buspirone (Buspar) | No addictive potential but onset delay (3–4 wk) |
| | Initial dosing should be tapered to avoid side effects |
| Beta blockers | Block sympathetic symptoms of anxiety, especially cardiac |
| | Good for performance anxiety (public speaking, musical performance) |
| Antihistamines | Diphenhydramine and hydroxyzine, for example |
| | Good for mild anxiety |
| | Nonaddicting, inexpensive |
| | Anticholinergic side effects |
| Psychological treatment | Repeated reassurance from primary care provider |
| | Directed counseling to practice problem-solving |
| | Psychotherapy (insight-oriented therapy, cognitive-behavioral therapy, anxiety management [relaxation, breathing exercises, distraction techniques]) |

SSRIs, selective serotonin reuptake inhibitors.

that just as many girls have ADHD, but female patients often are not as extreme on the motoric hyperactivity scale and therefore may go unidentified. The gender difference in diagnosed cases indicates a male:female ratio of about 9:1.

Adults with ADHD may be able to generally manage their lives and work but often have poorer job performance, more divorces, lower socioeconomic status, interpersonal problems, and more general distress. As many as half of the children with ADHD will continue to be significantly symptomatic as adults. People may be first diagnosed with ADHD as adults, after many years of frustration, low self-esteem, substance abuse, depression, and personal distress.

### Diagnosis

For decades, ADHD has been thought to have three primary symptom components: attention problems, impulsiveness, and hyperactivity. Under each of these primary symptom groups are numerous, more specific, observable problem behaviors that are characterized by individual variability in both children and adults. Additionally, each of these groups is characterized by a continuum of symptoms. Attention problems might include having difficulty listening, following instructions, or completing tasks; making careless errors on homework or other tasks; forgetfulness; and difficulty organizing tasks or activities. Impulsiveness is evidenced by blurting out answers before a question is completed, interrupting others, making judgments without evaluating all of the facts or consequences, acting without forethought, rudeness or immaturity, having trouble waiting in line, or being generally impatient. These problems contribute to poor academic or work performance.

Not every person with ADHD has gross motor hyperactivity; some are merely restless and squirmy. However, the degree of impairment is important when making an ADHD diagnosis. If symptoms observed were low on all three continuums (hyperactivity, attention, and impulsiveness), it is unlikely that they would meet the significant level of impairment criteria for an ADHD diagnosis.

The DSM-IV manual lists three types of ADHD:

1. Attention deficit/hyperactivity disorder combined type: includes criteria for inattention, hyperactivity, and impulsiveness
2. Attention deficit/hyperactivity disorder predominantly inattentive type: does not include criteria for hyperactivity or impulsiveness
3. Attention deficit/hyperactivity disorder predominantly hyperactive-impulsive type: includes criteria for hyperactivity and impulsiveness but not attention.

Each of these diagnoses is illustrated with a case scenario.

Children and adults with ADHD are considered to have a disabling condition. Attention deficit disorders have a childhood onset unless caused by a brain injury or encephalitis. Because of the Americans With Disabilities Act, individuals with ADHD sometimes are allowed academic accommodations such as untimed tests. Various licensing boards now require more rigorous documentation of level of impairment, childhood onset of the ADHD symptoms, and previous need for academic accommodations.

## Pathophysiology

### Glucose Utilization

One suggestion for the pathophysiology of ADHD is related to the rate of glucose metabolism in the brain. Studies show an abnormally low rate of glucose utilization in the frontal lobes, the site of the executive function control centers that are disturbed in ADHD. PET scans of the brain of a patient with ADHD compared with a normal patient can be viewed at *http://www.nimh.nih.gov/publicat/adhd.htm#adhd6*. Clearly, PET scans dramatically illustrate different patterns of glucose utilization. There also is evidence of neuroanatomical differences in the corpus callosum and the cortex.

### Bronowski's Theory of Delayed Response

In 1993, Russel Barkley used Bronowski's theory of delayed response and language to develop the disinhibition theory of ADHD. The patient with ADHD has a primary disturbance in the executive functions of the brain with disinhibition of emotions, reacting immediately, often lacking objectivity, and being unable to tolerate boredom or delayed gratification. Another aspect is the "in the moment" response of a person with ADHD, who often appears to be unable to look at past or future consequences. Their sense of time has been shown to be distorted (Barkley, 1994). The ability

---

### CLINICAL VIGNETTE 5.8

**ADHD: Predominantly Hyperactive-Impulsive Type**

Mr. Jones is a 50-year-old salesman whose wife has asked him to come in for an evaluation of his heart. He has not had any pain or symptoms, but he does have some risk factors. He is slightly overweight, is a self-professed type A personality, has slightly high blood pressure, and has quite a temper. Mr. Jones does not seem to be concerned and reports that he has been this way all of his life. He says that he is the top salesman in his company, but he admits to many problems when dealing with his staff. He gets behind in his paperwork, and this causes him a great deal of stress. His evaluations at work are negative in the areas of organization, timeliness, and being a team player. He continues to get good raises because his sales are so high.

As the clinician takes his history, she learns that his problem began when he started school. He was bored and had trouble staying in his seat and following the rules. He never did well in school and dropped out of college. He would start out great, then get bored, and sometimes quit going to class. He says he makes decisions quickly, which always has gotten him into trouble until he started his current job. If he makes a bad decision at the first of the month, he can make up for it by the end of the month. His restlessness makes it difficult for him to attend church, movies, or the school performances of his children. He says his "mouth" gets him in trouble, speaking before he thinks. He also informs the clinician that his son is on methylphenidate (Ritalin) but is quick to say, "He's just all boy."

---

### CLINICAL VIGNETTE 5.9

**ADHD: Predominantly Inattentive Type**

Susan is 25 years old and is requesting to have some testing done because she is worried about her poor memory. She tells you that she has always been forgetful. In elementary school, she would forget her homework and books and lose her purse and other things. She says her teachers told her parents that she was very bright but lazy. She was a daydreamer and reports that she continues to have problems concentrating. She describes herself as a disappointment to her parents because they had high expectations of her, but she had never been able to complete college. She had trouble completing assignments, would get behind, and lose her syllabi and sometimes completed assignments. She also tells you that she believes that she is going to get a bad evaluation at

work because she does her work so slowly and always makes careless errors. She reports that she was never a behavior problem in school and that she seldom feels restless or fidgety. Her history does not reveal a problem with impulsiveness. This type of ADHD has the significant impairment in the area of attentional problems but does not meet the criteria for impulsiveness or hyperactivity. These individuals often go undiagnosed because they are not disruptive. They are often daydreaming or lost in their own thoughts. It is not that they cannot attend; they focus on something, just not the right thing. It is more helpful to think of their problem as focused attention deficit and slowed cognitive processing (Barkley, 1990). They often do not complete their homework, finish timed tests, or hear all of the instruction and may appear like the "absent-minded professor types."

---

to retain a mental image of an event over time is necessary for reflection, comparison, learning from the past, or projecting into the future. This ability contributes to having a sense of time. A third aspect is the relative inability to internalize speech and perceive an inner voice for self-control. Language expressed to others allows for an exchange of ideas, for giving guidance to each other, and formulating rules in new situations.

Rule-governed (internal and external language-mediated) behavior is characteristically difficult for the ADHD patient. Finally, the ability to analyze parts of an event and reformulate the parts into new constructs is essential for problem solving. Problem solving is a complex process because it involves examining rules and making new rules to fit with new situations. This also is difficult for ADHD patients.

---

### CLINICAL VIGNETTE 5.10

**ADHD: Combined Type**

Steven is a 14-year-old whose parents have brought him into the clinic for a complete physical. It is obvious Steven does not want to be there. While his mother is giving the clinician some history, Steven fidgets with his socks, his chair, and his hat. He gets up and starts to pick up items in the examination room. His mother tells the clinician that he does not seem to care about his grades. A note was recently sent home from his school saying that Steven has several zeros for incomplete or missing work. Steven's mother learned at a parent-teacher conference that Steven often is unprepared and

comes to class without his books and homework. He has trouble following directions, does not complete assignments, and is disruptive in the classroom, both verbally and physically. She says he either interrupts the teacher to answer a question or has no idea what the question was when called on. On questioning, the clinician learns that he often loses his books, homework, and jackets and is disorganized. Steven seems to act without any thought of the consequences and does not seem to learn from his mistakes. These behaviors cause him a lot of problems at home and school, and socially, with his peers. His mother said that these problems have been present since he was a small child.

All of these necessary human capacities are dependent on the ability to delay a response to an event. This ability to delay response is the hallmark of self-control and is the primary deficit underlying all of the known symptoms of ADHD.

## Brain Structures

The similarity between the behaviors of prefrontal brain-injured patients and ADHD patients led to the original thought that ADHD was the result of brain injury. With the aid of PET scans and MRI, structural differences were found between ADHD and normal brains. The brains of ADHD subjects are 5.2% smaller on the right side than the brains of control subjects. Normal brains typically are larger on the right side (National Institute of Mental Health [NIMH], 1996). The three structures on the right that appear to be affected include the prefrontal cortex, the caudate nucleus, and the globus pallidus. The prefrontal cortex is the executive control center, and the caudate nucleus and the globus pallidus are thought to provide the inhibitory controls (NIMH, 1996). This area has numerous interconnections with the arousal mechanisms, located in the brainstem, and the emotional centers, located in the midbrain as well as the sensory cortex. These centers are illustrated in Figure 5-5.

### *Neurotransmitters*

The neurobiologic substrates of ADHD are unknown. Biologic factors that determine ADHD are a complex mix of homeostatic processes much like the homeostatic processes that control respiration (Wender, 1995), and it is doubtful that a single neurobiologic/chemical hypothesis will emerge. What is known about the mechanism of action of

medications that have given symptom relief to ADHD patients has significantly contributed to the current understanding of the etiology of ADHD. Approximately 60% to 80% of ADHD patients will have a paradoxical response to stimulant medications believed to be related to serontonergic transmission. The responses in ADHD to stimulants include improvement in the areas of attentiveness, concentration, distractibility, and motor restlessness. The symptoms of ADHD may result from increased amounts of DA in the right hemisphere and prefrontal cortex, thus leading to the characteristic feature of inattention; decreased levels of NE in the locus ceruleus and reticular formation, leading to hyperarousal; and decreased amounts of serotonin in the prefrontal cortex, leading to impulsivity. Generally, DA is stimulatory and serotonin is inhibitory within these systems.

The dopaminergic pathways are localized in the mesocortical, mesolimbic, nigrastiatial, and tuberoinfundibular structures. These structures all are located in the midbrain. The DA pathways innervate different structures at DA receptors, with the D2 and D4 receptors involved with ADHD. The D2 subtype is located in the striatum, nucleus accumbens (NA), substantia nigra, and olfactory bulb (Nihart, 1998). An overactive dopaminergic circuitry from the substantia nigra to the striatum is a possible cause of hyperactivity and impulsivity.

The prefrontal dopaminergic system shows a decreased susceptibility to the up-regulation and down-regulation of receptors by DA agonists or antagonists. PET scans show that the central tegmental region that innervates the frontal cortex of the brain seems to lack the autoreceptors found in the striatum (Castellanos, 1997). D4 is located in the frontal cortex, midbrain, and the medulla (Nihart, 1998). Abnormalities in the DA transporter and the D4 receptor have been suggested by some genetic theories (Castellanos, 1997).

Clearly, the interactions of DA and NE are significant in understanding the pathophysiology of ADHD. The dopaminergic system is related to basic emotions such as hunger, thirst, sexual drive, rage, and responses to social reinforcers. These emotions often are experienced immediately and intensely in ADHD, but responses to social reinforcers are not long lived. Individuals with ADHD often seem to behave without regard to social rules or consequences.

## Pharmacology Update

Stimulant medications improve symptoms in most people with ADHD. These include methylphenidate (Ritalin), amphetamine (Dexadrine,

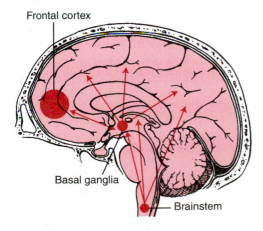

**FIGURE 5.5** ● Centers involved in attention deficit/hyperactivity disorder.

Adderall), or pemoline (Cylert) when given at high enough doses. The mechanism of action for stimulants involves increasing concentrations of NE, DA, or both. Similarly, bupropion (Wellbutrin) has been found to be effective in some children, adolescents, and adults with ADHD (Conners et al., 1996). Children with accompanying conduct disorder and oppositional defiant disorder seem to be even more responsive to bupropion (Simeon & Ferguson, 1986). Bupropion is similar to amphetamines because it causes reuptake of DA and blocks the uptake of serotonin and NE. Recent studies suggest that it acts on the noradrenergic system (Soorani & DeVincent, 1997).

Low-dose risperidone (Risperdal) is being used increasingly to treat ADHD (Weiss, 1996). Risperidone is an atypical antipsychotic medication that is thought to affect dopaminergic centers. It is primarily used with schizophrenic patients in doses of 8 to 10 mg. Cognitive impairments found in schizophrenia that overlap with ADHD symptoms include attention, memory, working memory, serial learning, and executive function. Schizophrenic patients on risperidone show improved frontal lobe functions, attention, memory, and planning. Currently, no studies have examined the cognitive outcome of ADHD patients being treated with risperidone. When used for ADHD, it controls the aggression. Risperidone has a high affinity for dopamine (D2), serotonin (5-HT$_2$), and adrenergic receptors. The use of risperidone with ADHD patients has not been approved by the Food and Drug Administration.

TCAs, specifically imipramine (Tofranil) and desipramine (Norpramine), have been found to decrease distractibility and improve attentiveness with ADHD patients. By blocking the reuptake of NE and DA, the TCA indirectly increases the available concentrations of these neurotransmitters. Another atypical antidepressant, venlafaxine (Effexor), works similarly by inhibiting the uptake of NE and 5-HT$_2$ at moderate doses; DA is inhibited at higher doses (George & Mortimer, 1998). Castellanos (1997) suggests a "hypodopaminergic state resulting in hypofunction of the prefrontal circuitry (p. 387)." When DA is increased at the synapse, the postsynaptic effect is increased.

### Common Myths About Attention Deficit/Hyperactivity Disorder

1. *Myth:* Allergies and refined sugar can cause ADHD. *Fact:* Controlled studies refute these ideas.
2. *Myth:* Children should take stimulant medication only during school hours, not in the evenings or during school vacations. *Fact:* Individuals who have ADHD will have problems with peers and family members because of their impulsiveness and hyperactivity. Dosing three times a day during school vacations helps ADHD patients to have more stable lives. Academia is not the only area of life affected by ADHD.
3. *Myth:* Ritalin will stunt growth. *Fact:* Controlled studies do not confirm this idea. Dose timing can minimize suppression of appetite. Avoidance of eating can stunt growth.
4. *Myth:* Children who take Ritalin are more likely to go on to do hard drugs later in life. *Fact:* Only the small portion of ADHD patients who have comorbid conduct disorder are likely to go on to use hard drugs. As a group, people with conduct disorder as a child, with or without ADHD, are more likely to use hard drugs later in life.
5. *Myth:* If parents would be consistent with their discipline, children with ADHD could learn to control their ADHD symptoms. *Fact:* Children and adults with ADHD are easily bored. Consequently, behavioral plans that are followed consistently are effective only for about 2 weeks before they have to be revamped with new rewards.
6. *Myth:* With proper treatment, ADHD can be cured. *Fact:* We only treat ADHD symptoms; we cannot yet cure ADHD. Perhaps when we know what it is, we will be closer to a cure.
7. *Myth:* Stimulant medication should be a last resort. *Fact:* All children deserve a stimulant trial unless contraindicated medically. Sixty percent to 80% of children respond positively to stimulant medication. Behavioral interventions and training in social skills are more effective when combined with medication and have poor transfer learning capability on their own.
8. *Myth:* Diets and biofeedback are worthwhile treatments for ADHD. *Fact:* Controlled studies have not confirmed these reports.
9. *Myth:* Children outgrow ADHD by adolescence. *Fact:* Most children continue to have ADHD symptoms through adolescence and adulthood, although their symptom pattern may change over time.
10. *Myth:* Stimulants are not effective for adolescents or adults. *Fact:* Stimulants work similarly for children, adolescents, and adults.

## ADDICTION DISORDERS

Substance abuse in the United States is a major, devastating, costly social and medical problem. It is the major preventable cause of illness and premature death in this country, with 100,000 deaths per year resulting from the use of drugs or alcohol (American Psychiatric Association [APA], 1999). The cost of substance abuse is over $300 billion per year (Gardner, 1997). Furthermore, the illicit use of injectable substances such as cocaine and heroin is the major mode of transmission of human immunodeficiency virus in the US. In this section, the neurobiology and pathophysiology of substance abuse are described, with special focus on alcoholism. Primary care providers will encounter substance abuse and addictive diseases frequently. They will frequently discover substance abuse as a comorbid condition with other psychiatric disorders. The strong relationship between alcohol and illicit drug abuse and automobile accidents, suicide, and domestic violence also is noteworthy. It is useful to understand the neurologic systems and processes involved in drug and alcohol craving and compulsive behaviors characterizing addiction, dependency, and relapse. Treatment strategies require a complete knowledge of these processes.

## Definition of Addiction

The various definition of addiction always includes similar elements. There is compulsive drug-craving, drug-seeking behavior, and drug use (Leshner & Koob, 1999). The compulsion to take the drug is associated with a loss of control in limiting the intake of the drug (Koob & Nestler, 1997). These compulsions become so overwhelming in the drug addict that a normal life becomes impossible, and the drug becomes the major motivator for all activities. Yet, in the early stages, the addict often leads a double life, hiding the habit and attempting to carry on normal social, occupational, and recreational activities. Often, substance abuse begins during the preadolescent years with experimental use of alcohol and marijuana. Later, children who will become substance abusers develop a predilection for a drug of choice, although some will continue to be multidrug users (APA, 1999).

The discovery of drug addiction may be made coincidentally by the primary health care provider in the course of completing the history or physical examination. Diagnostic criteria that must be met for drug addiction are tolerance; withdrawal; persistent desire or unsuccessful attempts to decrease use of the substance; use in amounts larger than intended; reduction in social, occupation, or recreational activities; an inordinate amount of time spent seeking the drug; and continued use of the substance despite recurrent problems. Three of these criteria must be met to make the diagnosis of substance abuse (Koob & Nestler, 1997). When the practitioner makes such a diagnosis, it carries with it many ramifications, since taking illicit substances is criminal behavior, and many drug addicts are engaged in felonious activities to support their habits. Alcoholism, on the other hand, is a chemical addiction that plays itself out within often-tenuous societal boundaries of propriety. The health care provider may be faced with a personal repugnance for the drug-addicted patient. Society generally has conveyed that drug addiction is the result of a flawed character, but the evidence discussed in this chapter emphasizes the role of biology in addiction and reinforces the concept that addiction is a brain disease and requires biologically based treatment.

The DSM-IV diagnostic criteria for substance dependence and abuse are provided in Tables 5-8 and 5-9 (American Psychiatric Association [APA], 1994).

Understandings of substance abuse and addiction have evolved from both animal and human studies. Most of the substances to which humans become addicted have the potential for evoking drug-seeking behavior and cravings in laboratory animals, most notably in laboratory rats. Addiction ultimately is considered a brain disease in that all elements of addiction involve neurologic substrates and are associated with changes in the nervous system. Most of the neurobiologic concepts presented in this chapter have been discovered through studies of animal behavior that mimics human drug abuse and dependence. Animals will avidly self-administer drugs or administer electric shocks through implantable electrodes in certain parts of the brain, and many aspects of human behavior are mirrored in their use of, craving for, and dependence on drugs.

## Epidemiology of Substance Abuse

An estimated 5.5 million individuals in the US have significant and disabling drug abuse disorders, and an additional 13 million need treatment for alcohol use disorders (Williams et al., 1989). On average in a single month, 10,000,000 people in the US use marijuana, 11,000,000 abuse alcohol, 200,000 use heroin, 1,500,000 use cocaine, and 800,000 use amphetamines. If nicotine and caffeine are considered to be drugs of abuse, then 61,000,000 people use nicotine and 130,000,000 use caffeine by drinking coffee (Nash, 1997). Two thirds of substance abusers are men, and African Americans are more likely

## TABLE 5.8

### Substance Dependence

A maladaptive pattern of substance use, leading to clinically significant impairment or distress, as manifested by three (or more) of the following, occurring at any time in the same 12-month period:

1. Tolerance, as defined by either of the following:
   a. A need for markedly increased amounts of the substance to achieve intoxication or desired effect
   b. Markedly diminished effect with continued use of the same amount of the substance

2. Withdrawal, as manifested by either of the following:
   a. The characteristic withdrawal syndrome for the substance
   b. The same (or a closely related) substance is taken to relieve or avoid withdrawal symptoms

3. The substance is often taken in larger amounts or over a longer period than was intended
4. There is a persistent desire or unsuccessful efforts to cut down or control substance use
5. A great deal of time is spent in activities necessary to obtain the substance (eg, visiting multiple doctors or driving long distances), using the substance (eg, chain-smoking), or recovering from its effects
6. Important social, occupational, or recreational activities are given up or reduced because of substance use
7. The substance use is continued despite knowledge of having a persistent or recurrent physical or psychological problem that is likely to have been caused or exacerbated by the substance (eg, current cocaine use despite recognition of cocaine-induced depression, or continued drinking despite recognition that an ulcer was made worse by alcohol consumption)

(From American Psychiatric Association [1994]. *Diagnostic and statistical manual of mental disorders* [4th ed.]. Washington, DC: American Psychiatric Association.)

to be afflicted than other races. The dimensions of the substance abuse problem in this country can be dramatically appreciated by logging on the worldwide web site *www.health.org/dynatable/ndu.asp?17580770*. This site provides a real time dynamic counting of first-time substance abusers.

It is a common misconception that seriously addicted people are homeless or live in shelters and are unemployed. However, national statistics indicate that 6.7 million illegal drug users were employed full time, which represents 6.5% of full-time workers aged 18 years and older (*www.whitehousedrugpolicy.gov*).

## TABLE 5.9

### Substance Abuse

A maladaptive pattern of substance use leading to clinically significant impairment or distress, as manifested by one (or more) of the following, occurring within a 12-month period:

1. Recurrent substance use resulting in a failure to fulfill major role obligations at work, school, or home (eg, repeated absences or poor work performance related to substance use; substance-related absences, suspensions, or expulsions from school; neglect of children or household)
2. Recurrent substance use in situations in which it is physically hazardous (eg, driving an automobile or operating a machine when impaired by substance use)
3. Recurrent substance-related legal problems (eg, arrests for substance-related disorderly conduct)
4. Continued substance use despite having persistent or recurrent social or interpersonal problems caused or exacerbated by the effects of the substance (eg, arguments with spouse about consequences of intoxication, physical fights)

The symptoms have never met the criteria for substance dependence for this class of substance.

(From American Psychiatric Association [1994]. *Diagnostic and statistical manual of mental disorders* [4th ed.]. Washington, DC: American Psychiatric Association.)

## Types of Addictions

There is evidence that all drugs of abuse ultimately interact with common neuroanatomic structures and chemistries. These mechanisms are reviewed in later sections of the chapter. The chemicals that produce drug addictions in this country include psychomotor stimulants such as amphetamines and cocaine, opiate drugs such as morphine and heroin, sedative hypnotics such as ethanol, nicotine, psychedelic drugs, and cannabinoids such as marijuana. Some also consider caffeine to be an addictive substance.

## Risk Factors

In childhood and adolescence, risk factors for substance abuse include behavioral problems (acting out, risk taking, ADHD), family problems, and environmental risk factors such as poverty, school failure, and rejection by peers. The risk increases if more than one of the factors is present and if the substance abuse begins early in life (*www.whitehousedrugpolicy.gov*). For adults, risk factors include dropping out of school, childhood misbehavior, ADHD, and psychiatric illnesses.

### Genetic Influences

Genetic influences governing substance abuse seem to be more important in alcoholism than in other drug-abusing conditions, but some evidence exists for genetic influences governing susceptibility to other drugs. The proenkephalin gene may be involved in opioid abuse (Comings et al., 1999). Genes coding for DA receptors D2 and D4, as well as genes responsible for clearing DA from the synapses, also have been suspected of being involved in susceptibility to drug abuse. An important theory is the existence of a genetic risk related to inadequate DA levels or responsiveness in the brain, creating a *reward-deficiency syndrome* (Blum et al., 1995). Individuals with this genetic defect seek ways to increase the brain's DA level, which includes ingestion of alcohol, drugs, and food (Noble, 1994). Other addictive behaviors such as gambling and binge eating also may increase brain DA in genetically at-risk persons. The D2 receptor is speculated to be involved in several neuro-psychiatric problems such as ADHD, obsessive-compulsive disorder, schizophrenia, and Tourette's syndrome.

The role of DA in addiction is important, and the next section of this chapter describes the dopaminergic pathways as well as other brain systems involved in substance abuse.

## Brain Pathways of Addiction

The pleasure produced by abused substances is powerful and produces cravings and compulsions for repeated use of the substance. Because these feelings and behaviors ultimately are produced through the biologic substrate of the brain, there is general agreement that the neuroanatomy and neurochemistry involved in substance abuse are normal physiologic reward systems. The function of these pathways would be to reinforce certain beneficial behaviors such as eating, drinking, or sexual activity by producing pleasurable brain states. The pleasurable sensations thus reinforce continuing the behaviors that produce them. Drugs of abuse appear to act through these primitive neuronal systems at various synapses and loci. The hedonic output produced by the interaction of drugs with this neurologic and chemical wiring seems to be exaggerated and addictive beyond what is normally produced through the natural activity of these systems.

Most of the current knowledge of the neurobiology of addiction comes from studies with the laboratory rat. Rats mimic many aspects of human drug seeking, drug use, and dependency. They self-administer drugs relentlessly while ignoring food, water, sleep, and sexual partners and become physically dependent. One behavioral measure thought to be similar to drug craving is *place preference*. Rats are given an addictive drug in one environment, and later, when drug free, are allowed the opportunity to choose a cage. They invariably choose the cage in which they received the drug. This is thought to be a behavior that is analogous to drug cravings exhibited by humans, even when detoxified and drug free, when they find themselves in environments associated with previous drug taking.

The neuroanatomy and neurochemistry of the laboratory rat can be studied and manipulated to a greater degree than human studies.

Researchers can place cannulae in the rat brain, inject tracers, use agonists and antagonists against neurotransmitter receptors, and surgically or chemically block parts of the systems. These type of studies have led to theories of drugs action, why they produce craving and dependence, and how relapse occurs. At the center of most of these theories is a brain structure known as the *mesolimbic system* and the neurotransmitter *dopamine*. DA seems to be a major common denominator molecule for the effects of all known drugs of abuse, although many other neurotransmitters also are involved. In fact, most mind-altering drugs have chemical structures that mimic known neurotransmitters. DA, however, is a molecule that produces reward reinforcement by affecting mood states and seems to be responsible for the "rush" or "high" produced by drugs such as cocaine and heroin. Table 5-10 summarizes how the major drugs of abuse affect brain DA.

If DA is the ultimate "pleasure" molecule, it is an important and ancient chemical, since reward reinforcing systems clearly have evolutionary benefit. In the drug addict, these systems sabotage the user into constantly seeking the rush of brain DA that the drugs produce. Brain DA acts, as do all neurotransmitters, by binding to synaptic membrane receptors that regulate ion channels. As high levels of DA occur in the user, the brain synaptic membranes down-regulate the numbers of DA receptors. This causes a "down" response when the drug is not present and a need for more drug to produce the high.

The mesocorticolimbic DA system in the midbrain plays an essential role as a normal, primitive reward reinforcer system and as a site of action for many drugs. This system is diagrammed in Figure 5-6). This system projects from the ventral tegmental area (VTA) to the nucleus accumbens (NA), olfactory tubercle, amygdala, and frontal cortex. Three relay systems are believed to be involved. The first is a nondopaminergic system that projects from the lateral hypothalamus onto the VTA. The dopaminergic cell bodies in the VTA then send axons to the NA. Finally, the third-stage neurons project from the NA to the ventral pallidum and use the endogenous opioid enkephalin as the primary neurotransmitter (Gardner, 1997). The second-stage dopaminergic neurons in this pleasure-reward circuitry appear to be a site of

action for many drugs, with the D1 receptors causing a tonic activation of this system. Disturbing the mesolimbic DA system results in aversive behavior (Herz, 1998). The third-stage neurons may be the site of action of opioid type drugs or may be involved in the production of pleasure and euphoria by drugs. The μ and δ opiate receptors are involved in pleasure signals, whereas the κ receptors are responsible for aversive states. The NA, in particular, is a sensitive site of action for drugs of abuse. If the DA receptors in this circuitry are blocked, the rewarding effects of drugs like cocaine are significantly reduced (Leshner & Koob, 1999).

Whereas initial drug use produces pleasure, the development of addiction ultimately is associated with many negative effects and is a highly distressful state. It is not clear what happens in the brain to transform drug taking into drug addiction. There is an apparent initial sensitization of the dopaminergic mesolimbic system by drugs such as morphine that can occur for months. Thus, the initial drug exposure causes an increased sensitivity to additional exposures, which may explain the drug craving and drug seeking experienced by some after taking a drug only once. With time, however, the sensitization process reverts to tolerance, so that more and more of the drug is needed to produce the hedonic effect. Over time, the drugs themselves may interrupt normal brain function. There also could be genetically endowed increased sensitivity to the action of the drug. There may be less DA present in the susceptible brain. Chronic administration of drugs of abuse produce a diminution in the reward effects of the drugs, perhaps reflecting changes in the projection

---

## TABLE 5.10  ● ● ●

### Effects of Drugs of Abuse on Brain Dopamine

| Drug | Effect on Brain Dopamine |
| --- | --- |
| Heroin | Causes release of dopamine; acts on μ opiate receptors in VTA and NA |
| Cocaine | Blocks dopamine reuptake |
| Marijuana | Causes release of dopamine in NA |
| Amphetamines | Causes release of excess dopamine; blocks reuptake of dopamine |
| Alcohol | Activates brain dopamine systems, GABAergic systems |
| Nicotine | Causes release of dopamine in mesolimbic dopamine system |
| Caffeine | May cause release of dopamine |

GABAergic, gamma-aminobutyric acid-ergic; NA, nucleus accumbens; VTA, ventral tegmental area.
(Modified from Nash, M. [1997]. Addicted. *Time, 149*, 1–8.)

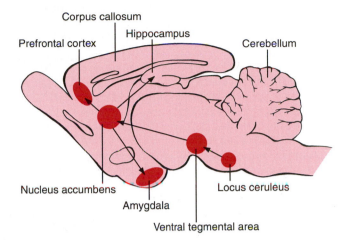

**FIGURE 5.6** ● Mesolimbic dopamine system in rat brain.

of impulses into the amygdala system from the VTA.

Another dimension of addiction is the loss of inhibitions and social controls when the person is craving and seeking drugs. As illustrated in the following clinical vignette, people act in socially unacceptable ways and steal or commit other crimes to attain the desired drug. A theory explaining this loss of impulse control and inhibition of normal behavior is related to serotonin, an inhibitory neurotransmitter. It is speculated that there is a deficiency in brain serotonin levels in the addict, producing the specific behaviors associated with drug craving and drug seeking (Ciccocioppo, 1999).

Withdrawal has been explained in several ways. One thought is that the drug produces certain opposing effects in the brain to the effects of pleasure, and when the drug is withdrawn, these oppositional responses produce the distressful psychological and physiologic effects of withdrawal. These negative effects may be long term and thus constantly induce a state of drug craving (Ciccocioppo, 1999).

Relapse also is a characteristic of drug addiction. There is evidence that taking a drug, with the resultant activation of the reinforcing reward neurologic circuitry, involves multisynaptic activation of many parts of the brain. The pleasure then becomes associated with time, place, and circumstances. This is seen in the place-preference activity of the laboratory rat. In humans, once drug use has been abolished, a susceptibility to relapse may be provoked by environmental stimuli associated with the taking of the drug. This could be a bar or another setting or social association with other users. In animals in which the drug-taking behavior has been extinguished, it is possible to quickly

reinstate this behavior by administering drugs that activate the mesolimbic DA system. There may be genetic loci that regulate one's vulnerability to relapse. Stress also is an important factor in relapse, with both animals and humans showing a susceptibility to relapse when faced with repeated stressors. Stress could sensitize the brain toward the effects of drugs of abuse. Stress has been shown to stimulate the mesolimbic DA system and thus may reactivate this system in the drug-free person, producing new craving. Of course, stress may result in affective states that are distressful, and the former addict may use drugs to "self-medicate" their emotional pain (Ciccocioppo, 1999).

In the next section, the most common substance abuse problem in the US is described in detail: alcoholism. Useful Internet sites for primary care providers to learn more about addiction include the American Psychiatric Association web site at *www.psych.org*. National policies can be learned about at the government site *www.whitehouse-drugpolicy.gov*. Patients and families will benefit from the information on *http://substanceabuse.tqn.com*. Recent information about mental health disorders, drugs, and treatment is available at *www.mentalhealth.com*.

## PATHOPHYSIOLOGY OF ALCOHOLISM

Evidence of the use and abuse of alcohol dates back to the beginning of civilization. Despite its history, a complete understanding of the pathogenesis of alcoholism has not been attained. The clinical diagnosis and treatment of alcoholism by primary care providers often is inadequate because of the various manifestations of alcoholism on the body, mind, and spirit. A correlation between the

---

### CLINICAL VIGNETTE 5.11

Mrs. Lyn Norris, a patient in the primary care practice, brings her 14-year-old son, Todd, to the clinic for a "drug test." Mrs. Norris has battled chronic alcoholism for many years and has been alcohol-free for 5 years. She informs the clinic staff that she is sure Todd is drinking and using drugs. Six months ago, Todd's parents divorced, and his father has moved to another state and recently remarried. Recently, his grades have plummeted, he stays in his room all of the time, he misses school, and a variety of unsavory characters have appeared at the door asking to see her son. His room smells of cigarette smoke and marijuana. She reports that money is missing regularly from her wallet. Today she found a stash of whiskey bottles behind the woodpile and a plastic bag in his room that she believes contains marijuana.

Todd is unkempt and uncommunicative. He appears to be highly distracted, tremulous, and angry at being brought to the clinic. He vehemently denies drug use and refuses to provide a urine specimen.

The nurse practitioner advises Mrs. Norris that she wishes to examine Todd in private. During the examination, the following findings are noteworthy. He has lost about 10 lb in the last month, his pulse is 100, and his blood pressure is 156/86. He has a fine tremor in both hands, and is highly agitated. His pupils are enlarged and his conjunctivae are injected. After being assured that the practitioner can be trusted, Todd divulges that he is experimenting, along with "all the other kids in his group," with marijuana, cocaine, and alcohol. All of his symptoms can be attributed to use and dependence on these drugs. Todd also smokes about one pack per day of unfiltered cigarettes. Further questioning reveals that Todd is using these substances on a daily basis and is stealing from his mother to buy the drugs. He agrees to a drug test if the practitioner will promise not to tell his mother the results. Since this is not acceptable, the practitioner convinces Todd that he needs further assessment, referral, and treatment. Todd is referred to a local psychiatrist who specializes in the treatment of drug dependency in children.

---

patient's presenting symptoms and alcohol abuse often is missed or purposefully avoided by the provider. Because alcohol remains a leading cause of morbidity and mortality in our culture, providers must become knowledgeable of the effects of alcoholism on the body, risk factors associated with the disease, appropriate screening techniques, and current treatment options for their patients.

## Epidemiology

Alcohol dependence is evidenced by either tolerance or symptoms of withdrawal. The essential feature of dependence on alcohol is a cluster of cognitive, behavioral, and physiologic symptoms indicating that the individual continues using alcohol despite significant and distressful alcohol-related problems (APA, 1994). Alcohol abuse and dependence affects more than 18 million people in the United States, making alcoholism one of our country's most expensive health problems. Twenty-five percent of all suicides and 67% of murders involve alcohol use (Hyman & Cassem, 1995). Alcohol continues to be the most abused

psychoactive drug in the US, with an average per-person annual consumption of 2.43 gallons of absolute alcohol by persons aged 15 years and older (Franklin & Francis, 1999). Despite a recent, slight decrease in alcohol consumption, alcohol-related deaths rank third among the leading causes of preventable mortalities in the United States (McGinnis & Foege, 1993). The two major risk factors for alcoholism are a family history of alcohol abuse and male gender. Sons of male alcoholics have the highest risk of becoming alcoholics. In general, it has been shown that men are more likely than women to drink alcohol and become an alcoholic. When both genetic and gender risk factors are present, there is a 25% chance that the individual will become an alcoholic (Hyman & Cassem, 1995).

## Causes of Alcoholism

### Genetic Theory

The basic premise of the pathogenesis of alcoholism is that it is an interaction between genetic predisposition and environmental factors such as parental influences, childhood experiences, and culture (Franklin & Frances, 1999). The genetic theory holds that no one is destined to become an alcoholic but certain genetic factors increase vulnerability to the disease. Studies performed on twin siblings adopted at early ages suggest that there is an approximately 60% concordance rate among identical twins (Schuckit, 1985). This genetic component is in females as well as males and is inherited independently of other psychiatric illnesses. Studies of at-risk men with a history of paternal alcoholism demonstrate a difference in their response to alcohol. These men had less subjective intoxication, less ataxia, and decreased levels of stress hormones than the control group when exposed to the same amount of ethanol, suggesting that at-risk individuals lack the warning signals that indicate intoxication (Hyman & Cassem, 1995).

The DA receptor gene has been investigated in the etiology of alcoholism because DA is the key transmitter in the brain that mediates the positive reinforcement of alcohol. Ethanol also has been shown to stimulate the activity of endorphins in the brain and pituitary. Therefore, it is hypothesized that individuals with a genetic predisposition to excessive ethanol consumption have inherited a sensitivity of the endogenous endorphin system to ethanol (Gianoulakis, 1996). These individuals would have an increased "reward" to drinking alcohol. The findings vary among studies, with some investigators reporting an association of a specific allele (A1) of the D2 dopamine receptor among alcoholics and other investigators finding no association between the allele and the disease (Hyman & Cassem, 1995). Currently, a specific

"alcogene" has not been discovered, but the research is considered a priority in the field of genetics. The neurobiologic model of alcohol dependence is illustrated in Figure 5-7.

### Glutamergic Theory

A glutamatergic theory for alcoholism also has been hypothesized. Recent data show that ethanol selectively affects the function of glutamate (Glu) and GABA receptors. The GABA receptor is the brain's major inhibitory neurotransmitter receptor, and standard pharmacologic management of alcoholism has been directed at activating these receptors. Glu is one of the brain's major excitatory neurotransmitters, with several glutamate receptors available for binding. The *N*-methyl-D-aspartate (NMDA) receptor is a subtype of the glutamate receptor, which is responsible for regulation of DA and NE release in the brain. Ethanol inhibits the depolarization generated by NMDA receptor activation, and acute exposure inhibits NMDA-triggered release of DA and NE. These indirect effects of alcohol on the catecholaminergic system may be responsible for the behavioral agitation and autonomic instability that occur during alcohol withdrawal (Tsai et al., 1995).

### Behavioral Theory

Although no particular personality type has been associated with alcoholism, certain characteristics of alcoholics have been identified through research. An early onset of problem drinking has been associated with greater dependence on alcohol, greater severity of related problems, and a more rapidly progressive clinical course (Hyman & Cassem, 1995). Familial alcoholics often have

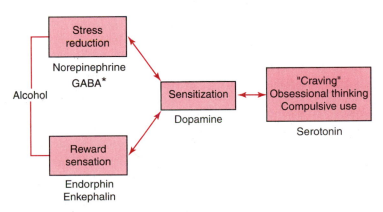

*GABA = γ-aminobutyric acid.

**FIGURE 5.7** ● Neurobiologic model of alcohol dependence.

poor academic and social histories, histories of antisocial behavior, and poorer prognosis with treatment. Children with aggression and impulsivity problems also have been found to have problems with alcohol in the future (Franklin & Frances, 1999).

## Adverse Physical Effects of Alcohol

The psychological changes or "buzz" that results from alcohol ingestion do not occur until blood alcohol levels reach 10 to 50 mmol/L. These are high levels compared with other psychoactive drugs because alcohol is a comparatively weak drug. The amount of alcohol that must be consumed to have even the slightest intoxicating effect is enough to alter all cell membranes within the human body. Thus, alcohol consumption to the point of intoxication affects every organ of the body, and chronic abuse of alcohol has deleterious effects on all body systems (Table 5-11).

### Hepatic Complications

Alcohol is absorbed in the small intestine and is metabolized in the liver. Alcohol dehydrogenase breaks down ethanol to toxic acetaldehyde, which is metabolized by aldehyde dehydrogenase to acetic acid. The byproducts of lactic acid, uric acid, and fat are damaging to the liver. It also has been demonstrated that cytochrome P450 in the liver plays a role in ethanol metabolism and tolerance. The involvement of the P450 system helps to explain the exacerbation of liver damage by selected chemical, environmental, and pharmaceutical agents.

Chronic alcohol abuse damages the liver in multiple ways. Fatty liver, early fibrosis, alcoholic hepatitis, and cirrhosis are the primary types of liver damage related to alcoholism. Fat accumulation in liver cells is the earliest response to alcohol overconsumption. The clinical presentation of fatty liver usually is nonsymptomatic hepatomegaly. Palpable hepatomegaly is present in 75% of clinical examinations of patients with fatty liver. Mild tenderness is common, and sometimes severe epigastric or right upper quadrant pain occurs (Lieber & Leo, 1992).

The symptoms associated with alcoholic hepatitis range from mild hepatomegaly to jaundice, ascites, hepatic coma, and all of the complications of severe hepatic insufficiency. Frequently, patients with mild hepatitis complain of anorexia, fatigue, fever, and right epigastric pain. Cirrhosis, without associated fatty liver or hepatitis, usually does not become symptomatic until around 50 years of age, and many cases are not diagnosed until autopsy. The classic symptoms of cirrhosis are hepatomegaly and jaundice. Low-grade or continuous fever also may be present in decompensated cirrhosis. Secondary symptoms include portal hypertension, splenomegaly, ascites, encephalopathy with asterixis, GI hemorrhage from esophageal or gastric varices, and bleeding abnormalities (Lieber & Leo, 1992).

### Gastrointestinal Complications

The ingestion of alcohol dissolves and irritates the gastric mucosa, resulting in gastritis, esophagitis, and ulcers. Acute alcohol ingestion may produce erosive or hemorrhagic gastritis, whereas chronic excessive alcohol intake usually results in atrophic, nonerosive gastritis. Bleeding of the upper GI tract is common in alcoholics because of the acute mucosal lesions. Esophageal varices, peptic ulcers, Mallory-Weiss lesions, duodenitis, and esophagitis also may cause GI bleeding associated with alcoholism. Diarrhea and weight loss are frequent manifestations of alcoholism. Steatorrhea, or "fatty stools," occur in 35% to 56% of alcoholics during a "binge," resulting from impaired pancreatic function. High ethanol concentrations have deleterious effects on the epithelial cells of the small intestine, resulting in malabsorption of proteins, vitamins, minerals, water, and electrolytes. In contrast, fat absorption is increased, further compromising the nutritional status of the alcoholic patient. The nutritional complications that accompany alcoholism have negative effects on the entire body, especially the musculoskeletal, neurologic, and cardiovascular systems (Feinman et al., 1992).

### Cardiovascular Complications

Chronic alcohol abuse creates a wide spectrum of cardiac problems. Controversy exists over the beneficial versus hazardous effects of ethanol on cardiac disease. However, ethanol administration at levels high enough to produce cardiac depression produces changes in lipid and protein metabolism, depresses mitochondrial function in cardiac tissue, reduces the activity of the sodium pump, and stimulates the formation of abnormal byproducts in the heart (Friedman, 1992). Alcohol has been shown to have a directly toxic effect on cardiac muscle tissue, with evidence of short- and long-term negative effects of alcohol ingestion (Urbano-Marquez et al., 1989). In a study of cardiac function of chronic alcoholics, long-term injury of myocardial tissue was proportional to the doses of ethanol consumed over time. The ejection fraction measurements of the alcoholic group were less than 60% of control group. The results of this study were inde-

## TABLE 5.11

### Medical Consequences of Alcoholism

| | |
|---|---|
| Nervous system effects | Intoxication: drunkenness, excitement, coma |
| | Abstinence or withdrawal syndromes, hallucinosis, seizures, delirium tremens |
| | Nutritional disease: Wernicke-Korsakoff syndrome |
| | Cerebellar degeneration |
| | Marchiafava-Bignami disease (rare) |
| | Central pontine myelinolysis (rare) |
| | Cerebral atrophy, ventricular enlargement |
| | Disorders secondary to liver disease: encephalopathy |
| | Psychiatric disorders: depression, antisocial behavior, anxiety |
| | Insomnia |
| | Peripheral neuropathies |
| Gastrointestinal effects | Esophagitis, gastritis, ulcer |
| | Increased incidence of cancer of the oral cavity, pharynx, larynx, and esophagus |
| | Disorders secondary to portal hypertension: esophageal varices and hemorrhoids |
| | Diarrhea |
| | Pancreatitis |
| | Liver disease: fatty degeneration, cirrhosis (in 10% of alcoholics) |
| Cardiovascular effects | Arrhythmias: tachycardia, ventricular premature contractions or conduction defects; ventricular tachycardia in delirium tremens |
| | Cardiomyopathy |
| | Worsened angina |
| | Hypertension |
| Metabolic effects | Carbohydrates: decreased gluconeogenesis (hypoglycemia) |
| | Proteins: decreased albumin and transferrin synthesis, increased lipoprotein synthesis |
| | Lipids: increased serum and liver triglycerides (fatty liver) |
| | Decreased serum magnesium and phosphate |
| | Ketoacidosis |
| Endocrine effects | Decreased plasma testosterone (impotence) |
| Musculoskeletal effects | Myopathy (weakness, wasting, swelling, pain) |
| | Osteoporosis, nontraumatic osteonecrosis of the head of the femur |
| Dermatologic effects | Rosacea, spider angiomas, nevi, pruritus |
| Hematologic effects | Thrombocytopenia |
| | Macrocytic anemias |
| | Coagulopathies (resulting from decreased hepatic synthetic function) |
| Effects on fetus | Growth retardation |
| | Mental retardation |
| | Fetal alcohol syndrome |
| Drug interactions | Increase in CNS depressant effects of benzodiazepines, antipsychotics, antidepressants, sedative-hypnotics |
| | Decrease in effectiveness of phenytoin (epileptics are more likely to have seizures), anticoagulants, tricyclic antidepressants |
| | Production of effects similar to mild disulfiram reaction (flushing, vomiting) when taken with oral antidiabetic agents or metronidazole |
| | Potentiation of hypoglycemic effects of oral antidiabetic agents and insulin |

CNS, central nervous system.
(From Hyman, S.E. & Cassem, N.H. [1995]. Alcoholism. In D.C. Dale & D.D. Federman [Eds.], *Scientific American Medicine*, New York: Scientific American.)

pendent of any nutritional deficiencies that might account for muscle weakness or atrophy.

The most common cardiac complication associated with chronic alcohol ingestion for longer than 10 years is congestive cardiac myopathy. Breathlessness and cough are the most frequent complaints. Patients may complain of exercise-induced chest pain and fatigue or anorexia and abdominal discomfort because of hepatic and intestinal congestion. Cardiomegaly is detected on physical examination by lateral displacement of the apical pulse. An $S_3$ heart sound is present in 80% to 100% of patients with cardiomyopathy. Auscultation commonly reveals a gallop rhythm, increased pulmonic closure sound, diminished $S_1$, and faint systolic murmur. As cardiac compromise worsens, pulmonary hypertension, right ventricular failure, hepatomegaly, edema, and eventually ascites may occur. Hypertension, especially systolic hypertension, may occur as a result of long-term alcohol abuse and is independent of age, weight, or smoking. In addition, the unfavorable effect of alcohol on lipid profiles greatly increases the risk for cerebrovascular incident. The cardiac arrhythmias accompanying acute alcohol ingestion further increase this risk because of the possibility of thrombus formation in the vascular tissue. Thus, although controversy exists, research shows that consuming greater than one to two alcoholic drinks per day has damaging effects on the cardiovascular system (Friedman, 1992).

## Neurologic Complications

The neurologic complications associated with alcoholism range from mild to fatal and may be permanent or reversible. Although not fully understood, researchers believe that ethanol acts on the CNS by directly dissolving into the plasma membrane of neurons at specific locations of the brain (Lehman, 1991). Ethanol appears to change neurotransmission through GABA and serotonin receptors. Acetaldehyde and the fatty acids produced from ethanol metabolism are neurotoxic. In addition, specific sites, such as the reticular activating system, are exceptionally susceptible to the effects of ethanol. Blood alcohol levels above 25 mg/dL usually produce clinical manifestations of mild intoxication. The level of intoxication and severity of neurologic depression increase as blood alcohol levels increase. Acute alcohol ingestion may lead to blackout spells with amnesia or short-term memory loss (Lehman, 1991).

The most profound neurologic complications of alcoholism become evident when withdrawal from alcohol is attempted. Seizures may occur at any time, most frequently during the 12 to 48 hours after detoxification begins. The most serious complication of alcohol withdrawal is delirium tremors, which can be described as an agitated, confusional state characterized by autonomic hyperactivity. Hospitalization is required for fluid replenishment and sedation (Lehman, 1991). Wernicke's encephalopathy in the alcoholic is thought to result from a deficiency of thiamine, a coenzyme necessary for carbohydrate metabolism. Clinically, patients with the condition present with encephalopathy, ophthalmoplegia, and ataxia. Typically, there is an abrupt onset of symptoms, but the condition also may develop insidiously (Reuler et al., 1985). In conclusion, manifestations of alcoholism such as peripheral neuropathy and myopathy benefit greatly from abstinence from alcohol; however, some effects on the neurologic system are irreversible and may be life-threatening.

## Pancreatic Complications

Alcoholism is a major cause of acute and chronic pancreatitis. Acute pancreatitis often follows a period of heavy alcohol consumption. The exact mechanism of pancreatic damage is not fully understood. Alcohol is highly toxic to pancreatic acinar cells, which leads to activation of intracellular trypsin by lysosomal enzymes, causing tissue injury through a mechanism not fully understood. It is also suspected that ethanol may produce inflammation of the sphincter of Oddi, causing retention of proteolytic enzymes in the duct and acini. Conversely, ethanol may cause relaxation of the sphincter, allowing reflux of bile or duodenal contents in the duct, causing injury (McPhee, 1997). The clinical manifestations of acute pancreatitis are acute upper abdominal pain, nausea, vomiting, and fever. Elevations of serum amylase and lipase are present on laboratory examination. Acute pancreatitis often recurs, and the gland may become permanently damaged (chronic pancreatitis) after several attacks. The prognosis of acute pancreatitis depends on the amount of inflammation in the gland. Pancreatitis ranges from a mild, self-limited illness to a medical emergency characterized by pancreatic necrosis, hemorrhage, and sepsis (1997).

## Screening and Treatment Options

Alcoholism is a chronic and progressive disease associated with numerous relapses and remissions. The primary care provider's role in treating alcoholism requires adept assessment and interpersonal skills to identify patients who require further screening. The provider needs a quick and straightforward screening tool on site to assist with the assessment. The Brief Michigan Alcoholism Screening Test (MAST) (Table 5-12) may be useful when confronting a patient with undiagnosed alcoholism. Since a defining characteristic of alcoholism is denial, the first step in the treatment of alcoholism is compassionately confronting the patient with the diagnosis and the implications on the individual's health.

## Physiologic Basis of Treatment

Treatment for alcoholism typically includes inpatient or outpatient treatment programs and pharmacologic therapy. Disulfiram (Antabuse) often is used as a deterrent from alcohol ingestion because of its inhibition of aldehyde dehydrogenase, the enzyme in the liver that aids in the metabolism of alcohol. Thus, the patient becomes sensitized to alcohol ingestion and feels sick after a small amount of ethanol. Naltrexone is a long-acting opioid antagonist that sometimes is used to decrease alcohol craving by blocking the pleasure of alcohol consumption. This stops the reward sensation or euphoria produced by alcohol. Both

disulfiram and naltrexone have conflicting reports in their efficacy of preventing relapse. Naltrexone has been shown to be more effective when combined with a comprehensive treatment program (O'Malley, 1996).

There is a considerable amount of comorbidity between alcoholism, anxiety, and affective disorders. Thus, it is important to assess, diagnose, and treat any coexisting conditions of the alcoholic patient. Depression and anxiety are the most common conditions associated with alcoholism. Drugs that affect NE and serotonin (5-HT) activity are being used to treat alcoholics who also have affective disorders. Also, 5-HT may play a role in the obsessive-compulsive aspect of alcohol use because of its effectiveness in treating obsessive-compulsive disorder (Anton, 1996). Future research is being directed toward the pharmacologic treatment of alcoholism from this neurobehavioral approach.

One web site that primary care providers may find useful for their patients is *http://alcoholism.about.com*, which provides patients with information, resources, and net links. Alcoholics Anonymous has a web page including links and messages to support recovery (*http://decaf.talkway.com/cgi-bin/cgi?request=enter&group=alt.recovery.aa*).

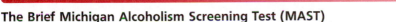

## TABLE 5.12

### The Brief Michigan Alcoholism Screening Test (MAST)

| Questions | Check One | |
|---|---|---|
| 1. Do you feel you are a normal drinker? | Yes (0) | No (2) |
| 2. Do friends or relatives think you are a normal drinker? | Yes (0) | No (2) |
| 3. Have you ever attended a meeting of Alcoholics Anonymous (AA)? | Yes (5) | No (0) |
| 4. Have you ever lost friends or girlfriends because of drinking? | Yes (2) | No (0) |
| 5. Have you ever gotten into trouble at work because of drinking? | Yes (2) | No (0) |
| 6. Have you ever neglected your obligations, your family, or your work for 2 or more days in a row because you were drinking? | Yes (2) | No (0) |
| 7. Have you ever had delirium tremors or severe shaking, heard voices, or seen things that were not there after heavy drinking? | Yes (2) | No (0) |
| 8. Have you ever gone to anyone for help about your drinking? | Yes (5) | No (0) |
| 9. Have you ever been in a hospital because of your drinking? | Yes (5) | No (0) |
| 10. Have you ever been arrested for drunk driving or driving after drinking? | Yes (2) | No (0) |

Alcoholism is indicated by a total score of greater than 5.
(From Selzer, M.L. [1971]. The Michigan Alcoholism Screening Test: The quest for a new diagnostic instrument. *American Journal of Psychiatry*, 127, 1653–1658.)

● **Case Study 5.1**

Mr. Joseph Blake is a 48-year-old white man who was seen recently by his medical doctor with complaints of an increased incidence of indigestion and a burning sensation in his stomach that usually occurs immediately after eating and is associated with nausea and vomiting. Mr. Blake reports that at times the vomitus looked as if it had blood in it. Currently, Mr. Blake denies any other physical symptoms.

During the initial interview, Mr. Blake casually mentioned that his wife of 24 years had recently left him and taken his children to live in another state because of his increased heavy drinking. Mr. Blake stated that not only had his marriage deteriorated over the last couple of years, but other problems also had occurred. He was recently fired for repeated absenteeism and tardiness at work. He also described that his children had withdrawn from him and did not want to be with him in public places. He indicated that he has not seen his children or wife since they left.

Mr. Blake reported that he grew up in a dysfunctional family. Both his father and his paternal grandfather were alcoholics and had disrupted marriages. His father died several years ago of cirrhosis of the liver after years of alcoholism. He recalls that his grandfather was stabbed to death after an argument outside of a bar where he had been drinking. Mr. Blake is the oldest of six children. He reports that he felt a tremendous responsibility to help raise his siblings and assist his mother with financial matters.

This is Mr. Blake's first visit to his medical doctor in 5 years. He reports that 3 years ago he tried to stop drinking, but his wife had to take him to the emergency room because he went through terrible withdrawal symptoms. He reports drinking approximately two six-packs of beer a day and sometimes a case of beer on the weekend. He denies any other drug abuse.

### Assessment

On palpation of the abdomen, Mr. Blake complained of mild epigastric pain with severe nausea and stated he felt as if he needed to vomit. There were no complaints of right upper quadrant pain on palpation. Physical examination did not reveal hepatomegaly. Results of musculoskeletal and neurologic examinations were normal. Chest was clear on auscultation. Cardiovascular examination revealed normal sinus rhythm, with no murmurs or extra heart sounds. The apical pulse was located at the left midclavicular line at the fifth intercostal space. The patient appeared slightly pale with no evidence of jaundice, lesions, or spider angiomia.

Vital signs                    T-98.2° F, P-98, BP-130/80

### Laboratory Studies

| Test | Result |
| --- | --- |
| Hgb | 12.3 g/dL |
| Hct | 41.6% |
| Alkaline phosphate | 2.6 |
| Bilirubin | 0.6 mg/dL |
| AST | 25 IU/L |
| ALT | 17 IU/L |
| Amylase | 82 IU/L |
| Lipase | 42 IU/L |
| PT | 11.5 seconds |
| PTT | 68 seconds |
| HIV | negative |

*(Case study continued on next page)*

### Diagnosis and Treatment

The nurse practitioner concludes that the patient has gastritis secondary to alcohol abuse. The practitioner explains to the patient that the illness is most likely due to alcohol abuse, and that an endoscopic examination is needed to determine the extent of the gastrointestinal damage. The patient states that he would like to stop drinking. The patient is scheduled for a gastroscopy the following morning. The practitioner prescribes omeprazole (Prilosec), 60 mg once daily, pending endoscopy results, to reduce the acid irritation of the gastric mucosa. A referral is made to an outpatient substance abuse treatment center where Mr. Blake can receive individual, group, and family counseling.

ALT, alanine aminotransferase; AST, aspartate aminotransferase; BP, blood pressure; Hct, hemotocrit; Hgb, hemoglobin; HIV, human immunodeficiency virus; P, pulse; PT, prothrombin time; PTT, partial thromboplastin time; T, temperature. (Contributed by Lisa Pullen, RN, PhD.)

## REFERENCES

Abelson, J.L., Glitz, D., & Cameron, O.G. (1991). Blunted growth hormone response to clonidine in patients with generalized anxiety disorder. *Archives of General Psychiatry, 25*, 141–152.

Adelman, S.A. & Scott, M.E. (1996). Depression. In H.L. Greene (Ed.), *Clinical medicine* (2nd ed., pp. 730–734). St. Louis: Mosby.

American Psychiatric Association. (1994). *Diagnostic and statistical manual of mental disorders* (4th ed.). Washington, DC: American Psychiatric Association.

American Psychiatric Association. (1999). Practice guideline for the treatment of patients with substance use disorders, alcohol, cocaine, opioids. Available at: *www.psych.org*.

Anton, R.F. (1996). Neurobehavioural basis for the pharmacotherapy of alcoholism: Current and future directions. *Alcohol & Alcoholism, 31*, (Suppl. 1), 43–53.

Arnold, L.E., Stroble, D., & Weisenberg, A. (1972). Hyperkinetic adult: Study of the paradoxical amphetamine response. *Journal of the American Medical Association, 222*, 693–694.

Barkley, R.A. (1990). *Attention deficit hyperactivity disorder.* New York: The Guilford Press.

Barkley, R.A. (1994a). More on the new theory of ADHD. *ADHD Report, 2* (2), 1–4.

Barkley, R.A. (1994b). It's about time. *ADHD Report, 6*, 1–2.

Birmaher, B., Ryan, N.D., & Williamson, D.E. (1996). Depression in children and adolescents: Clinical features and pathogenesis. In K.I. Shulman, M. Tohen, & Kutcher, S.P. (Eds.), *Mood disorders across the life span* (pp. 51–81). New York: Wiley-Liss.

Blum, K., Sheridan, P.J., Wood, R.C., Braverman, E.R., Chen, T.J., & Comings, D.E. (1995). Dopamine D2 receptor gene variants: Association and linkage studies in impulsive-addictive-compulsive behaviour. *Pharmacogenetics, 5*, 121–141.

Brawman-Mintzer, O. & Lydiard, R.B. (1996). Generalized anxiety disorder: Issues in epidemiology. *Journal of Clinical Psychiatry, 57*, 3–8.

Brawman-Mintzer, O. & Lydiard, R.B. (1997). Biological basis of generalized anxiety disorder. *Journal of Clinical Psychiatry, 58*, (Suppl. 3), 16–25.

Castellanos, F.X. (1997). Toward a pathophysiology of attention deficit hyperactivity disorder. *Clinical Pediatrics, 36*, 381–393.

Ciccocioppo, R. (1999). The role of serotonin in craving: From basic research to human studies. *Alcohol and Alcoholism, 34*, 244–253.

Comings, D.E, Blake, H., Dietz, G., Gade-Andavolu, R., Legro, R.S., Saucier, G., Johnson, P., Verde, R., & MacMurray, J.P. (1999). The proenkephalin gene (PENK) and opioid dependence. *Neuroreport, 10* (5), 1133–1135.

Conners, C., et al. (1996). Bupropion hydrochloride in attention deficit disorder with hyperactivity. *Journal of the American Academy of Child and Adolescent Psychiatry, 35*, 1314–1321.

Connor, T.J. & Leonard, B.E. (1998). Depression, stress and immunological activation: The role of cytokines in depressive disorders. *Life Sciences, 62* (7), 583–606.

Davis, W.M. (1998). New directions in treating depression. *Drug Topics, 142*, 85–90.

DeSimoni, M.G. & Imeri, L. (1998). Cytokine-neurotransmitter interactions in the brain. *Biological Signals and Receptors, 7*, 33–44.

Dougherty, D. & Rauch, S.L. (1997). Neuroimaging and neurobiological models of depression. *Harvard Review of Psychiatry, 5*, 138–159.

Feinman, L., Korsten, M.A., & Lieber, C.S. (1992). Alcohol and the digestive tract. In C.S. Lieber (Ed.), *Medical and nutritional complications of alcoholism: Mechanisms and management* (pp. 307–332). New York: Plenum Publishing.

Fibiger, H.C. (1995). Neurobiology of depression: Focus on dopamine. *Advances in Biochemical Psychopharmacology, 49*, 1–17.

Franklin, J.E. & Frances, R.J. (1999). Alcohol and other psychoactive substance use disorders. In R.E. Hales, S.C. Yudofsky, & J.A. Talbott (Eds.), *The American Psychiatric Press textbook of psychiatry* (3rd ed., pp. 363–424). Washington, DC: The American Psychiatric Press.

Friedman, H.S. (1992). Cardiovascular effects of ethanol. In C.S. Lieber (Ed.), *Medical and nutritional complications of alcoholism: Mechanisms and management* (pp. 359–395). New York: Plenum Publishing.

Gardner, E. (1997). Brain reward mechanisms. In J. Lowinson, P. Ruiz, R. Millman, & J. Langrod (Eds.), *Substance abuse: A comprehensive textbook*. Baltimore: Williams & Wilkins.

George, R.A. & Mortiner, D.B. (1998). Identification and medical treatment of ADHD in the juvenile justice setting. *ADHD Report, 6,* 1–9.

Georgotas, A. (1983). Affective disorders in the elderly: Diagnostic and research considerations. *Age and Aging, 12,* 1–10.

Gianoulakis, C. (1996). Implications of endogenous opiods and dopamine in alcoholism: Human and basic science studies. *Alcohol and Alcoholism, 31,* (Suppl. 1), 33–42.

Giedd, J.H. & Castellanos, X. (1994). Quantitative morphology of the corpus callosum in attention deficit hyperactive disorder. *American Journal of Psychiatry, 151,* 665–669.

Gray, J. (1988). The neuropsychological basis of anxiety. In C. Last & M. Herson (Eds.), *Handbook of anxiety disorders* (pp. 10–38). New York: Pergamon Press.

Herz, A. (1998). Opioid reward mechanisms: A key role in drug abuse? *Canadian Journal of Physiology and Pharmacology, 76,* 252–258.

Hyman, S.E. & Cassem, N.H. (1995). Alcoholism. In D.C. Dale & D.D. Federman (Eds.), *Scientific American Medicine.* New York: Scientific American.

Johnson, M.R. & Lydiard, R.B. (1995, December). The neurobiology of anxiety disorders. *The Psychiatric Clinics of North America, 18* (4), 681–725.

Katon, W., Von Korff, M., & Lin, E. (1990). Distressed high utilizers of medical care: DSM-III-R diagnoses and treatment needs. *General Hospital Psychiatry, 12,* 355–362.

Koob, G. & Nestler, E. (1997). The neurobiology of drug addiction. *The Journal of Neuropsychiatry and Clinical Neurosciences, 9,* 482–497.

Lehman, L.B. (1991). Neurologic complications of alcoholism. *Postgraduate Medicine, 90* (5), 165–172.

Leonard, B.E. & Song, C. (1996). Stress and the immune system in the etiology of anxiety and depression. *Pharmacology, Biochemistry, and Behavior, 54* (1), 299–303.

Leshner, A. & Koob, G. (1999). Drugs of abuse and the brain. *Proceedings of the Association of American Physicians, 111,* 99–108.

Lewinsohn, P.M., Clarke, G.N., Seeley, J.R., & Rohde, P. (1994). Major depression in community adolescents: Age at onset, episode duration, and time to recurrence. *Journal of the American Academy of Child and Adolescent Psychiatry, 33*(6), 809–818.

Lieber, C.S. (1988). Biological and molecular basis of alcohol-induced injury to liver and other tissues. *New England Journal of Medicine, 319* (25), 1639–1647.

Lieber, C.S. & Leo, M.A. (1992). Alcohol and the liver. In C.S. Lieber (Ed.), *Medical and nutritional complications of alcholism: Mechanisms and management* (pp. 185–239). New York: Plenum Publishing.

Manji, H.K. (1992). G proteins: Implications for psychiatry. *American Journal of Psychiatry, 149* (6), 746.

Mayberg, H.S. (1997). Limbic-cortical dysregulation: A proposed model of depression. *The Journal of Neuropsychiatry and Clinical Neurosciences, 9,* 471–481.

McGinnis, J. & Forge, W. (1993). Actual causes of death in the United States. *Journal of the American Medical Association, 270* (18), 2208.

McPhee, S.J. (1997). Disorders of the exocrine pancreas. In S.J. McPhee, V.R. Lingappa, W.F. Ganong, & J.D. Lange (Eds.), *Pathophysiology of disease: An introduction to clinical medicine* (2nd ed, pp. 356–373). Stanford, CT: Appleton & Lange.

Muller, N. & Ackenheil, M. (1998). Psychoneuroimmunology and the cytokine action in the CNS: Implications for psychiatric disorders. *Progress in Neuro-Psychopharmacology and Biological Psychiatry, 22,* 1–33.

Murphy, K. (1993). Effectively communicating adult ADHD diagnosis. *ADHD Report, 2,* 6–7.

Nash, M. (1997). Addicted. *Time, 149,* 1–8.

National Institute of Mental Health (1996). Subtle brain circuit abnormalities confirmed in ADHD. *http://www.nimh.gov/events/pradhd.htm.*

Noble, E.P. (1994). Polymorphisms of the D2 dopamine receptor gene and alcoholism and other substance use disorders. *Alcohol and Alcoholism,* (Supplement, 2), 35–43.

O'Malley, S.S. (1996). Opioid antagonists in the treatment of alcohol dependence: Clinical efficacy and prevention of relapse. *Alcohol and Alcoholism, 31,* (Suppl. 1), 77–81.

Pi, E.H., Gross, L.S., & Nagy, R.M. (1994). Biochemical factors in anxiety and related disorders. In B.B. Wolman & G. Stricker (Eds.), *Anxiety and related disorders: A handbook* (pp. 112–131). New York: John Wiley & Sons.

Raskin, A. (1979). Signs and symptoms of psychopathology in the elderly. In A. Raskin & L. Jarvik (Eds.), *Psychiatric symptoms and cognitive loss in the elderly* (pp. 3–18). Washington, DC: Hemisphere.

Reuler, J.B., Girard, D.E., & Cooney, T.G. (1985). Wernicke's encephalopathy. *New England Journal of Medicine, 312* (16), 1035–1038.

Risch, S. C. (1997). Recent advances in depression research: From stress to molecular biology and brain imaging. *Journal of Clinical Psychiatry, 58,* (Suppl. 5), 3–6.

Roy-Byrne, P.P. & Katon, W. (1997). Generalized anxiety disorder in primary care: The precursor/modifier pathway to increased health care utilization. *Journal of Clinical Psychiatry, 58,* (Suppl. 3), 34–38.

Safer, D. & Allen, R. (1975). Stimulant drug treatment of hyperactive adolescents. *Diseases of the Nervous System, 36,* 454–457.

Schildkraut, J.J. (1965). The catecholamine hypothesis of affective disorders: A review of supporting evidence. *American Journal of Psychiatry, 122,* 509–522.

Schuckit, M.S. (1985). Genetics and the risk for alcoholism. *Journal of the American Medical Association, 254* (18), 2614–2617.

Schuyler, D. (1998). *Taming the tyrant: Treating depressed adults.* New York: W.W. Norton.

Schweizer, E. & Rickels, K. (1997). Strategies for treatment of generalized anxiety in the primary care setting. *Journal of Clinical Psychiatry, 58,* (Suppl. 3), 27–31.

Simeon, J.G. & Fergusen H.B. (1986). Bupropion effects in attention deficit and conduct disorders. *Canadian Journal of Psychiatry, 31,* 581–585.

Soares, J.C. & Mann, J.J. (1997, August). The functional neuroanatomy of mood disorders. *Journal of Psychiatric Research, 31* (4), 393–432.

Soorani, E. & DeVincent, J. (1997). Bupropion may offset SSRI-induced sexual dysfunction. *Psychopharmacology Update, 1,* 1–6.

Thase, M.E. & Howland, R. H (1995). Biological processes in depression: An updated review and integration. In E.E. Beckham & W.R. Leber (Eds.), *Handbook of depression* (2nd ed., pp. 213–279). New York: The Guilford Press.

Tsai, G., Gastfriend, D.R., & Coyle, J.T. (1995). The glutamatergic basis of human alcoholism. *American Journal of Psychiatry, 152,* (3) 332–339.

Urbano-Marquez, A., Estruch, R., Navarro-Lopez, F., Grau, J.M., Mont L., & Rubin, E. (1989). The effects of alcoholism on skeletal and cardiac muscle. *The New England Journal of Medicine, 320* (7),409–415.

Viguera, A.C. & Rothschild, A.J. (1996). Depression: Clinical features and pathogenesis. In K.I. Shulman, M. Tohen,

& S.P. Kutcher (Eds.), *Mood disorders across the life span* (pp. 189–215). New York: Wiley-Liss.

Voeller, K. (1998). Right hemisphere deficit syndrome in children. *American Journal of Psychiatry, 143,* 1004–1009.

Weiss, M. (1996). Changes in the approach to pharmacotherapy dor ADHD. *Child and Adolescent Psychopharmacology News, 1,* 5–8.

Wender, P. (1995). *Attention deficit hyperactivity disorder in adults.* Oxford: University Press.

Williams, G.D., Grant, B.F., Harford, T.C., & Noble, J. (1989). Population projections using DSM-III criteria: Alcohol abuse and dependence, 1990–2000. *Alcohol Health Research World, 13,* 366–370.

Zametkin, A., et al. (1990). Cerebral glucose metabolism in adults with hyperactivity in childhood onset. *New England Journal of Medicine, 32,* 1361–1366.

Zametkin, A., et al. (1993). Brain metabolism in teenagers with attention deficit hyperactivity disorder. *Archives of General Psychology, 50,* 333–340.

# Ear, Nose, and Throat Disorders

Mary Kollar

## EAR, NOSE, AND THROAT

Ear, nose, and throat (ENT) disorders are among the most common reasons for patients to visit their primary care providers. Millions of office visits occur each year when patients experience common symptoms such as otalgia, decreased hearing, rhinitis, sinus pain, and sore throat. These symptoms cost millions of dollars not only for direct medical care, but also in terms of lost salaries and patient prescriptions. Antibiotics typically are prescribed for many of the common ENT etiologies. This widespread use of antibiotics has created an alarming national and worldwide situation in which bacterial organisms are becoming resistant to certain antibiotics.

For example, the occurrence of otitis media (OM) has been steadily increasing and now is the most common pediatric diagnosis in the United States. There were approximately 9.9 million visits for OM in 1975, which increased to approximately 24.5 in 1990 (Dowell et al., 1998). Currently, more than one fourth of all oral antibiotics are prescribed for the treatment of OM in children (Bluestone, 1998; Carlson & Fall, 1998).

### Common Organisms and Antibiotic Resistance

*Streptococcus pneumoniae*, *Haemophilus influenzae*, and *Moraxella catarrhalis*, the most common organisms responsible for causing infections in the ENT system, now are linked to a heightened antibiotic resistance. Specifically, *H. influenzae* and *M. catarrhalis* have become increasingly resistant to amoxicillin because of the microorganism's production of β-lactamase, an enzyme that

destroys the effectiveness of the antibiotic. *S. pneumoniae* also has become increasingly resistant to penicillin because of mutations that allow the bacteria to avoid the antibiotic's inhibitory effects on cell wall synthesis. Currently, second- and third-generation antibiotics may be required in the treatment of OM and sinusitis (Havens, 1998).

Primary care providers need to make accurate assessments and should not overprescribe antibiotics for ENT conditions. They also need to be aware of the pathophysiologic principles behind, and the recent findings regarding, the management of ENT problems in order to develop specific, effective, and comprehensive health plans with their patients.

### Common Disorders of the Ear

The ear is divided into the external, middle, and inner ear (see Fig. 6-1). The primary care provider must consider all of these anatomical areas when assessing a patient's ear problem. Otalgia and decreased hearing are the most common symtoms the patient will present in the primary care office. These symptoms may have etiologies in the external, middle, or inner ear. In addition, the primary care provider has to consider referred pain from other head and neck etiologies. For instance, otalgia may be referred from temporal mandibular joint dysfunction, impacted third molars, or malignant lesions of the oropharynx or larynx.

#### External Ear

The external ear is composed of the external ear lobe (pinna) and the external ear canal. The pinna is where multiple lesions and rashes can occur. Basal and squamous cell carcinomas especially

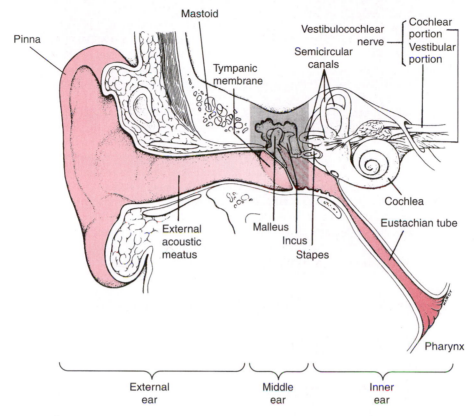

**FIGURE 6.1** ● Anatomy of the ear.

occur on the crest of the pinna, where it is exposed to sunlight. Keloids occur more commonly in African Americans after either an injury or earlobe piercing for earrings. The external ear is a common site for tophi, the deposition of urate crystals seen in patients with gout. Multiple other lesions that occur on other parts of the body also occur on the external ear, such as herpes zoster, contact dermatitis, and furuncles (Damjanov & Linder, 1996)

Otitis externa (OE) is one of the most common ear problems that primary care providers will see in places where it is hot and humid. It is likely to occur in those who participate in water sports or spend a lot of time in the water. In the warm summer months, as many as 20% of patients may present with this etiology (Cantor, 1999; Licameli, 1999). The usual symptoms are otalgia and otorrhea. In severe infection, the ear canal may occlude because of inflammation, with subsequent hearing loss. On examination, the ear canal usually is red and swollen, and discharge may be present. Movement of the auricle or tragal manipulation causes pain.

### Pathophysiology of Otitis Externa

The external ear canal has several functions: it protects the middle and inner ear, and it conducts and amplifies sound to the middle and inner ear. Cerumen is produced from the sebaceous and apocrine glands located in the medial portion of the external ear canal. The cerumen acts as a protective physical barrier. It is acidic (pH of 4 to 5) and bacteriostatic, creating a hostile environment for pathogens. Cerumen contains other factors that discourage infection such as immunoglobulins and lysozymes (Cantor, 1999; Damjanov & Linder, 1996).

The external ear canal normally is well protected against infection unless certain conditions exist. Major causes of OE are trauma to the canal and retained moisture within the canal. Trauma can occur from scratching the ear canal or attempting to remove ear wax with cotton-tipped applicators or sharper objects. The absence of cerumen and the presence of any factor that encourages an alkaline pH within the canal promotes secondary infection (Cantor, 1999). Both moisture in the canal and infection increase pH. Attempting to clean cerumen from the ear canals can cause trauma, and any retained moisture from the irrigation invites infection. Excessive swimming, especially in chlorinated pools where the water frequently is alkaline and contains chemicals that can kill the normal flora in the ears, also may make a person prone to OE (La Rosa, 1998).

The most common bacterial cause of OE is *Pseudomonas aeruginosa*. Rarely, fungi can be culprits. Treatment involves appropriate antibiotic or antifungal ear drops that usually clear the infection in 7 to 10 days. However, complications such as *malignant OE* can occur, particularly with diabetic or immunocompromised patients. Malignant OE involves the spread of the infection to the middle and inner ear, causing hearing loss, severe pain, and neurologic symptoms (if the cranial nerves become involved) (Cantor, 1999; Damjanov & Linder, 1996).

### Pathophysiology of Cerumen Impaction

Another common problem seen by primary care providers is cerumen impaction. The patient may come to the office with a chief complaint of sudden hearing loss. Normally, cerumen migrates out of the canal through the action of cilia and does not require any cleaning methods to be extruded. However, impacted cerumen may be a problem for certain people. Using cotton-tipped swabs and hearing aids may prevent the cerumen from normal migration, causing impaction.

The elderly have drier cerumen because the apocrine glands produce less moisture within the cerumen. In addition, the external ear canal cilia do not function as well. The elderly may find that the regular use of ear drops to soften the cerumen (ie, mineral oil, olive oil, baby oil) or periodic ear irrigations may prevent impacted cerumen.

## Middle Ear

The most common otologic problem seen in primary care patients is OM. OM is a general term referring to inflammation of the middle ear. Acute otitis media (AOM) is an acute infection of the middle ear characterized by otalgia, decreased hearing, fever, and a red, bulging tympanic membrane (TM) with diminished or absent landmarks (Bluestone & Klein, 1995).

Otitis media with effusion (OME) is the presence of fluid and negative pressure in the middle ear without evidence of infection. Other terms used synonymously with OME include serous OM, secretory OM, and mucoid OM. The major symptoms of OME are decreased hearing, discomfort, occasional otalgia, behavioral changes, and learning difficulties. The TM may appear normal or may be retracted or bulging with impaired

mobility. The practitioner may see fluid or bubbles behind a translucent TM (Bluestone & Klein, 1995). Because the signs of OME are so variable, pneumatic otoscopy and tympanometry are useful aids in determining the mobility of the TM and, therefore, the presence of fluid within the middle ear.

OM usually occurs after the onset of an upper respiratory infection (URI) or is an allergic ENT response. Both AOM and OME can cause conductive hearing loss. AOM usually presents with pain and therefore is treated rapidly with antibiotics. On the other hand, OME in children can go untreated for weeks or months because of its subtle presentation (hearing loss). Over time, the hearing loss may translate into learning deficits and behavioral problems. If OME occurs in the first 2 to 3 years of life, children are more likely to have speech and language delays. If OME occurs during the first year of school, the hearing deficit may interfere with schoolwork, resulting in stress and subsequent behavioral problems (Marchisio et al., 1998). Lindsay, Tomazic, Whitman, and Accardo (1999) found that social class was associated with different problems at school age. They found that a history of major ear problems was correlated with articulation disorders in children from a lower social class, hyperactivity in those from the middle class, and language problems in children from a high social class (Lindsay et al., 1999).

The earlier the onset of AOM (especially in infants before 6 to 9 months of age), the greater the possibility that the child will have recurrent problems with AOM. Researchers have found that other risk factors for AOM include the following: gender (males are at increased risk), family history of atopy, siblings or parents who have a history of AOM, increased exposure to URIs (eg, from day care centers), being bottle fed versus breast fed, exposure to secondary smoke at home, and anatomic disorders such as a cleft palate or submucous cleft palate. These findings indicate that the child who experiences allergies, an increased incidence of URIs, or anatomic problems may have more problems with OM (Kvaerner et al., 1997; Bluestone & Klein, 1995; Daley et al., 1999).

### Pathophysiology of Otitis Media

The primary factor contributing to OM is eustachian tube dysfunction (ETD). The eustachian tube drains fluid from the middle ear, protects the middle ear from infection, and regulates the pressure in the middle ear. One third of the eustachian tube, which connects to the middle ear, is osseous. The other two thirds of the eustachian tube, which connects to the nasopharyngeal orifice, is composed primarily of membrane and cartilage. The epithelium lining the eustachian tube contains ciliated and mucous cells that are involved in drainage and gas exchange within the tube (Prades et al., 1998). There is a normal narrowing of the orifice between the osseous portion and the membranous/cartilage portion. This area is called the isthmus or junctional portion (see Fig. 6-2). Drainage through the isthmus into the eustachian tube can be problematic if negative pressure exists in the middle ear or if mucous lodged in the isthmus is thick and, therefore, difficult to move. Several other factors involving the eustachian tube make a person more prone to OM: developmental factors, obstruction (opening failure), abnormal patency (closing failure), and other factors discussed later (Bylander-Groth & Stenstrom, 1998; Bluestone and Klein, 1995).

Important developmental factors make children more prone to OM. In adults, the eustachian tube is situated at a 45-degree angle, whereas in children, it lies more horizontally at about a 10-degree angle. In addition, the eustachian tube in adults is longer (usual range, 31 to 38 mm) than in children (average length, 18 mm) (see Fig. 6-2). The shorter eustachian tube also is seen in children with Down's syndrome and cleft palate (Tarlow, 1998). Children are more susceptible to infection because

these factors allow reflux of the nasopharyngeal secretions into the middle ear. Researchers have found that the cartilaginous portion of the eustachian tube has significant growth in both height and width from childhood to adolescence and hypothesize that this improves the basic three functions of the eustachian tube (Suzuki et al., 1998).

Eustachian tubes in children are less efficient than those of adults in regulating pressure in the middle ear. High negative pressure has been recorded in children who do not have any signs or symptoms of OM (Bluestone & Klein, 1995). Several explanations for this phenomenon have been offered. One is that the eustachian tube does not open efficiently enough to equilibrate the pressure. Another possibility is that some children are "sniffers," and this sniffing creates frequent higher negative pressure in the middle ear. The third explanation is that the normal gas absorption that occurs through the middle ear mucosa creates a negative pressure. If inflammation and excess mucus in the eustachian tube occurs, then the condition is aggravated and negative pressure may increase (Ovesen & Borglum, 1998). This negative pressure increases the likelihood that bacterial organisms that secondarily infect the middle ear are "sucked in from the nasopharynx into the middle ear cavity" (Tarlow, 1998), causing infection or

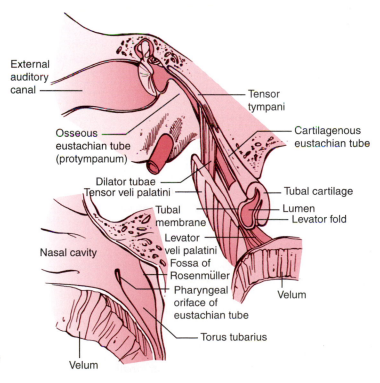

**FIGURE 6.2** ● Dissection of the eustachian tube.

External auditory canal

Tensor tympani

Osseous eustachian tube (protympanum)

Cartilagenous eustachian tube

Dilator tubae
Tensor veli palatini

Tubal cartilage

Tubal membrane

Lumen
Levator fold

Levator veli palatini

Nasal cavity

Fossa of Rosenmüller

Pharyngeal oriface of eustachian tube

Velum

Torus tubarius

Velum

AOM. When AOM occurs, the middle ear pressure rises as a result of the "transudation of serous fluid from subepithelial capillaries into the obstructed middle ear space that reduces the middle ear air volume, thereby increasing middle ear pressure" (Daley et al., 1999, p. 86).

OM may be caused by obstruction (opening failures) resulting from either functional or mechanical causes. In a normally functioning eustachian tube, intermittent opening of the tube occurs, primarily from contraction of the tensor veli palatini muscles on swallowing, yawning, or sneezing. This opening allows fluid to drain from the middle ear, regulating pressure in the middle ear. Research indicates that this active, opening function of the eustachian tube is impaired not only with children who have OME, but also in normal children (Bylander-Groth & Stenstrom, 1998). Takahashi, Hayashi, and Honjo (1996) found that children with OME have higher eustachian tube compliance, and adults with OME have a more rigid eustachian tube. The more compliant tube is more collapsible or floppy, which impairs the normal function of the eustachian tube, thereby increasing children's problems with OM. Further impairment of eustachian tube functioning in children with OME was found by researchers who observed that the cartilaginous portion of the eustachian tube contracts during swallowing (versus the normal dilating) (Takahashi et al., 1996). In less severe cases, the eustachian tube has a lower resistance to opening than normal. This may be seen in patients who have lost a large amount of weight or in adults who have unusually stiff eustachian tubes (Bluestone & Klein, 1995).

Tumors, enlarged adenoids, mucosal swelling, and lack of mucosal surfactants may cause mechanical obstruction of the patency of the eustachian tube (Bylander-Groth & Stenstrom, 1998). Enlarged tumors and adenoids can encroach on and obstruct the patency of the eustachian tube, increasing the likelihood of OM. Adenoidectomy and removal of the tumors is beneficial for this condition (Wright et al., 1998). Mucosal swelling can occur as a result of infection or an allergic response and can cause swelling of the mucosa in the eustachian tube and the mucosa in the nasal and nasopharyngeal area. This swelling further compromises the patency of an already potentially compromised eustachian tube. Eustachian tube and middle ear effusions contain mucosal surfactants, which reduce the surface tension. Lack of surfactant might promote eustachian tube collapse, causing ETD and OM. Lack of surfactant may occur

with inflammation of the eustachian tube (Miura et al., 1997). Animal studies indicate that eustachian tube function improves after topical application of surfactants (Nemechek et al., 1997). Researchers are investigating this method of treatment in humans, but it is not available yet.

Abnormal patency (closing failure) can increase the likelihood of ETD and subsequently OM. In severe cases, the eustachian tube remains open even at rest, increasing susceptibility to infection. Certain populations are more prone to this, specifically children with Down's syndrome and Native Americans (Tarlow, 1998). OM is caused by reflux of bacteria from the nasopharynx. Slight negative pressure normally occurs in the middle ear, but higher negative pressure can be produced by sniffing and, when followed by swallowing (thereby opening the ET), can cause reflux of the bacteria from the nasopharynx and subsequent infection. Data from several studies suggest that one third of normal adults and one fourth of children with histories of OM who can create a negative pressure in their middle ears by sniffing have a "relative closing failure of the tube" (Bylander-Groth & Stenstrom, 1998, p. 766).

Primary care providers should be aware of other factors that may make people more susceptible to OM. The ciliary function of the middle ear and eustachian tube may be impaired by smoking, viral infections (such as infection with influenza A) and bacterial endotoxins (ie, pneumolysin produced by *S. pneumoniae*) (Tarlow, 1998). When the cilia are impaired, mucous does not drain well from the middle ear, and infectious agents are more likely to enter, causing OME and AOM.

Bacterial endotoxins are an active bacterial product of lipopolysaccharide complexes, which originally are on the surface of Gram-negative bacteria. Endotoxins remain after antibiotic treatment, when the bacteria are no longer present, and even then can promote inflammation (Ovesen & Borglum, 1998). Ovesen and Borglum (1998) detected the presence of endotoxins in more than 90% of children who had had tympanostomy tubes inserted for OME. They found that endotoxins were difficult to inactivate and continued to produce and maintain mucosal inflammation. Researchers doing animal studies also found that after 3 months, endotoxins caused degeneration of the cilia and generation of goblet cells, which produce mucus. These researchers conclude that endotoxins have a significant role in chronic OME (Nell & Grote, 1999). In addition, bacterial toxins can diffuse through the oval or round window, causing a complication of OM, neural labyrinthitis, an inflammation of the inner ear (Tarlow, 1998).

## Nose and Paranasal Sinuses

The nose and paranasal sinuses are closely connected (see Fig. 6-3). The sinuses develop as out-pouchings of the nasal mucosa. Because of the close proximity and the drainage of the sinuses into the nose, problems within the nose can affect the functioning of the sinuses. Some of the common etiologies that a primary care provider may see related to the nose are allergic rhinitis (see Chapter 7), nonallergic rhinitis, vasomotor rhinitis, and sinusitis.

Nonallergic rhinitis is a condition that presents with symptoms similar to those of allergic rhinitis; however, although the nasal smear may display eosinophilia, results of skin testing for allergens are negative. Vasomotor rhinitis is caused by an exaggerated parasympathetic response to several stimuli, which produces nasal symptoms (Maltinski, 1998). The triggers may be a change in temperature, odors, irritants, or other substances that do not ordinarily affect people. The nasal smear of a patient with vasomotor rhinitis does not show eosinophilia, and skin tests for allergens produce negative results.

### Sinusitis

Sinusitis frequently is diagnosed by primary care providers. In 1996, about 26.7 million people visited primary care providers for illness attributable to sinusitis, with expenditures of approximately $5.78 billion for the treatment of sinusitis and its complications (Ray et al., 1999). Sinusitis is an inflammation of the sinus mucosa caused by viral, bacterial, or fungal etiologies. Acute sinusitis, by definition, usually lasts less than 4 weeks, whereas chronic sinusitis lasts longer than 3 months. Sinusitis is subacute if the symptoms last between 1 and 3 months.

Viral inflammation of the sinuses, resulting in thickening of the sinus mucosa, can be seen in patients with the common cold or influenza (Hueston et al., 1998; Puhakka et al., 1998). It usually lasts a short time, may or may not involve signs and symptoms of sinusitis, and does not require antibiotics to resolve it. Finnish researchers studying 200 young, healthy adults with common viral URIs found that 40% had radiologic findings consistent with acute sinusitis, 95% had purulent rhinitis, and all recovered without treatment with antibiotics (Puhakka et al., 1998).

Bacterial sinusitis can be a complication of viral rhinosinusitis or an URI, allergic rhinitis, or several other factors that are discussed later. Historically, it has been difficult to distinguish between viral URI, allergic rhinitis, and viral sinusitis from bacterial sinusitis because they share similar signs and symptoms. Multiple studies have tried to identify the symptoms and signs of bacterial sinusitis. Because antibiotics are used

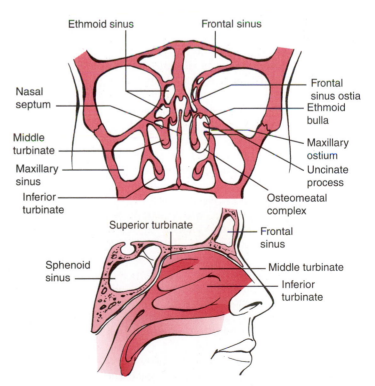

**FIGURE 6.3** ● Anatomy of the nose *(top)* and paranasal sinuses *(bottom)*.

only to treat sinusitis with a bacterial etiology, sinusitis must be diagnosed correctly to prevent overprescribing antibiotics.

Symptoms more consistently associated with bacterial sinusitis are maxillary toothache, sinus pressure or pain, poor response to nasal decongestants, purulent rhinitis, cough, halitosis, history of the illness worsening after it seemed to be abating (called "double sickening"), and a longer duration of illness. Common signs are purulent rhinitis (although a lack of drainage could indicate occlusion of the ostia); red, swollen nasal mucosa; and abnormal transillumination. Facial pain or tenderness on percussion, considered a classic sign used to diagnose bacterial sinusitis, has not been found to be a reliable indicator (Hueston et al., 1998; Poole, 1999; Slavin, 1993). The diagnosis of bacterial sinusitis is even more problematic in children than adults because of a child's inability to localize symptoms. There is also a lack of agreement about the appropriate symptoms to diagnose pediatric sinusitis. In children, the symptoms of sinusitis may be less specific than in adults. Additional symptoms seen in children may be snoring, mouth breathing, feeding problems, nasal speech, and fever (Jones, 1999). Children typically do not present with headache or facial pain.

Fungal sinusitis rarely is seen and is categorized into four categories: acute/fulminant, chronic indolent, fungus ball, and allergic fungal sinusitis. The acute/fulminant and fungus sinusitis ball occurs primarily in immunocompromised patients. The chronic/indolent form rarely is seen in the United States but is more common in Sudan and Northern India. Allergic fungal sinusitis occurs in approximately 7% of patients with chronic sinusitis. These patients may have problems with nasal polyps and asthma. Signs and symptoms of fungal sinusitis may be similar to sinusitis in general, except neurologic signs and symptoms may develop, especially with the fulminant fungal varieties seen in immunocompromised patients (Gungor, 1998).

### Pathophysiology of Sinusitis

Three paired sinuses are involved in sinusitis: the maxillary, frontal, and ethmoid sinuses. The fourth paired sinus is the sphenoid sinus, which rarely is involved. The maxillary and ethmoid sinuses are present at birth and become functional around 6 months of age. The frontal sinuses do not fully develop until adolescence and are not a locus for sinusitis until that time. In a small percentage of patients, the frontal sinuses never develop or develop on only one side.

The sinuses are air-filled, sterile cavities that are lined by ciliated epithelium and mucus. The functions of the sinuses are to (1) reduce the weight of the skull, (2) buffer the shock in case of head trauma, and (3) improve vocal resonance. The sinuses are lined with mucosa, which produces mucus and cilia that sweep the mucus toward the ostia, or drainage ducts. The ostia drain into the superior meatus (ethmoid and sphenoid sinuses) and middle meatus (frontal and maxillary sinuses). The region of sinus drainage in the nose is termed the osteomeatal complex (Fagan, 1998; Maltinski, 1998). Failure of mucus to drain normally and ventilation of the sinuses are the main factors that result in sinusitis.

The osteomeatal complex is susceptible to inflammation from reduced mucociliary clearance, retention of secretions, and decreased sinus ventilation. When mucosal swelling occurs, the ostia becomes obstructed, and drainage is impaired (Poole, 1999). When there is nasal mucosal swelling, the turbinates enlarge and impinge on the ostia, preventing mucous from draining from the sinuses. The stasis in the sinuses, along with inflammation, sets the stage for sinusitis. Typically, the patient with sinusitis has had an antecedent URI; allergic, nonallergic, or vasomotor rhinitis; or a condition creating mucosal edema and subsequent ostial obstruction. A negative pressure can develop within the sinus cavity, and when the patient sneezes, coughs, or blows the nose, bacteria are drawn into the sinus cavity. Organisms that typically cause acute bacterial sinusitis are the same components of the normal flora involved in OM: *S. pneumoniae, H. influenzae,* and *M. catarrhalis.* Other factors may cause nasal mucosal swelling and subsequent sinusitis, including increased temperature and humidity, hormonal and emotional status, and medications such as beta blockers, reserpine, and oral contraceptives. Rhinitis medicamentosa is associated with the overuse of topical nasal decongestants and may cause swelling of the nasal mucosa, inhibiting the ostia from draining (Cunha, 1998; Lund, 1997; Poole, 1999).

Occlusion of the ostia is caused not only by inflammation, but also by anatomic or mechanical causes. Anatomic problems include concha bullosa, septal deformities, paradoxic middle turbinates, Haller (infraorbital ethmoidal) cells, pneumatization of the agger nasi, and deformed uncinate processes (Lund, 1997). Patients with anatomic problems typically have chronic or repetitive episodes of sinusitis. Computed tomography (CT) may help to detect these abnormalities.

Anything that impinges on the ostial drainage in the nose may set the stage for sinusitis. This includes foreign bodies in the nose (typically a small object placed by children, nasal packing, or intranasal tubes), tumors, and nasal polyps. For instance, researchers found that most (95%) patients who had nasogastric tubes had radiographic evidence of sinusitis (Lund, 1997; Poole, 1999).

Proper sinus drainage depends not only on patency of the osteomeatal complex, but on the mucociliary transport system. Infection in the sinuses produces an environment that impairs this function. Oxygen tension is decreased, and pH is reduced under these circumstances. Anaerobic glycolysis becomes the favored metabolic pathway for infiltrating neutrophils, and L-lactic acid is produced as a result (Lund, 1997). L-lactic acid lowers pH, causing ineffective ciliary function. Cilia usually beat at approximately 700 beats per minute, but this is reduced to approximately 300 beats per minute with infection. Ciliary action also is inhibited by viruses, bacterial toxins, smoking, and certain medications such as atropine, phenylephrine, antihistamines, and certain intranasal medications. Maxillary sinusitis is particularly problematic because the cilia have to transport the mucus superiorly through the osteomeatal complex to the nasal meatus, and if the cilia are not functioning well, then sinusitis is more likely to occur (Fagan, 1998; Lund, 1997).

Thickened mucus also inhibits the transport of the mucous from the sinuses. In cystic fibrosis, patients produce mucus with increased viscosity, making it harder to remove; thus, these patients are more prone to sinusitis. In fact, 92% to 100% of patients with cystic fibrosis have radiographic evidence of sinusitis. These patients also have more problems with nasal polyps, which can impinge on the drainage of the osteomeatal complex.

Bacteria may gain entry to the sinuses by means other than the osteomeatal system. Dental disease has been associated with 5% to 10% of patients with sinusitis. Typically, an oro-antral fistula may develop as a result of dental extractions, periodontal disease, dental fillings, and stumps of roots being pushed into the maxillary sinus. Infection can spread to the maxillary sinuses from dental abscesses or implants. Fracture of the sinuses from trauma is a rare cause for sinusitis (Lund, 1997).

The individual in Case Study 6-1 appears to have sinusitis that has progressed from an acute to a subacute sinusitis (since the symptoms have continued for about 4 weeks). Sinusitis is an infection of the paranasal sinuses that follows an URI, dental infection, allergies, or mechanical obstruction. This patient has a history of seasonal allergies and frequent colds. Because it is difficult to distinguish "cold" symptoms from allergic symptoms, there

---

### ● Case Study 6.1

A 45-year-old construction worker presents to the primary care practice with complaints of hoarseness, facial pain, constant postnasal drip, and morning headache. He recalls having a severe cold about 1 month ago that was associated with the development of the current symptoms. The symptoms have become worse within the last few days.

#### History

##### Past Medical History

| | |
|---|---|
| Allergies | Seasonal |
| Current medications | No over-the-counter medications; no prescription medications |
| Surgeries | None |
| Injury/trauma | Head injury 5 years ago after fall from scaffolding. Hospitalized × 3 days. No fractures and no sequelae. |
| Childhood illness | Immunizations current. No history (hx) influenza or pneumonia, +Hepatitis B vaccines |

##### Social History

| | |
|---|---|
| Marital status | Divorced 2 years ago; three children in custody of wife. Currently in a monogamous relationship, sexually active |
| Tobacco | Smokes 1 pack/day |

*(Case study continued on page 108)*

| | |
|---|---|
| Alcohol | Beers on weekend, occasional alcoholic beverage during week |
| Social drugs | Denies |
| Caffeine | 3 cups of coffee every morning, several Cokes every day |
| Exercise | Lots of exercise on the job |
| Employment | Construction worker, outside most of the time. Has been employed by same company for 30 years |

*Family History*

| | |
|---|---|
| Mother | Died, age 40, breast cancer |
| Father | Died, age 60, stroke |

## Review of Systems

| | |
|---|---|
| General | Feels unwell, doesn't sleep well, wakes frequently feeling like "cement is in my nose" |
| Skin | No problems. No hx rash, pruritus, lesions |
| HEENT | Wears corrective lenses for reading. Occasionally feels dizzy on arising in AM. Frequent "pounding" AM headache. Throat is slightly sore all the time |
| | Needs to blow nose frequently, drainage thick and yellow |
| | No hx thyroid disease |
| Lungs | Denies SOB at rest or on exertion. No PND. No hx asthma, pneumonia, or bronchitis. Frequent colds |
| Cardiac | Denies chest pain or palpitations at rest or on exertion |
| | No hx MRG. No prior ECG |
| GI | No nausea and vomiting |
| GU | Denies dysuria, retention, hesitancy in starting a stream |
| MS | Denies pain, tenderness, swelling of joints |
| Neurologic | Denies numbness, tingling, blackouts, seizures |

## Differential Diagnoses

1. Chronic sinusitis
2. Upper respiratory infection
3. Allergic rhinitis

## Physical Examination

| System | Findings |
|---|---|
| Vital signs | T–99.2°F, P–54, R–12 |
| | BP–130/86 sitting, 120/80 standing |
| | Height 6'2" Weight 220 lb |
| General | Alert and oriented, in no acute distress |
| | Mildly overweight adult male in NAD |
| HEENT | Normocephalic. Vision 20/20 OU corrected |
| | Cranial nerves intact. Funduscopic examination without hemorrhage or AV nicking. Optic disc margins well defined. Neck supple, no thyromegaly, no bruit, no palpable nodes. TMs clear, hearing normal at conversational levels. Throat mildly erythematous without exudate, tonsils 1+. Nose, red with yellow drainage. Sinus pain on palpation of maxillary sinuses. Frontal and maxillary sinuses do not transilluminate |

*(Case study continued on next page)*

| Lungs | CTA bilaterally. Breath sounds equal |
| Cardiac | HRRR. No MRG |
| Abdomen | Nontender. No masses. No HSM. BS in 4 quadrants |
| GU | Deferred |
| Extremities | Pulses 2+ bilateral lower and upper. No pedal edema. Skin warm, dry, and intact. Sensation intact |

### Laboratory Studies

| Test | Result |
| --- | --- |
| CBC | WBC 12,000, neutrophils 52%, monocytes 20%, lymphocytes 25%, eosinophils 2%, basophils 1% |
| CT scan of sinuses | Evidence of enlargement, fluid filled |

### Impression

Subacute sinusitis

### Physiologic Basis of Treatment Plan

Mucolytic agents such as guaifenesin, often must use the highest doses tolerated to thin the secretions and facilitate their removal

Steam vaporizers, especially in the winter, when the humidity may drop to 20% to 30%, to help liquefy secretions by adding humidity to inspired air

Intranasal steroids to reduce obstruction by decreasing inflammation of the mucosa (once-a-day dosing)

Initial antibiotic treatment can include amoxicillin, trimethoprim-sulfamethoxazole, or erythromycin. Patients with chronic sinusitis often have resistant organisms. Patients typically respond within 4 to 5 days; if they do not, the antibiotics may need to be changed (Tichenor, 1997).

AV, anterioventricular; BP, blood pressure; BS, bowel sounds; CBC, complete blood count; CT, computed tomography; CTA, clear to auscultation; ECG, electrocardiogram; GI, gastrointestinal; GU, genitourinary; HEENT, head, eye, ear, nose, and throat; HRRR, heart regular, rate and rhythm; HSM, holosystolic murmur; hx, history; MRG, murmur, rub, or gallop; MS, musculoskeletal; NAD, not in distress; P, pulse; PND, paroxysmal nocturnal dyspnea; R, respiration; SOB, shortness of breath; T, temperature; TM, tympanic membrane; WBC, white blood count.

may be some overlap. This man also smokes. Smoking can be an allergen and also can affect the proper physiologic functioning of the nose and sinuses. He is a construction worker who may be exposed to allergens or irritants (ie, dust, dirt, molds) in his work environment. This needs further investigation. Immunotherapy may be a consideration.

Patients should be advised of complications that can occur from sinusitis. Although the infection is of the sinusoidal mucosal epithelium, it may spread into surrounding tissue, including the periorbital area, leading to an acute cellulitis; to bone, causing an osteomyelitis; or to the brain, causing abscess formation of meningitis. Subacute sinusitis can progress to a chronic infection if not treated effectively. Chronic sinusitis is diagnosed when symp-

toms have been present for 3 months or longer. Therefore, follow-up of this patient is mandatory to prevent chronic sinusitis or complications from occurring, and to provide effective, holistic primary care for preventing future acute or chronic health problems. Table 6-1 depicts the recommended antibiotics, their advantages and disadvantages, and coverage provided for OM and sinusitis.

### Pharynx and Tonsils

Sore throat is a common presenting complaint of patients. Primary care providers are faced with determining whether the cause is infectious or noninfectious. Infectious causes are bacterial, viral, and fungal. Noninfectious causes include irritants such as postnasal drip, smoke, mouth

## TABLE 6.1

### Recommended Antibiotics for Otitis Media and Sinusitis

| Antibiotic | Advantages | Disadvantages | Coverage |
|---|---|---|---|
| **First-line antibiotics** | | | |
| Amoxicillin (Amoxil, Trimox, Wymox) | Inexpensive Pleasant taste | Rash in patients with mononucleosis | +Coverage *S. pneumonia* −Coverage β-lactamase–producing organisms +Anaerobic coverage |
| TMP-SMZ (Bactrim, Septra) | Inexpensive BID dosing Good if allergic to PCN | May cause rash, blood dyscrasia in susceptible patients Not for use in infants < 2 mo Poor taste | +Coverage of common ENT organisms −Anaerobic coverage |
| Erythromycin-sulfisoxazole (Pediazole) | Inexpensive Good if allergic to PCN | Primarily for children (same disadvantages as for TMP-(SMZ) Poor taste | +Coverage of common ENT organisms and anaerobes |
| **Second-line antibiotics** | | | |
| Amoxicillan and clavulanate potassium (Augmentin) (7:1) | BID dosing Pleasant taste | Expensive | ++Coverage of common ENT organisms and anaerobes |
| Cefuroxime (Ceftin) | BID dosing | Expensive Poor taste Not for use in infants < 3 mo | ++Coverage of common ENT organisms and anaerobes |
| Cefpodoxime (Vantin) | BID dosing | Expensive Poor taste Not for use in infants < 6 mo ↑ risk of *Clostridium difficile* | +Coverage of common ENT organisms and anaerobes |
| Cefproxil (Cefail) | BID dosing | Expensive Poor taste Not for use in infants < 6 mo | ++Coverage of common ENT organisms and anaerobes |
| Azithromycin (Zithromax) | Primarily once daily Dosing (1st d BID) × 5 d Good tasting | Expensive Not for use in infants < 6 mo | +Good coverage of common ENT organisms and anaerobes |
| Clarithromycin (Biaxin) | BID dosing | Expensive Poor taste Not for use in infants < 6 mo | +Coverage of common ENT organisms and anaerobes |
| **Third-line antibiotics** | | | |
| Quinolones   Levofloxacin    (Levaquin)   Trovafloxacin    (Trovan) | Once-daily dosing | Not for use in children < 18 y | ++Coverage of common ENT organisms and anaerobes |

(continued)

## TABLE 6.1 (continued)

### Recommended Antibiotics for Otitis Media and Sinusitis

| Antibiotic | Advantages | Disadvantages | Coverage |
|---|---|---|---|
| Clindamycin (Cleocin) | QID dosing | Good tasting | ++Coverage of *Streptococcus pneumoniae* and anaerobes −Coverage of β-lactamase–producing organisms |
| Ceftriaxone (Rocephin) (for otitis media only) | One dose | IM injection only Expensive | Useful in refractory cases +Coverage of common ENT organisms and anaerobes |

BID, twice daily, ENT, ear, nose and throat; IM, intramuscular; PCN, penicillin; QID, four times per day; TMP-SMZ, trimethoprim-sulfamethoxazole; +, good; ++, excellent; −, poor.
Dr. Tichenor provides a valuable web site, which is a useful resource for the primary care provider *(http://www.sinuses.com)*.

breathing, or hot food. Viral infection is the most common cause of acute pharyngitis or tonsillitis.

It is important for primary care providers to diagnose sore throats caused by the bacteria group A β-hemolytic streptococcus (GABHS). The potential sequelae from untreated streptococcal infection include rheumatic heart disease, glomerulonephritis, and suppurative complications such as mastoiditis, peritonsillar abscess, and cervical lymphadenitis. The practitioner does not want to unnecessarily treat sore throats with antibiotics. Typically, GABHS presents with a sore throat, fever, cervical adenopathy, exudative tonsillitis/pharyngitis, and occasionally petechiae on the palate. There usually is a lack of other upper respiratory symptoms and signs such as rhinitis and cough. If primary care providers use these criteria, they have a 50-50 chance of being correct in their diagnosis. Therefore, providers use rapid *Streptococcus* tests or throat cultures to help in more definitively diagnosing this condition (Perkins, 1997).

### Pharyngitis/Tonsillitis

Tonsils are composed of lymphoid tissue. However, unlike lymph nodes, they do not filter lymph. Tonsillar anatomy comprises a system of endothelium-covered channels that mediate antigen uptake and present antigen to the immune system (Richardson, 1999). The tonsils play a role in inducing secretory immunity during childhood between 3 and 10 years of age. The tonsils are ideally located to encounter foreign material and transport it to lymphoid cells. Because children are exposed to and experience multiple infections, their tonsils usually enlarge as a result of increased immunologic activity.

Although the tonsils seem to be involved immunologically, removal of the tonsils does not seem to result in a significant immune problem. Of interest, however, are findings that children who had tonsillectomies and adenoidectomies show diminished immunologic responsiveness to the poliovirus (Richardson, 1999).

### Pathophysiology of Pharyngitis/Tonsillitis

The high exposure to antigens of the tonsils stimulates B cell proliferation, antibody secretion, and T cell secretion of cytokines (Richardson, 1999). Acute pharyngotonsillitis is associated with the presence of numerous bacteria and neutrophils on the tonsillar surface. Phagocytosis occurs, and as the disease progresses, the number of bacteria and neutrophils decreases (Ebenfelt et al., 1998). The bacteria do not invade the parenchyma of the tonsillar tissue but primarily cause inflammation on the tonsillar and pharyngeal mucosa. However, with chronic or recurrent tonsillitis caused by GABHS, the bacteria eventually invade the parenchyma or core of the tonsil and participate in the development of a mixed aerobic-anaerobic flora.

Researchers theorize that the presence of more than one species of bacteria may be necessary for chronic or repeated infection. Antibiotics (penicillin) typically have been used to treat acute pharyngitis, but when it recurs, penicillin-resistant organisms become entrenched inside the tonsils (Bieluch et al., 1989; Brook et al., 1995). A longitudinal study over 16 years examining patients who had recurrent tonsillitis demonstrates a significant increase over time in the rates and types of β-lactamase–producing bacteria (BLPB) (Brook et al., 1995). With recurrent tonsillitis, penicillin is ineffective, and other second- and third-generation antibiotics are required against BLPB. The BLPB may protect the GABHS by inactivating penicillin (Brook, 1998). Other explanations are increased penicillin tolerance, reinfection, and noncompliance by the patients with their antibiotic therapy, contributing to more antibiotic resistance (Brook, 1998; Pichichero, 1998).

Vaccination may be the primary preventative strategy for recurrent tonsillitis. Brook, Yocum, and Foote (1995) noted that the rate of recovery from infection with *H. influenzae* (the primary BLPB) increased over the period ex-cept for *H. influenzae* type b. The decline in recovery of this organism was thought to result from prior immunization with *H. influenzae* type b vaccine (HiB).

The following case study demonstrates the common problems encountered in patients with ENT problems.

This child initially may have had either an URI or allergic rhinitis. The symptoms of both conditions may be similar. Initially, there was no history of fever, which suggests allergy rather than URI. However, Tim attends a preschool where he could easily have contracted an URI from other sick children.

Tim has a strong family history of allergies. His mother and sister have allergic rhinitis, and his

---

● **Case Study 6.2**

A 5-year-old white boy, Tim, presents with the chief complaint of otalgia for 1 day. His mother relates that Tim first became sick about 10 days ago with clear rhinitis and a scratchy throat. She thought it was a "cold" and treated him with Tylenol and Triaminic. He seemed to be improving until 2 days ago, when she noted the clear rhinitis had turned greenish-yellow and was thicker, and then today he woke up with his left ear hurting and difficulty hearing. He also complained of a scratchy throat and a nonproductive cough that kept him awake at night. Tim denied headaches, sinus pressure, eye drainage or redness, ear drainage or problems with his right ear, dizziness, or fever, although his mother said he felt warm last night. His mother denies that Tim has nausea, vomiting, and diarrhea. For the last day, Tim has had a decreased appetite, although he has continued to drink plenty of fluids.

### Pertinent Medical History

#### History of a Similar Illness

Tim has a history of two to three episodes of otitis media per year for the last 2 years, occurring primarily during the winter. The last episode was 1 month ago. He was treated with amoxicillin for 10 days. He did not return for a recheck.

#### Neonatal and Developmental History

Tim was the product of a full-term pregnancy and is one of three children. Birth weight was 7 lb 2 oz. Pregnancy and neonatal period were without complication, and well-child examinations conducted at this office demonstrate appropriate achievement of developmental milestones. Childhood immunizations are current. Tim attends a local preschool. Both parents work outside of the home.

#### Family History

| | |
|---|---|
| Father | Age 35; asthma; smokes × 15 years |
| Mother | Age 32; allergic rhinitis |
| Female sibling | Age 10; asthma/allergic rhinitis |
| Male sibling | Age 4; no known health problems |

Denies family hx atopic dermatitis, food allergies, recent streptococcal infection

*(Case study continued on next page)*

*Present Medications*

Tylenol for ear pain
Discontinued using Triaminic when Tim seemed to be improving

*Allergies*

None known

## Differential Diagnoses

1. Viral upper respiratory infection
2. Acute otitis media
3. Otitis media with effusion
4. Otitis externa
5. Allergic rhinitis
6. Acute bronchitis/asthma
7. Sinusitis
8. Streptococcal pharyngitis
9. Viral pharyngitis

## Objective Information

| | |
|---|---|
| Vital signs | T–100°F, P–100, R–18, BP–90/60<br>Weight 40 lb Height 45 inches |
| General | Alert, oriented to person, place, and time; active and playful |
| Ears | Auricle and tragus: Nontender with movement<br>Mastoid: Nontender; small amount yellow cerumen; no drainage<br>Left TM: Bulging; red; no landmarks visible; no mobility noted<br>Right TM: Landmarks visible, light reflex diffuse; retracted; no redness |
| Sinuses | Nontender maxillary sinuses |
| Nose | Nonpatent; mouth breathing; yellow discharge visible; turbinates enlarged and red |
| Throat | Slight redness, cobblestoning; slight postnasal drainage seen; tonsils 2+ enlarged, no redness or exudates |
| Neck | Tonsillar lymph nodes enlarged and tender; several shotty, movable, tender cervical lymph nodes palpated; supple |
| Chest | No use of accessory muscles, retractions; respirations symmetrical; resonant; no adventitious sounds |
| Heart | Normal sinus rhythm; no murmurs, gallops, or extra sounds |
| Abdomen | Soft, nontender; bowel sounds normal; no organomegaly or masses |
| Genitourinary | Deferred |

## Assessment

1. Left acute otitis media
2. Sinusitis
3. Secondary exposure to smoke
4. Strong family history of allergies/asthma

*(Case study continued on page 114)*

### Plan

1. Auralgan ear gtts: fill ear canal and insert cotton plug; repeat every 1–2 h PRN for the 1–2 d
2. Tylenol for fever and pain
3. Saline nose spray to use every 4 h; education regarding nose blowing and other methods to thin and remove secretions
4. Amoxicillin-clavulanate 250 mg TID × 14 d
5. Sudafed 30 mg every 4–6 h
6. RTC if the signs and symptoms become worse at any time or they do not improve in 48–72 h
7. RTC in 2 weeks for a recheck
8. Work with the family to have the father cease smoking or at the very least to go outside of the house to smoke, not smoke in the car, or around the children
9. Give pneumococcal and influenza vaccine on return visit if appropriate time of year and history reveals the need for these immunizations

BP, blood pressure; gtts, drops; P, pulse; R, respiration; RTC, return to clinic; T, temperature; TM, tympanic membrane.

father and sister have asthma. He does not seem to have a personal history of allergies, although he has been having two to three episodes of AOM in the winter, which might be precipitated by either URIs or allergic rhinitis. He is exposed to a known allergen: his father's smoking.

In this illness, Tim seemed to be improving, and then he worsened, as evidenced by the change from clear to greenish yellow rhinitis and the start of his fever, cough, and earache. These factors may indicate double sickening, or a secondary bacterial infection of his left middle ear and sinuses. AOM and sinusitis do occur simultaneously, since similar pathophysiologic mechanisms and the same bacterial organisms can cause infections in both areas (Lindbaek et al., 1996; O'Brian et al., 1998; Van Buchem et al., 1997).

The diagnosis of acute OM was fairly straightforward. Tim presented with otalgia after having upper respiratory symptoms. This is a typical presentation for acute OM; however, it is important to keep other etiologies that can cause pain in the differential diagnoses and remember that there may be multiple etiologies present. The physical findings of a red, bulging TM immediately suggested the diagnosis of acute OM.

Children may not present with the usual history and physical findings found in adults with sinusitis. For instance, children may not have a headache or sinus pressure. Tim's major subjective findings related to sinusitis were the change in color and consistency of his nasal drainage and his cough (usually more bothersome in the supine position with postnasal drainage from sinusitis), and the objective findings included his enlarged, red turbinates plus a slightly elevated temperature (indicating infection).

The diagnosis of bacterial sinusitis typically is made from the subjective and objective data. Radiologic testing may be needed if the history reveals recurring episodes of sinusitis or chronic sinusitis, if complications are suspected, or the if diagnosis is unclear. This was the first episode of sinusitis for this patient, who will be treated with antibiotics for AOM and sinusitis. Follow-up is important to be sure that the conditions resolve. If not, then radiology might be needed to determine the extent and location of the sinusitis and to look for anatomic abnormalities.

Radiology is an important diagnostic aid for sinusitis; however, in addition to being expensive, the results may be confusing. Sinus x-rays and CT can be misleading because both can be abnormal in asymptomatic patients. This may result from the fact that mucosal changes in the sinuses occur after most URIs and may not resolve for a variable length of time (Jones, 1999). Researchers found that 90% of patients with a viral respiratory illness had an abnormal finding from CT of the maxillary sinuses in the first 48 to 96 hours of their illness. All recovered without antibiotics, with radiologic clearing of the sinuses after approximately 2 weeks.

## Physiologic Basis for Treatment

### Antibiotics

Remember that the treatment of acute viral URIs, allergic rhinitis, and acute viral sinusitis will not benefit from antibiotics. Several studies show that antibiotics offer little or no additional benefit to the symptomatic or placebo treatment of acute viral sinusitis (Lindbaek et al., 1996; O'Brian et al., 1998; Van Buchem et al., 1997). Only a small percentage (0.5% to 5%) of adults with URIs have the complication of bacterial sinusitis; however, with children, this increases to 5% to 10%. Bacterial sinusitis usually is treated with antibiotics and adjunctive therapy.

Most cases of AOM and bacterial sinusitis (approximately 60%) resolve spontaneously without antibiotics. Researchers find that complications do occur in a few of these patients. Because patients with illness that will resolve spontaneously cannot be distinguished from those who may have problems, the usual treatment for AOM and bacterial sinusitis involves using antibiotics. Antibiotics usually are chosen empirically by knowing the common organisms that typically cause sinusitis and AOM, and knowing the bacterial resistance present in the patient's community. First-line drugs are amoxicillin and trimethoprim-sulfamethoxazole (if the patient is allergic to penicillin). Second-line drugs should be used if there are penicillin-resistant organisms or β-lactamase–producing organisms in the community, if there is a lack of response in 48 to 72 hours, or if a patient has used antibiotics frequently or has chronic sinusitis. Chronic sinusitis may be caused by anaerobic bacteria (see Table 6-1 for common antibiotics used to treat sinusitis).

Because of the increase in antibiotic resistance, researchers are investigating the use of shorter courses of antibiotics rather than the usual 10-day course for the treatment of OM. A shorter course would facilitate the use of the antibiotic because patients are more likely to take an antibiotic once a day for 5 days (usual dosage for azithromycin) rather than three times a day for 10 days (usual dosage for amoxicillin). Also, findings indicate that the shorter courses may not increase antibiotic resistance as much as the 10-day course (Cohen et al., 1999).

With most antibiotics, a longer duration of treatment (10 to 14 days or longer) is standard practice for acute sinusitis (Cunha, 1998; Ferguson & Johnson, 1999; Poole, 1999). Tim was treated with a second-line antibiotic because he had been treated a month ago with an antibiotic for AOM. He did not return for his follow-up appointment, so the first episode of AOM may not have cleared completely and he may have had a bacterial organism that was resistant to amoxicillin. Follow-up of this episode is important to ensure that the etiologies are properly treated. Sometimes the patient may need longer therapy or a change in therapy. For instance, a change in antibiotics may be needed if the AOM or sinusitis has not resolved. OM with effusion can be a sequela after the patient has been treated for AOM, and if this occurs, then further follow-up is needed.

### Adjunctive Treatment

Once the diagnoses have been made, several non-pharmacologic methods can aid the mucociliary system in removing the excess mucus from the nose and sinuses. Simple methods involve nose blowing and saline sprays or irrigation. Saline may temporarily decrease the size of the mucous membranes and thin the mucus, thereby aiding in drainage through the ostia and eustachian tube. Both methods can be repeated as often as needed without causing harm. Steam inhalations, warm compresses, plenty of oral fluids, astringents (pine oil and menthol), spicy foods, and mucoevacuants such as guaifenesin also may be used to aid in mucus removal.

Both topical and systemic decongestants may be used to improve eustachian and ostiomeatal drainage by vasoconstricting the vascular mucosa and reducing the congestion. Topical nasal decongestants can be effective in local improvement without systemic side effects; however, use is limited to 3 to 4 days because of rebound congestion and swelling of the mucosa, known as rhinitis medicamentosa. If longer use is needed, then oral decongestants may be needed; however, systemic side effects with the oral medications may occur. These symptoms may be nervousness, insomnia, tachycardia, and hypertension. Controversy exists about the benefit of treating with decongestants because of conflicting research results.

Antihistamines generally are contraindicated for patients with sinusitis and acute OM because of their anticholinergic side effects, which can impede the clearance of secretions by increasing the viscosity, and their affect on the proper functioning of the cilia. Allergic patients, however, may need topical or oral antihistamines and topical nasal steroids. Avoiding the allergen is paramount, but if avoidance is impossible, immunotherapy may be needed (see Chapter 7 for further details).

Although it is uncertain that Tim is an allergic child, it is known that exposure to his father's smoking is a potential allergen/irritant in Tim's environment. Talking with Tim's father would be important to explain the impact of his smoking on

Tim's health and explore the father's feelings about quitting. Realizing the repercussions that smoking has on his own health along with his son's health may inspire him to quit. At that point, different methods to help him quit may be discussed.

Analgesics can be prescribed to relieve otalgia. Acetaminophen (Tylenol) helps to relieve the pain and reduce the fever, therefore making Tim feel better. Auralgan contains a topical analgesia and anesthetic, which relieves the pain associated with AOM. It also contains glycerin, which uses hygroscopic activity to decrease the middle ear pressure because of fluid osmosis through the TM. Research reveals that Auralgan reduces moderate to severe otalgia more effectively than olive oil or sweet oil (placebo) in patients with AOM (Hoberman et al., 1997).

Rarely, complications occur as a result of either AOM or sinusitis. Educating the patient and family about the signs and symptoms of these complications is important so that they can alert the primary care provider if they occur. Complications of AOM may be mastoiditis and meningitis; complications of sinusitis may be abscesses and meningitis. These may present with symptoms such as fever, mastoid tenderness, headache, nuchal rigidity or tenderness, and altered mental status.

As more organisms become resistant, administering vaccines against the most common pathogens causing health problems such as OM and sinusitis may be the best preventative measure. Currently available are the pneumococcal vaccine, HiB, and influenza immunization directed against *S. pneumoniae* and *H. influenzae*. However, multiple strains of these organisms have not been identified and are not covered by immunization. Research is ongoing in vaccine development.

Another preventative measure for allergic patients is immunotherapy, especially for patients having chronic problems with sinusitis and OM. Only the present episode of sinusitis was documented for Tim, but he has had multiple episodes of OM and has a strong family history of allergies. If he continues to have problems, he may need further workup to determine if he is an allergic child and would benefit from immunotherapy.

## EYE

### Conjunctivitis

The primary care practitioner generally should refer eye injuries and most eye disease to ophthalmologic specialists. However, one common inflammation is diagnosed and managed often in primary care. Conjunctivitis (by common parlance, pink eye) is an inflammation of the conjunctiva, usually caused by bacterial or viral infection, although allergic conjunctivitis is common in atopic individuals.

A bacterial conjunctivitis leads to purulent drainage, redness, and itchiness. Common organisms are *H. influenzae*, *S. pneumoniae*, and *Staphylococcus aureus*. Prompt treatment with an antibacterial eye ointment is necessary. Poor hygiene and improper care and wearing of contact lenses are risk factors, and corneal ulceration may occur, leading to eye damage and visual problems. Viral conjunctivitis is less common, and conjunctivitis often is associated with other viral illness symptoms. The eye is red, itchy, and painful with photophobia. Whereas adenoviruses are the most common origin, the practitioner should be aware of herpes simplex as a potential cause, since this virus can lead to blindness. Allergic conjunctivitis causes people to experience redness, tearing, and itchiness from atopic reactivity. This type of conjunctivitis is seasonal and usually is associated with allergic rhinitis.

## REFERENCES

Bieluch, V.M., Chasin, W.D., Martin, E.T., & Tally, F.P. (1989). Recurrent tonsillitis: Histologic and bacteriologic evaluation. *Annals of Otological and Rhinological Laryngology, 98*, 332–335.

Bisno, A.L., Gerber, M.A., Gwaltney, J.M., Kaplan, E.L., & Schwartz, R.H. (1997). Diagnosis and management of Group A streptococcal pharyngitis: A practice guideline. *Clinical Infectious Diseases, 25*, 574–583.

Bluestone, C.D. (1998). Otitis media: To treat or not to treat? *Consultant, 38* (6) 1421–1433.

Bluestone, C.D. & Klein, J.O. (1995). *Otitis media in infants and children* (2nd ed.). Philadelphia: WB Saunders.

Brook, I. (1998). Microbiology of common infections in the upper respiratory tract. *Primary Care, 25* (3), 633–647.

Brook, I., Yocum, P., & Foote, P.A. (1995). Changes in the core tonsillar bacteriology of recurrent tonsillitis: 1977–1993. *Clinical Infectious Diseases, 21*, 171–176.

Bylander-Groth, A. & Stenstrom, C. (1998). Eustachian tube function and otitis media in children. *Ear, Nose, and Throat Journal, 77* (9), 762–769.

Cantor, R.M. (1999). Otitis externa: Not always simple. *Emergency Medicine, 31* (2), 40–60.

Carlson, L.H. & Fall, P.A. (1998). Otitis media: An update. *Journal of Pediatric Health Care, 12* (6), 313–319.

Cohen, R., Naval, M., Grunberg, J., Boucherat, M., Geslin, P., Derriennie, M., Pichon, F., & Goehrs, J.M. (1999). One dose ceftriaxone vs. ten days of amoxicillan/clavulanate therapy for acute otitis media: Clinical efficacy and change in nasopharyngeal flora. *Pediatric Infectious Disease, 18* (5), 403–409.

Cunha, B.A. (1998). Acute sinusitis. *Emergency Medicine, 30* (2), 134–141.

Daley, K.A., Hunter, L.L., & Glebink, G.S. (1999). Chronic otitis media with effusion. *Pediatrics in Review, 20* (3), 85–93.

Damjanov, I. & Linder, J. (1996). *Anderson's Pathophysiology* (10th ed.). St. Louis: Mosby.

Dowell, S.F., Marcy, S.M., Phillips, W.R., Gerber, M.A., & Schwartz, B. (1998). Principles of judicious use of antimicrobial agents for the pediatric upper respiratory tract infections. *Pediatrics, 101* (1), 163–174.

Ebenfelt, A., Ericson, L.E., & Lundberg, C. (1998). Acute pharyngitis is an infection restricted to the crypt and surface secretion. *Acta Oto-Laryngology (Stockh), 118* (2), 264–271.

Fagan, L.J. (1998). Acute sinusitis: A cost-effective approach to diagnosis and treatment. *American Family Physician, 58* (8), 1795–1801.

Ferguson, B.J. & Johnson, J.T. (1999). Allergic rhinitis and rhinosinusitis. Is there a connection between allergy and infection? *Postgraduate Medicine 105* (4), 55–64.

Gungor, A. (1998). Fungal sinusitis: Progression of disease in immunosuppression. A case report. *Ear, Nose, and Throat Journal, 77* (3), 207–215.

Havens, P.L. (1998). Acute otitis media in children: What next when first-line therapy fails? *Consultant, 38* (11), 2681–2690.

Hueston, W.J., Eberlein, C., Johnson, D., & Mainous, A.G. (1998). Criteria used by clinicians to differentiate sinusitis from viral upper respiratory tract infection. *The Journal of Family Practice, 46* (6), 487–492.

Hoberman, A., Paradise, J.L., Reynolds, E.A., & Urkin, J. (1997). Efficacy of auralgan for treating ear pain in children with acute otitis media. *Archives of Pediatric and Adolescent Medicine, 151,* 675–678.

International Rhinosinusitis Advisory Board (1997). Infectious rhinosinusitis in adults: Classification, etiology and management. *ENT Journal, 76* (12 Suppl.), 1–22.

Jones, N.S. (1999). Current concepts in the management of paediatric rhinosinusitis. *The Journal of Laryngology and Otology, 113,* 1–9.

Kvaerner, K., Nafstad, P., Hagen, J.A., Mair, I.W.S., & Jaakkola, J.J.K. (1997). Recurrent acute otitis media: The significance of age at onset. *Acta Oto-Laryngology (Stockh), 117* (4), 578–584.

La Rosa, S. (1998). Primary care management of otitis externa. *The Nurse Practitioner, 23* (6), 125–133.

Licameli, G.R. (1999). Diagnosis and management of otalgia in the pediatric patient. *Pediatric Annals, 28* (6), 364–368.

Lindbaek, M., Hjortdahl P., & Johnson U.L. (1996). Randomized, double blind, placebo controlled trial of penicillin V and amoxicillan in treatment of acute sinus infections in adults. *British Medicine Journal, 313,* 325–329.

Lindsay, R., Tomazic, T., Whitman, B.Y., & Accardo, P.J. (1999). Early ear problems and developmental problems at school age. *Clinical Pediatrics, 38* (3), 123–131.

Maltinski, G. (1998). Nasal disorders and sinusitis. *Primary Care, 25* (3), 663–681.

Marchisio, P., Principi, N., Passali, D., Salpietro, D.C., Boschi, G., Chetri, G., Caramia, G., Longhi, R., Reali, E., Meloni, G., De Santis, A., Sacher, B., & Cupido, G. (1998). Epidemiology and treatment of otitis media with effusion in children in the first year of primary school. *Acta Oto-Laryngology (Stockh), 118* (4), 557–562.

Miura, M., Takahashi, H., Honjo, I., Hasebe, S., & Tanabe, M. (1998). Influence of the upper respiratory tract infection on tubal compliance in children with otitis media with effusion. *Acta Oto-Laryngology (Stockh), 117* (4), 574–577.

Nell, M.J. & Grote, J.J. (1999). Structural changes in the rat middle ear mucosa due to endotoxin and eustachian tube obstruction. *European Archives of Otorhinolaryngology, 256* (4), 167–172.

Nemechek, A.J., Pahlavan, N., & Cote, D.N. (1997). Nebulized surfactant for experimentally induced otitis media with effusion. *Otolaryngology—Head and Neck Surgery, 117* (5), 475–479.

O'Brian, K.L., Dowell, S.F., Schwartz, B., Marcy, S.M., Phillips, W.R., & Gerber, M.A. (1998). Acute sinusitis: Principles of judicious use of antimicrobial agents. *Pediatrics, 101,* 174–177.

Ovesen, T. & Borglum, J.D. (1998). New aspects of secretory otitis media, eustachian tube function, and middle ear gas. *Ear, Nose, and Throat Journal, 77* (9), 770–776.

Perkins, A. (1997). An approach to diagnosing the acute sore throat. *American Family Physician, 55* (1), 131–137.

Pichichero, M. (1998). Group A beta-hemolytic streptococcal infections. *Pediatrics in Review, 19* (9), 291–302.

Poole, M.D. (1999). A focus on acute sinusitis in adults: Changes in disease management. *The American Journal of Medicine, 106* (5A), 38S–47S.

Puhakka, T., Makela, M.J., & Alanen, A. (1998). Sinusitis in the common cold. *Journal of Allergy and Clinical Immunology, 102,* 403–408.

Prades, J.M., Dumollard, J.M., Calloc'h, F., Merzougui, N., Veyret, C., & Martin, C. (1998). Descriptive anatomy of the human auditory tube. *Surgical and Radiologic Anatomy, 20* (5), 335–340.

Ray, N.F., Baraniuk, J.N., Thamer, M., Rinehart, C.S., Gergen, P.J., Kaliner, M., Josephs, S., & Pung, Y.H. (1999). Healthcare expenditures for sinusitis in 1996: Contributions of asthma, rhinitis, and other airway disorders. *Journal of Allergy and Clinical Immunology, 103* (3), 408–414.

Richardson, M.A. (1999). Sore throat, tonsillitis, and adenoiditis. *Medical Clinics of North America, 83* (1), 75–83.

Slavin, R.G. (1993). Ten questions physicians often ask. *Consultant, 33* (2), 65–68.

Suzuki, C., Balaban, C., Sando, I., Sudo, M., Ganbo, T., & Kitagawa, M. (1998). Postnatal development of eustachian tube: A computer-aided 3-D reconstruction and measurement study. *Acta Otolaryngology, 118* (6), 837–843.

Suzuki, M., Watanabe, T., Suko, T., & Mogi, G. (1999). Comparison of sinusitis with and without allergic rhinitis: Characteristics of paranasal sinus effusion and mucosa. *American Journal of Otolaryngology, 20* (3), 143–150.

Takahashi, H., Miura, M., & Honjo, I. (1996). Cause of eustachian tube constriction during swallowing in patients with otitis media with effusion. *Annals of Otology and Laryngology, 105,* 724–728.

Takahashi, H., Hayashi, M., & Honjo, I. (1986). Compliance of the eustachian tube in patients with otitis media with effusion. *American Journal of Otoloaryngology, 3,* 154–156.

Tarlow, M. (1998). Otitis media: Pathogenesis and medical sequelae. *Ear, Nose, and Throat Journal, Supplement, 77* (6), 3–5.

Tichenor, W. (1997). Sinusitis: A practical guide for physicians. *Medscape Respiratory Care 1* (7). Available at: http://www.medscape.com.

Van Buchem, F.L., Knottnerus, J.A., Schrijnmaekers, V.J., & Peeters, M.F. (1997). Primary care based randomized placebo-controlled trial of antibiotic treatment in acute maxillary sinusitis. *Lancet, 349,* 683–687.

Wright, E.D., Pearl, A.J., & Manoukian, J.J. (1998). Laterally hypertrophic adenoids as a contributing factor in otitis media. *International Journal of Pediatric Otorhinolaryngology, 45*(3), 207–214.

# Allergic Rhinitis

Timothy L. Jones

Allergic rhinitis is an immunologic disease that significantly impacts the lives of those with allergy. Allergic rhinitis usually is a lifelong disease, peaking between 20 and 50 years of age, with some variability (Naclerio & Solomon, 1997). Allergic rhinitis costs over $5 billion dollars per year in medications alone, 26.1 million cases of allergic rhinitis are reported annually, and it is a significant cause of lost productivity and missed school days (Georgitis et al., 1997; Hulisz & Fillwock, 1996; Adams & Marano, 1995). According to the National Center for Health Statistics, allergic rhinitis is a chronic condition in 10.1% of the population (all ages and sexes) (Adams & Marano, 1995). Misery is the true high cost of allergic rhinitis unless it is treated effectively. Primary symptoms of allergic rhinitis are ocular itching and tearing, rhinorrhea, repetitive and paroxysmal sneezing, nasal pruritus, nasal congestion, sinus tenderness, postnasal drainage (PND), and palatal itching. Common associated symptoms occurring secondary to the primary symptoms include headaches, conjunctivitis, earaches, cough, hoarseness, sore throat, nausea, halitosis, malaise, and fatigue (Lierl, 1995; Naclerio, 1991; Druce, 1993). Cough, hoarseness, sore throat, and nausea often result from PND. Symptoms may be seasonal or perennial but still are considered chronic rhinitis (Druce, 1993). Perennial allergic rhinitis results primarily from allergy to house dust, dust mites, molds, animal proteins, and cockroaches (Lierl, 1995; Druce, 1993). Common signs of allergic rhinitis include allergic shiners (bluish discoloration under the eyes from venous congestion), allergic nasal crease, the allergic salute (constant hand-wiping of the nose), mouth breathing, posterior pharyngeal wall lymphatic hyperplasia (cobblestoning), pale nasal mucosa (irregular mucosal surface is seen with chronic disease), and clear and watery nasal discharge (Naclerio, 1991). The key symptoms of allergic rhinitis that differentiate it from other causes include those caused by the release of histamine and other mast cell granulation products, such as itching and sneezing. In addition, symptoms noticed after exposure to an identified allergen also are hallmark signs of allergic rhinitis (Naclerio, 1991).

Allergic rhinitis can be managed within primary care practices; however, board-certified allergists are highly recommended for patients with perennial allergic rhinitis, patients with asthma when therapy fails, or when immunotherapy may be beneficial. Wherever allergic rhinitis is managed, the care provider must be knowledgeable regarding the common trees, grasses, molds, the abundance of ragweed, and their seasonal peak levels. Features of the local climate (humidity, temperature changes, pollution, rainfall, temperature) also are of great use in managing allergic rhinitis.

Complications often associated with allergic rhinitis include nasal polyps, anatomic abnormalities (concha bullosa, facial bone maldevelopment), acute sinusitis, chronic sinusitis, epistaxis, asthma, atopic dermatitis, conjunctivitis, eustachian tube dysfunction, recurrent serous otitis media, sleep disturbances, impaired concentration, and a diminished quality of life (Lierl, 1995; Georgitis et al., 1997). Secretory otitis media may cause hearing loss and impaired learning and speech (Lierl, 1995). Acute sinusitis is common because of chronic inflammation of the nasal mucosa, which can interfere with mucociliary clearance of the sinuses. Chronic sinusitis is a chronic inflammation of the mucosa of any sinus (ethmoid, sphenoid, maxillary, frontal) or blockage of the osteomeatal units. This complication often is overlooked in primary care, but it should be included as a high priority in the differential diagnosis of any patient with recurrent acute sinusitis with a history of allergic rhinitis. Because chronic sinusitis is present in 13.4% of the population, this complication must be considered and monitored for in patients with allergic rhinitis (Adams & Marano, 1995).

Chronic sinusitis is diagnosed by history and computed tomography (limited coronal of paranasal sinuses) (Slavin, 1993; Ransom, 1997). Computed tomography is the gold standard because it detects sinus mucosal thickening by the millimeter and visualizes bony anatomy, sinus opacification, and the osteomeatal units (Lierl, 1995; Corren et al., 1996; Slavin, 1993). Chronic sinusitis is defined as mucosal thickening of greater than 6 to 8 mm or blockage of the osteomeatal unit, which drains the sinus into the nasal cavity (Lierl, 1995; Slavin, 1993). Chronic sinusitis often requires 3 to 8 weeks of antibiotics for cure, and it is best to use an antibiotic with good anaerobic coverage because of the low $Po_2$ within inflamed sinuses (Lierl, 1995; Slavin, 1993) (Table 7-1).

## PATHOGENESIS

### Genetics

The genetic influence in allergy is not clear. Some studies have determined that specific IgE responsiveness (major histocompatibility complex [MHC] linked) and the control of the production (non-MHC linked) of IgE antibodies is under genetic control. These studies suggest an autosomal dominant trait for transmission of atopy, but that is probably too simple an explanation for the marked heterogeneity of expression of atopy as a trait. Candidate genes are being identified on chromosomes 5, 11, and 14 (Lemanske & Busse, 1997). The interaction of environmental and genetic influences need to be delineated in future research (Huang & Marsh, 1993).

### Aeroallergens

Inhaled allergens (aeroallergens) are the inflicting substances that induce symptoms. Aeroallergenic proteins are relatively large and are multivalent in binding to IgE (Li, 1998). Allergic diseases are increasing, partially because of industrialization (Takenaka et al., 1995). For example, ragweed spores are stirred up with industrialization, spread by the air, and settle on the ground (Naclerio & Solomon, 1997). The ragweed spores then can remain on the surface of the ground for up to 8 years (Naclerio & Solomon, 1997). Specific characteristics of certain allergens make them highly allergenic. The ragweed allergen has the appearance of a ball covered with spikes, which allows it to easily attach to nasal mucosa in a mechanical fashion. Studies show that polyaromatic hydrocarbons from diesel exhaust increase IgE antibody production (once sensitization has occurred) (Takenaka et al., 1995). This adds to the overall clinical and pathophysiologic responses to IgE (Takenaka et al., 1995).

Certain inhaled allergens have seasonal patterns. Ragweed season is in the fall, beginning in August and extending until early October (Hulisz & Fillwock, 1996). Trees bloom from March through May (Hulisz & Fillwock, 1996). Various plants and grasses bloom in May until July (Hulisz & Fillwock, 1996). Airborne mold spores are prevalent in the middle of March and extend until November (Hulisz & Fillwock, 1996).

Inhaled allergens may cause perennial allergic rhinitis. House dust and dust mites are the most notorious for year-round symptoms. *Dust mites* are about $1/3$ mm long (which is not visible with the naked eye) and require water (from humidity) to survive (Platts-Mills & Chapman, 1987). Humans are allergic to the feces (in house dust) of dust mites and may be allergic to the dust mite itself. *Cockroaches* also may cause perennial symptoms. Even in a home without cockroaches, decayed cockroach exoskeleton proteins are spread by wind and may settle within the home. *House dust* may be a combination of fibers, dust mite feces, dead dust mites, cockroach proteins, mold spores, pollen, and other rodent droppings. *Mold* also can cause perennial symptoms if the residence has areas of mold growth (basements, plants, carpet, and plasterboard that has been wet).

### Sensitization

Sensitization must first occur for the allergic response to take place. Generally, it takes about 3 years to become sensitized to a specific allergen (Adelman & Saxon, 1995). On exposure to an allergen (after the allergen penetrates through nasal mucosa), macrophages process and then present the allergen (antigen-MHC complex) to CD4 T-lymphocytes (Shames & Adelman, 1997; Adelman & Saxon, 1995). B-lymphocytes then are stimulated, or activated, by activated type 2 T-helper ($T_H2$) cells and cytokines, most notably interleukin-4 (IL-4), IL-5, and IL-13 (Lierl, 1995; Adelman & Saxon, 1995; Naclerio & Solomon, 1997). B cells then differentiate into antibody-producing cells (plasma cells) (Adelman & Saxon, 1995; Naclerio & Solomon, 1997). Plasma cells produce IgE specific for that antigen (Adelman &

## TABLE 7.1  ● ● ●

### Allergic Rhinitis: Differential Diagnoses

| | |
|---|---|
| Allergic rhinitis | Seasonal vs perennial |
| Vasomotor (nonallergic) rhinitis | Gustatory, especially with alcohol ingestion, aromatic, changes in air temperature, weather fronts, irritants, hypersensitivity, other (lying down, allergic rhinitis, or other conditions causing chronic nasal inflammation) (Li, 1998; Lierl, 1995; Naclerio & Solomon, 1997) |
| Infectious rhinitis | Viral, bacterial, fungal (Michelini, 1996) |
| NARES (Lierl, 1995) | In adults, about 15% of chronic rhinitis that is not a result of anatomy is caused by NARES (Lierl, 1995) |
| Nasal polyposis (Michelini, 1996) | |
| Rhinitis medicamentosis (Michelini, 1996) | Including nasal sprays such as Migranal and Miacalcin (USP DI, 1997) |
| Asthma (Hulisz & Fillwock, 1996) | Asthma often is associated with allergic rhinitis; sometimes allergic rhinitis can develop into asthma (discussed in Chapter 8) |
| Chronic sinusitis (Georgitis et al., 1997) | |
| Acute sinusitis (Naclerio & Solomon, 1997; Georgitis et al., 1997) | |
| Drug-induced rhinitis | Many older antihypertensive agents, beta blockers, vasodilators, alpha blockers, ACE inhibitors (Druce, 1993; Hulisz & Fillwock, 1996) |
| Septal deviation (Michelini, 1996) | |
| Choanal atresia (Naclerio & Solomon, 1997) | |
| Nasal obstruction | Concha bullosa, foreign body (Lierl, 1995) |
| Nasal mastocytosis (Druce, 1993) | |
| Atrophic rhinitis (Druce, 1993) | |
| Tumor (Michelini, 1996) | |
| Granulomatous rhinitis | Wegener's granulomatosis, sarcoidosis, rhinoscleromatosis, polychondritis (Michelini, 1996; Druce, 1993) |
| Cystic fibrosis (Naclerio & Solomon, 1997; Georgitis et al., 1997) | |
| Hypothyroidism (Michelini, 1996) | |
| Pregnancy (Druce, 1993) | |

ACE, angiotensin-converting enzyme; NARES, nonallergic rhinitis with eosinophilia.

Saxon, 1995). IgE synthesis is further supported by IL-4 most notably, but IL-5, IL-6, and tumor necrosis factor (TNF) also support its synthesis (Leung, 1996). IgE antibodies then attach to high-affinity receptors on mast cells and basophils (also monocytes, eosinophils, and platelets) (Naclerio, 1991; Adelman & Saxon, 1995).

### Early-Phase Reaction

Within minutes of reexposure to an allergen, a cascade of immunologic events occurs. Within 15 to 60 minutes, clinical evidence of the allergic response becomes evident, mainly because of histamine (Shames & Adelman, 1997; Leung, 1996).

The inciting allergen or antigen attaches to bound IgE antibodies on mast cells (Naclerio, 1991). Mast cells, by virtue of their residence in tissue and plentiful numbers, are the key cells in allergic inflammation. The binding of allergen to the IgE causes these complexes to aggregate on cell surface, and this produces a signal for the cell to become activated and then to degranulate. This process is illustrated in Figure 7-1. The mast cell acutely degranulates, releasing histamine, proteases, tosyl-L-arginine methyl ester esterase (TAME-esterase), leukotrienes, prostaglandins, kinins, and other intragranular substances (Lierl, 1995; Shames & Adelman, 1997; Adelman & Saxon, 1995). The preformed mediators (histamine, proteases, TAME-esterase, kinins) have immediate activity within the nasal mucosa and vascular system, producing rhinitis symptoms (Druce, 1993). Chemotactic factors also are released by mast cells and basophils, which recruit neutrophils and eosinophils (Adelman & Saxon, 1995). The increase of neutrophils and eosinophils into the nasal tissues increases the intensity of symptoms in the early phase (Iliopoulos et al., 1990). New mediators are formed from arachidonic acid, such as leukotrienes, prostaglandin $D_2$ ($PGD_2$), platelet-activating factor (PAF), and other arachidonic acid metabolites. Most of these mediators play a larger role in the late-phase reaction (Shames & Adelman, 1997; Adelman & Saxon,

1995). Basophils also are involved by releasing kininogens (Shames & Adelman, 1997). In the early-phase reaction, there is also a mild influx of granulocytes into the involved tissues (Shames & Adelman, 1997). Epithelial cells also contribute to the allergic reaction by secreting the cytokines IL-6, IL-8, and granulocyte-macrophage colony-stimulating factor (GM-CSF). These cytokines promote B-cell differentiation, regulate histamine release, attract neutrophils (chemotaxis), stimulate basophil histamine release, enhance eosinophil's toxic effects, and increase granulocytes, macrophages, and eosinophils (Naclerio & Solomon, 1997; Adelman et al., 1995). After about 30 to 90 minutes, this phase of the allergic response begins to dissipate (Leung, 1996).

These immunologic mediators cause smooth muscle contraction, vasodilation, and vascular permeability, resulting in mucosal edema (Lierl, 1995; Shames & Adelman, 1997). Prostaglandins and thromboxanes have little known clinical significance in allergic rhinitis (Barnes, 1993). Histamine is responsible for most clinical symptoms. Erythema, itching, sneezing, and rhinorrhea are caused by the irritation of nerve endings and secretory glands by histamine (Shames & Adelman, 1997). Bradykinin and serotonin also promote rhinorrhea, congestion, and a sore throat (Naclerio, 1991; Proud et al., 1988). Leukotrienes may promote edema, vascular leakage, and chemotaxis (Busse, 1996). The parasympathetic nervous system is activated by these mediators, resulting in the release of acetylcholine, causing the secretion of mucus (Shames & Adelman, 1997; Naclerio & Solomon, 1997). Other actions of these mediators include promoting the generation of prostaglandins, activation of suppressor T-lymphocytes, and chemotaxis (Wasserman, 1997).

To summarize the early phase of allergy, mast cell degranulation causes the release of immunologic mediators (most notably histamine), which affects blood vessels, nerves, and glands in the respiratory tract. This reaction causes sneezing, rhinorrhea, mucus production, congestion, and pruritus (Naclerio, 1991; Shames & Adelman, 1997). The pathophysiologic effects and presence of histamine, leukotrienes, adenosine, $PGD_2$, and PAF are enough to produce the clinical responses seen in the early-phase reaction (Wasserman, 1997).

### Late-Phase Reaction

The early-phase reaction is associated with the breakdown of the phospholipid layer of the mast cell, releasing arachidonic acid (Frazee et al.,

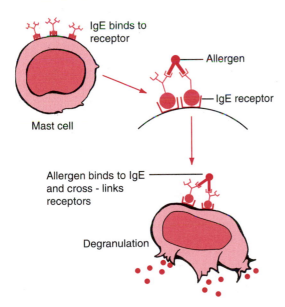

IgE binds to receptor

Allergen

IgE receptor

Mast cell

Allergen binds to IgE and cross - links receptors

Degranulation

**FIGURE 7.1** ● Early phase sensitization reaction. The binding of the allergen to the IgE starts the degranulate process in the cell.

1997). The arachidonic acid forms several immunologic mediators through two complex pathways: the cyclooxygenase (COX)/peroxidase pathway and 5-lipooxygenase pathway (FLAP) (Frazee et al., 1997; Demoly et al., 1998). The COX pathway results in prostaglandins and thromboxanes (Frazee et al., 1997). The FLAP results in the production of leukotrienes (Frazee et al., 1997). Other arachidonic acid metabolites include PAF, cytokines, and chemotactic factors, which recruit more proinflammatory cells for the late-phase response (Shames & Adelman, 1997; Frazee et al., 1997). By direct experimental observation, the products of the COX pathway, prostaglandins, have not been shown to be major mediators causing symptoms in the nasal mucosa (Demoly et al., 1998). The use of drugs that block the COX pathway or receptors of the mediators do not have any clinical effects on rhinitis symptoms (Naclerio, 1991; Simons, 1996; Brooks et al., 1985). Preliminary studies show some benefit using anti-leukotrienes in allergic rhinitis. These mediators are important in airway diseases, as is discussed in Chapter 8 on asthma (O'Brien, 1998). Arachidonic acid metabolite actions cannot be negated, however, based on their physiologic actions on blood vessels and chemotaxis in rhinitis (Adelman & Saxon, 1995).

In the late-phase response, eosinophils and basophils release mediators (eg, IL-1, IL-6, and IL-8; GM-CSF, TNF, RANTES, PAF) (Shames & Adelman, 1997; Naclerio & Solomon, 1997; Barnes, 1993). Most of the mediators in the early-phase reaction are released again by basophils (and possible other cells) in the late-phase reaction, most significantly, histamine (Naclerio, 1991; Shames & Adelman, 1997). Histamine also may be responsible for coordinating and causing many of the immunologic events of the late-phase response (Barnes, 1993; Hamano et al., 1998). Numerous other cells are recruited to the area of inflammation, including T-helper cells (CD4), eosinophils, basophils, mononuclear cells, and especially neutrophils (Naclerio, 1991; Adelman & Saxon, 1995; Leung, 1996). Numerous eosinophils accumulate within nasal tissues during the late phase (Iliopoulos et al., 1990). Eosinophils become activated by various cytokines, which then allow the eosinophils themselves to secrete cytokines (Barnes, 1993). Eosinophils are the most crucial cells responsible for late-phase inflammation because of their release of toxic substances (Leung, 1996; Barnes, 1993). Mast cells and T cells produce cytokines that help maintain the presence and proliferation of eosinophils in inflamed tissues (Leung, 1996). Cytokines (IL-1,

TNF) are the regulators of the influx of the inflammatory cells into tissues under allergenic attack (Leung, 1996; Adelman et al., 1995). $PGD_2$ is the only mediator not found in the late-phase reaction, although it is an arachidonic acid metabolite (Shames & Adelman, 1997; Druce, 1993). Because $PGD_2$ is released only by mast cells, it is suspected that basophils are the major cells responsible for the release of mediators, specifically histamine and IL-4, in the late-phase response (Shames & Adelman, 1997; Naclerio & Solomon, 1997; Druce, 1993).

At 2 to 4 hours, the late-phase reaction begins, peaking between 6 and 12 hours, and resolution occurs within 24 hours (Shames & Adelman, 1997). The degree and number of symptoms is relative to that of the early-phase reaction (Iliopoulos et al., 1990). The major immunologic characteristic of the late phase is acute inflammation (Leung, 1996). The nasal mucosal epithelium becomes thickened, proliferation of connective tissue occurs, and the adjacent periosteum hypertrophies (Lierl, 1995). Chronic late-phase reactions lead to hyperresponsiveness (priming) and destruction of respiratory tract epithelium (Shames & Adelman, 1997; Naclerio & Solomon, 1997). Priming is a result of repeated exposure to antigens, which results in hypersensitization to that antigen (Iliopoulos et al., 1990). Fewer antigens then are needed to elicit another allergic response (Iliopoulos et al., 1990). There also is the increased deposition of mast cells (with IgE-bound antibodies) and other proinflammatory cells into tissues (Naclerio & Solomon, 1997; Leung, 1996). These mast cells and other proinflammatory cells become chronically stimulated, resulting in degranulation and inflammation (Naclerio & Solomon, 1997; Leung, 1996). The increased levels of eosinophils and neutrophils in nasal tissues are associated with the levels of mediators released (Iliopoulos et al., 1990). This association is characterized by an increase in vascular permeability (Iliopoulos et al., 1990). Major basic protein, released by eosinophils, is thought to cause epithelial destruction (Shames & Adelman, 1997; Leung, 1996). Fibroblasts and connective tissue cells also are formed, contributing to the long-term changes in nasal tissues (Naclerio, 1991). The hyperresponsiveness partially results from prolonged inflammation (Shames & Adelman, 1997). This IgE-mediated late-phase response is the cause of chronic allergic states (eg, allergic rhinitis, asthma) (Leung, 1996).

A hyperresponsive state can cause the production of symptoms that are not allergic, such as exposure to irritants (eg, tobacco smoke, dust)

(Naclerio, 1991). These reactions to nonspecific stimuli are a result of the destruction of the epithelium and chronic inflammation (Naclerio & Solomon, 1997). Exposure to these nonspecific irritants also can decrease mucociliary clearance of the sinuses, which protects the sinuses from infection (Corren et al., 1996).

To summarize the late phase, because the same mediators (from the early response) are released again in the late-phase response, most of the same symptoms of the immediate-phase response recur. Histamine is again responsible for these symptoms. The most notable and significant symptoms in the late-phase response are inflammation and mucus hypersecretion. Hyperresponsiveness of nasal mucosa to allergens and irritants occurs as a result of chronic inflammation and epithelial destruction in nasal tissues. Figure 7-2 illustrates the early and late phases of the allergic response.

A subsequent reexposure to the same antigen may result in an increase in allergic mediator levels, possibly from unresolved inflammation from the initial reaction (Iliopoulos et al., 1990). Because of hyperresponsiveness of the immune system, mediator levels (high or low) do not correspond with the degree or presence of a clinical reaction (Iliopoulos et al., 1990). This suggests that the degree of clinical symptoms may not correspond with the level of serum mediators, IgE, or reaction to diagnostic skin testing (Iliopoulos et al., 1990). Continual exposure to allergens result in unrelenting nasal symptoms (Iliopoulos et al., 1990). Allergic rhinitis, like all allergic manifestations, therefore is a disease of *inflammation*.

Increased levels of $T_H2$ cells are present in patients with chronic allergic diseases (Leung, 1996). Repeated and continuous exposure to allergens, causing allergic responses, cause increasing numbers of $T_H2$ lymphocytes (Leung, 1996). The secretion of IL-4 (from basophils in the late-phase response) also recruits more helper T-lymphocytes to specialize as $T_H2$ cells (Naclerio & Solomon, 1997). $T_H2$ cells (once differentiated and functioning has been established) also may impair type 1 T-helper ($T_H1$) cell functioning in allergic disease by the actions of IL-4 and IL-10 produced by $T_H2$ cells (Leung, 1996). Chronic inflammation may result from cytokine-promoted existence of effector cells (Leung, 1996). $T_H2$ cells, when exposed to allergens, secrete IL-3, IL-4, IL-5, IL-6, and GM-CSF (Leung, 1996). These cytokines promote the migration, differentiation, and survival of the two major cellular components of allergic disease: IgE B cells and eosinophils (Leung, 1996). This is evidenced by eosinophilia and increased IgE levels in people with chronic allergic rhinitis (Leung, 1996).

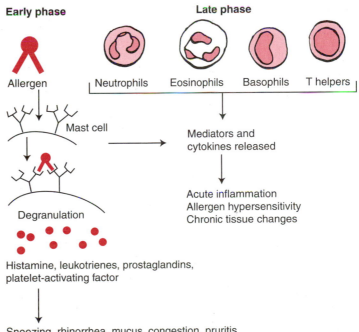

**FIGURE 7.2** ● Early and late phases of the allergic response.

## Circadian Rhythms

Circadian rhythms may have some significant affect on allergic rhinitis, just as they have critical physiologic actions in asthma. Circadian rhythms play important roles in immune function, hormone secretion, and in physical and psychologic functions. Serum cortisol levels begin to decline after 10 PM and reach their trough after midnight (McPhee, 1997; Donohue, 1997; Haus & Touitou, 1997; Martin, 1993). A peak of cortisol occurs between 6 and 8 AM (Haus & Touitou, 1997). The peak functioning and increased levels of lymphocytes and eosinophils occur during sleep (Lawlor & Tashkin, 1995; Ritchie et al., 1983). Other endogenous actions occurring during sleep include an increased vagal tone, trough of sympathetic tone, trough of ciliary activity, and possibly an increase in the secretion of mucus (Donohue, 1997; Martin, 1993). Circadian rhythms may affect mediators such as histamine and bradykinin by increasing their levels from midnight until morning (Barnes et al., 1997). Histamine peaks at about 4 AM (Barnes et al., 1980). In the late evening (after 7 PM), histamine receptor activity and the number of binding sites decrease (Reinberg, 1997). Alterations in circadian rhythms cause lower secretion of catecholamines (Smolensky & D'Alonzo, 1993). In the early morning, around 6 AM, a surge in catecholamines and cortisol is seen (Barnes et al., 1980). Catecholamines reach a trough at 4 AM and peak in the afternoon (Barnes et al., 1980). Even with the surge of catecholamines and cortisol in the early morning, patient symptoms may be at their worst at this time (Reinberg, 1997). This probably results from increased histamine levels, overnight exposure to allergens, late-phase responses, and increase pollen in the morning. Chronobiology still requires more investigation and correlation with chronotherapeutics in allergic rhinitis.

Circadian rhythms of allergic symptoms need to form the basis for designing treatment plans (Lee et al., 1977). Reactivity or responses to common allergens (grasses, dust mites) and histamine peak between 7 and 11 PM in cutaneous testing (Lee et al., 1977). Nasal symptoms generally are highest in the morning (Reinberg, 1997). The symptoms of sneezing, nasal pruritus, rhinorrhea, and congestion are increased in the morning (increasing after midnight) (Reinberg et al., 1988). Pollen may be at peak levels in the morning, in addition to concurrent late-phase reaction from dust mite exposure during sleep. Dosing of antihistamines in the evening may provide better alleviation of morning symptoms (Reinberg, 1997). In addition, bedtime dosing of intranasal corticosteroids may be more beneficial because of decreased cortisol levels and the high incidence of morning symptoms. These factors are highly significant in asthma; however, their role in allergic rhinitis also has been shown to be significant.

## PHYSIOLOGIC BASIS OF DIAGNOSTIC ALLERGY TESTING

### Skin Testing

Prick, scratch, and intradermal skin testing are the most commonly used diagnostic tests for allergy determination. These tests are more specific than any other form of diagnostic testing. Intradermal testing is less specific but more sensitive (Li, 1998). A decrease in the specificity of intradermal injection tests results because the allergens are being introduced to the cells responsible for the diagnostic reaction (Li, 1998). This causes a decreased specificity with the intradermal injections (Li, 1998). Scratch tests are performed initially for specific allergens (eg, oak tree, *Candida*, dust mites). If no reaction or a low-level response occurs, intradermal testing is performed with general classes of allergens (eg, early trees, mold mix), which is less specific but more sensitive to immunologic reaction.

Allergy skin testing has some drawbacks. Allergy skin testing is less sensitive for food allergens, since food proteins generally are not inhaled. A double-blind food challenge is the best diagnostic method for determining food allergy (Li, 1998). Also, note that about 15% of the population, if tested, would have positive test results without any clinical presentation of atopy (Li, 1998).

### In Vitro Allergy Testing

This form of diagnostic testing involves serum testing with radioimmunoassay testing (RAST). This involves exposing IgE antibody (serum) to allergenic protein molecules (Li, 1998). RAST testing is less sensitive, more expensive, and takes longer to receive results than allergy skin testing (Li, 1998).

## DEVELOPMENTAL CONSIDERATIONS

In children, anatomical deformities and delayed learning abilities may result from allergic rhinitis or its complications. With persistent, chronic mouth breathing, children may develop abnormalities of facial structures (Lierl, 1995). These abnormalities include a narrow, high-arched palate; elongated and flat maxilla bone; and a recessed chin, which causes a dental overbite from a caudally angulated mandible (Lierl, 1995). Sinusitis may occur frequently in children with allergic rhinitis and may progress to chronic sinusitis (Brady, 1996). Allergic rhinitis often results in secretory otitis media in children (Lierl, 1995). Chronic and persistent secretory otitis media may cause developmental delays in speech and cognition (Lierl, 1995). Deafness may result from chronic secretory otitis media (Lierl, 1995). If nasal polyps are found in children with allergic rhinitis, the possibility of cystic fibrosis must be investigated (Naclerio & Solomon, 1997). Consider foreign bodies as a cause of rhinitis in children. Traditional antihistamines may cause a paradoxical reaction of stimulation rather than sedation (Hulisz & Fillwock, 1996).

While it generally takes 3 years to develop sensitization to an allergen, infants may develop perennial allergic rhinitis before 2 years of age (Brady, 1996). Choanal atresia or stenosis, cystic fibrosis, vasomotor rhinitis, and foreign body obstruction become higher considerations in the differential diagnosis for children (Brady, 1996). Pharmacotherapy remains essentially the same as in adults; however, not all medications are indicated in certain ages of children (Brady, 1996). As children develop, nasal passages become more patent anatomically (Brady, 1996). Allergic symptoms from seasonal allergy may increase during adolescence (Brady, 1996). Female patients may exhibit an increase in symptoms or worsening of disease after puberty (Hamano et al., 1998). Children with allergic rhinitis frequently develop sensitization to other allergens after moving to other parts of country (Brady, 1996).

Changes in the pattern of allergic rhinitis may occur during pregnancy. Release of histamine may be affected, cortisol production may increase, and IgE production may decrease as a result of increased chorionic gonadotropin (Lawlor & Tashkin, 1995). Pregnancy may provide a period of remission of symptoms in many women (Lierl, 1995). However, some studies have found increased $H_1$ receptors in nasal endothelium during pregnancy (Hamano et al., 1998). An increase in the female hormones estradiol and progesterone (as in pregnancy and onset of puberty) may be responsible for the increase in $H_1$ receptors, resulting in an increase in symptoms and nasal hyperreactivity (Hamano et al., 1998).

Pregnancy brings on therapeutic challenges. Drug therapy may be limited; however, the use of intranasal cromolyn is considered safe, especially considering the misery of the allergic symptoms. Immunotherapy may be continued if maintenance doses have been achieved. Some antihistamines are pregnancy category B (loratadine, cetirizine, chlorpheniramine) (Ellsworth et al., 1998).

In the elderly, special consideration should be given to the type of treatment. Sedation, orthostatic hypotension, and anticholinergic side effects may be harmful because of comorbid diseases and the risk of falls. Mixture of antihistamines with antihypertensives, diuretics, and sedatives could lower blood pressure, leading to syncope. Allergic rhinitis tends to decrease in symptom intensity after 65 years of age (Naclerio & Solomon, 1997; Adams & Marano, 1995).

The financial expense of treatment, outlined in the following section on treatment, can be an area of concern for health care providers, patients, and managed care organizations. Implementing the primary treatment, avoidance (eg, buying air cleaners, installing air conditioning, and replacing carpeting), can be very expensive to the patient, and these items are not covered by insurance (generally). The health care provider can assist patients who are at the point of being disabled (especially those with asthma) by obtaining community resources to assist (although these types of resources may be scarce). If the patient can tolerate traditional antihistamines, there is little justification for using the second-generation antihistamines, which are relatively expensive.

## PHYSIOLOGIC BASIS OF TREATMENT

### Approach to the Patient

Treatment for allergic rhinitis must be individualized. After diagnosis (seasonal or perennial), a care plan should be designed to attack the pathophysiologic mechanisms underlying the symptoms and the disease. Avoidance always is the first-line defense in allergic rhinitis. Pharmacologic therapeutics should be directed at (1) reducing inflammation (Lierl, 1995), (2) preventing another reaction (Naclerio, 1991), (3) altering immune functioning, and (4) alleviating symptoms. These goals overlap, but therapy still is the same. Patients are most concerned with goal 4, immediate relief. This may be provided pharmacologically with intramuscular corticosteroids, antihistamines, and topical decongestants. However, achieving the goal of reducing inflammation and preventing future reactions takes time and requires full engagement from the patient. Education then may be the most powerful tool for treating allergic rhinitis.

## Avoidance

Avoidance is the first and the most important treatment for allergic rhinitis. It is the major way to *control* allergic rhinitis. Although not all allergens can be avoided, steps can be taken to limit exposure.

### House Dust and Dust Mites

Because house dust and the house dust mite frequently are the cause of allergic rhinitis, the following steps are essential for *control* (Spieksma, 1991). However, these steps must be aggressively undertaken to have any effect on the numbers of dust mites in the home and the symptoms resulting from dust mite allergy (Platts-Mills & Chapman, 1987). Particular attention needs to be given to the bedroom because this room needs to be the cleanest of all rooms for patients allergic to dust mites (Platts-Mills & Chapman, 1987).

- Special pillow and mattress covers with membranes are needed to prevent the passage of skin cells and dust particles and dust mites. Dust mites feed on human skin cells (Spieksma, 1991; Platts-Mills & Chapman, 1987). These vinyl membranes cut off food for the dust mite plus limit exposure to the dust mite. Unless dust is stirred up (eg, using fans, dusting, vacuuming), the only significant exposure to dust and dust mites occurs at night, when the patient's face is buried in the pillow or sheets. Bed linens and Dacron pillows should be washed weekly in extremely hot water (130°F or greater is optimal) (Lierl, 1995; Michelini, 1996). All bed linens, blankets, and toys should be washable (Lierl, 1995).
- No feather pillows should be used. Dust mites also thrive within feather pillows (Platts-Mills & Chapman, 1987). Dacron, polyester-filled, or hypoallergenic foam is recommended, but these still need regular changing and an impermeable cover, as mentioned earlier (Platts-Mills & Chapman, 1987).
- Removing carpet and curtains significantly reduces dust mite populations (Platts-Mills & Chapman, 1987). Hardwood floors are preferred because they harbor significantly fewer dust mites (Platts-Mills & Chapman, 1987). Shampooing the carpet and using detergents have no effect on the dust mites, but they may remove some of the superficial dust (Platts-Mills & Chapman, 1987). However, if excess water is applied to the carpet, dust mite growth may be promoted. Wet carpet also can harbor mold. If carpet is on concrete flooring, dust mites may be more abundant within the carpet than on the bedding (Li, 1998). Some allergy practitioners sell products to kill molds and dust mites in the carpet.
- Keep the humidity down. Optimal indoor humidity is 35% to 50% to reduce dust mite and fungi growth, although a humidity level lower than 40% is best for dust mite control (Fischer et al., 1995). Dust mites grow best at about 70% humidity but also grow at 60% with a temperature of 70°F (Platts-Mills & Chapman, 1987; Michelini, 1996). Do not use humidifiers for this reason. Humidifiers also promote fungi growth. Air conditioning helps to control humidity in the home (Platts-Mills & Chapman, 1987). Dehumidifiers may be necessary if humidity exceeds 40%.
- Dusting frequently with products such as Pledge, followed by thorough vacuuming of all upholstery and carpets, reduces house dust. Some vacuums have high efficiency particulate air (HEPA) filters, which confine the dust and allergens that are stirred and spread by the vacuum's exhaust (Fischer et al., 1995). Notice that this measure does not have a significant effect on dust mites (Platts-Mills & Chapman, 1987).
- Air cleaners, such as portable HEPA room air filters, are helpful in removing dust and other allergens up to the size of 0.3 μm (Fischer et al., 1995). Portable HEPA air cleaners should be positioned at least 3 ft off of the ground (so that the dust on the ground is not stirred up), they should be efficient enough to perform six air changes per hour in the room, and the filters should be changed routinely according to the manufacturer's instructions. *Only* HEPA air cleaners are proven to be beneficial. No credible evidence exists for other air cleaners, including ozone cleaners.
- Central HEPA filter systems are available for the home air conditioner uptake. Electrostatic filters for all exhaust ducts and air vents may also be enough for beneficial air cleaning.

### Pollens and Other Allergens

Most of the measures just discussed, such as HEPA filters, dusting, and vacuuming, also apply to controlling pollen. Dusting is especially important, since in peak seasons, house dust consists primarily of pollen (Platts-Mills & Chapman, 1987). The following measures should be considered:

- Use air conditioning and keep doors and windows closed (Lierl, 1995).
- Use pollen masks when outdoors—it may be beneficial.

- Houseplants do not provide a significant source of allergens, except under greenhouse conditions (Burge et al., 1982).
- Use pest control measures to kill cockroach populations (Kang, 1990).
- Avoid tobacco smoke (because of high irritant effects). Prohibit smoking in the home.
- Avoid using products with strong odors (eg, bug sprays) (Lierl, 1995).

## Pets

If a patient is allergic to pets, getting rid of the animal is best, but it has been said that the patient would rather get rid of the allergist than the cat (Georgitis et al., 1997). Cat and dog fur is not allergenic. Feline saliva (which is spread over their coat) and sebaceous gland secretions contain proteins (*Fel d* I) that are allergenic. Horses and other animals have dander that is allergenic (Li, 1998). Rodent urine is another allergenic substance (Li, 1998). To control pet allergens:

- Keep pets indoors if possible (since they may bring in outdoor allergens within their hair or fur). Although it may be best to keep pets outdoors, it is important that they always stay outdoors (Lierl, 1995). Definitely keep pets out of the bedroom (Lierl, 1995).
- Bathe the pet every other week if possible; ask your veterinarian for safe products to bathe your pets. Some recommend 3% tannic acid solution to denature cat allergens (Fischer et al., 1995). It is questionable if any products actually denature the protein *Fel d* I on the coats of cats (Klucka et al., 1995). It has not been studied as to whether products affect other allergenic proteins on animals, which may be significant because some products sold through allergy offices have subjectively improved tolerance to pets (Klucka et al., 1995).

## Molds and Fungi

To control molds and fungi, the following measures should be used:

- Control humidity. Use a dehumidifier if necessary.
- Keep household temperature less that 72°F (Lierl, 1995).
- Clean bathrooms thoroughly and frequently with fungicides. A solution of 1 cup of chloride bleach in 1 gal of water kills mold on household surfaces and probably is the cheapest method.
- Use the air vent during showers to reduce the humidity produced during showering (Michelini, 1996).

- No plants should be permitted in the bedroom (Michelini, 1996). Some studies have found that most common houseplants are not a significant source of allergens (even mold) unless they exist under greenhouse conditions (Burge et al., 1982)
- No live Christmas trees should be permitted, since they may host a large amount of mold.
- Avoid mowing the grass, raking leaves, and walking through leaves, since this stirs up mold spores.
- Use air cleaners, as described earlier.
- Avoid allowing carpets, carpet pads, walls, and upholstery to become wet.
- Avoid areas of stagnating water around the outside of the house.
- Allow as much natural sunlight as possible into the house.

## Outdoors

- Watch pollen counts. The pollen count generally is lower in conditions of high humidity, light rain, lower temperatures, and between 8 PM and 4 AM (Hulisz & Fillwock, 1996). High pollen counts usually occur with low humidity, windy days, warmer temperatures, and from 5 PM to 1 AM (Hulisz & Fillwock, 1996). The pollen hot line number is 1-800-POLLEN.

## Systemic Corticosteroids

Systemic corticosteroids may be needed on an occasional basis, usually during peak seasonal periods, to relieve exacerbation of allergic symptoms. They also may be necessary to reduce nasal inflammation to allow intranasal corticosteroid sprays to penetrate the nasal mucosa (Li, 1998). The most important concept in using systemic corticosteroids is to use a sufficient *dose* (eg, prednisone 40 to 60 mg daily in adults) for a sufficient period of *time* (usually 5 to 7 days) (Li, 1998). It also is not necessary to taper oral steroid bursts, since this will not cause adrenal insufficiency (Li, 1998). Intramuscular injection of long-acting corticosteroids (usually dexamethasone) is another alternative. Intramuscular injections usually are limited to twice a year and may be a better choice because of guaranteed compliance. Patients need thorough education on the side effects of systemic corticosteroids. Systemic corticosteroids are safe for their short-term use in allergic rhinitis, with the benefits outweighing the risks (Hulisz & Fillwock, 1996).

Systemic corticosteroids work on the late-phase reaction only. Corticosteroids reduce the release and responses of proinflammatory mediators and cytokines from mast cells, eosinophils, lymphocytes, and fibroblasts (Frazee et al., 1997; United States Pharmacopeial Convention [USP DI], 1997; Shlom, 1996). This action also decreases the influx of proinflammatory cells into nasal and bronchial tissues, most importantly, eosinophils (USP DI, 1997; Iliopoulos et al., 1990). Mast cell numbers are reduced; however, this action is better achieved with topical administration of intranasal steroids (Schleimer, 1993). The activation of eosinophils is suppressed by corticosteroids (USP DI, 1997). The actions of mediators released by the inflammatory cells, including histamine, bradykinin, serotonin, and some arachidonic metabolites, are reduced (Shlom, 1996). Other actions, with respect to the immune response, include inhibiting antigen processing, reducing serum levels of lymphocytes, reducing adhesion molecules, and reducing transcription of the $COX_2$ pathway (Shlom, 1996; Lemanske & Busse, 1997). Transcription of the macrophage inhibitory factor, secretory leukocyte inhibitory protein, is increased (Lemanske & Busse, 1997).

## Intranasal Corticosteroids

Intranasal corticosteroids are perhaps the key and most important part of pharmacologic treatment of allergic rhinitis. Patients with chronic rhinitis have intense inflammation; therefore, interventions such as corticosteroids to reduce inflammation are essential (Shames & Adelman, 1997). Intranasal corticosteroids may be first-line treatment for some patients. If used on a daily basis, nasal inflammation and drainage can be diminished, and, in a way, they heal the nose (Simons, 1996). Little corticosteroid is absorbed systemically, and, therefore, corticosteroids are safe for regular use (Li, 1998). Adverse side effects seen with systemic corticosteroids (eg, suppression of the hypothalamic-pituitary-adrenal axis; increased risk of osteoporosis) are not seen with the intranasal steroids (Simons, 1996). Intranasal steroids may be used year-round and indefinitely, without altering the risk of nasal infection (Li, 1998). Even upper respiratory infections (URIs) are unaffected by intranasal steroids; therefore, discontinuation during an URI is not necessary (Li, 1998).

Intranasal corticosteroids have a variety of effects on the allergic state: they decrease mast cells, basophils, eosinophils, and neutrophils and inhibit histamine release from basophils (Simons, 1996). The responses of these cells in the early- and late-phase response to allergen exposure are reduced (Simons, 1996). Overall, the entire spectrum of primary allergic rhinitis symptoms is reduced. In patients with allergic rhinitis,

intranasal corticosteroids have better effectiveness than systemic corticosteroids (Simons, 1996).

Mast cells become more numerous after repeated exposure to allergens within the nasal mucosa (Naclerio & Solomon, 1997). Treatment with intranasal corticosteroids decreases the numbers of mast cells recruited to the nasal mucosa (Naclerio & Solomon, 1997). By reducing the release of cytokines, corticosteroids also reduce the numbers of eosinophils from airway and nasal mucosa (Barnes, 1993).

Compliance with intranasal steroids may be hampered because of cost, epistaxis, and delivery vehicles and systems. Choosing the lowest cost brand can help because no single topical nasal corticosteroid can make adequate claims as to having a better efficacy than the others. Epistaxis sometimes can be controlled by discontinuing the corticosteroid for 1 week or until the epistaxis ceases, then restarting the medication. Proper selection of a brand with a more tolerable delivery system on an individual basis also may improve compliance (eg, aqueous solutions generally are more tolerable, especially if there is less aromatic scent to the solution). Aerosols (eg, Nasacort, Rhinocort, Vancenase Pockethaler) cause nasal dryness and headaches in some patients (USP DI, 1997). Some of the intranasal steroids can be used once daily, which may improve compliance. Based on the circadian rhythm secretion of cortisol (trough at bedtime hours), if the inhaled corticosteroid is a once-daily formulation, dosing at bedtime theoretically is more beneficial. Septal perforation has been associated with aerosol preparations, so aqueous solutions (eg, Nasacort AQ, Nasonex, Vancenase AQ, Flonase) are recommended (Li, 1998; USP DI, 1997). Patients also must be educated to avoid spraying onto the septum, since septum perforation also may occur, although rarely (Georgitis et al., 1997).

Inhaled nasal corticosteroids should be used every day, usually year-round. However, in patients with seasonal allergic rhinitis, therapy should be initiated at least 1 week before the season and used throughout the season (Li, 1998). It is crucial that patients be educated to know that these nasal sprays do not work immediately and to expect at least 2 weeks before improvement in symptoms (Li, 1998). If symptoms are not adequately reduced, then a temporary increase in the dose (number of sprays) may be required (Lierl, 1995). A topical decongestant may be applied in cases of severe mucosal edema, to allow the intranasal corticosteroids to penetrate the nasal mucosa (Lierl, 1995). Other conditions (possibly comorbid) can be improved by intranasal cortico-steroids, such as nasal polyposis, nasal eosino-philia, and vasomotor rhinitis (Li, 1998). Caution should be used in prescribing any corticosteroid in patients with active or quiescent tuberculosis (Lierl, 1995).

## Antihistamines

There are three types of histamine receptors: $H_1$, $H_2$, and $H_3$. The brain, gastrointestinal (GI) tract, and respiratory tract are the major locations of $H_1$ receptors (Simons & Simons, 1993). $H_1$ receptors are primarily involved in allergic symptoms. The actions of $H_1$ receptors include functions such as increasing prostaglandin production, stimulating afferent vagal nerves, increasing capillary perme-ability, releasing mediators, and recruiting inflam-matory cells (Simons & Simons, 1993). Clinical signs of $H_1$ receptor activation include hypoten-sion, flushing, pruritus, and headache (Simons & Simons, 1993). $H_2$ receptors are found predomi-nantly in the gut (also brain and uterus) but may be present in the nasal tissues and skin (Li, 1998; Simons & Simons, 1993). Antagonism of $H_2$ receptors along with $H_1$ receptor antagonism may provide an improvement in allergic symptoms, especially urticaria (Simons & Simons, 1993). $H_2$ receptors have a variety of immunologic functions, such as stimulating T-suppressor cells, inhibiting natural killer T cells, and inducing basophil hista-mine release (Simons & Simons, 1993). Clinical effects of $H_2$ receptors include increased mucus production, gastric acid production, flushing, relaxation of bronchial smooth muscle, and hypotension (Simons & Simons, 1993).

Antihistamines work by competitively block-ing $H_1$ receptor sites, which are abundant in respi-ratory mucosa and ocular tissues. Antihistamines may be used routinely or as needed. Since antihis-tamines compete for histamine receptors, it makes sense that they should be taken before histamine is released. Histamine-induced symptoms are the most predominant in the early-phase reaction. Therefore, peak allergen exposure must be consid-ered when dosing antihistamines so that the peak serum levels coincide with peak exposure. When serum levels of antihistamines drop, histamine receptors become desaturated, allowing any hista-mine present to attach to the histamine receptor (Bernstein, 1997). In prolonged allergic seasons or with perennial allergic rhinitis, patients would benefit by having continuous serum levels of anti-histamines to keep $H_1$ receptors blocked. Bedtime dosing may be optimal, since most symptoms occur early in the morning; however, the individ-

ual and his or her history must guide the dosing regimen. Antihistamines may improve symptoms of nasal congestion, nasal itching, and sneezing (Li, 1998). The effects of antihistamines on nasal congestion are limited and poor, which may require the addition of a decongestant and defi-nitely an anti-inflammatory agent (Shames & Adelman, 1997; Naclerio & Solomon, 1997). Some cases of rhinitis may be relieved by the anti-cholinergic effects of traditional antihistamines (first generation) (Li, 1998). Some antihistamines (eg, azelastine), in addition to the $H_1$ receptor blockade, have anti-inflammatory mechanisms that are not fully understood (Bernstein, 1997). Cyproheptadine and azatadine have antiserotonin effects (Facts and Comparisons, 1998). Antihista-mines generally have more effectiveness in the early-phase response.

Tolerance or a loss of clinical effectiveness may occur with antihistamines (Lierl, 1995). However, other authorities believe that tolerance to antihista-mines does not occur and their clinical effective-ness remains unchanged in allergic rhinitis, regard-less of chronicity of use (Bernstein, 1997). However if the symptoms begin to increase, switching to a different class of antihistamines may be of benefit, regardless if tolerance truly develops (Table 7-2) (Lierl, 1995). Different classes of anti-histamines have a different spectrum of activity and side effects (Facts and Comparisons, 1998). For severe allergic rhinitis, an antihistamine regi-men of a low-dose traditional antihistamine at bed-time and a second-generation antihistamine in the morning may comprise optimal antihistamine management (Druce, 1993). This approach can provide exceptional results (see Table 7-2).

Traditional antihistamines have good efficacy but may be limited by their side effects. These agents, in addition to sedation, can be a cause of significant anticholinergic side effects. This limits their use in patients with conditions that are wors-ened by inhibition of the parasympathetic system (eg, glaucoma, benign prostatic hypertrophy). Some of the traditional antihistamines (eg, chlor-pheniramine) have a long half-life, exceeding 24 hours (Simons, 1996). Generally, people can become tolerant to these side effects after several days of therapy and these drugs are usually less expensive (Lierl, 1995). Giving an antihistamine with a decongestant can offset some of the seda-tive effects with stimulant effects (Hulisz & Fill-wock, 1996). Low-dose combination formulations (eg, Lodrane LD, D.A. chewable) of these antihis-tamines, often with a decongestant, taken at bed-time can be of particular benefit, especially if an allergy to dust or dust mites is present.

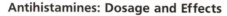

## TABLE 7.2       ● ● ●

### Antihistamines: Dosage and Effects

| Antihistamine | Dose* (mg) | Dosing Interval[†] (h) | Sedative Effects | Antihistaminic Activity | Anticholinergic Activity | Antiemetic Effects |
|---|---|---|---|---|---|---|
| *First-generation (nonselective)* | | | | | | |
| Ethanolamines | | | | | | |
|   Clemastine | 1 | 12 | ++ | + to ++ | +++ | ++ to +++ |
|   Diphenhydramine | 25–50 | 6–8 | +++ | + to ++ | +++ | ++ to +++ |
| Ethylenediamines | | | | | | |
|   Tripelennamine | 25–50 | 4–6 | ++ | + to ++ | +/− | B |
| Alkylamines | | | | | | |
|   Brompheniramine | 4 | 4–6 | + | +++ | ++ | B |
|   Chlorpheniramine | 4 | 4–6 | + | ++ | ++ | B |
|   Dexchlorpheniramine | 2 | 4–6 | + | +++ | ++ | B |
| Phenothiazines | | | | | | |
|   Promethazine | 12.5–25 | 6–24 | +++ | +++ | +++ | ++++ |
| Piperazines | | | | | | |
|   Hydroxyzine | 25–100 | 4–8 | +++ | ++ to +++ | ++ | +++ |
| Piperidines | | | | | | |
|   Azatadine | 1–2 | 12 | ++ | ++ | ++ | B |
|   Cyproheptadine | 4 | 8 | + | ++ | ++ | B |
|   Phenindamine | 25 | 4–6 | +/− | ++ | ++ | B |
| Phthalazinone | | | | | | |
| Azelastine[‡] | 0.5 | 12 | +/− | ++ to +++ | +/− | B |
| *Second-generation (peripherally selective)* | | | | | | |
| Piperazine | | | | | | |
|   Cetirizine | 5–10 | 24 | +/− | ++ to +++ | +/− | B |
| Piperidines | | | | | | |
|   Astemizole | 10 | 24 | +/− | ++ to +++ | +/− | B |
|   Fexofenadine | 60 | 12 | +/− | B | +/− | B |
|   Loratadine | 10 | 24 | +/− | ++ to +++ | +/− | B |

++++, very high; +++, high; ++, moderate; +, low; +/−, low to none; B, no data.
*Usual single adult dose.
[†]For conventional dosage forms.
[‡]Some effects may be enhanced or reduced as a result of administration through the nasal route.
(From Drug Facts and Comparisons [1998 ed.]. St. Louis: Facts and Comparisons.)

Second-generation antihistamines include fexofenadine (Allegra), loratadine (Claritin, Claritin Reditabs), cetirizine (Zyrtec), and astemizole (Hismanal). Loratadine (Claritin D, Claritin D 24-hour) and fexofenadine (Allegra D) also have preparations combined with decongestants. The second-generation antihistamines bind to $H_1$ receptors in a noncompetitive manner, and they are slow to release from these receptors (Bernstein, 1997; Simons, 1996). These antihistamines generally are no more effective than the traditional antihistamines, but they are associated with fewer side effects (most notable is a relative lack of sedation and anticholinergic effects) (Simons, 1996). The relative lack of sedation and anticholinergic side effects is a result of their inability to cross the blood-brain barrier (Lierl, 1995). Binding to peripheral $H_1$ receptors is predominant with these nonsedating antihistamines (Facts and Comparisons, 1998). Second-generation antihistamines also have more convenient dosing regimens (eg, cetirizine is once daily).

Since allergic conjunctivitis can be a common part of the allergic response, ophthalmic antihistamines can be beneficial. Most over-the-counter ocular antihistamines also contain decongestants, which can cause rebound redness (similar to rebound congestion with intranasal decongestants). The prescription ophthalmic antihistamine olopatadine (Patanol) blocks histamine and also has some mast cell–stabilizing properties (Alcon, 1997).

Since asthma and allergic rhinitis commonly are comorbid conditions, antihistamine therapy often is a necessary part of treatment. Antihistamines were previously thought to worsen asthma because of the drying effect of some antihistamines (anticholinergic effects) (Li, 1998). Contrary to old popular belief, antihistamines are safe in asthma (especially the newer agents, which produce less anticholinergic side effects, such as loratadine, cetirizine, and fexofenadine) (Li, 1998). Antihistamines may be of benefit to asthmatics because of their effects on bronchial inflammation (Li, 1998).

It should be noted that astemizole (Hismanal) has been associated with life-threatening arrhythmias (because of increased serum levels of astemizole by inhibition of CYP3A4, which prolongs the Q-T interval, increasing the risk of torsades de pointes and ventricular fibrillation) when taken with erythromycin, clarithromycin, cisapride, and azole-type antifungals. With the newer agents, such as loratadine, cetirizine, and fexofenadine, this interaction has not occurred (Facts and Comparisons, 1998).

## Mast Cell Stabilizers

Mast cell stabilizers have late- and early-phase reaction effectiveness (Simons, 1996). These agents, cromolyn and nedocromil, stabilize the cell membrane of the mast cell. Cromolyn (Nasalcrom) is the only agent available in an intranasal spray. Because mast cells degranulate in both the immediate- and late-phase reactions, cromolyn can be the most crucial part of preventative treatment. On inhalation, cromolyn binds to mast cells (Gopal & Fletcher, 1997). Degranulation and the resultant release of mediators from mast cells are inhibited by cromolyn (Simons, 1996). It is not known if this effect of cell stabilization occurs with basophils in vivo (Simons, 1996). Cromolyn also works through a reduction of the inflammatory properties and an inhibition of the chemotaxis of eosinophils, monocytes, and neutrophils (Lierl, 1995; Simons, 1996). Mediator release caused by nonallergenic substances is inhibited by cromolyn (Simons, 1996).

Cromolyn nasal spray should be a first-line pharmacotherapeutic agent in any form of allergic rhinitis. Cromolyn must be used every day, 3 to 6 times per day, and benefits may not be seen for up to a month (Lierl, 1995; USP DI, 1997; Simons, 1996). This poses a compliance problem with multiple dosing requirements. However, some practitioners advise patients who have symptoms on exposure to a known aeroallergen to use cromolyn before the exposure. For chronic rhinitis, daily use is recommended for therapeutic benefits (Lierl, 1995). Clinical effects include a reduction in sneezing, rhinorrhea, and nasal pruritus (Simons, 1996). Cromolyn is poorly absorbed, producing limited systemic absorption (USP DI, 1997). Cromolyn also comes in an ophthalmic form (Opticrom, Crolom) to ameliorate the symptoms of allergic conjunctivitis. There are no known toxic effects or drug interactions with medications used in ambulatory care, and it remains the safest drug used in allergic rhinitis (Simons, 1996).

## Sympathomimetic Amines

Sympathomimetic amines (decongestants) used in allergic rhinitis include pseudoephedrine, phenylpropanolamine, and phenylephrine (other imidazoline intranasal decongestants are available) (Simons, 1996). Decongestants may not have any effectiveness in the late-phase response (Druce, 1993). These three main decongestants vary in their actions. Pseudoephedrine has effects on $alpha_1$, $alpha_2$, $beta_1$, and $beta_2$ receptors (Simons, 1996). Phenylephrine has actions only on $alpha_1$ receptors by agonist effects (Simons, 1996). Stimulation of $alpha_1$ and $alpha_2$ receptors results in vasoconstriction of vascular smooth muscle. In the nasal mucosa, this action on the sinusoids results in a decreased volume of blood flow in the nasal mucosa (Simons, 1996). These effects are achieved by oral and topical administration (Simons, 1996).

Clinical effects of oral decongestants include decreased nasal congestion and mucosal edema (Simons, 1996; Hulisz & Fillwock, 1996). Oral phenylephrine has little effect because of poor bioavailability (Simons, 1996). Patients who are not used to the effects of common stimulants (caffeine, decongestants) may be sensitive to the stimulant effects of decongestants (eg, insomnia, tremors, increased heart rate and blood pressure, excitability). Pseudoephedrine probably is the least likely agent to cause these side effects (Simons, 1996). Extreme caution should be exerted in patients with hypertension, diabetes mellitus, hyperthyroidism, and ischemic heart disease, and decongestants should be absolutely contraindicated with treatment using monoamine oxidase inhibitors (Hulisz & Fillwock, 1996). Oral decongestants have a limited response in allergic rhinitis and possibly a better response in vasomotor rhinitis (Lierl, 1995).

Intranasal agents are notorious for addiction and rhinitis medicamentosa from overuse. This occurs because chronic stimulation of alpha receptors in the blood vessel walls results in depressed responsiveness of alpha receptors to endogenous sympathetic outflow. As a result, rebound vasodilation occurs (Gopal & Fletcher, 1997). Dilute preparations provide effective relief (Gopal & Fletcher, 1997). Use should be limited to 3 to 5 days for intranasal decongestants.

## Drying Agents and Anticholinergics

Drying agents and anticholinergics include intranasal ipratropium bromide, oral scopolamine, and methscopolamine. These agents inhibit parasympathetic activity on muscarinic receptors, which decreases secretions from submucosal glands. Intranasal ipratropium bromide (Atrovent nasal spray) can be used as needed for rhinorrhea. Ipratropium bromide is poorly absorbed from nasal and GI mucosa, so minimal side effects are seen (Simons, 1996). Ipratropium bromide blocks the parasympathetic neurotransmission and stimulation of submucosal glands (Simons, 1996). This action results in a decrease in rhinorrhea only, with no effects on sneezing, postnasal drip, or sinus congestion (Simons, 1996; Hulisz & Fillwock, 1996). The use of ipratropium bromide in allergic rhinitis is of limited value and benefit (Lierl, 1995). Scopolamine and methscopolamine, found in several combinations with antihistamines with or without decongestants (eg, Duravent DA, Atrohist), decrease rhinorrhea and PND. Caution should be used if secretions are thick.

## Mucolytics

Mucolytics are commonly used in allergic rhinitis patients, but their efficacy is questionable. The proposed mechanism of action is a decrease in the thickness of secretions. Dosages must be sufficient, usually 1200 to 2400 mg/day, to achieve desired effects. A full glass of water should accompany each dose for further thinning of secretions (which may be the actual mechanism of action).

## Saline Nasal Sprays

Saline nasal sprays may be useful in removing dried secretions, which could block the ostium (Corren et al., 1996). They also may remove pathogens and allergens by mechanical mechanisms (Lierl, 1995). Saline sprays may improve symptoms of congestion. Saline nasal sprays probably are underused and may help to treat epistaxis caused by dry nasal mucosa or intranasal corticosteroids.

## Immunotherapy

Immunotherapy (hyposensitization) affects the early- and late-phase responses. Immunotherapy may be a first-line treatment in selected patients with allergic rhinitis (Li, 1998). Peripheral blood and nasal mucosa immunity is affected by immunotherapy. Immunotherapy involves administering increasing doses of allergens that have been identified as significant allergens for the patient (see section on the physiologic basis of diagnostic testing). Immunotherapy is efficient in reducing the allergic state by several mechanisms. $T_H2$ cells may be converted to $T_H1$ cells by decreasing the cellular influx of the late-phase response, therefore possibly decreasing IgE antibody production (Shames & Adelman, 1997; Naclerio & Solomon, 1997). A decrease in IL-4 has been noted in vitro after provocation with a specific antigen (Shames & Adelman, 1997). Mast cell populations may be reduced, in addition to the decrease in IgE antibody production (Gopal & Fletcher, 1997). Production of mononuclear cell-derived histamine-releasing factor is decreased with immunotherapy (Naclerio, 1991). Immunotherapy induces the production of allergen specific IgG-blocking antibodies, which lowers specific IgE antibodies for specific allergens (Shames & Adelman, 1997; Fischer et al., 1995; Gopal & Fletcher, 1997). Mast cells and basophils are less sensitive to antigen-induced degranulation (Fischer et al., 1995). This type of therapy works in about 80% to 85% of patients (some estimate up to 90%) in reducing overall symptoms and severity of disease (Druce, 1993; Gopal & Fletcher, 1997).

## Pathophysiology and Treatment of Reactions to Immunotherapy Injections

- Reactions usually occur within 20 to 30 minutes after injection but may occur within 1 hour, and risk extends for 24 hours (Fischer et al., 1995).
- Local reactions of swelling may occur after subcutaneous injection of allergen extract. Most allergy practices have standards for adjusting doses of serum, depending on the size of the reaction. A reaction greater than 2 cm (of swelling, not erythema) is considered significant and should be reported to the ordering allergist. Treatment includes oral antihistamines and cold packs, and reducing the dose of the next injection is required (Fischer et al., 1995). This reaction results from a local release of vasodilators, causing edema, pruritus, and erythema at the injection site.
- Severe anaphylaxis results from antigen-IgE binding, which causes mediator release (O'Brien, 1998). Atypical symptoms may be present such as back pain and syncope (O'Brien, 1998). Acute and systemic release of potent vasodilators (histamine, kinins) and chemotoxins, results in angioedema, bronchospasms, shock, hypotension, and cardiac arrest (Fischer et al., 1995).

Treatment includes epinephrine (0.01 mL/kg of 1:1000 solution) intramuscularly (IM), subcutaneously, or intravenously (IV); diphenhydramine (1.25 mg/kg) IV or IM, and hydrocortisone (5 mg/kg) IV (Fischer et al., 1995). Do not forget the ABCs: Administer oxygen (100% by mask), albuterol by aerosol for Bronchospasms, and Crystalloids (normal saline, lactated Ringers) for hypotension, and use electrocardiogram monitoring (O'Brien, 1998). Additional measures include infiltrating the allergen injection site with epinephrine after placing a tourniquet above the site (Fischer et al., 1995). The patient should be watched for at least 4 hours because a late-phase reaction may occur (O'Brien, 1998).

### Exercise

Exercise can be of some benefit by the induction of the sympathetic nervous system (Lierl, 1995). Sympathetic stimulation of nasal tissues causes vasoconstriction, resulting in less edema and extravasation. Effects last for 15 to 30 minutes (Lierl, 1995). However, exercise may induce vasomotor rhinitis, especially during a late-phase reaction (Georgitis et al., 1997).

---

### ● Case Study 7.1

A 12-year-old male patient accompanied by his mother presents to the primary care provider with complaints of allergies and a sinus infection.

#### *History*

The patient is well known to the clinic, with history of a sinus infection diagnosed and treated with a 2-week course of amoxicillin about 2 months ago, and allergic rhinitis diagnosed at the age of 6. Allergic symptoms have been worse over the last month (May), and for the last week, he has complained of sinus pressure over the maxillary and frontal sinuses, a frequent morning headache, cough, and hoarseness, particularly in the morning. The allergic symptoms include rhinorrhea, postnasal drainage, and sinus congestion, which is worse in the morning. Has occasional paroxysms of sneezing, particularly after being outdoors. Medications include: OTC Tylenol Allergy Sinus as needed; he has not been using the prescription intranasal steroid prescribed at the last visit.

*(Case study continued on page 134)*

*Past Medical History*

No major childhood illness incurred. Mom states he had frequent ear infections, never required PE tubes. Immunizations up to date

*Family Medical History*

Mom has a positive history of allergies. One sister has mild intermittent asthma

*Environmental History*

No allergy-prevention measures; two indoor cats, one outdoor dog. Has lived in a carpeted house without a basement for the last 8 years

## Physical Examination

Normal vital signs; well-developed male with no obvious deformities. Tenderness over frontal and maxillary sinuses; nasal mucosa erythematous, irregular surface, yellow mucoid discharge, with 3+/3+ edema; a clear coating of clear drainage over posterior pharynx with cobblestoning. No other abnormalities detected on physical examination

## Impression

Allergic rhinitis with seasonal and perennial characteristics, and acute sinusitis

## Plan

Septra DS[7] 1 BID × 14 days, Claritin D BID, and Nasacort AQ 2 pEN QHS

## Follow-Up

One month later, the patient returns complaining of a sinus infection. He states the infection improved some after taking the prescribed antibiotics, but complete resolution never occurred. Sneezing has improved, but he still has all other symptoms, worse particularly in the morning. States the nasal spray has not helped. A limited coronal CT scan is ordered, which reveals blockage of the osteomeatal units on the left, 10 mm of mucosal thickening in the sphenoid, 8 mm in the frontal sinuses, and 11 mm in the maxillary sinuses. Based on this information you diagnose: chronic sinusitis. You order prednisone 20 mg BID × 5 days, continue intranasal steroids, and Cedax 400 mg qd × 3 weeks, Nasalcrom 1 pEN before going outdoors, and change to Zyrtec 10 mg QHS. You recommend referral to a board-certified allergist for diagnostic allergy testing and immunotherapy.

The morning symptoms are indicative of allergic exposure during sleep, which is commonly produced by animal dander, dust mites, and mold. This chronic exposure to allergens produces a prolonged late-phase characteristic reaction, resulting in chronic inflammation. The lack of frequent sneezing, profuse rhinorrhea, and pale nasal mucosa indicate a chronic inflammation (late phase). The intranasal steroids probably were ineffective because the inflamed nasal mucosa prevented adequate penetration of the intranasal steroids. The oral prednisone should reduce the inflammation, allowing penetration of the intranasal steroids and alleviation of symptoms. Seasonal allergic rhinitis also is present, based on the incidence of sneezing on acute exposure to outdoor allergens, particularly in May (trees, grasses). This produces an acute mast cell degranulation, resulting in a histamine-driven reaction (early phase).

CT, computed tomography; PE, pressure equalization; pEN, spray each nostril; OTC, over-the-counter.

● **Case Study 7.2**

A 20-year-old woman presents to the clinic for the first time with the complaint that her allergies have been out of control.

## History

She states that the symptoms began around August and has been dealing with this over the last 2 years. Her primary symptoms include profuse rhinorrhea, paroxysms of sneezing, and unrelenting nasal and ocular pruritus. Symptoms are exacerbated by mowing the grass and dusting and generally are worse in the fall. She has been taking Tavist-D OTC without adequate relief; she states that she tried Nasalcrom for a few days but did not notice any relief.

### Past Medical History

No major acute or chronic illnesses. No drug allergies. Tonsillectomy as a child. Immunizations up to date

### Environmental History

Has one dog, lives outside. No other indoor pets. Wall-to-wall carpeting, central heat/air, no basement or areas of mold. House is 10 years old.

## Review of Systems

| | |
|---|---|
| General | No weight changes |
| Skin | Negative |
| Neurologic | Negative |
| HEENT | See HPI |
| Cardiovascular | Negative |
| Respiratory | Negative |
| Gastrointestinal | Negative |
| Musculoskeletal | Negative |
| Endocrine | Negative |
| Hematologic | Negative |
| Psychosocial | Negative |

## Physical Examination

Conjunctiva injected; pale, boggy nasal mucosa with 3+/2+ edema and clear-water discharge. Throat negative, lungs negative

## Impression

Seasonal allergic rhinitis probably caused by ragweed, since her symptoms and physical examination results are characteristic of acute degranulation, resulting in histamine.

## Plan

Claritin 1 PO QD, Nasalcrom 1 spray EN QID, Nasonex 2 sprays EN QD for duration of ragweed season, Patanol 1–2 gtts OU BID (at 6- to 8-hour intervals), and Dalalone (dexamethasone), 1 mL IM. The primary goal is to prevent histamine release and block histamine receptors.

EN, each nostril; gtts, drops; HEENT, head, eyes, ears, nose and throat; HPI, history of prior illness; OTC, over-the-counter; PO, orally.

# REFERENCES

Adams, P.F. & Marano, M.A. (1995). Current estimates form the National Health Interview Survey, 1994. National Center for Health Statistics. *Vital and Health Statistical Series, 10* (193), 83–84.

Adelman, D. & Saxon, A. (1995). Immediate hypersensitivity: Approach to diagnosis. In G. Lawlor, Jr., T. Fischer, & D. Adelman (Eds.), *Manual of allergy and immunology* (3rd ed.). On *MAXX: Maximum access to diagnosis and therapy: The electronic library of medicine* (CD-ROM). Philadelphia: Lippincott-Raven.

Adelman, D., Kesarwala, H., & Fischer, T. (1995). Introduction to the immune system. In G. Lawlor, Jr., T. Fischer, & D. Adelman (Eds.), *Manual of allergy and immunology* (3rd ed.). On *MAXX: Maximum access to diagnosis and therapy: The electronic library of medicine* (CD-ROM). Philadelphia: Lippincott-Raven.

Alcon (1997). Patanol [package insert]. Fort Worth, TX: Alcon Laboratories.

Barnes, P., Fitzgerald, G., Brown, M., & Dollery, C. (1980). Nocturnal asthma and changes in circulating epinephrine, histamine and cortisol. *New England Journal of Medicine, 303* (5), 263–267.

Barnes, P. (1993). Pathophysiology of allergic inflammation. In E. Middleton, C. Reed, E. Ellis, N. Adkinson, Jr., J. Yunginger, & W. Busse (Eds.), *Allergy: Principles and practice* (4th ed.). St. Louis: Mosby-Year Book.

Bernstein, J. (1997). Antihistamines. In R. Patterson, L.C. Grammar, & P. Greenberger (Eds.), *Allergic diseases: Diagnosis and management* (5th ed.). Philadelphia: Lippincott-Raven.

Brady, M. (1996). Atopic disorders and rheumatic diseases. In C. Burns, N. Barber, M. Brady, & A. Dunn (Eds.), *Pediatric primary care*. Philadelphia: W.B. Saunders.

Brooks, C.D., Nelson, A.L., & Metzler, C. (1985). Treatment of ragweed hay fever with flurbiprofen, a cyclooxygenase-inhibiting drug. *Annals of Allergy, 55* (4), 551–562.

Burge, H., Solomon, W., & Muilenberg, M. (1982). Evaluation of indoor plantings as allergen exposure sources. *Journal of Allergy and Clinical Immunology, 70* (2), 101–108.

Busse, W. (1996). The role of leukotrienes in asthma and allergic rhinitis. *Clinical and Experimental Allergy, 26* (8), 868–879.

Corren, J., Rachelefsky, G., Shapiro, G., & Slavin, R. (1996). Sinusitis. In C.W. Bierman, D. Pearlman, G. Shapiro, & W. Busse (Eds.), *Allergy, Asthma, and Immunology from Infancy to Adulthood.* (3rd ed.). Philadelphia: W.B. Saunders.

Demoly, P., Crampette, L., Lebel, B., Campbell, A.M., Mondain, M., & Bousquet, J. (1998). Expression of cyclooxygenase 1 and 2 proteins in upper respiratory mucosa. *Clinical and Experimental Allergy, 28* (3), 278–283.

Donohue, J. (1997). Asthma. In L. Dornbrand, A. Hoole, & C. Pickard (Eds.), *Manual of clinical problems in adult ambulatory care* (3rd ed.). On *MAXX: Maximum access to diagnosis and therapy: The electronic library of medicine* (CD-ROM). Philadelphia: Lippincott-Raven.

Druce, H. (1993). *Allergic and nonallergic rhinitis*. In E. Middleton, C. Reed, E. Ellis, N. Adkinson, Jr., J. Yunginger, & W. Busse (Eds.), *Allergy: Principles and practice* (4th ed.). St. Louis: Mosby-Year Book.

*Drug facts and comparisons* (1998). St. Louis: Facts and Comparisons.

Ellsworth, A., Witt, D., Dugdale, D., & Oliver, L. (1998). *Mosby's 1998 medical drug reference*. St. Louis: Mosby-Year Book.

Fischer, T., O'Brien, K., & Entis, G. (1995). Basic principles of therapy for allergic disease. In G. Lawlor, Jr., T. Fischer, & D. Adelman (Eds.), *Manual of allergy and immunology* (3rd ed.). On *MAXX: Maximum access to diagnosis and therapy: The electronic library of medicine* (CD-ROM). Philadelphia: Lippincott-Raven.

Frazee, L., Wissuchek, J., & Ziegler, J. (1997). Antileukotrienes in the management of asthma. *U.S. Pharmacist, 22* (7), 101–110.

Georgitis, J., Kaiser, H., & Kaliner, M. (1997). Allergic rhinitis: Taming the troubled nose. *Patient Care, 30*, 51–60.

Gopal, H., & Fletcher, R. Rhinitis. (1997). In L. Dornbrand, A. Hoole, & C. Pickard (Eds.), *Manual of clinical problems in adult ambulatory care* (3rd ed.). On *MAXX: Maximum access to diagnosis and therapy: The electronic library of medicine* (CD-ROM). Philadelphia: Lippincott-Raven.

Hamano, N., Terada, N., Maesako, K., Ikeda, T., Fukuda, S., Wakita, J., Yamashita, T., & Konna, A. (1998). Expression of histamine receptors in nasal epithelial cells and endothelial cells: The effects of sex hormones. *International Archives of Allergy and Immunology, 115* (3), 220–227.

Haus, E. & Touitou, Y. (1997). Chronobiology of development and aging. In P.H. Redfern & B. Lemmer (Eds.), *Physiology and pharmacology of biological rhythms*. New York: Springer.

Huang, S. & Marsh, D. (1993). Genetics of allergy. *Annals of Allergy, 70* (5), 347–358.

Hulisz, D. & Fillwock, L. (1996). Management of allergic rhinitis. *U.S. Pharmacist, 21* (7), 49, 50, 53–56, 58–60.

Iliopoulos, O., Proud, D., Adkinson, N., Norman, P., Kagey-Sobotka, A., Lichtenstein, L., & Naclerio, R. (1990). Relationship between the early, late, and rechallenge reaction to nasal challenge with antigen: Observations on the role of inflammatory mediators and cells. *Journal of Allergy and Clinical Immunology, 86* (6), 851–862.

Kang, B. (1990). Cockroach allergy. *Clinical Reviews in Allergy, 8* (1), 87–98.

Klucka C., Ownby, D., Green, J., & Zoratti, E. (1995). Cat shedding of *Fel d* I is not reduced by washings, Allerpet-C spray, or acepromazine. *Journal of Allergy and Clinical Immunology, 95* (6), 1164–1171.

Lawlor, Jr., G., & Tashkin, D. Asthma. (1995). In G. Lawlor, Jr., T. Fischer, & D. Adelman (Eds.) *Manual of allergy and immunology* (3rd ed.). On *MAXX: Maximum access to diagnosis and therapy: The electronic library of medicine* (CD-ROM). Philadelphia: Lippincott-Raven.

Lee, R., Smolensky, M., Leach, C., & McGovern, J. (1977). Circadian rhythms in the cutaneous reactivity to histamine and selected antigens, including phase relationship to urinary cortisol excretion. *Annals of Allergy, 38* (4), 231–236.

Lemanske, R., Jr. & Busse, W. (1997). Primer on allergic and immunologic diseases: Asthma. *Journal of the American Medical Association, 278* (18), 1855–1873. Available at: http://www.amaassn.org/special/asthma/library/readroom/pr7002.htm.

Leung, D. (1996). Allergic immune responses. In C.W. Bierman, D. Pearlman, G. Shapiro, & W. Busse (Eds.), *Allergy, asthma, and immunology from infancy to adulthood* (3rd ed.). Philadelphia: W.B. Saunders.

Li, J. (1998). Allergy. In U. Prakash (Ed.), *Mayo internal medicine board review 1998–99*. Philadelphia: Lippincott-Raven.

Lierl, M. (1995). Allergy of the upper respiratory tract. In G. Lawlor, Jr., T. Fischer, & D. Adelman (Eds.), *Manual of allergy and immunology* (3rd ed.). On *MAXX: Maximum access to diagnosis and therapy: The electronic library of medicine* (CD-ROM). Philadelphia: Lippincott-Raven.

Martin, J. (1993). Nocturnal asthma: Circadian rhythms and therapeutic interventions. *American Review in Respiratory Disease, 147* (6 Pt. 2), S25–S28.

McPhee, S. (1997). Disorders of the adrenal cortex. In S. McPhee, V. Lingappa, W. Ganong, & J. Lange (Eds), *Pathophysiology of disease: An introduction to clinical medicine* (2nd ed.). Stamford, CT: Appleton & Lange.

Michelini, G. (1996). Allergic rhinitis. In R. Rakel (Ed.), *Saunders manual of medical practice.* Philadelphia: W.B. Saunders.

Naclerio, R. (1991). Allergic rhinitis. *New England Journal of Medicine, 325* (12), 860–869.

Naclerio, R. & Solomon, W. (1997). Rhinitis and inhalant allergens. *Journal of the American Medical Association, 278* (22), 1842–1849.

O'Brien, J. (1998). Allergic reactions: 10 question physicians often ask. *Consultant, 38* (4), 851–854, 859–861, 865–866.

Platts-Mills, T. & Chapman, M. (1987). Dust mites: Immunology, allergic disease, and environmental control. *Journal of Allergy and Clinical Immunology, 80* (6), 755–774.

Proud, D., Reynolds, C., Lacapra, S., Kagey-Sobotka, A., Lichtenstein, L., & Naclerio, R. (1988). Nasal provocation with bradykinin induces symptoms of rhinitis and a sore throat. *American Review of Respiratory Disease, 137* (3), 613–616.

Ransom, J. (1997). Sinusitis: Diagnosis and treatment. *Medscape, 1* (8) [on-line]. Available at: http://www.medscape.com/Medscape/RespiratoryCare/1997/v01.n08/mrc3087.ransom/mrc3087.ransom.html.

Reinberg, A., Gervais, P., Levi, F., Smolensky, M., Del Cerro, L., & Ugolini, C. (1988). Circadian and circannual rhythms of allergic rhinitis: An epidemiologic study involving chronobiologic methods. *Journal of Allergy and Clinical Immunology, 81* (1), 51–62.

Reinberg, A. (1997). Chronopharmacology of H$_1$-receptor antagonists. In P.H. Redfern & B. Lemmer (Eds.), *Physiology and pharmacology of biological rhythms.* New York: Springer.

Ritchie, A., Oswald, I., Micklem, H., Boyd, J., Elton, R., Jazwinska, E., & James, K. (1983). Circadian variation of lymphocyte subpopulations: A study with monoclonal antibodies. *British Medical Journal, 286* (6380), 1773–1775.

Schleimer, R. (1993). Glucocorticosteroids: Their mechanisms of action and use in allergic diseases. In E. Middleton, C. Reed, E. Ellis, N. Adkinson, Jr., J. Yunginger, & W. Busse (Eds.), *Allergy: Principles and practice* (4th ed.). St. Louis: Mosby-Year Book.

Shames, R. & Adelman, D. (1997). Disorders of the immune system. In S. McPhee, V. Lingappa, W. Ganong, & J. Lange (Eds.), *Pathophysiology of disease: An introduction to clinical medicine* (2nd ed.). Stamford, CT: Appleton & Lange.

Shlom, E. (1996). Adrenocortical dysfunction and clinical use of steroids. In E. Herfindal & D. Gourley (Eds.), *Textbook of therapeutics: Drug and disease management* (6th ed.). Baltimore: Williams & Wilkins.

Simons, F.E. & Simons, K.J. (1993). Antihistamines. In E. Middleton, C. Reed, E. Ellis, N. Adkinson, Jr., J. Yunginger, & W. Busse (Eds.), *Allergy: Principles and practice* (4th ed.). St. Louis: Mosby-Year Book.

Simons, F.E. (1996). Pharmacology and therapeutics. In C.W. Bierman, D. Pearlman, G. Shapiro, & W. Busse (Eds.), *Allergy, asthma, and immunology from infancy to adulthood* (3rd ed.). Philadelphia: W.B. Saunders.

Slavin, R. (1993). Nasal polyps and sinusitis. In E. Middleton, C. Reed, E. Ellis, N. Adkinson, Jr., J. Yunginger, & W. Busse (Eds.), *Allergy: Principles and practice* (4th ed.). St. Louis: Mosby-Year Book.

Smolensky M. & D'Alonzo, G. (1993). Medical chronobiology: Concepts and applications. *American Review of Respiratory Disease, 147* (6 Pt. 2), S2–S19.

Spieksma, F. (1991). Domestic mites: Their role in respiratory allergy. *Clinical and Experimental Allergy, 21* (4), 655–660.

Takenaka, H., Zhang, K., Diaz-Sanchez, D., Tsien, A., & Saxon, A. (1995). Enhanced human IgE production results from exposure to the aromatic hydrocarbons from diesel exhaust: Direct effects on B-cell IgE production. *Journal of Allergy and Clinical Immunology, 95* (1), 103–115.

United States Pharmacopeial Convention (USP DI). (1997). *United States pharmacopeial convention drug information* (Vol. 1). On *MAXX: Maximum access to diagnosis and therapy: The electronic library of medicine* (CD-ROM). Philadelphia: Lippincott-Raven.

Wasserman, S. (1997). Biochemical mediators of allergic reactions. In R. Patterson, L.C. Grammar, & P. Greenberger (Eds.), *Allergic diseases: Diagnosis and management* (5th ed.). Philadelphia: Lippincott-Raven.

# Asthma and Other Allergic Disorders

Drema Phelps

Maureen Groer

This chapter describes the pathophysiology of additional allergic disorders, including asthma, anaphylaxis, and skin and food allergies. The primary care provider has many patients with allergies, and the range of severity and disability is wide. We have described the common allergic disorder, allergic rhinitis. Some individuals have rhinitis as only one manifestation of the pathophysiology of atopy. They may have other manifestations, depending on the season, their age, previous treatment, and type of allergen. Other patients manifest only one type of allergic response to a well-defined number of allergens. The heterogeneity of the allergic response has been previously noted and should be remembered by primary care providers. This chapter reviews common allergic disorders seen in primary care practices. Notice that patients with allergies often get worse or have flare-ups when they are under stress. Asthma is particularly noteworthy in this regard. Whereas psychoneuroimmunologic mechanisms may impact the expression of atopic disease in those who already are affected, they also may play a role in the genesis of allergy. A review of possible mechanisms through which stress can impact asthma is provided by Wright, Rodriguez, and Cohen (1998).

## ASTHMA

Asthma is a chronic obstructive inflammatory disorder of the airways characterized by airway hyperreactivity. The incidence of the disease has increased markedly in much of the world over the last 30 years (Crater & Platts-Mills, 1998).

In 1990, almost 10 million people in the United States had asthma (Grayson & Bochner, 1998). In that same year, the health care costs from the disorder were estimated at a little over $6 billion. The mortality rate from asthma increased by 40% between 1982 and 1991 (Barnes et al., 1997).

Many studies have been undertaken to explain the marked increase in both incidence and severity of this disorder. Dietary changes (decreased antioxidant intake, increased sodium intake, increased intake of saturated fatty acids) have been speculated to cause the increased incidence of asthma (Crater & Platts-Mills, 1998). Another theory suggests that air pollution is the culprit. However, for over 30 years, government regulations in industry have resulted in improvements in air quality in the United States, so air pollution does not necessarily explain the trend. The theory that seems to hold the most merit is that because of economic and societal changes over the last 4 decades, the amount of time that the average person spends indoors has increased greatly. This trend leads to greater exposure to indoor allergens, such as dust mites, and to a decrease in exercise. Dust mites have long been implicated in the development and exacerbation of asthma, and the improved construction and airtightness of homes provides a better environment for dust mite habitation. Another factor is that children and adults have become more sedentary. In parts of the world where walking still is the mode of transportation, such as New Guinea, asthma is relatively rare. Regardless of the cause, clinicians must deal with the increase in asthmatic patients.

## Diagnosing Asthma

The diagnosis of asthma is made on symptomatology and pulmonary function testing (Barnes et al., 1997). Asthma is characterized by wheezing, cough, dyspnea, and chest tightness. The severity of the symptoms depends on the degree of hyperresponsiveness and reversibility of the bronchial airway obstruction. The severity of the symptoms is not always a good indicator of the progression of the inflammation and obstruction. When airways become dangerously constricted or obstructed, the cough and wheezing may be markedly diminished (McPhee et al., 1997).

A classification for asthma based on severity of symptoms before treatment has been developed by the National Institutes of Health (NIH) and is presented in Table 8-1.

Airflow obstruction in the asthmatic occurs after an initial insult from an irritant. Bronchoconstriction, airway edema, and mucus hypersecretion result from the ensuing inflammatory process.

This interferes with the passage of air out of the lungs, causing air trapping and hyperinflation. The spirometry pulmonary function tests that best demonstrate these changes are (1) peak expiratory flow rate (PEF), (2) forced expiratory volume in the first second ($FEV_1$), and (3) ratio of forced expiratory volume in the first second to forced vital capacity ($FEV_1/FVC$). These spirometric tests measure the amount of air that the lungs can expel in a given amount of time. The normal ranges for these test results depend on age, sex, race, and height (NIH, 1997). In the asthmatic, reversibility of the abnormal spirometry results helps to diagnose the disorder. After spirometry tests are done, the patient inhales a short-acting $beta_2$ agonist, and the tests are repeated. The degree of reversibility of the initial results helps to determine the severity of the asthmatic response. A simple method of measuring the PEF is the portable spirometer, which is a small, inexpensive device that the patient can use at home to demonstrate trends in peak flow volume by recording

## TABLE 8.1   ● ● ●

### Severity of Asthma

| | Symptoms | Nightime Symptoms | Lung Function |
|---|---|---|---|
| Step 1: Mild intermittent | Symptoms 2 times/wk<br>Asymptomatic; normal PEF between exacerbations<br>Exacerbations brief; varying intensity | 2 times/mo | $FEV_1$ or PEF about 80% predicted value<br>PEF variability < 20% |
| Step 2: Mild persistent | Symptoms > 2 times/wk but < 1 time/d<br>Exacerbations may affect activity | > 2 times/mo | $FEV_1$ or PEF about 80% predicted value<br>PEF variability 20%–30% |
| Step 3: Moderate persistent | Daily symptoms<br>Daily use of inhaled short-acting $beta_2$ agonist<br>Exacerbation after activity<br>Exacerbation about 2 times/wk; may last days | > 1 time/wk | $FEV_1$ or PEF > 60% to < 80% predicted value<br>PEF variability > 30% |
| Step 4: Severe persistent | Continual symptoms<br>Limited physical activity<br>Frequent exacerbation | Frequent | $FEV_1$ or PEF 60% predicted value<br>PEF variability > 30% |

$FEV_1$, forced expiratory volume in first second; PEF, peak expiratory flow rate.
(Adapted from National Institutes of Health: National Heart, Lung, and Blood Institute [July 1997]. *Expert panel report 2: Guidelines for the diagnosis and management of asthma* [NIH Publication No. 97-4051]. Bethesda, MD: National Institutes of Health.)

morning and afternoon readings. Because of the variability in technique and accuracy, the primary care provider should supply ongoing patient education concerning its proper use.

## Risk Factors

Asthma does not respect age or socioeconomic status (Barnes et al., 1997). It affects people of all ages and in every socioeconomic class. Because asthma has symptoms similar to those of other illnesses, it can be difficult to diagnose, particularly in infants and young children (NIH, 1997). Asthma is diagnosed based on symptoms and results of pulmonary function tests, which limits the ability for diagnosis in this age group (Barnes et al., 1997). Pulmonary function tests are difficult or impossible to perform on the infant and young child, leaving only symptomatology for diagnosis. Many illnesses in infants cause wheezing, which, along with cough and dyspnea, are the hallmarks of asthma. Martinez (1997) studied the presence of wheezing in infants as they progressed to the age of 6 years. A correlation existed in persistent wheezing during infancy and the incidence of wheezing at 6 years of age. The presence of narrowed air passages may predispose infants to later airway hyperresponsiveness. Atopy has not been implicated as a cause of airway hyperresponsiveness in infants (Barnes et al., 1997), and bronchodilators have not been shown to be effective in infancy.

During childhood, asthma is the most common chronic illness (Barnes et al., 1997). Hospitalizations for children with asthma increased by 200% between 1965 and 1985, with African American children admitted at a much higher rate than white children. Asthma and atopy in children are strongly correlated. Atopy is known to be strongly influenced by genetic predisposition, and the likelihood of childhood asthma is 23 times greater if both parents have asthma. Increased exacerbation of asthma between the ages of 8 and 14 years is a strong predictor for chronic asthma lasting into adulthood. Much of the current effort is directed toward determining the cause and optimal treatment of childhood asthma because of the increases in morbidity and mortality.

Adult asthma is closely associated with childhood asthma (Barbee & Murphy, 1998). Studies show that having asthma in childhood, regardless of severity, increases the risk for developing the disorder in adulthood. Atopy is found in most adult asthmatics. In the elderly, atopy may not be as prevalent; however, the aging process is thought to affect the ability of the immune system to mount a response (Quadrelli & Roncoroni, 1998). Symptoms of asthma generally are more severe in the elderly population, and the elderly have an increased use of corticosteroids and shorter intervals between asthma exacerbation. The worsening severity with age is thought to result from the duration of asthma and the aging process. Asthma, regardless of the age, is a potentially fatal disorder that must be monitored closely.

## Intrinsic and Extrinsic Asthma

Asthma was once considered and treated as a disease primarily of airway reactivity and bronchospasm, instigated by allergic mechanisms. Current thinking, however, is that asthma is primarily an inflammatory disease that may be provoked by a number and variety of stimuli. Two general categories of asthma exist: one with clear evidence of atopy (extrinsic asthma) (Ying et al., 1998); and intrinsic asthma, which may occur without exposure to an external allergen. A person with extrinsic asthma also can develop airway obstruction in response to the stimuli known to provoke intrinsic asthma. Most patients with childhood-onset asthma have extrinsic asthma, and these children often have other allergic manifestations such as allergic rhinitis and eczema (Martinez, 1997). Intrinsic asthmatics seem to have no identifiable allergens that initiate the symptoms of asthma (Ying et al., 1998). These typically are female individuals who have adult-onset asthma. Generally, IgE levels are normal, whereas in an allergic response, the IgE level is elevated. Because of the similar cascade of events in extrinsic and intrinsic asthma, some researchers believe that an unidentified allergen is responsible for intrinsic asthma (Barnes et al., 1997).

## Pathophysiology of Asthma

The symptoms of asthma are coughing, wheezing, dyspnea, and chest tightness (Grayson & Bochner, 1998). These symptoms are a result of the cascade of events that take place after the airways have been exposed to an allergen or other stimuli (Barnes et al., 1997). These changes are illustrated in Figure 8-1. Although these stimuli mostly involve inhalation, asthma also may appear in response to food allergens and injected substances. Once initiated, both an early and a late phase follow. The early phase is characterized by bronchial smooth muscle spasm, edema of the airway mucosa from leakage of serum proteins through permeable capillaries, increased mucous production, and development of mucous plugs. The late

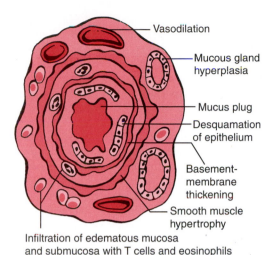

— Vasodilation

— Mucous gland hyperplasia

— Mucus plug

— Desquamation of epithelium

— Basement-membrane thickening

— Smooth muscle hypertrophy

Infiltration of edematous mucosa and submucosa with T cells and eosinophils

**FIGURE 8.1** ● Acute and chronic airway changes seen in asthma.

phase is characterized by inflammation of the airways leading to epithelial denudation, cellular infiltration, submucosal edema, and increased collagen deposition under the epithelial basement membrane (Lemanske & Busse, 1997). These pathophysiologic events cause airway hyperresponsiveness (bronchoconstriction) and, usually, reversible airway obstruction. Chronic changes include airway remodeling, leading to permanent fibrotic effects. The cascade of events in the inflammatory process is complex and is initiated mainly by IgE-allergen binding on the membrane surfaces of mast cells.

The previous chapter discusses the tendency of the atopic person to produce higher levels of IgE than normal in response to antigens. The same pathophysiologic processes occur in asthma or any other type of allergic manifestation. However, in asthma, the allergens usually are inhaled into the airways, and the allergic inflammatory response thus is confined to the respiratory passages, whereas in allergic rhinitis, the disease process involves the nasal mucosa.

When a stimulus (inhaled allergen or chemical irritant) initiates the process, structural and biologic changes occur in the airways. The mast cell is largely responsible for the clinical response that initially occurs in asthma. It usually is the first type of cell on the scene in an inflammatory response because it is a resident cell in the tissues. Numerous naturally occurring tissue mast cells normally are found in the nasal mucosa, conjunctiva, and lung. The location of these cells helps to explain the manifestations of allergy as watery eyes, nasal discharge, and bronchial edema. Once

the mast cell has been stimulated by membrane-bound allergen-IgE binding, degranulation occurs, releasing the mediators that are stored in mast cell granules. Other inflammatory cells that are later arrivals include basophils, lymphocytes, neutrophils, and eosinophils. These cells are largely responsible for the prolonged allergic response in asthmatics. The basophil originates in the bone marrow, with interleukin (IL)-3 stimulating the differentiation of the cell. Basophils and mast cells bind IgE through cell Fc receptors. Unlike mast cells, basophils also bind IgG. The basophilic granules contain histamine and IL-4. Histamine causes bronchoconstriction, bronchospasm, mucus secretion, and airway edema. IL-4 is responsible for increasing IgE production, which facilitates and prolongs the allergic response.

Mast cells degranulate when allergen binds to bound IgE on the cell surface, as described in Chapter 7. Mediators released by degranulation include histamine, tryptase, and chymase. Histamine is produced through the action of the enzyme histidine decarboxylase. Histamine's effects on lung tissue depend on whether the $H_1$, $H_2$, or $H_3$ receptor is stimulated. The $H_1$ receptors on the bronchial smooth muscle cause bronchospasm, bronchoconstriction, and airway edema. The $H_2$ receptors cause increased mucus production. The $H_3$ receptor works as a negative feedback to regulate the release of histamine. Another role of histamine is as a messenger to the other components of the inflammatory process. Histamine can cause increased production of prostaglandins and antibodies. This may partly explain the prolonged bronchoconstriction in some asthmatics.

Tryptase is a serine protease that is made and released by mast cells (Barnes et al., 1997). Tryptase is released in such abundance after mast cell activation that it often is measured in studies to evaluate the asthmatic response. Tryptase is a larger molecule than histamine, moving more slowly to the inflamed site and exhibiting its effect after histamine already has been activated. The clinical effects of tryptase include worsening of bronchoconstriction by enhancing the effects of histamine on the airway and by degrading bronchoactive peptides (smooth muscle relaxants). Other roles of tryptase include the basement membrane thickening and fibrotic changes of the airways in asthmatics. This occurs because tryptase is thought to be a growth factor for smooth muscle cells in the airway. Also, as mentioned earlier, tryptase degrades the bronchoactive peptide, vasoactive intestinal peptide (VIP). Under normal circumstances, VIP prevents overproliferation of airway epithelium to preserve the integrity of the airway. The combination of the inhibited VIP and abundance of tryptase results in significant changes in the structure of the airway. After combining with heparin, tryptase may be involved in the transport of other inflammatory cells to the site of injury by acting as an anticoagulant.

Another serine protease that is released on mast cell activation is chymase (Barnes et al., 1997). Chymase, like tryptase, is made and stored in the granules of the mast cell. Chymase is not as abundant as tryptase, and only a few mast cells throughout the lung contain chymase; however, most are in the bronchial airways. The actions of chymase are similar to tryptase and include increased vascular permeability, breakdown of neuroactive peptides, airway tissue remodeling, and, possibly, airway repair. Increased vascular permeability allows the movement of proteins and fluid across the endothelium, increasing inflammation. Neuroactive peptides promote bronchial smooth muscle relaxation. The destruction of these peptides prevents relaxation, enhancing bronchoconstriction caused by the other mediators. A major change caused by chymase is the breakdown of the matrix proteins that compose the epithelial lining of the airways. This results in epithelial damage and, after repeated episodes, may cause permanent airway remodeling, leading to fibrosis and thickening.

Other mediators that are activated when mast cells degranulate are products of the arachidonic acid pathway and cytokines, as has been described previously. Phospholipases release arachidonic acid from membrane phospholipids. Arachidonic acid, after exposure to certain enzymes, releases mediators that are involved in the inflammatory response of asthma. The enzymes that act on the arachidonic acid determine the end product (mediator). The enzyme cyclooxygenase (COX) acts on arachidonic acid to produce mainly prostaglandin $D_2$ (PGD$_2$). PGD$_2$ is an aggressive bronchoconstrictor. The enzyme 5-hydroperoxyeicosatetraenoic acid acts on arachidonic acid to produce leukotrienes, mainly LTC$_4$. LTC$_4$ causes chemotaxis and bronchoconstriction. The chemotaxis occurs through specific receptors that are activated during the process, activating other components of the inflammatory process. The leukotriene LTC$_4$ becomes a contractile agonist at the CysLTs receptor, which is located on the smooth muscle of the human airway. This results in marked bronchoconstriction and airway obstruction.

Cytokines are released when mast cells are activated. Tumor necrosis factor-alpha (TNF-$\alpha$), IL-4, IL-5, and IL-6 are cytokines that are important in the propagation of the asthmatic attack. TNF-$\alpha$

plays a major role in facilitating the other inflammatory components of the asthmatic lung. For other inflammatory cells to be recruited, vasoactive effects must take place. TNF-$\alpha$ increases the levels of adhesion molecules, which cause the adhesion of leukocytes to endothelium. The leukocytes then move through the endothelium to the injury site.

The ILs affect the asthmatic lung in various ways (Barnes et al., 1997). IL-4 is thought to increase the production of IgE by influencing the specificity of the T$_H$2 lymphocytes. These T-helper cells promote B-cell synthesis and release of IgE, which is the immunoglobulin responsible for the atopic response in asthmatics. IL-5 is involved in the production and survival of the eosinophil. The eosinophil is a leukocyte that is critical in the prolonged response of the asthmatic. IL-6 is similar to IL-4 in its effect on IgE synthesis; however, IL-6 is thought to have an anti-inflammatory role in asthmatics as well. It is believed to be involved in a negative feedback mechanism that reduces the effects of the cytokines involved in the inflammatory process. Although much of the knowledge concerning the mediators is speculation, the importance of the mast cell in the inflammatory process is clear.

One of the hallmarks of asthma is the infiltration of eosinophils into the site of inflammation. For eosinophil maturation and activation to occur, the T lymphocyte must release IL-3, IL-5, and granulocyte-macrophage colony-stimulating factor (GM-CSF). These cytokines also are powerful chemoattractants, causing eosinophils to migrate to the site of injury. This accumulation of eosinophils leads to cell damage and airway edema.

Eosinophils have been recognized as abundant cells in the reactive airway of the asthmatic. The recruitment of these cells to the site of injury is mediated mostly by T cells. The effects of eosinophils on the asthmatic airway are epithelial denudation, airway edema, and bronchial smooth muscle contraction. The denudation is caused by the major basic protein (MBP), which is housed in the granules of the eosinophil. Animal studies demonstrate airway epithelial damage (Plager & Gleich, 1998), reduced ciliary action, and histamine release on exposure to MBP (Barnes et al., 1997). The airway edema is thought to result from the epithelial damage from the MBP. The bronchoconstriction also may be caused by MBP, which enhances the effect of cholinergic contraction of the airways. Eosinophils are abundant in bronchoalveolar lavage fluid. The inflammatory cells responsible for most of the clinical symptoms in asthma are mast cells, basophils, eosinophils, and lymphocytes.

Another cellular component of the inflammatory process in asthmatic disease is the macrophage. The macrophage originates from blood monocytes. The release of the growth factor GM-CSF during the inflammatory process stimulates the increased maturation and release of macrophages. This cell has several roles in inflammation, although its role in asthma is not understood as well. The macrophage is an important antigen-presenting cell. For T cells to become activated and release cytokines, the antigen-presenting cell (macrophage, among others) must be present for activation. This occurs through a signal passed between the B7 molecule located on the macrophage and the CD28 molecule located on the T cell. The macrophage also secretes cytokines when activated, including IL-1, IL-6, and TNF-$\beta$. IL-1 causes enhanced proliferation and activation of the T and B cells, which are imperative in the immune response. IL-1 also increases capillary permeability, allowing inflammatory components to migrate to the site. Oxidant levels increase as a result of neutrophil exposure to IL-1. Oxidants potentiate the airway hyperresponsiveness and obstruction by causing airway epithelium damage, bronchoconstriction, and decreased ciliary action. IL-1 also causes the increased production of other cytokines. IL-6 may be a necessary component in the production of IgE through the IL-4 pathway. TNF-$\beta$ stimulates cytokine production and increases permeability of the endothelium to facilitate movement of blood cells to the injured site. Each of these components increases the effects of the inflammatory process.

Another component of the asthmatic response involves the autonomic nervous system (Barnes et al., 1996). The adrenergic, cholinergic and non-adrenergic, noncholinergic (NANC) innervation must maintain a delicate balance to ensure a normally functioning airway. The adrenergic effect on the airway, through the release of catecholamines, is bronchodilation and mucus secretion. The cholinergic effect is the opposite, through acetylcholine, causing bronchoconstriction, increased mucus secretion, and bronchial vasodilation. When the airways are not hyperresponsive, the cholinergic effect maintains airway tone through the vagus nerve. During the inflammatory process, the cholinergic innervation is exposed through eosinophilic denudation of the airway epithelium. After exposure, several irritants cause activation, including cold air, citric acid, and inflammatory mediators (prostaglandins, bradykinin). Another stimulus that may

activate the cholinergic effect is increased vagal output. This occurs during emotional stress or at night, with no known cause. It is assumed that during an asthmatic response, the cholinergic effect overrides the adrenergic effect with resulting bronchoconstriction, mucus production, and circulatory congestion. The sympathetic beta-adrenergic system may be hyporesponsive, thus allowing the vagus to override. Studies have found a variety of genetic defects in the beta-adrenergic receptors of asthmatics (Lemanske & Busse, 1997). NANC innervation is a new discovery. Little is known about the function of NANC innervation, except that it stimulates bronchodilation and mucus secretion. If NANC innervation malfunctions, bronchoconstriction may result.

## Triggers for Asthma

The causes of asthma attacks include exposure to an allergen; exposure to cold air (Skowronski et al., 1998); viral illness, particularly rhinovirus (Suzuki et al., 1998); exercise (Barnes et al., 1998); and ingestion of aspirin in those with aspirin sensitivity. Asthma usually is exacerbated in the early morning (Barnes et al., 1997). This occurs because of the natural rhythm of the body's chemical balance and is referred to as nocturnal asthma. The degree of hyperresponsiveness of the airways corresponds to this rhythm; however, it is not limited to this phenomenon. Asthma can be triggered at any time of the day.

Although the mechanism of nocturnal asthma exacerbation is not known, several circadian rhythms during the early morning contribute to the problem. Hormonal changes include the decrease in cortisol and epinephrine levels in the early morning. Normally, cortisol is thought to protect the airways through its anti-inflammatory effect. Epinephrine acts on the beta$_2$ receptors to cause bronchial smooth muscle relaxation and, thus, bronchodilation. These early morning changes may cause the airways to become inflamed and constricted, with less stimulation than is needed normally to initiate an asthmatic response. Also, the cholinergic response (increased bronchial airway tone) increases late at night and early in the morning. In asthmatics, the cholinergic tone is increased at all times, worsening the response during the early morning hours. Along with increased tendency for bronchoconstriction, histamine levels rise at the same time. The increased histamine levels are specific to asthmatics. As discussed earlier, histamine promotes bronchoconstriction, mucus secretion, and airway edema. In the early morning, when the cortisol and epinephrine levels decrease, the cholinergic airway tone increases, and histamine release increases, the asthmatic is predisposed to have an asthmatic attack.

Allergen exposure is thought to cause most of the extrinsic asthma exacerbations. Although all asthmatics do not have positive results from skin tests, many researchers believe that the asthmatic response is mounted in response to allergens, some of which may be unidentified. Once the exposure has occurred, the inflammatory process mobilizes fluids, proteins, and inflammatory cells to the injured site. Some common allergens include the house dust mite, cat dander, the cockroach, fungi, pollen from any source, and environmental irritants such as cigarette smoke (Eisner et al., 1998). In some studies, the house dust mite has been implicated as the most prevalent allergen in asthmatics (Duffy et al., 1998). Sensitization to the mites may take several years. This phenomenon is reflected in the increasing prevalence of asthma in persons of all ages. Another important environmental issue is exposure to secondhand cigarette smoke. The controversial issue of environmental cigarette smoke and its effect on asthmatic outcome was examined by Eisner, Yelin, Henke, Shiboski, and Blanc (1998). They found that asthmatics who were constantly exposed to environmental tobacco smoke presented to the health care system more often, the severity of the asthma worsened, and their state of health declined. When these individuals were removed from the exposure to tobacco smoke, all of these conditions improved. Health care providers must stress smoking cessation and avoidance of environmental tobacco smoke to the asthmatic person and the family.

The exacerbation of asthma from exercise and cold air exposure is poorly understood (Barnes et al., 1997). This phenomenon affects asthmatics of all ages, with about half of all asthmatics experiencing exacerbation of asthma during exercise. The mechanisms of irritation of the airways are thought to be similar for exercise-induced and cold air–exposure asthma. The normal response of the bronchial tree to exercise is bronchodilation, which is seen in both normal and asthmatic individuals at the start of an exercise session. Colder or dryer air reduces the humidification of the air reaching the bronchia and exacerbates the obstructive process in the asthmatic. Catecholamines are released as sympathetic nervous system activity increases during exercise. However, in the susceptible asthmatic, progressive bronchospasm begins to occur and reaches maximal obstruction 5 to 10 minutes after the exercise is completed. The intensity of the exercise (minute ventilation) is related to the degree of bronchospasm (Lemanske & Busse, 1997).

Cooling the airway by exposure to cold air does not seem to directly narrow the airway. This is supported by a study by Skowronski, Nelson, and McFadden (1998), who examined the effect of cooling the head and chest of asthmatic subjects who had been given a methacholine challenge. The results suggest that cooling had little effect on bronchoconstriction. Osmolarity changes in the airways during exercise or exposure to cold air could cause a decrease in the caliber of the airway (Barnes et al., 1997). Normally, the bronchial airway warms and humidifies the air before it reaches the terminal bronchioles (McPhee et al., 1997). During increased demand such as exercise or cold air exposure, this causes a change in the osmolarity of the epithelium in the bronchial airway (Barnes et al., 1997). When this occurs in the asthmatic individual, airway narrowing and asthma exacerbation occur. Another theory suggests that continued cooling and warming of the bronchial airway causes an increase in the blood flow to the area. This increase in blood flow causes airway obstruction.

Viral infections that cause upper and lower respiratory tract illnesses (particularly rhinoviruses) can exacerbate asthma (Barnes et al., 1997). This can affect all asthmatics, regardless of age. The mechanism for this is not completely understood. Animal studies suggest that bronchial denudation or beta-adrenergic inhibition may cause airway hyperresponsiveness, although these results should not be generalized to humans.

Another irritant for about 10% to 20% of asthmatics is aspirin (Barnes et al., 1997). Aspirin sensitivity usually has an adult onset in asthmatics, starts with signs and symptoms of an upper respiratory infection, and does not resolve. Generalized sinusitis may develop along with nasal polyps, chronic rhinorrhea, and worsening asthma. The physical examination may reveal polyps or mucosa suggestive of rhinitis (pale, boggy). Unfortunately, no test can detect aspirin sensitivity except the oral aspirin challenge. An oral aspirin challenge can be administered by a physician; however, depending on the degree of sensitivity to aspirin, a severe reaction can occur. It is difficult to distinguish aspirin sensitivity from other forms of sinus infections, and the tests available are not definitive. Therefore, the general advice to asthmatics is to avoid aspirin and nonsteroidal anti-inflammatory drugs (NSAIDs).

Normally, aspirin and NSAIDs are used to reduce inflammation and pain. This occurs through the interruption of the arachidonic pathway. Arachidonic acid is released from cell membrane phospholipids through the action of phospholipase. Mediators then can be formed from the arachidonic acid. The mediators that are formed are determined by one of the four known enzymes that react with arachidonic acid: (1) COX, (2) 5-lipooxygenase (5-LO), (3) 12-lipooxygenase, and (4) 15-lipooxygenase. Aspirin and NSAIDs interrupt the COX pathway, which forms prostaglandins and thromboxane. In asthmatics who take these medications, blocking the CO pathway is thought to cause the arachidonate molecules to be diverted to the 5-LO pathway. The end products of arachidonic acid and 5-LO are the leukotrienes $LTA_4$, $LTB_4$, $LTC_4$, $LTD_4$, and $LTE_4$. These leukotrienes cause bronchoconstriction and inflammation and are responsible for recruiting other components of the inflammatory process to the injured site. The other components of the inflammatory process, including mast cells, may be responsible for the continued exacerbation of the initial sensitivity reaction. Because of the difficulty of making this diagnosis and the importance of avoiding the sequelae from aspirin sensitivity, asthmatics should avoid taking aspirin and NSAIDs.

Exacerbation of asthma can be triggered by many irritants (Barnes et al., 1997). Most irritants are inhaled, but some can be ingested. The triggers mentioned earlier are some of the most common causes of exacerbations. Many unidentified irritants of asthma exist. Occupational exposure to allergens develops with time, and sensitization may occur to environmental chemicals after industrial spills (Lemanske & Busse, 1997).

## Categorizing Asthma for Diagnosis and Treatment

An important note about people with asthma is that they often have a flawed perception of the severity of their illness. If symptoms develop quickly and the degree of obstruction is acute, they will seek immediate treatment in most cases. However, if they are slowly progressing to an increasingly limited pulmonary function, they may not be aware of these responses or may ignore them. They may not seek health care until seriously ill. Asthma can be fatal, and the health care provider should have some method of assessing the seriousness of the illness.

For years, health care providers have treated asthmatics on an individual basis, without evidence-based standard protocols (NIH, 1997). Set boundaries, rules, and regulations for the management of asthma did not exist. The NIH recognized the need for consistency in diagnosis and management of the disorder and in 1991 released an expert panel report detailing recommendations for the diagnosis and management of asthma. This report revolutionized the attitudes and treatment of asthma, providing a source of uniformity to health care providers. Research was generated from the expert panel's report. As further data were provided, a new report became necessary and was released in 1997. This report gave specific guidelines for categorizing the severity of asthma (see Table 8-1).

## Physiologic Basis for Medications and Treatment of Asthma

The NIH places asthma medications into two categories, quick relief and long-term control, depending on the action of the drug (NIH, 1997). The quick-relief medications have an immediate effect on the airways and include the short-acting inhaled $beta_2$ agonist ipratropium (anticholinergic) and oral steroids. The long-term controllers must be used with regularity for effectiveness and include cromolyn or nedocromil (mast cell stabilizers), theophylline, inhaled steroids, and zafirukast or zileuton (leukotriene antagonists). A complete guide to the management of asthma is available through the NIH web site at *http://www.nhlbi.nih.gov/nhlbi/nhlbi.com*. The address is the National Heart, Lung, and Blood Institute Information Center, P.O. Box 30105, Bethesda MD 20824-0105.

## Developmental Considerations

### Asthma in Children Younger Than 5 Years

The diagnosis of asthma in the child younger than 5 years of age can be difficult (NIH, 1997). The pulmonary function tests usually performed in the diagnostic phase are difficult or impossible to perform in the infant or young child. In addition, because of the pulmonary structure and immune status of the young child, the patient may be predisposed to many upper respiratory infections that cause wheezing and cough that is not an asthmatic response. Clinicians are confused regarding how to diagnose asthma in the young child, and many cases of asthma may be missed in childhood. The NIH recommends that a young child who is symptomatic and requires medical treatment more than twice a week should be considered a candidate for anti-inflammatory treatment. Unfortunately, few studies have been done on younger children's responses to anti-inflammatory medications. Any treatment that is initiated must be closely monitored. Some evidence shows that inhaled or oral corticosteroids may cause developmental delay in young children. This must be considered when weighing benefit and risk of treatment.

### Asthma in the School-Aged Children

As a child enters the school system, issues of socialization and self-image emerge. When teaching the child and the family about asthma management, independence should be considered and encouraged, as is appropriate. As the child enters adolescence, these issues become of paramount importance and should be considered on every encounter. Another problem that may arise is the child using the asthma medications at school. It is not always possible to schedule the child's medication administration during out-of-school hours. A note from the provider addressed to the school may be necessary to ensure that the child can continue taking the necessary medications. The NIH recommends that the clinician prepare an action plan for the child, which should be placed in the child's file at school. The plan outlines necessary emergency information.

Other issues of importance when dealing with the older child are pulmonary function testing and exercise (NIH, 1997). When testing the older child or adolescent for pulmonary function, use appropriate guidelines for pulmonary function ranges. The ranges differ from those of adults and, if not referenced properly, may result in unnecessary treatment. Even if the child is on a treatment regimen for asthma, exercise should be encouraged. It is a myth that the child cannot participate in sports and other physical activities. Exercise should be discussed with the child and the parents, with specific instructions on use of a short-acting $beta_2$ agonist inhaler before strenuous physical activity. Asthma is a manageable disorder, and the older child must understand this.

### Asthma and Pregnancy

Controlled asthma in pregnancy is essential for maternal and fetal well-being (Barnes et al., 1997). Many studies have been done on pregnancy and the effect of asthma and related medications on maternal and fetal outcomes. Close observation and management of the pregnant asthmatic results in better outcomes. Continued asthmatic exacerbation and large doses of asthma medications may cause fetal hypoxia. Adverse outcomes that can occur in the pregnant asthmatic include low birth weight newborns, preterm labor, preeclampsia, and miscarriage.

Unfortunately, little is known concerning the effects of the asthma medications on pregnancy (NIH, 1997). Because of the magnitude of the possible consequences of misinformation to the pregnant asthmatic, explicit information concerning management, medications, and alternative treatments must be addressed throughout the pregnancy (Barnes et al, 1997). For more complete information concerning the treatment recommendations for the pregnant asthmatic, contact the NIH (NIH, 1997).

### Asthma in the Elderly Person

The management of any chronic illness in the elderly person is a challenge because of the effects of the aging process (Noble, 1996). Liver and kidney functions decrease, affecting the metabolism of medications. These patients may have more than one disease process, with multiple drugs producing polypharmacy, increasing the likelihood of adverse reactions. Many older asthmatics also have other pulmonary diseases such as emphysema or chronic bronchitis. These disorders can be exacerbated by the same irritants as asthma, making differentiation and management difficult.

Medication administration must be carefully monitored, especially with medications that can become toxic such as theophylline (NIH, 1997). The clearance rate of medications may be slowed in the older patient, and toxicity levels occur at a lower dose than normal (Noble, 1996). Polypharmacy for multiple chronic illnesses also can be a problem. NSAIDs and aspirin are used to treat arthritis and heart disorders (NIH, 1997). These medications are contraindicated in the asthmatic patient because of the threat of aspirin sensitivity. In addition, beta blockers are used to treat heart disease and some optic conditions. These medications can precipitate an asthmatic response by causing bronchoconstriction (Barnes et al., 1997).

Another consideration in the elderly is the presence of sensory deficits (Noble, 1996). Vision and hearing changes occur that can hinder effective communication. Education and repeat demonstration is important when discussing the medication regimen for the elderly patient. Although the patient may have someone to assist with administering medications, encouraging independence as appropriate is beneficial for the patient's sense of self-worth. Because of the developmental changes in the elderly, careful management is necessary to preserve quality of life.

Asthma is a disorder that, in its mild state, can be easily dismissed as an upper respiratory infection. The following case study is a about a real patient who presented to the clinical setting with vague complaints. Carefully consider the patient's history and his family history and try to understand how the diagnosis of asthma had been missed so often.

### ● Case Study 8.1

A 30-year-old white man presents to the clinic with complaints of coughing and wheezing throughout the night. He thinks he has "come down" with an upper respiratory infection because this has happened before. States the mild, nonproductive cough started at about 9 PM last evening. He lay down about midnight, after watching the news about the forest fires that had continued for the second week in the Smoky Mountains, which are close to his home. The cough worsened, becoming productive with moderate amount clear-to-white sputum, and he reports intermittent sleep. The patient woke up about 3 AM with continued cough and wheezing. He states that he "feels better" this morning, still coughing, and feels "tight" in his chest. Denies taking any medications for relief. States had shortness of breath during the night but has resolved somewhat. Clear nasal drainage × 2 days. Denies headache, otalgia, facial tenderness, sore throat, lymphadenopathy, fever/chills, chest pain, nausea/vomiting, or constipation/diarrhea. Works in an office. Has had similar episodes that kept him from going to work. States usually worse in the early spring and fall. Was occurring once a month; however, episodes increasing to 2 to 3 times per month. When exacerbated, would present to walk-in clinic and be treated for upper respiratory infection.

### History

#### Past Medical History

| | |
|---|---|
| Allergies | NKDA |
| Current medications | No prescription medications. Takes OTC Benadryl for a frequent "runny nose" |
| Surgeries | Had right kneecap removed 1979 |
| Injuries/Trauma | Had MVA in 1979—kneecap removal |
| Childhood illness | Had immunizations, chicken pox age 7, mumps age 9 |

#### Social History

| | |
|---|---|
| Married | Monogamous |
| Employment | Employed by a firm and in charge of public relations—stressful, travels a lot for job |
| Tobacco | Smokes 2 ppd × 12 y |
| Alcohol consumption | 2 beers/d |
| Caffeine intake | 6–8 C/d |
| Illegal drug use | Denies |
| Exercise | Daily, walks 3 miles/d unless bothered by an "upper respiratory infection" |

#### Family History

| | |
|---|---|
| Father | 60 y, HTN |
| Mother | 58 y, healthy except for eczema on both arms |
| Brother | 28 y, childhood asthma, allergic rhinitis |

### Review of Systems

| | |
|---|---|
| General | Denies weight changes, night sweats, or fatigue |
| Skin | States episodic pruritis on forearms, resolves in 1–2 d. Denies dry skin, lesions, rashes |
| HEENT | Wears glasses. Denies headaches, dizziness, sore throat, hoarseness, or dysphagia |

*(Case study continued on page 148)*

| | |
|---|---|
| Respiratory | States occasional wheezing, shortness of breath. Occasional coughing at night worsened by "upper respiratory infection." Denies history of emphysema, bronchitis, TB, or chest pain with coughing or breathing. Does not know when last chest x-ray done |
| CV | Denies chest pain, pedal edema, history of HTN or heart murmurs |
| GI | Denies change in appetite, dyspepsia, or reflux |
| GU | Denies pain/irritation/urgency on urination |
| MS | Denies joint pain, swelling, history of arthritis |
| Neurologic | Denies weakness, seizure disorders, numbness or tingling |

## Physical Examination

| System | Findings |
|---|---|
| Vital signs | T–98.8°F, P–88, R–18, BP–135/78 Height 6'0", Weight 175 lb |
| General | Alert and oriented, well-groomed, no acute distress |
| Skin | Warm/dry. No scaling, rashes, or lesions noted |
| HEENT | Head: normocephalic without scaling or lesions Eyes: sclera slightly erythematous, without discharge or crusting. Funduscopic—no AV nicking, hemorrhages, or exudate noted Ears: external auditory canals without erythema, discharge; TMs pearly gray with visible landmarks; hearing normal Nose: boggy, pale, scant amount clear discharge, no crusting or lesions noted, septum midline, no sinus tenderness noted Throat: without erythema, exudate or lymphadenopathy |
| Neck | Thyroid midline without nodularity |
| Respiratory | Breath sounds clear except for a few wheezes heard throughout lung fields, breathing even/unlabored, lung fields resonant, no rales or crackles noted |
| CV | RRR. No murmurs/rubs/gallops noted |
| GI | Abd soft, BS 2+, no masses or tenderness palpated, no bruits noted |
| GU/rectal | Deferred to complete physical exam on next visit |
| Neurologic | CN II–XII intact, DTRs 2+, muscle tone and strength bilaterally equal |

## Laboratory Results

| Test | Result |
|---|---|
| CBC | WNL |
| Chem profile | WNL |
| UA | WNL |
| Chest x-ray | Normal |
| Spirometry | 12% variability in $FEV_1$ after albuterol treatment |

*(Case study continued on next page)*

### Impression

Asthma, mild intermittent

### Discussion

Asthma is diagnosed based on the entire assessment of the patient. The family history, the patient's past medical history, and his current subjective and objective information must be considered. This patient has family history of allergic disease. Although it isn't necessary to determine a familial link in the diagnosis of asthma, it is common to find that link. The patient has a positive history of an allergic disorder with seasonal clear nasal discharge, which may indicate allergic rhinitis, and pruritic forearms, which may indicate eczema. An important part of diagnosis is the spirometry testing. Many illnesses mimic the signs and symptoms of asthma. Pulmonary function testing, demonstrating reversibility in the diminished lung function, is helpful in the diagnosis of asthma. This was achieved by determining that this patient had a positive spirometry test. He has been treated for upper respiratory infections instead of being diagnosed with asthma.

Asthma is exacerbated by irritants. Until allergy testing is done, the clinician will not know the triggers for this patient; however, some obvious problems may be the forest fires causing wood smoke, the patient's personal habit of smoking 2 ppd, and the pollen from the blooming plants. The patient could be sensitized to any of these irritants because sensitivity can occur after years of exposure (Barnes et al., 1997).

With education and medication management, this patient can return to a normal routine without constant interruption from asthmatic flare-ups. Although this patient's asthma is mild, close monitoring is important. Sensitization can worsen and become life threatening.

Abd, abdomen; AV, arterioventricular; BP, blood pressure; BS, bowel sounds; CBC, complete blood count; Chem, chemistry; CN, cranial nerve; CV, cardiovascular; DTRs, deep tendon reflexes; exam, examination; $FEV_1$, forced expiratory volume in first second; GI, gastrointestinal; GU, genitourinary; HEENT, head, eyes, ears, nose, and throat; HTN, hypertension; MS, musculoskeletal; MVA, motor vehicle accident; NKDA, no known drug allergies; OTC, over the counter; P, pulse; ppd, packs per day; RRR, regular rate and rhythm; T, temperature; TB, tuberculosis; TMs, tympanic membranes; WNL, within normal limits; UA, urinalysis.

## ANAPHYLAXIS

Anaphylaxis can occur in any setting, including the primary care clinician's office. Anaphylaxis is a nearly immediate (usually within 10 minutes) and systemic hypersensitivity response to an allergen that produces instant, dramatic, and sometimes life-threatening responses to allergen exposure. It also manifests as a bizarre reaction to a food or drug to which the person had never been allergic before. Common foods that can suddenly produce anaphylaxis are seafood and nuts. Urticaria and angioedema are the most common anaphylactic reactions, but the most severe are bronchospasm, airway edema, and shock. Most patients with anaphylaxis have cutaneous symptoms that are important clues (urticaria, edema, and flushing).

The pathophysiology of anaphylaxis is the same as in any other allergic response: degranulation of mast cells, usually in response to an IgE-mediated allergen binding. Common provokers of anaphylaxis are foods, insect stings, and medications. Anaphylactoid reactions appear to be similar to anaphylaxis but are not mediated by an allergen and an IgE response. Common causes of anaphylactoid reactions are drugs that directly stimulate mast cell degranulation (opiates), drugs that interfere with arachidonic acid pathways (NSAIDs), injection of immune complexes (intravenous gamma globulin), transfusion reactions, and non-immune complement activation (radiocontrast dyes) (Lieberman, 1997).

Histamine is the major, immediate cause of the symptoms in anaphylaxis. $H_1$ and $H_2$ are responsible for the cardiovascular and respiratory reactions. Binding of histamine to $H_1$ receptors results in increased vascular permeability, smooth muscle contraction, vasodilatation, increased heart rate and excitability, stimulation of sensory nerve endings, and increased viscosity of mucus. $H_2$ receptors cause cardiac effects, vasodilatation, and increased mucus secretions (Lieberman, 1997).

Because the arteriolar dilatation and increased vascular permeability result in a decrease in effective circulating volume, there is a compensatory tachycardia accompanied by a severe hypotension. Shock can be profound, since up to half of the intravascular volume can be lost into the tissue spaces within as little as 10 minutes of anaphylactic shock (Fisher, 1989). Bronchoconstriction can result in hypoxemia, which contributes to coronary vasospasm and myocardial depression.

The immediate recognition and treatment of anaphylaxis or an anaphylactoid reaction in critical. Included in the differential are vasodepressor reactions such as a vasovagal syncope; Chinese restaurant syndrome, which is a nonallergic reaction to monosodium glutamate; flushes such as the postmenopausal patient might experience; and several other conditions associated with dropping blood pressure, wheezing, or flushing. The history of allergen exposure is the most critical piece of information for practitioner, along with the immediacy of the onset of clinical symptoms. Patients must be treated aggressively and immediately with attention to the adequacy of the airway; a tourniquet should be placed proximal to the site of an injected drug or insect sting and released every 5 minutes for at least 3 minutes during the treatment. Oxygen should be administered, and epinephrine should be given subcutaneously or intramuscularly. Antihistamines, corticosteroids, beta-adrenergics, vasopressors, atropine and glucagon, intravenous fluids, and oxygen all need to be available in the office for the management of anaphylaxis (Lieberman, 1997).

## ATOPIC DERMATITIS

Atopic dermatitis is a common and apparently increasing problem that ranges in severity from mild to debilitating. Up to 20% of the population in the United States has this disorder, and, therefore, it is commonly encountered in primary care practice. It is often seen in families with a strong history of atopy, and the parental history of atopic dermatitis is the most powerful predictor of the disorder in children (Beyer & Wahn, 1999). There is a relationship between nickel in the diet and the development of atopic dermatitis, although nickel may act as a hapten rather than as a true allergen. Other contact allergens include fragrances, skin lotions, lanolin, neomycin, and metals. Atopic dermatitis can develop through skin contact with allergenic substances and should be differentiated from contact dermatitis, which is a delayed hypersensitivity reaction. IgE is a major factor in allergy, and the patient usually is atopic, whereas contact dermatitis occurs through T-cell–mediated processes and is present in the absence of atopy.

---

## *CLINICAL VIGNETTE 8.1*

Mr. Baxter is brought to the office by his wife after he complained of feeling "strange" at dinner. They were eating at a local restaurant, and Mr. Baxter had eaten two or three shrimp as an appetizer. Within 5 minutes, he began to experience swelling of his lips, hives over his trunk and face, and tightness in his chest. He had been seen previously in the office for allergic rhinitis. Currently, he presents with flushing, wheezing, and swelling—all classic signs of anaphylaxis, particularly in relationship to ingesting seafood. His blood pressure is 80/60, his pulse is 120, and his respirations are labored at 40, with pronounced expiratory wheezing. Mr. Baxter needs immediate treatment to avoid shock. He is given epinephrine intramuscularly, 0.5 mL of a 1:1000 aqueous solution, oxygen at 4 L/min by nasal cannula, and intravenous Ringer's lactate. He shows immediate improvement and does not require additional epinephrine. His blood pressure rises, pulse decreases, and his respirations return to normal without wheezes. He will require an antihistamine for the treatment of the angioedema and urticaria and close follow-up in the office for delayed reaction, which may occur 2 to 24 hours after the initial event (Lieberman, 1997). The patient should be stabilized and transferred to the hospital for careful observation, and instructed to avoid shrimp in any form for the rest of his life.

A genetic tendency toward atopy in infancy often is expressed by the development of eczema. The erythematous, dry, extremely pruritic lesions of infantile eczema appear early in life, often on the cheeks, and eczema used to be considered an allergy to cow's milk. However, eczema can arise as a reaction in breast-fed infants in response to allergens ingested by the mother. Common allergens that produce eczema include eggs, soy protein, and cow's milk. Children who are allergic to cow's milk during infancy may later develop eczema, allergic rhinitis, and asthma (Hill & Hosking, 1995). Eczema usually does not resolve totally with time, and as adults, the patient who had childhood eczema often has exacerbations of eczema when physically or emotionally stressed. Early introduction to solid foods also increases the risk of eczema in children. In a study of more than 1200 young subjects, children exposed to an early and diverse solid food diet had risks of eczema 2.5 times greater than children not introduced to early solid feeding (Fergusson & Horwood, 1994). Other potent dietary allergens that can produce responses in both atopic children and adults are nuts and legumes—particularly peanuts—fish, and cereals. Whereas allergies to eggs and milk often disappear over time in childhood, peanut allergy does not (Burks & James, 1997). Anaphylactic reactions to small amounts of peanuts have occurred in school-aged children.

Eczema and atopic dermatitis (these terms often are used interchangeably) can develop through food allergies, as described earlier. The general prevalence of food allergy is lower than is popularly perceived: only about 1% in adults, and 2% to 8% in children (Burks & James, 1997). Whereas a skin reaction can be a manifestation of food allergy, other possible effects are on the respiratory system and gastrointestinal tract. In a study of nearly 400 children with food allergies, almost half demonstrated their allergies in the form of atopic dermatitis, 18% had urticaria, 14% had edema, 8% had asthma, 5% had anaphylaxis, and only 2% had gastrointestinal symptoms (Rance et al., 1999).

In atopic dermatitis, a population of skin-associated lymphocytes seems to be specifically involved in the pathophysiology. These are the cutaneous lymphocyte-associated antigen T (CLAT) cells, which appear to be an expanded lymphocyte subset in patients with atopic dermatitis. These T cells spontaneously release IL-5 and IL-13, induce IgE secretion from B cells, and increase the survival of eosinophils by inhibiting apoptosis (programmed cell death). They therefore support a $T_H2$ cytokine pattern and humoral IgE responses (Akdis et al., 1999). A general finding in food-allergic patients is that their lymphocytes have an altered cytokine pattern, producing little interferon gamma (IFN-$\gamma$) when stimulated and greater amounts of the type 2 cytokines IL-4 and IL-5. The pathophysiologic basis of the atopic response therefore may involve decreased ability to secrete IFN-$\gamma$.

IgE has a dominant role in producing symptoms in food allergy. In atopic dermatitis, evidence indicates that the symptoms also are produced through mast cell and basophil degranulation after IgE-allergen reactions on the cell membranes. There is infiltration of the skin with T cells and eosinophils, hypertrophy of the epidermis and dermis, and expression of cytokines. Intestinal mucosal IgE secreting plasma cells and serum IgE levels are increased in gastrointestinal reactions to food allergy (nausea, vomiting, diarrhea, flatulence). In addition, foods can produce respiratory symptoms and anaphylaxis through IgE-mediated mechanisms.

Atopic dermatitis often is colonized by *Staphylococcus aureus*. Because the rash is so pruritic and people scratch the lesions until they open, the weeping lesions become subject to infection by skin microorganisms. When the skin has been damaged over time, chronic eczema, which is refractory to treatment, may develop. An example of this is hand eczema, which can develop on one hand while the other is spared.

## Physiologic Basis of Treatment

The hallmark of treatment for atopic dermatitis, or any of the symptoms of food allergies, is avoidance. This follows identification of the offending agents by testing and elimination diets. Topical corticosteroid ointments are widely used, especially when the dermatitis is in an acute phase. Solutions that decrease itching also help at this time, and some patients may require antihistamines. For chronic atopic dermatitis, tar compounds may be useful either alone or in conjunction with topical corticosteroid ointments. Occasionally, systemic corticosteroids are used in acute situations, but not for chronic disease. Phototherapy may be recommended for chronic conditions, and infections should be treated with appropriate antibiotics.

## REFERENCES

Akdis, C.A., Akdis, M., Simon, H.U., & Blaser, K. (1999). Regulation of allergic inflammation by skin-homing T cells in allergic eczema. *International Archives of Allergy and Immunology, 118* (2–4), 140–144.

Barbee, R.A. & Murphy, S. (1998). The natural history of asthma. *Journal of Allergy and Immunology, 102,* S65–S72.

Barnes, P.J., Grunstein, M.M., Leff, A.R., & Woolcock, A.J. (1997). *Asthma.* Philadelphia: Lippincott-Raven.

Beyer, K. & Wahn, U. (1999). Is atopic dermatitis predictable? *Pediatric Allergy and Immunology, 10,* (Suppl. 12), 7–10.

Crater, S.E. & Platts-Mills, T.A. (1998). Searching for the cause of the increase in asthma. *Current Opinion in Pediatrics, 10,* 594–599.

Duffy, D.L., Mitchell, C.A., & Martin N.G. (1998). Genetic and environmental risk factors for asthma. *American Journal of Respiratory Critical Care Medicine, 157,* 840–845.

Eisner, M.D., Yelin, E.H., Henke, J., Shiboski, S.C., & Blanc, P.D. (1998). Environmental tobacco smoke and adult asthma. *American Journal of Respiratory Critical Care Medicine, 158,* 170–175.

Fergusson, D.M. & Horwood, L. (1994). Early solid food diet and eczema in childhood: A 10-year longitudinal study. *Pediatric Allergy and Immunology, 5,* (Suppl. 6), 44–47.

Fisher, M. (1989). Clinical observations on the pathophysiology and implications for treatment. In J.L. Vincent (Ed.), *Update in intensive care and emergency medicine* (pp. 309–316). New York: Springer-Verlag.

Grayson, M.H. & Bochner, B.S. (1998). New concepts in the pathogenesis and treatment of allergic asthma. *Mt. Sinai Journal of Medicine, 65* (4), 246–256.

Hill, D.J & Hosking, C.S. (1995). The cow milk allergy complex: Overlapping disease profiles in infancy. *European Journal of Clinical Nutrition, 49,* (Suppl. 1), S1–S12.

Klein, J. & Horejsi, V. (1997). *Immunology.* Malden, MA: Blackwell Science.

Lemanske, R. & Busse, W. (1997). Asthma. *Journal of the American Medical Association, 278,* 1855–1873.

Lieberman, P.L. (1997). Anaphylaxis. *Medscape Respiratory Care, 1* (7), 1–17.

Martinez, F.D. (1997). Definition of pediatric asthma and associated risk factors. *Pediatric Pulmonology, 15,* S9–S12.

McPhee, S.J., Lingappa, V.R., Ganong, W.F., & Lange, J.D. (1997). *Pathophysiology of disease: An introduction to clinical medicine.* Stamford, CT: Appleton & Lange.

National Institutes of Health: National Heart, Lung, and Blood Institute. (July 1997). *Expert panel report 2: Guidelines for the diagnosis and management of asthma* (NIH Publication No. 97-4051). Bethesda, MD: National Institutes of Health.

Noble, J. (1996). *The textbook of primary care medicine.* St. Louis: Mosby.

Plager, D.A. & Gleich, G.J. (1998). Human eosinophil granule major basic protein and its novel homolog. *Allergy, 53,* 33–40.

Quadrelli, S.A. & Roncorone, A.J. (1998). Is asthma in the elderly really different? *Respirations, 65,* 347–353.

Rance, F., Kanny, G., Dutau, G., & Moneret-Vautrin, D. (1999). Food allergens in children. Archives of Pediatrics, 6 (Suppl. 1), 61S–66S.

Sano, S.F., Sole, D., & Naspitz, C.K. (1998). Prevalence and characteristics of exercise-induced asthma in children. *Pediatric Allergy and Immunology, 9,* 181–185.

Skowronski, M.E., Nelson, J.A., & McFadden, E.R. (1998). Effects of skin cooling on airway reactivity in asthma. *Clinical Science, 94,* 525–529.

Suzuki, S., Suzuki, Y., Yamamoto, N., Matsumoto, Y., Skirai, A., & Okubo, T. (1998). Influenza A virus infection increases IgE production and airway responsiveness in aerosolized antigen-exposed mice. *Journal of Allergy and Clinical Immunology, 102,* 732–740.

Wright, R.J. & Rodriguez, M., Cohen, S. (1998). Review of psychosocial stress and asthma: An integrated biopsychosocial approach. *Thorax, 53* (12), 1066–1074 .

Ying, M.G., Durham, S.R., Corrigan, C.J., Robinson, D.S., Hamid, Q., Humbert, P.R., & Humbert, M.K. (1998). Molecular concepts of IgE-initiated inflammation in atopic and nonatopic asthma. *Allergy, 53,* 15–21.

# Common Respiratory Disorders

Maureen Groer

This book has previously discussed upper respiratory problems such as the common cold and sinusitis, as well as allergic respiratory diseases such as asthma. In this chapter, lower respiratory tract conditions that are commonly encountered in primary care practice are described. These include influenza, pneumonia, tuberculosis (TB), chronic obstructive pulmonary disease (COPD), and lung cancers. Patients with these conditions may need referral to specialists or acute care facilities, but the primary care provider often is the patient's first contact with the health care system. Recognition of signs and symptoms and diagnostic skills and reasoning based on an understanding of the pathophysiology of respiratory diseases is prerequisite for prompt diagnosis and management.

## INFLUENZA

One of the most common respiratory infections diagnosed and managed by primary care providers is influenza (flu). Whereas respiratory symptoms always are a part of the clinical picture, influenza is a systemic illness. We describe influenza in this chapter, while acknowledging that for some people, the respiratory symptoms are not the most distressful aspect of being sick with the flu. A serious complication of flu, and the cause of most of the mortality from flu, is pneumonia, which is discussed later in the chapter under the sections on viral pneumonia.

### Characteristics of the Viruses

The influenza viruses are RNA viruses that are classified into types A, B, and C. Two identifying proteins on the outer envelopes of both type A and B influenza viruses, H (hemagglutinin) and N (neuraminidase), are used to further subtype flu viruses. The nomenclature of viruses relates to the type of H or N identified, the place of origin, the laboratory in which the viruses was isolated, and the year that it was isolated. Type A influenza viruses infect both animals and humans, which gives rise to the potential for genomic exchange between animal and human strains, so that possible harboring of lethal influenza strains by animals becomes a real threat. Type C causes mild infections, without epidemics, but types A and B occur in an epidemic-type pattern. During epidemics, primary care providers may see many patients who are very sick and unable to work or go to school. In 1994, 90 million people in the United States contracted the flu. This translated to 170 million days in bed and 69 million lost workdays (Laver et al., 1999). These ubiquitous viruses continue to cause high rates of infection and even worldwide pandemics, although most people have been exposed to them and have developed effective titers of antibodies.

The viruses are able to baffle the immune system because of the phenomena of *antigenic drift* and *antigenic shift* in both type A and type B influenza viruses (Treanor & Hall, 1996). The viruses mutate frequently, particularly at the H and N genes, and the minor changes that occur lead to amino acid changes in the protein products and significant subtype differences. This antigenic drift results in new strains of the virus appearing frequently, to which previously influenza antibody has reduced effectiveness. Occasional major changes in the viral genome, antigenic shift, results in significant changes at the H or N loci, and an entirely new subtype arises to which the population has no immunologic protection. This phenomenon occurs only with the type A viruses, resulting in extremely virulent new viruses capable of causing catastrophic pandemics with high mortality rates. The "Spanish flu" of 1918 was the result of an antigenic shift, and the new viral strain spread like wildfire across the world, killing 20 million people in about 4 months. The virus spread across the entire United States in 7 days. The Hong Kong flu in 1968 was another such pandemic in which there was a reassortment of viral genes with genes of animal origin in the H gene. The medical community expressed concern over the appearance of a new influenza virus that appeared in Hong Kong in 1997, killing six people. The virus infected poultry and jumped *directly* from infected birds to 18 people, a phenomenon that never had been reported before. All of the poultry in Hong Kong was destroyed to ward off the possibility of an epidemic or pandemic with a new strain of flu (Laver et al., 1999). Figure 9-1 illustrates the changes that occur in antigenic drift and antigenic shift.

### Symptoms of Infection

Influenza spreads through droplets sneezed or coughed by infected persons. The virus enters the upper respiratory tract, and the hemagglutinin on the outer envelope binds to cell membrane sialic acid. This initiates entry of the virus into the cell, where it uncoats and begins viral replication. The new virions formed in the cell have sialic acid incorporated into the outer envelope. However, because neuraminidase is able to cleave the sialic acid, the virus recovers its ability to infect other cells. Neuraminidase also cleaves proteins in mucus so that the viral particles can travel easily through mucus (Laver et al., 1999).

There usually is an incubation period of 1 to 2 days, followed by onset of respiratory and systemic symptoms. The upper respiratory infection is characterized by rhinitis, cough, and sore throat. Systemic manifestations usually include headache, malaise, anorexia, severe myalgia, high fever, and ocular symptoms (photophobia, pain on eye movement). The course of the uncomplicated illness consists of up to 5 days of fever; 8 to 9 days of respiratory symptoms, with cough sometimes continuing for longer and representing the most disturbing symptom; and continuing weakness and lack of energy lasting for up to 2 weeks (Treanor & Hall, 1996). A major concern in influenza is the development of viral pneumonia or secondary bacterial infections.

### Physiologic Basis of Treatment

One of the major goals of primary care is to prevent disease, and flu vaccination programs are effective at preventing influenza. Flu vaccines are inactivated whole virus, H and N, or split-product, immunogenic vaccines (Treanor & Hall, 1996). Individuals at risk require yearly vaccination because the strains of virus change, and last year's flu vaccine does not necessarily protect against this year's strains. Persons who should receive vaccination include adults and children with chronic cardiac or respiratory diseases requiring medical care; residents of nursing homes and other types of long-term care facilities; every healthy person older than 65 years of age; any patient with health problems or who has been admitted to a hospital for kidney disease, cystic fibrosis, diabetes, anemia, or severe asthma; any immunosuppressed patient; medical staff or family members who provide care for high-risk patients; travelers to foreign countries where there is flu; groups of

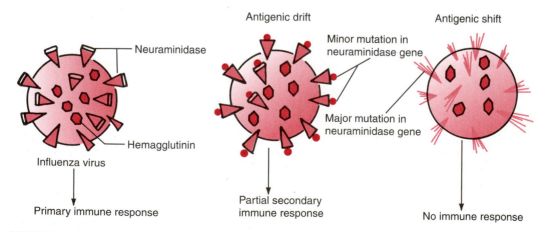

**FIGURE 9.1**  •  Antigenic shift and drift.

individuals living in close quarters; and any person who requests flu vaccination.

Another approach to influenza therapy is the development of antiviral drugs. Two drugs are available: amantadine and rimantadine. A problem with these drugs is that they do not cover type B influenza, and the viruses develop resistance quickly. A new approach is to block neuraminidase, which then would be unable to cleave the sialic acid on the virion's envelopes, thus inhibiting infectivity. Zanamivir and a newer drug, GS4104, do exactly that, and several clinical trials are testing newer neuraminidase inhibitors. These drugs do not prevent flu but decrease the infectivity of the virus after infection, thus decreasing symptoms and length of illness. Primary care practitioners may be able to detect flu virus by using a strip inserted on the tongue that detects flu; thus, in the future, they could prescribe appropriate antivirals before infection becomes established (Laver et al., 1999).

The general approach to treatment for influenza is use of symptomatic therapy to reduce discomfort and careful observation and early intervention for complications.

Web sites that are useful for primary care providers include the Centers for Disease Control and Prevention (CDC) site, which monitors the incidence of flu-like illness across the country and provides information about possible epidemics and new treatment options (*http://www.cdc.gov/ncidod/diseases/flu/fluvirus.htm*). Another site for information is the National Foundation for Infectious Diseases (*http://www.nfid.org/library/influenza/virus/index.html*).

## TUBERCULOSIS

### Epidemiology

Tuberculosis continues to be the major human respiratory infection throughout the world, causing greater mortality than any other infection. This is not true in Western countries, and worldwide statistics reflect the extremely high incidence and lethality of TB in the Third World. There are 20 million active cases of TB in the world, with an annual mortality of 3 million per year, most of which occurs in developing countries (Stead & Dutt, 1994). One third of the world population (1.7 billion persons) are infected with the TB bacillus (McDonald & Reichman, 1998).

In the United States, the overall case rate is roughly 10 per 100,000, a rate that, until recently, had been declining, probably as the result of better medical care for patients with TB. A decline in

medication-resistant organisms also has occurred, which had been a major problem in the 80s and early 90s because of incomplete compliance with medication leading to the establishment of resistant strains. However, a recent epidemiologic shift in rates is occurring in some parts of the country, such as New York City, showing a significant upward trend and a rise in medication-resistant disease. The case rate in New York City is over 50/100,000. The overall US incidence is 2.8 cases per 105 population for whites, 14.5 cases per 105 population for Native Americans, 17 cases per 105 population for Hispanics, 22.3 cases per 105 population for African Americans, and 41.6 cases per 105 population for Asians and Pacific Islanders. Males are more commonly infected than females by a 2:1 ratio, and there is a disproportionate incidence of TB in immigrants. Thirty-six percent of the cases of TB in the US occurred in immigrants in 1996. Risk for TB increases with age. Developing TB is also a major risk for patients infected with HIV. When people are in crowded and unsanitary conditions, the risk for TB increases, since the disease is spread by airborne transmission of tiny droplets, which usually contain one to three bacilli coughed up by infected persons. These droplets can become suspended in the air in enclosed environments for long periods (Snider, 1994). Such environments include homeless shelters, prisons, and nursing homes. It has become a disease of the minority population in the United States. TB was declared a global emergency by the World Health Organization in 1993.

TB has been present in humans for thousands of years; evidence for its existence goes back to the time when cattle were domesticated (Iseman, 1995). It has achieved notoriety as the killer of many famous people (eg, Emily Brontë, Frédéric Chopin, Edgar Allen Poe, and Vivien Leigh). The tubercle bacillus (*Mycobacterium tuberculosis*) is a hardy microbe, resisting acid and chemical disinfectants; it has been discovered surviving for thousands of years in the wrappings of mummies.

### Characteristics of *Mycobacterium tuberculosis*

*M. tuberculosis* is an acid-fast bacillus that is not motile and does not form spores or secrete toxins. A group of mycobacteria species has been identified as causing mammalian TB. These include *M. tuberculosis*, *M. bovis*, and *M. africanum*. Strains of *M. tuberculosis* vary in virulence throughout the world. *M. tuberculosis* has a resistant, waxlike cell wall that is difficult for the host to penetrate and destroy. The microbe is an intracellular, aerobic, hydrophobic bacillus. It grows best in tissues with high $P_{O_2}$, and the lungs are ideal in this regard. It can survive inside the cytoplasm of infected cells as an intact organism for years. It reproduces slowly and requires high levels of oxygen to divide and metabolize. Without oxygen, it can enter a dormant state, either inside the cytoplasm of macrophages, or extracellularly in the caseous material that forms in pulmonary infection.

An important characteristic of *M. tuberculosis* is its ability to develop resistant strains. This property was discovered early, when a soil-derived antibiotic, streptomycin, was discovered to be bactericidal for *M. tuberculosis*. Although effective, some mutant strains that were resistant to streptomycin always developed when this antibiotic was used alone (Iseman, 1995). This resulted in the resistant strain quickly dominating and surviving. Drug resistance occurs much less readily when two antibiotics are given together, since the probability for resistant mutants to two drugs developing simultaneously is small. If isoniazid and streptomycin are given together, the streptomycin-resistant strains that develop are killed by the isoniazid and vice versa (Iseman, 1995). A problem for clinicians is the new, multidrug-resistant strains that have developed because of incomplete treatment, malabsorption of drugs, or poor compliance. The rate of resistance differs according to population characteristics, such as sanitation, poverty, poor health care, and drug abuse, but is as high as 33% of strains being resistant to one drug and 19% being resistant to two drugs in New York City (Iseman, 1995). The overall rate of resistance in the United States was 14.2% (13.4% in new cases and 26.6% in chronic disease) in 1994 (Bloch et al., 1994).

## The Infectious Process

Once the inhaled droplets enter the airways, alveolar macrophages phagocytose the bacilli. This is both a blessing and a curse, since macrophages have the ability to destroy or inhibit the microbes. On the other hand, if the macrophages do not destroy the bacilli, the organisms can survive inside these host cells and retain their infectivity. Often, the macrophage seems to be unable to fully phagocytose the microbe, and the phagosome does not fuse with the lysosome, as is usual in phagocytosis (see Chapter 2). This results in a state of "suspended animation." The host can protect itself by killing infected macrophages, which produces a cheeselike solidification in infected tissue, leading to *caseous tissue*. The tubercle bacilli are not able to divide and multiply in solid caseous tissue, but

they can multiply extracellularly within the liquefied cavity that often forms in caseous tissue. There is a constant battle between host defenses and the evasive properties of the microorganism in TB (Dannenberg, 1994). It is thought that variation exists in the killing ability of alveolar macrophages and differences in the hardiness of the microorganisms, so that the disease results when the microbes are hardy and the host macrophages are weak (Dannenberg, 1994). The lesions are exudative, proliferative, or combinations of both (Moulding, 1994). Exudative lesions are inflammatory lesions heavily infiltrated with polymorphonuclear leukocytes, monocytes, and lymphocytes and producing a fibrinous exudate. Proliferative lesions are the classic tubercles, which are granulomatous lesions.

Whereas alveolar macrophages are the most likely to become infected and the lung is the most common site of infection, TB can occur in any tissue or organ. It is well known for its predilection for vertebral bones, causing Pott's disease. It can become disseminated by spreading from the lungs through the blood or lymphatic drainage. TB can occur in organs as diverse as the liver and the middle ear. This chapter, however, focuses on its most common manifestation: pulmonary TB.

## Diagnosis

A case definition of TB requires that the *M. tuberculosis* organism is cultured, or if not cultured, a positive acid-fast bacilli smear must be obtained. It also can be made clinically if all of the following are present: positive tuberculin skin test, presence of signs and symptoms of TB, treatment with two or more TB drugs, and complete diagnostic evaluation (MMWR, 1997).

There are four stages in pulmonary TB (Dannenberg, 1994), as diagrammed in Figure 9-2. Stage 1 (days 1 to 7 after infection) is characterized by destruction or inhibition of the organism by resident alveolar macrophages and no microbial growth. The bacilli inside alveolar macrophages may be destroyed and the infectious process arrested at this point. The macrophages may, on the other hand, rupture, releasing living microbes, which then initiates stage 2 (days 7 to 21). In stage 2 (symbiosis), immature, nonactivated macrophages from the blood enter the pulmonary tissue, initiate a granulomatous reaction, and form the tubercle. The bacteria divide and replicate at this point. Stage 3 occurs when the bacterial growth is slowed because of both cell-mediated immunologic activities and delayed-type

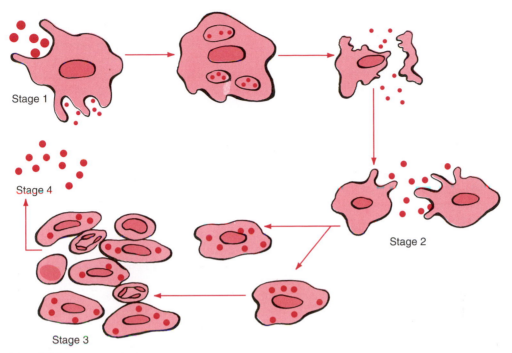

Stage 1

Stage 4

Stage 2

Stage 3

***FIGURE 9.2*** ● Stages of tuberculosis.

hypersensitivity responses. The tubercle becomes a solid, caseous lesion. Because there is a relative anoxia in the solid, caseous granuloma, the tubercle bacilli no longer can multiply, but they are able to survive. Because the bacilli are more or less dormant in this stage, the anti-TB drugs are not effective (Dannenberg, 1994). Macrophages are present in rings around the granuloma, providing a protective barrier for the uninfected tissue. Up to half of the solid caseous lesions that form in primary TB are completely sterile. The tubercles that become calcified and fibrotic are even less likely to contain living bacilli (Moulding, 1994). Finally, in stage 4, liquefaction of the center of the caseous granuloma occurs, which permits extracellular multiplication of the bacilli and an ineffective immune response to the large number of microorganisms produced during this stage. Cavitation then occurs, and the bacteria emerge to infect additional lung and bronchial tissue. Liquefaction is the most significant factor in predicting clinical symptoms of TB (Moulding, 1994). Fistulas carrying the infected material can form from the lungs to other areas such as the skin and musculature. Cavities form in the bronchi, leading to blood in the expectorated sputum. These cavitations are filled with bacilli, and the patient is highly contagious at this point. The bacteria also can disseminate into the blood during stage 4.

Diagnosis of infection is made by the criteria listed previously. However, in stages 1 and 2, the tuberculin skin test is negative, since up to 10 weeks of infection may pass before there is a positive skin test. A positive TB test indicates that exposure and infection has occurred, but it does not indicate the stage of the disease or whether living microorganisms are present. Providers also must realize that false-negative reactions can occur in infected people. Infants, immunodeficient patients, and persons receiving immunosuppressive drugs frequently have false-negative reactions. The size of the response also is not necessarily a good indicator of resistance or stage of disease.

*Primary TB* is that resulting from the initial infection. It may produce symptomatic disease in children, but often the disease progression is insidious, with chronic development of pulmonary pathophysiology and symptoms not appearing until adulthood. However, 95% of people infected with the TB bacillus never develop symptoms of the disease. Adult TB has had several terms attached to it, but it is *postprimary* and most often results from reactivation of chronic, latent disease and, less commonly, from reinfection. In HIV disease, the high prevalence of TB is thought to result from the former mechanism, with dropping CD4 counts being the primary mechanism through which *M. tuberculosis* becomes activated.

## Immune Responses to the *Mycobacterium tuberculosis*

The host defenses to tubercle bacilli are important deterrents to both local spread and dissemination, but they often are incompletely effective. Figure 9-3 diagrams the cellular responses, beginning with antigen ingestion of the bacillus by alveolar macrophages in the middle or lower lung lobes, which then travel to regional lymph nodes. As is true for other bacteria, the macrophage digests some of the microbes into smaller antigenic fragments and presents antigen in association with major histocompatibility complex I on the cell surface. However, as noted previously, some of the TB bacilli remain intact and alive within the macrophage cytoplasm because of inefficient phagocytosis. Antigen presentation results in activation of the macrophage, release of cytokines such as interleukin (IL)-1, and recruitment and activation of CD4 lymphocytes of the $T_H1$ class. The $T_H1$ cells become activated and proliferative, releasing IL-2, interferon gamma (INF-γ), and other proinflammatory cytokines. These cytokines stimulate resting macrophages within the tissues, a process that requires vitamin $D_3$ metabolites. (Perhaps this is the basis of the fresh air and sunshine treatment of TB advocated in the past). The activation of the resting macrophage results in further macrophage phagocytosis of *M. tuberculosis*. These macrophages then release cytokines such as IL-1, IL-6, IL-8, and tumor necrosis factor-alpha (TNF-α) particularly in response to the cell wall constituents of the bacilli (lipo-arabino-mannose). These cytokines transform monocytes into the epithelioid cells and Langerhans cells, which are typical of the developing granuloma. TNF-α is an important cytokine, causing the caseous necrosis in the center of the tubercle (Fine, 1994).

Other inflammatory and immune cells are involved in the production of the tubercle. These include $T_H2$ cells, natural killer cells, and neutrophils.

## Clinical Presentation

Tuberculosis is a chronic disease characterized by periods of illness and then, sometimes, long periods of apparent good health. The clinical symptoms of TB are nearly always pulmonary, with cough, hemoptysis, and chest pain being the most frequent symptoms. Early in the disease, the cough may not be productive, but eventually blood-streaked sputum is produced. The systemic manifestations of TB include fever and chills, night sweats, weight loss and anorexia, and fatigue. Most of the systemic symptoms can be explained through the effects of cytokines released by

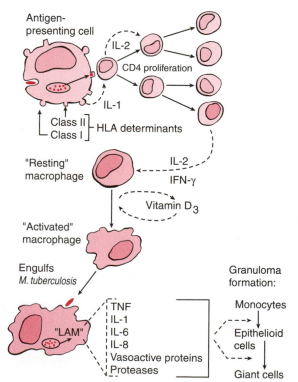

**FIGURE 9.3**  ●  Inflammatory and immune responses to infection with *M. tuberculosis*. APCs process and present microbial antigens and then present them to CD4 cells, secreting IL-1. CD4 cells proliferate and secrete IL-2 and IFN-γ. Resting macrophages become activated in the presence of cytokines and vitamin $D_3$ metabolites. The macrophages then phagocytose microbes, releasing a large number of cytokines that perpetuate the development of the granuloma. (Adapted from Fine, P.E. [1994]. Immunities in and to tuberculosis. In J. Potter & K. McAdams [Eds.]. *Tuberculosis: Back to the Future.* West Sussex, England: John Wiley & Sons, Ltd. Publishers.

macrophages. TNF-α particularly is known for its systemic effects. Depending on whether bacteria are disseminated to other sites, additional symptoms may be present.

Up to 30% of healthy elderly individuals harbor the tubercle bacillus. The elderly are a difficult group to diagnose. They may have concurrent COPD and other pathophysiologic conditions that obfuscate the signs and symptoms of TB. Symptoms may be nonspecific and atypical (McDonald & Reichman, 1998).

Figure 9-4 is a typical x-ray of the patient with pulmonary TB. There are no pathognomonic signs by radiography, although typical findings include pleural effusions, infiltrates, consolidations, and nodules.

## Physiology of Treatment

Primary care providers play an important role in preventing the spread of TB and in identifying those who are infected so that they can be treated. Table 9-1 indicates the groups of individuals who should be screened by tuberculin skin testing.

### The Positive Tuberculin Skin Test

The preferred skin test for TB is the Mantoux PPD (purified protein derivative), which is the most accurate and determines whether delayed-type hypersensitivity to the bacilli is present. A two-step procedure for testing may be required for elderly patients who are initially negative. The second test may be positive, since the first test produces a recall boost to the immune system that subsequently shows a positive reaction. When a test is

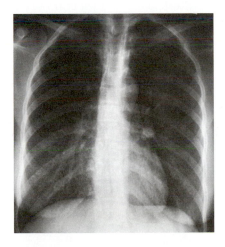

**FIGURE 9.4** ● Miliary tuberculosis in patient with AIDS showing fine diffuse nodular pattern throughout both lower lobes.

---

**TABLE 9.1**

### Groups That Should Be Screened With the Tuberculin Skin Test

Persons with or at risk for HIV infection

Close contacts of persons with infectious tuberculosis

Persons with certain medical conditions

Persons who inject drugs

Foreign-born persons from areas where tuberculosis is common

Medically underserved, low-income populations, including high-risk racial and ethnic groups

Residents of long-term care facilities

Locally identified high-prevalence groups (eg, migrant farm workers or homeless persons)

(From McDonald, R. & Reichman, L. [1998]. Tuberculosis. In G.L. Baum, J.D. Crapo, B.R. Celli, & J.B. Karlinsky [Eds.], *Textbook of pulmonary diseases* [6th ed., p. 613]. Philadelphia: Lippincott Williams & Wilkins.)

---

positive, it generally means that the person has been exposed to *M. tuberculosis* bacilli and has become infected. However, as described earlier, infection usually is a lifelong process of dormancy in that the bacilli are not reproducing and the body's immune system is actively protecting the host. Nevertheless, since a positive TB skin test indicates infection, the person is at risk for developing *active* TB and therefore requires treatment.

### Other Diagnostic Tools

Diagnosis of TB has relied on the chest x-ray, which still is useful in the patient with a positive skin test to rule out active disease. Examination of sputum and culturing for acid-fast bacilli are more definitive tests for active disease, and determination of drug sensitivity is standard.

## Pharmacology Updates

Because drug resistance is a major concern in treating TB, antibiotic therapy for TB needs vigilant and careful attention by the primary care provider. Three factors are critical: patient compliance, use of multidrug therapy, and length of time that the antibiotics are taken. In geographic areas in which drug-resistant strains are endemic, the choice of drugs may differ. Guidelines for treatment of TB are provided in Table 9-2.

Several web sites can be found on the World Wide Web. One address that enables health profes-

## TABLE 9.2

### Treatment Guidelines for Tuberculosis

| Clinical Presentation | Therapy |
|---|---|
| Positive skin test with negative chest x-ray Household contacts of patients with active TB | Isoniazid prophylactic therapy (300 mg/d) for 6–12 mo |
| Active TB with negative sputum smear and culture | Isoniazid and rifampin therapy for 4 mo |
| Patients with positive cultures | Initial phase: isoniazid, rifampin, and pyrazinamide for 2 mo, followed by isoniazid and rifampin for 4 mo. Minimal length of treatment is 6 mo |
| Patients who have failed therapy or have relapsed | Repeat susceptibility testing for resistance Retreatment with an initial daily phase of isoniazid, rifampin, pyrazinamide, ethambutol, and streptomycin for 2 mo followed by the same drugs minus streptomycin for an additional 1 mo, then 5 mo of therapy with isoniazid, rifampin, and ethambutol given 3 times per wk or daily |

TB, tuberculosis.

sionals to find many other links is *http://www.cpmc.columbia.edu/resources/tbcpp/extres.html*.

## PNEUMONIA

In the age of antibiotics, it is easy to overlook the significant contribution of pneumonia to morbidity and mortality. Yet pneumonia is the sixth leading cause of death in the United States and affects people of all ages. The greatest mortality is seen in the very young and the very old. All types of organisms cause pneumonia, and the treatment of pneumonia often is a therapeutic challenge. This section discusses the pathophysiology of pneumonia and describes the most common causes of pneumonia seen in the primary care setting.

Pneumonia is an acute, usually infectious, inflammation of the parts of the lower lung involved in gas exchange (alveolar units and respiratory bronchioles). Community-acquired pneumonia (CAP) is described in this chapter. By definition, CAP is pneumonia acquired outside of hospitals. Over 3 million cases occur each year, with up to 10% of the patients becoming ill enough to require hospitalization. The mortality rate ranges from 3% to 30%, with the greatest mortality occurring in the elderly, patients who are immunosuppressed, and in those who require hospitalization.

### Pathogenesis

Community-acquired pneumonia is more likely to develop in a person who has deficient host defenses than in a healthy person. Groups at risk include alcoholics, patients with COPD or HIV infection, immunocompromised patients, elderly patients, and patients with mental status alterations (seizures, drug abuse, stroke). Whereas CAP can be spread through the hematogenous route, it mostly results from colonization of the lower respiratory tract with microorganisms that previously colonized and infected the upper respiratory tract. Over half of patients with CAP report having had an upper respiratory infection within the 2 weeks preceding the onset of CAP symptoms. CAP rarely occurs as the result of direct inhalation of microbes, although *Legionella* organisms are transmitted this way. CAP can be classified according to the infecting organisms, with the most common bacterial infection being caused by *Streptococcus pneumoniae*. Other causes of CAP include viruses and mycoplasmas.

Contamination of the lower passages is the result of pathophysiologic mechanisms. Causes of impaired pulmonary defenses include a weak, suppressed, or ineffective cough reflex; decreased level of consciousness; airway obstruction; decreased epiglottal and glottal protection;

## CLINICAL VIGNETTE 9.1

Mary Nelson is a 27-year-old graduate student in nursing at a local college of nursing who comes to the primary care clinic for a physical examination before starting her clinical experiences. She has had no significant illnesses or hospitalizations and previously has been well. After graduation from college, she traveled extensively in the Middle East and Africa for about 1 year. She had routine immunizations before travel but did not take bacille Calmette-Guérin vaccine. Her purified protein derivative (PPD) has always been negative, but today she has a 10-mm induration 48 hours after her PPD skin test. She reports a frequent, dry cough for the last 2 months, which she attributes to allergies. She also has been tired lately, has lost about 5 lb, and has occasional night sweats. She does not think she has had fevers.

Mary's chest film shows bilateral infiltrates and a left upper lobe consolidation, but no cavitations, and her sputum is positive for acid-fast bacilli. Sensitivity indicates that she has developed a multidrug-resistant TB infection, probably because of her exposure in a Third World country. The organisms are isoniazid (INH) and rifampin resistant. Her HIV test is negative.

The physical examination reveals fine rales over the left anterior middle lobe, a fever of 100, heart rate of 90, respiratory rate of 20 breaths/minute, an increased sedimentation rate (50 mm/h), and mild anemia (hematocrit 32%, hemoglobin 11 g/dL). The rest of her physical examination is normal.

Mary is hospitalized and referred to a specialist in multidrug-resistant TB. INH and rifampin resistance is a difficult problem, and many of these patients have relapses. Most patients require a drug regimen with four to six drugs for at least 6 months of treatment.

---

immune deficiency; abnormality of mucociliary clearance mechanisms; and recent viral infection, which affects mucosal function, pneumocyte integrity, and phagocytosis.

The steps in the pathogenic process are illustrated in Figure 9-5. First, there is colonization of the oropharynx with pathogenic organisms, which may be facilitated by bacterial adhesin molecules, which allow attachment to the epithelium. Second, there is aspiration of upper airway secretions containing these microbes. The amount of aspirate and the virulence of the organisms are determining factors in this step. Third, there is invasion of the distal alveoli with replication of the organisms, which depends on host surveillance, immune integrity, and niches for infection. Finally, infection is established. Damage from infection generally does not result from toxins elaborated from the bacteria but from the inflammatory and immune reactions that are localized to the alveoli and lung parenchymal tissues.

### Host Factors

Figure 9-6 illustrates the defense mechanisms of the lung. The upper airway has a filtration function, trapping larger inhaled particles in the mucus and along the nasal hairs, turbinates, epiglottis, and larynx (Chaudhry & San Pedro, 1999). These particles then are expelled into the oropharynx through the mucociliary escalator. The material then is either swallowed or coughed out. Smaller particles that remain suspended in the inhaled air may reach the alveoli, which have several biochemical, immune, and cellular forms of protection. Protective molecules elaborated by pulmonary cells include comple-

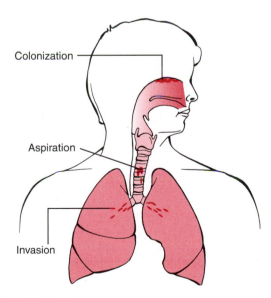

**FIGURE 9.5** ● Stages of pneumonia development.

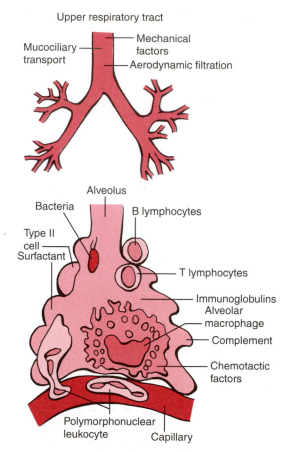

Upper respiratory tract

Mucociliary transport — Mechanical factors — Aerodynamic filtration

Alveolus

Bacteria

B lymphocytes

Type II cell Surfactant

T lymphocytes

Immunoglobulins

Alveolar macrophage

Complement

Chemotactic factors

Polymorphonuclear leukocyte

Capillary

**FIGURE 9.6** ● Airway defenses. Upper airway mechanisms provide filtration. Salivary IgA binds potentially harmful material. The mucociliary escalator moves particles away from the lungs that may be swallowed or coughed out. Material that reaches the lungs is destroyed biochemically or by alveolar macrophages. (Adapted from Fishman, A, et al [1988]. *Pulmonary diseases and disorders.* New York: McGraw-Hill.)

ment and surfactant. Surfactant is the first layer encountered by pathogens and is bactericidal for several bacteria. Another protective molecule is secretory IgA. These immunoglobulins are produced by migrating B cells within the salivary glands and are secreted in high concentration into the saliva, specifically binding to antigenic material in the oropharynx and neutralizing it, so that it is unable to penetrate the mucus into the respiratory epithelium.

If penetration into the alveolar unit occurs, resident lung macrophages are strategically positioned to engulf bacteria. Their antigen-processing and antigen-presenting function is enhanced by proteins in the alveolar lining fluid (Chaudhry & San Pedro, 1999). The activated macrophages then call forth vigorous inflammatory processes, dominated by neutrophil migration and typical cellular and humoral immune responses.

Local protective defenses ensure that the lower respiratory tract is essentially sterile, whereas parts of the upper respiratory tract are heavily colonized with normal flora, which protects the host by occupying adherence sites, thus displacing more virulent microbes.

## Microbial Factors

The organisms that cause CAP are listed in Table 9-3. Notice the differences in susceptibility for young versus elderly individuals.

### Pneumococcal Pneumonia

*Streptococcus pneumoniae*, also termed pneumococcus, is the leading cause of CAP. This organism is a leading cause of upper respiratory infections. *S. pneumoniae* is a Gram-positive, spherical diplococcus that often is a component of the normal flora in the oropharynx. It is more likely that an introduction of a new serotype into the normal flora will predict risk of infection than for CAP to develop from the organisms that have been long-time members of the flora. Most people carry four different *S. pneumoniae* serotypes in their normal flora (Blinkhorn, 1998). There are more than 80 serotypes of the organism, with virulence associated with those serotypes having a lower number. Serotype 3 has the highest level of virulence for human infections, and some serotypes are more likely than others to have developed penicillin resistance, which is becoming a major treatment problem for clinicians and their patients (Blinkhorn, 1998). Two common upper respiratory infections caused by *S. pneumoniae* include sinusitis and otitis media. The organisms must be aspirated into the lungs to cause infection, and most people aspirate small amounts of secretions during sleep (Chaudhry & San Pedro, 1999). However, this is not a common cause of pneumonia except in the elderly or comatose patient, and aspiration of large amounts of highly infected material, especially in an immunocompetent host, is required.

The mechanism through which *S. pneumoniae* causes pulmonary, meningeal, and blood infection is its ability to evade host phagocytosis. It is coated with a polysaccharide capsule, which makes it difficult for macrophages to ingest it, and the capsule is the major line of defense for the microorganism. The capsule, however, is antigenic to the host, and immunoglobulins and complement will react against it. Persons with titers of immunoglobulin to pneumococcal capsular polysaccharides are immune to infection. The capsule components differ among the serotypes, and the capsular polysaccharides of several

## TABLE 9.3  ● ● ●

**Organisms Causing CAP in Young and Old Patients**

| Organism | Percentage in Younger | Incidence in Elderly (>65 y) |
|---|---|---|
| *Streptococcus pneumoniae* | < 50 | Higher |
| *Haemophilus influenzae* | < 7 | Higher |
| *Legionella* | < 7 | Lower |
| *Staphylococcus aureus* | < 2 | Lower |
| Gram-negative bacilli | < 1 | Lower |
| Atypical (*Mycloplasma pneumoniae, Chlamydia psittaci*) | < 7 | Lower |
| Influenza viruses | < 7 | Lower |
| Viral | < 6 | Lower |
| Other | < 2 | Lower |
| No pathogen identified (probably many are *S. pneumoniae*) | < 30 | Higher |

CAP, community-acquired pneumonia.

serotypes are used for the pneumococcal pneumonia vaccine.

Once the cell wall is penetrated, the bacterial cell wall constituents, such as *teichoic acid* and *peptidoglycan*, provoke the inflammatory response primarily by increasing the secretion of IL-1, and numerous, but not yet well characterized, virulence factors are released from the pathogens. The microbes then enter alveolar pneumocytes, a process that is facilitated by cytokines, which may increase the expression of receptors to which the bacteria bind. As long as the organism is not phagocytosed, it is able to cause damage. Therefore, any deficits in macrophage and neutrophil functions allow the bacteria to cause the most disease. Patients who are neutropenic, alcoholic, or have undergone splenectomy thus are at higher risk for infections because of defective phagocytic abilities.

The clinical effects of pneumococcus depend on host defenses. The organism can be confined to the alveoli and distal airways, can spread into the lung parenchyma, and can even invade the pleura. The initial response is characterized by infiltration of many neutrophils and edema. This produces protein-rich alveolar fluid in which the microorganisms rapidly divide and grow. Macrophages and neutrophils attempt to phagocytose the microbe. Opsonization of the microbes, which facilitates phagocytosis, requires immune activation, which may take up to 5 days to effectively

occur (Blinkhorn, 1998). Macrophages process and present antigen to T lymphocytes, which elaborate proinflammatory cytokines and stimulate humoral immunity to bacterial antigens. As bacteria, inflammatory cells, and exudate fill the alveoli and invade the lung tissue, the tissue becomes thick and *consolidated*. This reduces pulmonary function significantly, causing overall reduction in alveolar ventilation, ventilation–perfusion mismatches, and shunting, leading to hypoxemia. Although cellular necrosis occurs in the lung, if the pneumonia resolves, damage is repaired and normal function is restored. If the disease has progressed to cause significant parenchymal tissue destruction, then resolution will be accompanied by fibrosis and scar formation, which leads to chronically decreased pulmonary function.

### *Clinical Picture*

The patient with pneumococcal pneumonia presents a typical clinical picture of illness. The exception to this is in the elderly, whose response is described later. There usually is a fever, which can be high, and may be accompanied by shaking chills, tachypnea, tachycardia, cough, and chest pain. Systemic symptoms include fatigue, anorexia, and often severe myalgia. The elderly may have "rusty" sputum, indicating the presence of blood in the distal airways. The physical examination may reveal dullness to percussion, diminished breath sounds, bronchial breath sounds, tactile fremitus, decreased thoracic excursion, inspiratory rales, and rhonchi. Some patients also have a pleural friction rub. These patients are extremely sick, yet most are treated outside of the hospital. Concern about development of bacteremia and significant hypoxemia and hypercapnia, especially in an elderly person, requires hospitalization in about 10% of patients. The more common complications of pneumococcal pneumonia include empyema, pericarditis, endocarditis, lung abscess, atelectasis, and meningitis. Most patients with CAP from infection with *S. pneumoniae* have radiographic clearing at 5 weeks, and most are completely clear within 2 to 3 months. Resolution of CAP is affected by the number of lobes involved and the patient's age.

### Physiologic Basis of Treatment

Diagnosis of pneumococcal pneumonia relies on the clinical picture, complete blood count, radiography, sputum Gram stain, and culture and sensitivity. A Gram stain of the sputum specimen demonstrating the organisms is definitive. However, culture studies may take several days, and treatment must be initiated immediately, so the results of the Gram stain generally are used for initial choice of antibiotic treatment. The treatment includes antibiotics and supportive therapy to restore the individual to wellness.

A growing concern for clinicians is the development of antibiotic-resistant strains of *S. pneumoniae*. A study by Ewig, Ruiz, Torres, Marco, Martinez, Sanchez, and Mensa (1999) found that over 50% of a group of patients with culture-proven pneumococcal pneumonia were resistant to penicillin, cephalosporin, or a macrolide drug. Resistance to beta-lactam antibiotics in *S. pneumoniae* infection results from mutations that decrease the binding of drug to the bacterial cell wall. Because of resistance, some clinicians do not use penicillin, whereas others consider it the first-line antibiotic. Erythromycin often is recommended for CAP as an empiric therapy because it covers *S. pneumoniae* as well as *Mycoplasma*, *Chlamydia*, and *Legionella*. However, erythromycin-resistant strains have been reported. Cefotaxime or ceftriaxone often is recommended for CAP because they provide coverage against *S. pneumoniae*, *Escherichia coli*, *Haemophilus influenzae*, *Moraxella catarrhalis*, and *Proteus mirabilis*. The practitioner should know the epidemiologic characteristics of the community because some areas of the country have remarkable rates of resistance to *S. pneumoniae* (eg, New York City).

Decision to hospitalize depends on the age of the patient, coexisting conditions, and extent and degree of illness. Elderly patients may require hydration and electrolyte therapy, oxygen therapy, nutritional management, and intensive nursing care. All patients with pneumococcal pneumonia require careful follow-up to ensure treatment efficacy. An algorithm quick test is available at *http://www.medscape.com/Medscape/features/calculators/CAP/CAPCalculator.html*. It allows a quick calculation of the risk for the patient managed as an outpatient compared with those who require hospitalization.

One of the most important aspects of care for patients at risk for CAP is immunization. It is recommended for all individuals older than 65 years of age; for immunocompromised patients; and for patients with diabetes, cancer, or renal disease. The protection offered by the vaccine is on the order of about 56% to 70%, and it provides protection for most people for several years. Revaccination every 6 years is an option for high-risk patients. Vaccination in this country is underused; it could prevent a significant number of illnesses and deaths (Ely, 1997).

## Other Types of Community-Acquired Pneumonia

Table 9-3 indicates the causes of CAP. Often, the clinician must determine the etiology based on a variety of factors. *Legionella pneumoniae* gained notoriety as the cause of Legionnaires' disease at a Legionnaires' convention in Philadelphia in 1976. The organism grows in water, and the disease was spread through contaminated air-conditioning systems. This organism can be aerosolized and inhaled deep into the lungs. The organism is a Gram-negative bacillus, which occurs seasonally in outbreaks during the summer and early fall. It causes an acute-onset, rapidly progressive bacterial pneumonia and produces both systemic and hepatic effects.

Another important organism in the etiology of CAP is *Mycoplasma pneumoniae*. The genus *Mycoplasma* consists of organisms that are the smallest free-living microbes. Their cell walls contain both RNA and DNA and have receptors that allow them to attach to human cell membranes. In the lungs, attachment to respiratory epithelium causes denudation of the cilia and death of the cells (O'Handley & Gray, 1997). *M. pneumoniae* is a resident of the normal flora in many individuals. It can cause upper respiratory infections such as pharyngitis and otitis media. The organism is spread through direct contact with respiratory droplets from an infected host. It is more common in populations living in close quarters, such as in the army, and it also occurs in case clusters.

Symptoms of *Mycoplasma* pneumonia, sometimes termed atypical pneumonia, have led to its occasional designation as "walking pneumonia." Patients may become ill suddenly or may develop symptoms slowly. Usually, there is a preceding upper respiratory infection, and its onset is heralded by an often nonproductive, hacking cough; fever; headache; and other systemic symptoms such as myalgia. The physical examination may reveal minimal signs in comparison with the degree of illness. Sometimes, the chest is clear or exhibits only minimal rales. The white blood cell count usually is elevated during the illness. X-ray of the chest often shows variable and non-pathognonomic signs of interstitial infiltration. The course of the disease also is variable, with patients continuing to slowly resolve, with the generalized symptoms and fever abating but the cough persisting, sometimes for weeks.

Diagnosis of infection with *M. pneumoniae* often is based on exclusion. This organism is extremely sensitive to killing by complement, therefore complement fixation may be used in the diagnosis. The standard for diagnosis is the rising titer of specific antibodies.

A third type of microorganism that causes CAP is viruses. Hundreds of viruses are capable of causing CAP, but varicella, adenoviruses, and influenza viruses are the most important. Children are more likely to develop viral pneumonia than adults. Influenza causes its major pathophysiologic effect through the CAP it can produce, particularly in elderly or immunocompromised persons. The occurrence of secondary bacterial infection in patients with influenza pneumonia is a major concern. Influenza viruses invade respiratory epithelial cells, which results in infected cells being recognized by macrophages and cellular cytotoxicity responses. The damage is related to the inflammatory and immune mechanisms that contain the virus. There have been several pandemics of influenza with high mortality rates in patients with pneumonias (Blinkhorn, 1998). The clinical presentation is similar to what has been described. The patient has leukocytosis, fever, nonproductive cough, and dyspnea. The chest x-rays show patchy infiltration, but consolidation is rare. The treatment of viral pneumonia is supportive. Antiviral agents do not seem to be effective.

## Developmental Considerations

### Pneumonia in the Elderly Patient

The elderly are susceptible to pneumonia and are more likely to become seriously ill and die than younger persons. Many factors contribute to this predisposition (Ely, 1997). There may be coexisting chronic illnesses such as cardiac disease or COPD. The elderly are more likely to have oral hygiene problems related to dental care, false teeth, and medications that dry out the mucosal membranes of the mouth. This allows an opportunity for upper airway colonization with pathogens, which usually is a prerequisite for the development of pneumonia. There is also a decline in cellular immunity with aging, which may contribute to risk. Older persons may have an ineffective cough mechanism, thus reducing the clearance ability of the airways. The lungs are less elastic, and the mucociliary escalator is less effective. If the elderly person is institutionalized in a nursing home or long-term care facility, they may be exposed to more virulent organisms and are at increased risk for developing TB and infection with drug-resistant *S. pneumoniae* and *S. pyogenes*.

Another important contributing factor to risk is nutritional status. Malnourished elderly are at greater risk, as determined by indices such as body mass index, serum albumin, and arm-muscle area (Bulbin & Simberkoff, 1995).

The elderly person with pneumonia often presents a subtly different clinical picture compared with younger persons. Table 9-4 illustrates the diagnostic challenge presented by the elderly patient with pneumonia. These differences are most pronounced in those older than 75 years of age. The diagnostic algorithm for pneumonia is not particularly useful in elderly patients. Only two thirds of elderly patients with pneumonia have an elevated white blood cell count, and many do not have the usual shift to the left, which is expected in a bacterial infection (MacLennan et al., 1994). Diagnosing pneumonia therefore may be made based on signs such as confusion or falling.

Nursing home patients are at the greatest risk, with the following factors being important: malnutrition or recent weight loss, history of aspiration or use of suctioning, altered level of consciousness or confusion, difficulty with clearing oropharyngeal secretions, presence of nasogastric or gastric tube, presence of upper respiratory tract infection, or use of inhalation therapy (Bulbin & Simberkoff, 1995). Once an elderly patient develops pneumonia, the risk of mortality is related to advanced age, number of lobes infected, whether the patient is a nursing home resident, whether ventilatory support is required, and the number of complications that occur in the hospital (Bulbin & Simberkoff, 1995).

The primary care practitioner working with elderly patients can play a significant role in preventing CAP in the elderly by providing both influenza

## TABLE 9.4

### Signs and Symptoms of Pneumonia in the Elderly

| Sign or Symptom | Comments |
| --- | --- |
| Fever | 25% to 50% have no fever |
| Pulmonary symptoms (cough, sputum, dyspnea, wheezing, orthopnea) | Often absent; symptoms are not good predictors of seriousness of disease |
| Tachycardia and tachypnea | Often the only early manifestation; important clinical feature |
| Confusion | Sudden onset of change in mental status may be early sign of pneumonia |
| Rales and rhonchi | Not a regular feature |
| Leukocytosis | No difference between young and old |
| Gram stain | Often negative because of nonproductive cough, previous antibiotic treatment |

(Modified from Ely E.W. [1997] Pneumonia in the elderly: Diagnostic and therapeutic challenges. *Infections in Medicine, 14,* 643–654.)

and pneumococcal vaccination (pneumovax). Once pneumonia is diagnosed, the elderly patient requires empiric antibiotic therapy to be instituted immediately. The Gram stain may not provide the diagnosis in over half of the patients. The initial empiric therapy generally is erythromycin, 3 to 4 g/day, since it is inexpensive and has good coverage for common CAP-causing organisms. A complete guide to decisions about the use of antibiotics for CAP in the elderly can be found at *http://www.medscape.com/SCP/IIM/1995/v12.n08 /m877.bulbin/m877.bulbin.html#Tab2.*

### ● Case Study 9.1

Mrs. Lorene Smyth is a 73-year-old widow who lives alone in a retirement village apartment and receives routine medical care through the primary care clinic. She has been generally well, although in the last year she was diagnosed with atrial fibrillation and placed on Coumadin. She is brought into the clinic by a neighbor because of a fall in her bedroom that morning. She has a large hematoma over her right hip and a small laceration on her forehead, which requires several stitches.

#### History

##### Past Medical History (from medical record)

| | |
| --- | --- |
| Allergies | NKDA |
| Current medications | Coumadin |
| | Hydrothiazide |
| Surgeries | Hysterectomy at age 55 for uterine polyps |
| Injury/Trauma | No significant injuries |
| Childhood illness | Doesn't know for sure; thinks had immunizations |

*(Case study continued on next page)*

*Social History*

|  | Widowed 5 years ago; moved into retirement village 4 years ago; active in community and church affairs |
|---|---|
| Tobacco | Never smoked |
| Alcohol | Occasional glass of wine with friends |
| Social drugs | Negative |
| Caffeine | 1 cup of coffee every morning |
| Exercise | Walks with friends and goes to water aerobics |
| Employment | Never employed outside of home. Lives on husband's pension and Social Security, and has a small portfolio of stocks and bonds, as well as savings. Is financially secure |
| Sleep | Sleeps 6 hours at night and naps for an hour every day |

*Family History*

| Mother | Deceased, breast cancer at age 60 |
|---|---|
| Father | Deceased at age 50 of heart attack |
| Children | Two male children, ages 50 and 48, living and well |

## Review of Systems (Difficult to elicit, and neighbor helps answer questions, since patient appears dazed and confused)

| General | Recent weight loss of about 5 lb
Feels okay, except for pain in left hip from fall |
|---|---|
| Skin | Abrasion on forehead and hematoma on hip today; no rashes or lesions, except for many actinic keratoses |
| HEENT | Wears glasses. Had cataracts diagnosed recently |
| Lungs | Experienced a little SOB while walking to clinic from parking lot. No cough |
| Cardiac | Has noticed palpitations and a little generalized chest pain today. Says this might be due to her "heart problems." Hurts to inhale deeply |
| GI | No N&V; no diarrhea, constipation |
| GU | No dysuria, urgency; no increase in urination |
| MS | Denies joint pain, or swelling; states she is feeling "shaky" today and that is why she fell |
| Neurologic | Denies numbness, tingling, fainting, seizures, weakness |

## Physical Examination

| System | Findings |
|---|---|
| Vital signs | T–99°F, P–105, R–18, BP 130/88
Height 5'4", Weight 110 lb |
| General | Appears tremulous and shaky; confused about time of day and not sure of her memory about today's incident
Thin extremities, skin warm and dry |

*(Case study continued on page 168)*

| HEENT | Normocephalic, cranial nerves intact; TMs intact; Rinne and Weber sign negative; hearing normal; throat negative; no adenopathy; thyroid not palpable; no carotid bruits; funduscopic exam indicates bilateral cataracts; no retinopathy |
| Lungs | Clear to auscultation; respiratory excursion 3 cm on left, 5 cm on right; percussion indicates small area of dullness over right lower lobe |
| Cardiac | Heart rate irregular; no murmurs |
| Abdomen | Soft, nontender, no masses; BS in all 4 quadrants; no CVA tenderness |
| GU | Deferred |
| Rectal | Deferred |
| Extremities | All pulses 2–3+<br>Grip strength weak bilaterally 10 cm hematoma over left hipbone, with moderate swelling; able to ambulate although she states that it hurts |
| Neurologic | DTRs 2+ in upper and lower extremities; Romberg sign negative; sensations and range of motion intact; fine hand tremor bilaterally; disoriented to time and place; both long-term and recent memory impaired; confused and unable to follow simple directions |

## Laboratory Results

| Test | Result |
| --- | --- |
| CBC | WBC 9000, differential: neutrophils 60%, lymphocytes 22%, monocytes 14%, basophils 3%, eosinophils 1% |
| Urine | WNL |

## Differential Diagnosis

1. Rule out myocardial infarction
2. Rule out TIA or seizure
3. Rule out fracture
4. Rule out head injury
5. Rule out pneumonia

BS, bowel sounds; CBC, complete blood count; CVA, costovertebral angle; DTR, deep tendon reflexes; exam, examination; GI, gastrointestinal; GU, genitourinary; HEENT, head, eyes, ears, nose, and throat; MS, musculoskeletal; NKDA, no known drug allergies; N&V, nausea and vomiting; SOB, shortness of breath; TIA, transient ischemic attack; TMs, tympanic membranes; WBC, white blood cell count; WNL, within normal limits.

The patient in Case Study 9-1 is a diagnostic challenge, as are many elderly patients seen in primary care. She has experienced a fall, with potential injuries that could be producing her symptoms. She also could have fallen because of a preceding pathologic condition. Any elderly, hypertensive patient who complains of chest pain needs to be evaluated for myocardial infarction. A head injury could produce the confusion and disorientation that she exhibits. The possibility of fracture in an elderly woman needs to be ruled out. Her fall at home may have resulted from a temporary loss of consciousness or decreased brain blood flow. Finally, her physical findings, although not striking, suggest the possibility of pneumonia. Whereas her white count and differential do not provide clues and her lack of pulmonary symptoms may seem surprising, dullness to percussion always is an abnormal finding and suggests significant infiltrate and possibly consolidation.

The chest x-ray showed left lower lobe pneumonia. Her electrocardiogram did not indicate ischemia, and results of her hip and head films were negative. Her $PaO_2$ was 68, indicating severe hypoxemia. She was admitted to the hospital, and since no sputum for culture was produced, she was treated empirically with vancomycin, oxygen, and intravenous fluids.

## LUNG CANCERS

### Epidemiology and Risk Factors

Whereas primary care providers rarely manage the treatment of cancer patients, they clearly play a significant role in cancer screening, detection, and referral. Lung cancer is one of the most common cancers. In 1997, there were 160,400 deaths from bronchogenic carcinoma, and the number of lung cancer cases and lung cancer deaths has increased every year during the last 50 years (Strauss, 1998). The incidence of lung cancer is rising, and it has become a greater cause of mortality for women than breast cancer. Like all other cancers, lung cancer is thought to be caused by an interaction of genetic factors and environmental influences. Ultimately, though, all cancers are diseases involving cellular DNA.

Environment repeatedly has been shown to be important in causing cancers. Cancer risk can change in just one generation, when a previously low-risk group moves to a higher cancer risk environment. Most notable is a disease like breast cancer, which is low in the Japanese, but in one generation after immigration to the United States, breast cancer risk mirrors that of the US in Japanese women. There are many examples of this phenomenon, so we know that environment is important. Environment is an all-encompassing term that refers to many components: lifestyle, diet, chemical exposure, living conditions, culture, sexual activity, and health habits. Many of these components have been shown to influence cancer rates. For lung cancer, the most prominent influence is the carcinogenic contaminants that an individual inhales into the lungs and to which the bronchopulmonary epithelium is exposed. Carcinogenic compounds that produce lung cancers include cigarette smoke, air pollutants (carbon particles and sulfur dioxide), radon, and asbestos. The risk for developing lung cancer increases dramatically in cigarette smokers who are exposed to additional environmental carcinogens. Environmental carcinogenic chemicals are thought to combine with DNA, forming DNA-chemical adducts, which is one of the first steps in the multistage carcinogenic process. This leads to a somatic mutation, which is required for carcinogenesis to proceed. The targets for environmental carcinogens include cellular regulatory proteins, which control cell growth, DNA repair, and apoptosis (programmed cell death). Carcinogens may directly mutate genes that code for these various proteins or may act *epigenetically*. This means that carcinogenic agents may act at promoter regions of certain genes, causing a mutation that then could interrupt the normal regulation of certain gene expression. Another possibility is that chemical carcinogens may act directly on proteins themselves, affecting their functions. For example, cell membrane receptors may be altered by carcinogens so as to disturb growth regulatory processes, and when combined with a germline or somatic mutation in a critical gene, cancer is the result. The ultimate effects of carcinogens are to disturb normal growth, cell cycle, and programmed cell death kinetics of affected cells.

Genetic factors are important in determining risk for some cancers. Many lines of research and the accumulated information from the human genome project has led to the identification of more than 20 genes in the human gene pool that are involved in the development of cancer (Minamoto et al., 1999). Many of these genes are either proto-oncogenes or tumor suppressor genes.

### Carcinogenesis

Lung cancer is an epithelial cancer and develops through multiple stages, as illustrated in Figure 9-7. The first event, initiation, involves cellular DNA and is mutagenic. After this initial, irreversible alteration, other carcinogenic events produce promotion. These result from environmental agents acting on the initiated cell to alter the growth and reproductive aspects of cell physiology. These events are believed to occur over time, thus accounting for the lengthy progression of cells from initiation to malignancy. Unlike initiation events, they are reversible effects. Finally, the transformed cell undergoes irreversible progression to the anaplasia of cancer.

One important gene that is mutated in a variety of cancers, including lung cancers, is the p53 gene, which is a tumor suppressor gene that blocks entry of the cell into the S phase of the cell cycle. Normally, p53 prevents cell division, and if it is mutated, cell growth can be excessive, a character-

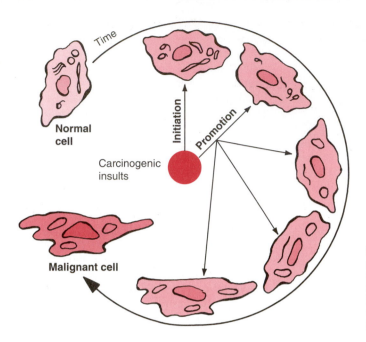

**FIGURE 9.7** ● Berenblum's theory of carcinogenesis: initiation and promotion. Several events are required for a normal cell to become transformed into a cancer cell. Initial event, initiation, will not cause cancer unless several promoting events occur over time.

istic of cancer cells. Table 9-5 indicates the known oncogenes and tumor suppressor genes involved in the etiology of lung cancer.

## Cigarette Smoking

The primary care practitioner will have the greatest impact on lung cancer by helping patients to either stop smoking or by working with younger populations to discourage developing a smoking habit. Advocating clean air and decreasing exposure to secondhand smoke in the home and workplace is another important role. Cigarette smoking is the major risk factor for lung cancer, with heavy smokers (more than 25 cigarettes/day) experiencing a risk 20 times greater than that of nonsmokers (Fedullo, 1996). Exposure to secondhand smoke also increases risk of lung cancer. The numerous carcinogens found in cigarette smoke include aromatic hydrocarbons, nitrosamines, nitrosonormicotine polonium, and arsenic.

## Types of Lung Cancers

There are four major types of lung cancer: squamous, adenocarcinoma, large cell, and small cell (SCLC). The division of lung cancer into SCLC and non-SCLC types typically is used for predicting the course of the malignancy. Squamous cell carcinomas comprise about 30% to 40% of all lung cancers, are more common in men, and are strongly associated with cigarette smoking. They tend to be slow growing, centrally located tumors

that progress from epithelial dysplasia through carcinoma in situ. It may take as long as 4 years for squamous carcinoma tumors to develop into a mass large enough to cause symptoms (Strauss, 1998). Patients with these tumors also have the highest 5-year survival rate (50%). Adenocarcinomas are the most common lung tumors in nonsmokers and women. They also are slow growing and arise from the bronchial glandular epithelium. Small cell carcinomas comprise 20% of lung cancers and are the most strongly related to cigarette smoking. They tend to occur proximally and arise from small cells of neuroendocrine origin. Finally, large cell carcinomas, which make up 10% of lung cancers, are large tumors located peripherally in the lungs and have microscopic features in common with both adenocarcinomas and squamous cell carcinomas.

Lung cancer mortality continues to be high (87%) despite the many new therapeutic approaches. Part of the problem is that lung cancer tends to be diagnosed late in the malignant progression. Therefore, primary care providers can contribute enormously to prevention and early treatment by understanding the carcinogenic process and learning ways to identify risk and early disease.

## Diagnosis and Symptoms

Lung cancer is clinically staged depending on the tumor characteristics, the extent of metastatic dis-

| TABLE 9.5 |
| --- |

**Known Oncogenes and Tumor Suppressor Genes Involved in the Etiology of Lung Cancer**

| Gene | Histology |
| --- | --- |
| *Dominant oncogenes* | |
| K-*ras* | NSCLC (adenocarcinoma) |
| c-*jun* | NSCLC/SCLC |
| cyclin D1 | NSCLC |
| *myc* family | SCLC |
| HER-2/*neu* | NSCLC |
| bcl-2 | NSCLC |
| c-*raf* | SCLC/NSCLC |
| c-*myb* | SCLC |
| *Tumor suppressor genes* | |
| p53 | SCLC/NSCLC |
| Retinoblastoma | SCLC |
| FHIT | SCLC/NSCLC |
| p16 | NSCLC |

FHIT, fragile histidine triad; NSCLC, non-small cell lung cancer; SCLC, small cell lung cancer.
(From Szabo, E. & Shaw, G. [1997]. Intermediate markers and molecular genetics of lung carcinogenesis. *Cancer Control: Journal of the Moffitt Cancer Center, 4* [2], 109–117.)

ease, and the lymph node involvement. Early diagnosis is important in preventing progression of the disease, particularly in slow-growing forms, but less than 40% of newly diagnosed lung cancers are resectable at the time of diagnosis (Fedullo, 1996).

It is not uncommon for a patient to be diagnosed with lung cancer from a chest radiograph and, at the time of diagnoses, to have no symptoms. Chronic cough is the most common presenting symptom in lung cancer, and a large amount of sputum may be produced. In patients with other chronic pulmonary disorders, a change in their chronic cough may be the presenting symptom. The presence of some degree of dyspnea also is seen in up to half of patients. Bloody sputum may be present, and some patients complain of chest pain (Strauss, 1998). As the tumor enlarges, it causes obstructive symptoms such as wheezing, atelectasis, decreased lung volume, and abscess formation. Later disease usually is characterized by fatigue, anorexia and weight loss, nausea and vomiting, and weakness. Common metastatic sites are prescalene lymph nodes, brain, liver, adrenal glands, and bone.

Diagnosis usually is made based on findings from x-ray, sputum cytologic study, bronchoscopy, computed tomography scan, endoscopy, and fine-needle aspiration, depending on the site of the lesion.

## Physiology of Treatment

Lung cancer is treated surgically, with radiation, and with chemotherapy, depending on the stage and extent of disease. The primary care provider is most interested in ways to prevent the disease from developing or in slowing its progression. One approach for the primary care practitioner is to encourage all patients to eat a diet high in vegetables and fruit. The results from several studies suggest that vitamins A and E may act as antioxidants, protecting cancer cells from malignant conversion. This would be especially important for patients who smoke cigarettes.

## CHRONIC OBSTRUCTIVE PULMONARY DISEASE

Included in the category of chronic obstructive pulmonary disease are chronic bronchitis, emphysema, and asthma. Asthma has been discussed previously and therefore is not included here. COPD patients rarely have only chronic bronchitis or only emphysema. Typically, both diseases are present to varying degrees in the same patient. Emphysema primary involves the alveolar duct and alveoli, whereas chronic bronchitis involves the airways. However, clinically, both disorders result in dyspnea and in similar limitations in airway flow.

## Epidemiology

Primary care providers can expect to have many patients in their practices with COPD. The disease is four times more common in men, and many men (65%) will have some degree of emphysema on postmortem examination of the lungs, most of whom never had symptoms. There are 15 million people living with COPD in the United States, which translates to about 6% of the population (Hafner & Ferro, 1998).

The personal, family, and community burden of COPD is enormous. The 10-year survival rate after diagnosis is about 50%, and the quality of life progressively declines as pulmonary function deteriorates. The mortality rate continues to rise, and COPD is the fifth leading cause of death. The financial cost of this disease was about $12 billion dollars in 1990 (Hafner & Ferro, 1998).

## Chronic Bronchitis

Chronic bronchitis has been characterized and defined in many different ways, leading to diagnostic confusion. The best clinical definition uses the following diagnostic criteria as provided by Moser and Bordow (Moser & Bordow, 1996):

1. Essentially normal lung volume with minimum elevation of the residual volume–total lung capacity ratio
2. Some degree of expiratory and inspiratory flow obstruction (both flows are abnormal because airway narrowing is fixed anatomically)
3. Flow obstruction not acutely improved by bronchodilator administration
4. Normal elastic recoil and compliance
5. Significant disturbances of gas exchange producing hypoxemia without, in the stable state, hypercapnia (from ventilation–perfusion imbalance)
6. Normal diffusing capacity for carbon monoxide.

## Emphysema

Emphysema is a disease of the portions of the airways distal to the terminal bronchioles. There is enlargement and destruction of the walls of the alveoli. Centriacinar or panacinar emphysema can occur (Fig. 9-8). The former is caused by enlargement of the respiratory bronchioles, which are the airway structures immediately distal to the bronchiolar ducts and which participate to some degree in air exchange. The alveoli supplied by these ducts initially are preserved in centriacinar emphysema. The panacinar type involves the entire acinus and tends to be widespread throughout the entire lung.

Cigarette smoking is a major etiologic factor for both emphysema and chronic bronchitis. A hereditary form of emphysema also occurs, and many patients with these genetic mutations are never diagnosed. If a person with the hereditary form smokes cigarettes or is exposed to second-hand smoke, they will develop COPD much earlier in life and the disease will progress more rapidly.

### The Role of Alpha₁-Antitrypsin Deficiency

The hereditary form of emphysema causes 2% to 3% of all cases of COPD and results from a genetically endowed deficiency in the enzyme alpha$_1$-antitrypsin (AAT). People with this genetic deficiency are more likely to develop emphysema and asthma. AAT inactivates elastase, which is an enzyme released by neutrophils in the lung. Elastase acts on lung elastin, breaking down the elastic

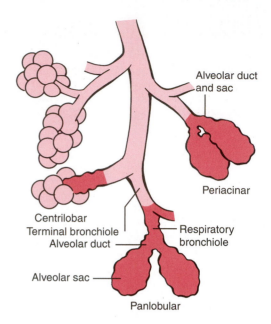

**FIGURE 9.8**  ●  Diagram of the two common types of emphysema. Panacinar type is seen in hereditary form, while centriacinar type is seen in smokers.

fibers in the lung, and thus producing a loss of structural integrity in the pulmonary matrix. This leads to a panacinar form of emphysema in affected individuals. If affected persons do not smoke, they may never develop the disease, but typically, smokers with the genetic defect will have COPD in their 40s (Eden, 1998).

Cigarette smokers develop emphysema through a similar pathophysiologic pathway. Cigarette smoke oxidizes the elastin binding site, causing AAT to have much less of a binding affinity to neutrophil elastase. This frees the elastase to act on elastin fibers, breaking them down. The interactions between elastase, AAT, and cigarette smoke are illustrated in Figure 9-9. Notice that any condition that tips the balance toward elastase accelerates pulmonary tissue damage. For example, inflammatory conditions associated with the influx of neutrophils and the irritating and inflammatory effects of smoke itself increase lung elastase concentration.

Another important effect of elastase is that it stimulates pulmonary macrophages to release pro-inflammatory cytokines such as IL-1 and TNF-α. These and other cytokines cause further neutrophil chemotaxis and accumulation in the lungs (Eden, 1998).

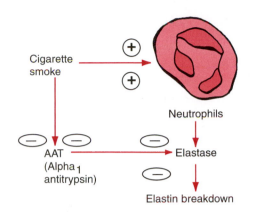

**FIGURE 9.9** ● Interaction between elastase, AAT, and cigarette smoke.

## Pathophysiologic Changes in the Lung

The breakdown of elastase is a critical event in the development of emphysematous changes. In emphysema, there is enlargement of the air spaces distal to the terminal bronchioles. This enlargement results from elastin breakdown and leads to loss of lung elasticity. Enlargement also is produced through the processes that obstruct the airways, such as the changes that occur in chronic bronchitis. Alveoli adjacent to each other lose their individual structural integrity, and then higher-pressure, smaller alveoli collapse into larger alveoli, forming progressively larger air sacs (*bullae*). This leads to decreasing functional surface area and ventilation–perfusion mismatches. Expiratory airflow obstruction leads to progressively worsening dyspnea. The expiratory airflow obstruction is caused by loss of elastic recoil with increasing airflow resistance (Niewoehner, 1998). The unsupported airways tend to collapse on expiration, causing dyspnea.

## Symptoms

The symptoms of COPD depend on the relative contributions of the chronic bronchitis (type B) and emphysema (type A) components. The patient with predominantly type B COPD is bothered more with chronic coughing and has less progressive dyspnea than the patient with type A disease. Since it is rare for a patient to have exclusively chronic bronchitis or emphysema, but rather a combination of both, the symptoms are on a continuum and depend on the relative proportion of one or the other. The typical picture is for a patient to develop symptoms after at least 20 pack-years of smoking, which results in most patients being older than 40 years of age. The pathophysiologic changes associated with bronchitis lead to a productive cough. These changes include hyperplasia and hypertrophy of the bronchial mucous glands, small airway mucus plugging, fibrosis of the bronchioles, and infiltration of inflammatory cells (Moser & Bordow, 1996). Type-B–predominant patients may have mild dyspnea or dyspnea on exertion, and mild obstruction. There may be some hypoxemia from ventilation–perfusion mismatches. This patient is likely to develop infections, at which time the symptoms become much worse. The patient can become severely hypoxemic and hypercapneic and may develop acidosis, which causes pulmonary arteriolar vasoconstriction and precipitates right ventricular failure. All of this is reversible, however. Between exacerbations, the patient may be only mildly impaired (Moser & Bordow, 1996).

The patient who is type A predominant will have major problems with progressive dyspnea but may not cough or produce sputum. The dyspnea can become crippling, and even mild exertion eventually produces severe symptoms (Celli, 1998). Hypoxemia results in erythropoiesis with the development of a polycythemia. Cyanosis may develop, along with cachexia and cor pulmonale, but usually this occurs fairly late in the disease after an acute chest infection has tipped the balance. These patients are considered "fighters" in that they hyperventilate and maintain $P_{O_2}$ values even in the face of remarkable parenchymal lung damage.

The patient with COPD has a reduced ratio of forced expiratory volume in the first second ($FEV_1$) to forced vital capacity, and the disease progression can be staged by the declining $FEV_1$. Table 9-6 indicates this staging system.

## Clinical Presentation

The patient with COPD learns to manage the complex pathophysiologic outcomes of their disease in several ways. They tend to hunch over, which helps the accessory muscles of respiration to function best. They also often develop a pattern of pursed lip breathing, which causes them to slow the rate at which breath is expired, preventing the pressure drops that may cause airways to collapse. Many also learn to adapt their lives to their disease by using energy efficiently to preserve calories needed for the work of breathing. The thoracic cage is enlarged and rounder, with an increased anteroposterior diameter, decreased respiratory excursion, hyperresonance to percussion, and distant heart sounds (Bardow & Moser, 1996). The chest x-ray shows hyperinflation, hyperlucency

# TABLE 9.6

## Staging System of Patients With COPD

|  | Stage 1 | Stage 2 | Stage 3 |
|---|---|---|---|
| $FEV_1$ | > 50% | 36–49% | < 35% |
| Clinical findings | Most patients; many patients do not have symptoms; may have mild dyspnea on exertion; managed by primary care providers | Few patients; dyspnea at rest; may have hypoxemia | Fewest patients; severe dyspnea at rest; hypoxemic and may be hypercapneic; requires specialist care |

COPD, chronic obstructive pulmonary disease; $FEV_1$, forced expiratory volume in the first second.
(Modified from Celli, B. [1998]. Clinical aspects of chronic obstructive pulmonary disease. In G.L. Baum, J.D. Crapo, B.R. Celli, & J.B. Karlinsky [Eds.], *Textbook of pulmonary diseases* [6th ed., p. 848]. Philadelphia: Lippincott Williams & Wilkins.)

(from bullae), and a low diaphragm. Although these patients are subject to respiratory acidosis, they often compensate remarkably through both metabolic means and through respiratory alkalosis (hyperventilation). They may be hypoxemic, but can have a normal blood pH and be hypocapnic between infectious exacerbations of the disease.

## Physiologic Basis of Treatment

### Smoking Cessation

The continuation of smoking in the patient with COPD is a major concern. The changes in chronic bronchitis can be partially reversed by smoking cessation, although the emphysematous component of the disease is not reversible. However, smoking cessation halts the further progression of changes in the lungs, which makes an ultimate difference in quality of life, morbidity, and mortality. Unfortunately, many patients with COPD continue to smoke, challenging the resources and skills of the primary care provider. The Agency for Health Policy and Research has established guidelines for clinicians to help patients stop smoking. These are summarized and can be reviewed at *http://www.physiciansguide.com/smoke1.html*.

### Prevention of Infection

Pulmonary infections sometimes are fatal to patients with COPD. Primary care providers need to be vigilant with these individuals. Concerns include ensuring influenza and pneumococcal pneumonia vaccination; early recognition and treatment of purulent sputum; avoidance of crowds, especially during flu season; and complete compliance with antibiotic therapy to avoid developing resistant organisms.

### Medications

Bronchodilation is a major goal of the pharmacotherapy of COPD, and $beta_2$ agonists are one choice. However, these drugs may cross-react with $beta_1$ receptors, causing tachycardia in elderly patients, and the dose must be decreased to reduce this effect, thus limiting the drug's ability to cause bronchodilation. Therefore, these drugs often are not a good choice, especially in the elderly person with COPD (Hafner & Ferro, 1998).

The current bronchodilator used most in COPD is ipratropium, which is an anticholinergic drug that can be inhaled into the lungs. Occasionally, patients require both the anticholinergic and a $beta_2$ agonist inhaler for adequate bronchodilation. Another bronchodilator that occasionally is used is theophylline.

Systemic steroids also are used for COPD during acute exacerbations but usually are not prescribed on a long-term basis.

### Oxygen Therapy

Supplemental home oxygen therapy can be used for severely hypoxemic patients. It is expensive and inconvenient therapy, and the practitioner needs to weigh many factors when deciding to prescribe it. An algorithm for this decision is provided in the report by Hafner and Ferro (1998) at *http://www.medscape.com/quadrant/HospitalMedicine/1998/v34.n01/hm3401.02.hafner/hm3401.02.hafn.html#Table2*.

---

### CLINICAL VIGNETTE 9.2

John Elgin is a 60-year-old patient who arrives at the primary clinic complaining of cough and generally not feeling well. He has noticed some shortness of breath on stair climbing over the last 2 days. The latter symptom he attributes to lack of conditioning. He reports having a chronic "smoker's cough," which is productive of large amounts of sputum, and in the last few months, the cough has become increasingly bothersome. It is worse in the morning, and it takes him about an hour to clear mucus from his lungs after a night's sleep. Over the last 2 days, John has developed a fever, increased severity and frequency of his cough, and purulent sputum. He reports having frequent bouts with bronchitis, although he never has had pneumonia.

John's medical history is unremarkable except that he has a 50 pack-year history of smoking cigarettes. Currently, he smokes about one pack per day of filtered cigarettes. He expresses a desire to quit smoking but states that he has tried to quit at least 10 times in the last year without success. The physical examination reveals slight hyperresonance of the lung fields and an increased anteroposterior diameter. There is no dullness to percussion. There are expiratory rhonchi throughout and no rales. He has a regular heart rate without murmurs or irregularities. His heart sounds are somewhat distant. His throat is not infected and his tonsils are 2+. There is mild lymphadenopathy of the cervical lymph nodes. The $FEV_1$ is 60%, and the $Po_2$ is 80 mm Hg. He has a fever of 102°F. A sample of sputum appears greenish-brown, but is not blood streaked. He coughs paroxysmally and loses his voice for a few moments after coughing. The white blood cell count is 14,000, with 72% neutrophils, 20% lymphocytes, 6% monocytes, 0 eosinophils, and 2% basophils. There are 5% bands present. Chest x-ray shows mild hyperinflation, areas of bronchiectasis, and a flattening of the diaphragm.

---

### Pulmonary and Nutritional Rehabilitation

Teaching patients proper breathing techniques, exercise management, sleep strategies, and avoidance of fatigue is helpful in improving quality of life for the patient. Nutritional therapy may help the cachectic patient but is difficult and laborious, as the number of calories needed often exceeds what the patient can consume.

### Surgery

Recent surgical approaches have helped some patients with COPD. Wedges of hyperinflated lung tissue can be surgically resected, leading to considerable improvement in $FEV_1$ and quality of life. This type of surgery is thought to restore elastic recoil forces of the lungs and the length–tension relationship of the respiratory muscles and the diaphragm (Celli, 1998). (See Clinical Vignette 9-2.)

In this clinical vignette, the patient has been in stage 1 COPD, with a predominant type B pattern. However, now that a superimposed acute infection has occurred, he is moving into a deteriorating state with a reduction in $FEV_1$ and an acute inflammatory process in the bronchial tree, which is causing dyspnea for the first time. He requires antibiotic therapy for the acute infectious bronchitis and follow-up for treatment with bronchodila-tors. He also needs encouragement to stop smoking and should be evaluated, advised, and aided in the selection of an appropriate smoking cessation program.

### REFERENCES

Hafner, J.P. & Ferro, T.J. (1998). Recent developments in the management of COPD. *Hospital Medicine, 34* (1), 29–30, 32–38.

Blinkhorn, R.J. (1998). Community acquired pneumonia. In G.L. Baum, J.D. Crapo, B.R. Celli, & J.B. Karlinsky (Eds.), *Textbook of pulmonary diseases* (6th ed.). Philadelphia: Lippincott Williams & Wilkins.

Bloch, A. Canthen, G., Onorato, I., Dansbury, K., Kelly, G., Driver, C., and Snider, D. (1994). Nationwide survey of drug resistant tuberculosis in the United States. *Journal of the American Medical Association, 271,* 665.

Bordow, R.A. & Moser, K.M. (1996). *Manual of clinical problems in pulmonary medicine.* On *MAXX: Maximum access to diagnosis and therapy: The electronic library of medicine.* [CD-ROM]. Philadelphia: Lippincott-Raven.

Bulbin, A. & Simberkoff, M. (1995). Prevention of pneumonia in the elderly. *Infections in Medicine, 12,* 385–394.

Cassiere, H.A. & Niederman M.S. (1998). Community-acquired pneumonia. *Disease of the Month, 44,* 613–675.

Celli, B. (1998). Clinical aspects of chronic obstructive pulmonary disease. In G.L. Baum, J.D. Crapo, B.R. Celli, & J.B. Karlinsky (Eds.), *Textbook of pulmonary diseases* (6th ed.). Philadelphia: Lippincott Williams & Wilkins.

Chaudry, M. & San Pedro, G. (1999). Respiratory infections. In J. Ali, W. Summer, & M. Levitsky (Eds.), *Pul-*

*monary pathophysiology.* New York: McGraw-Hill.

Dannenberg, A. (1994). Pathogenesis and immunology. In D. Schlossberg (Ed.), *Tuberculosis* (3rd ed.). New York: Springer Verlag.

Eden, E. (1998). Alpha$_1$-antitrypsin deficiency in COPD: Clinical implications. *Medscape Respiratory Care 2* (2).

Ely, E.W. (1997). Pneumonia in the elderly: Diagnostic and therapeutic challenges. *Infections in Medicine, 14,* 643–654.

Ewig, S., Ruiz, M., Torres, A., Marco, F., Martinez, J.A., Sanchez, M., & Mensa, J. (1999). Pneumonia acquired in the community through drug-resistant *Streptococcus pneumoniae. American Journal of Respiratory Critical Care Medicine, 159,* 1835–1842.

Fedullo, P.F. (1996). Lung cancer: Classification, pathology, and epidemiology. In R.A. Bordow & K. Moser (Eds.), Manual of clinical problems in pulmonary medicine. On *MAXX: Maximum access to diagnosis and therapy: The electronic library of medicine.* [CD-ROM]. Philadelphia: Lippincott-Raven.

Fine, P.E. (1994). Immunities in and to tuberculosis. In J. Potter & K. McAdam (Eds.), *Tuberculosis: Back to the future.* New York: John Wiley & Sons.

Iseman, M. (1995). Evolution of drug-resistant tuberculosis: A tale of two species. In Roizzman, B. (Ed.), *Infectious diseases in an age of chance.* Washington, DC: National Academy Press.

Laver, W., Bischofberger, N., & Webster, R. (1999). Disarming influenza viruses. *Scientific American, 280* (1), 78–87.

MacLennan, W., Watt, B., & Elder, A. (1994). *Infections in elderly patients.* London: Edward Arnold.

McDonald, R. & Reichman, L. (1998). Tuberculosis. In G.L. Baum, J.D. Crapo, B.R. Celli, & J.B. Karlinsky (Eds.), *Textbook of pulomonary diseases* (6th ed.). Philadelphia: Lippincott Williams & Wilkins.

Minamoto, T., Mail, M., & Ronai, Z. (1999). Environmental factors as regulators and effectors of multistep carcinogenesis. *Carcinogenesis, 20* (4), 519–527.

*Morbidity and Mortality Weekly Report.* (1997). 46 (No. RR-10), 40–41.

Moser, K. & Bordow, R. (1996). Chronic obstructive pulmonary disease: Clinical and laboratory manifestations, pathophysiology, and prognosis. In K. Moser & R. Bordow (Eds.), Manual of clinical problems in pulmonary medicine. On *MAXX: Maximum access to diagnosis and therapy: The electronic library of medicine.* [CD-ROM]. Philadelphia: Lippincott-Raven.

Moulding, T. (1994). Pathophysiology and immunology: Clinical aspects. In D. Schlossberg (Ed.), *Tuberculosis* (3rd ed.). New York: Springer-Verlag.

Niewoehner, D. (1998). Anatomic and pathophysiological correlates in COPD. In G.L. Baum, J.D. Crapo, B.R. Celli, & J.B. Karlinsky (Eds.), *Textbook of pulmonary diseases* (6th ed.). Philadelphia: Lippincott Williams & Wilkins.

O'Handley, J. & Gray, L. (1997). The incidence of *Mycoplasma pneumoniae* pneumonia. *Journal of the American Board of Family Practice, 10,* 425–429.

Snider, D. (1994). Tuberculosis: The world situation. In J.D. Porter & K.P. McAdam (Eds.), *Tuberculosis: Back to the future.* New York: John Wiley & Sons.

Stead, W.W. & Dutt, A.K. (1994). Epidemiology and host factors. In D. Schlossberg (Ed.), *Tuberculosis* (3rd ed.). New York: Springer-Verlag.

Strauss, G.B. (1998). Bronchogenic carcinoma In G.I. Baum, J.D. Crapo, B.R. Celli, & J.B. Karlinski (Eds.), *Textbook of pulmonary diseases* (6th ed.). Philadelphia: Lippincott Williams & Wilkins.

Szabo, E. & Shaw, G. (1997). Intermediate markers and molecular genetics of lung carcinogenesis. *Cancer Control: Journal of the Moffitt Cancer Center, 4* (2), 109–117.

Treanor, J.T. & Hall, C.B. (1996). Influenza and infections of the trachea, bronchi, and bronchioles. In R. Reese & R. Betts. A practical approach to infectious disease. On *MAXX: Maximum access to diagnosis and therapy: The electronic library of medicine.* [CD-ROM]. Philadelphia: Lippincott-Raven.

# Thyroid and Endocrine Disorders

Patricia Coulson Shivers

## ENDOCRINOPATHIES

Endocrinopathy is the study of abnormal levels of endocrine hormones. These secretions are chemical substances that are synthesized by one tissue, carried in the bloodstream or body fluids, and bind to specific receptors at another site. An expanded view of endocrinology also takes into account chemical messengers that act on cells local to their synthesis site and are considered autocrine and paracrine substances.

The classic hormones can be divided into two major chemical types: (1) the peptide/amino acid derivatives include single amino acid hormones (catecholamines, serotonin, and dopamine), the dipeptides (thyroxine [$T_4$], triiodothyronine [$T_3$]), the short amino acid chains or peptides (insulin and glucagon), and the complex polypeptides, which frequently have sugar (carbohydrate) side chains attached (luteinizing hormone, thyrotropin [TSH], follicle-stimulating hormone); and (2) the steroid-cholesterol hormones include those with an intact four-ring steroid such as cholesterol (eg, cortisol, aldosterone, estrogen, progesterone, testosterone) and those that originate from cholesterol but are metabolized or converted and have one of their ring structures opened (eg, vitamin D and its metabolites).

Hormones exert complex controls on all tissues of the body, in conjunction with the nervous system controls, to coordinate the physiologic processes of the body. Most hormones have multiple target tissues; multiple effects; and multiple, distinct receptors located in these various tissues. In certain situations, hormones also play a "permissive role"; that is, their presence is required for a specific normal function but is not the primary driving or control-

ling force. For example, thyroid and cortisol hormones are not the principle controlling factors for development and growth, but they are necessary for the normal processes to take effect. Without thyroid and cortisol, even in the presence of normal growth hormone, growth is retarded.

Feedback control loops have been identified for most of the hormone systems studied. These "servo" mechanisms usually are paired controls (described as yin-yang combinations) with the end product inhibiting further production of one while giving positive feedback to the other (eg, insulin-glucagon influenced by glucose levels, or parathyroid hormone [PTH]–calcitonin influenced by calcium [$Ca^{2+}$] levels). Endocrine feedback systems may involve metabolic *substrates* (eg, increasing glucose stimulates increased insulin and decreased glucagon); *cations* (eg, increasing calcium causes decreased PTH but increased calcitonin); *tonicity* or extracellular *fluid volume* (eg, increasing plasma osmolality stimulates decreased vasopressin [ADH] but increased aldosterone concentrations).

Endocrinopathies may be genetically based (inherited) and are present from the moment of conception, or they may be congenital (eg, induced after fertilization) and develop as a result of some external (eg, nutritional, physical, or autoimmune) exacerbation. The appearance or manifestation of a particular endocrinopathy can be evident at birth. Frequently, however, it does not manifest itself until later in life. For instance, hypothyroidism may first appear in a pediatric, juvenile, adolescent, adult, or geriatric patient. Individual patients may exhibit some but not all of the symptoms listed for any particular hormonal disorder.

With regard to treatment of the common endocrinopathies, since several permissive hormones may be required for any specific tissue to function correctly, it is essential to correct the primary or permissive endocrine systems first (eg, thyroid, adrenal) and not be sidetracked by a single, specific symptom. The key to successful treatment is diagnosing the "basic" problem.

## THYROID PATHOPHYSIOLOGY

### Thyroid Anatomy

The two lobes of the thyroid gland are located on either side of the trachea at the level of the cricoid thyroid cartilage and are connected by a bridge of tissue called the isthmus. The thyroid gland weights approximately 15 to 20 g (Kettyle & Arky, 1998). The parathyroid glands (usually four) are buried within the thyroid tissue with two on each side of the trachea. Occasional ectopic loci can occur anywhere in the lingual or mediastinal regions. The follicle is the structural unit of the thyroid and provides both synthesis and storage functions (Fig. 10-1).

Control of thyroid hormone involves a three-tiered hierarchy (Fig. 10-2). Thyrotropin-releasing hormone (TRH) is a modified tripeptide from the hypothalamus; it represents tertiary (3°) control factors that integrate the neural controls with the endocrine. These releasing factors are small molecular weight compounds that are carried to the anterior pituitary through the portal system to induce release of the anterior pituitary hormone TSH. TSH is the secondary (2°) level of control. It is a large glycoprotein (alpha and beta subunits) synthesized by thyrotrope cells located in the anterior pituitary gland. TSH is carried in the bloodstream to the thyroid gland where it stimulates both synthesis and release of thyroid hormones. The diurnal pattern of TSH release is highest at

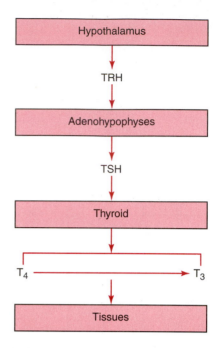

**FIGURE 10.2** ● The hypothalamus releases TRH, which causes TSH to be released. TSH stimulates the thyroid to release both $T_3$ and $T_4$, which then act on target tissues.

night (nocturnal surge) and lowest in the afternoon and evenings. This pituitary trophic hormone, TSH, is a large glycoprotein hormone with a molecular weight of 28,000 d with three sugar side chains attached to two separate subunits (McPhee & Bauer, 1997). The follicles of the thyroid gland contain enzymes capable of iodinating the amino acid tyrosine to form monoiodotyrosine and diiodotyrosine molecules, which are used as $T_4$ precursors. Two diiodotyrosine molecules are combined to form tetraiodothyronine ($T_4$), which is the primary (1°) hormone of the thyroid gland. $T_4$ has some metabolic activity and is very stable. Normally, when one of the iodine molecules is removed from $T_4$, either within the thyroid or at extra thyroidal sites, the molecule becomes tri-iodothyronine ($T_3$) or reverse triiodothyronine ($rT_3$) which is more effective compared to $T_4$ but has a shorter half-life. Large amounts of $T_3$ and $T_4$ are stored within the thyroid follicles for rapid release on demand, with about a 1% turnover per day.

***Clinical Alert***: Activity of the deiodinase enzyme, human iodothyronine seleno deiodinase, decreases with age, causing a continuous decline in blood $T_3$ levels after 30 years of age (Larsen et al., 1998).

To remain euthyroid, the dietary intake of iodide should exceed 150 µg/day. Under normal

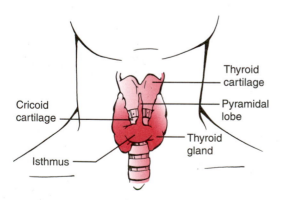

**FIGURE 10.1** ● The thyroid gland is located just below the cricoid cartilage, extending bilaterally from the midline of the trachea.

dietary conditions, an individual in the United States consumes 500 to 800 μg/day of iodine, primarily from seafood or artificially iodized salt and flour (Reed & Pangaro, 1995).

   *Clinical Alert*: Individuals on diets severely restricted in sodium (limiting intake of iodized salt), such as cardiac and hypertensive patients, and those avoiding carbohydrates (limiting intake of iodized flour), such as obese or diabetic patients, may be at increased risk for deficient intake of dietary iodine. Dietary hypothyroidism can be induced by either too little or too much iodine (iodide myxedema) (Larsen et al., 1998).

## Thyroid Hormones ($T_3$ and $T_4$)

$T_3$ and $T_4$ are transported in the plasma bound to serum proteins such as thyroxine-binding globulin (TBG), transthyretin, and albumin, which bind $T_4$ more avidly than $T_3$. Partial dissociation from the binding globulins at the distant tissue sites allows free thyroid hormones to diffuse across the cell membranes. Levels of free thyroid hormones are considered better for diagnosis of pathologic conditions but usually are more expensive to measure. Decreased levels of TBG (from malnutrition or liver disease) may cause low values of total $T_3$ and $T_4$, whereas high plasma levels of TBG (during pregnancy or estrogen therapy) may give abnormally high $T_3$ and $T_4$ values. Target tissues contain receptors specific for $T_3$ and $T_4$; however, nuclear receptors have a 10-fold greater avidity for $T_3$ compared with $T_4$ and thus it is considered more biologically active.

   Low blood levels of $T_3$ and $T_4$ serve as a positive feedback to stimulate the release of TRH and TSH and thus maintain homeostasis. In contrast, dopamine (including L-DOPA or the dopamine agonist bromocriptin) and somatostatin (somatotropin release inhibiting hormone) inhibit TSH secretion in a negative feedback manner.

   Thyroid hormones act on other tissues in two major fashions: (1) $T_4$ functions as a permissive hormone to set the stage for the action of numerous other hormones; and (2) $T_4$ is primarily responsible for thermogenesis, or heat production, by muscular tissues. In this capacity, it can uncouple oxidative phosphorylation, which diverts adenosine triphosphate (ATP) and oxygen consumption from pathways leading to fat storage. It moves these high-energy compounds into metabolic pathways that primarily release heat while the high-energy ATP molecules are broken down (this results in elevation of body temperature).

   Identification of thyroid disorders frequently is made in the clinical setting by a patient itemizing symptoms and physical findings that suggest too much or too little hormone (see the following web site for information on thyroid for medical students: *http://www.medinfo.ufl.edu/year4/imi/projects/thyroid/thyroid.html*). However, definitive identification of the specific basic pathology requires a careful correlation of the patient history and laboratory data before optimum treatment can be selected. Because of factors such as diurnal variation and the effects of stress or infection, relying on a single thyroid hormone level sometimes can be misleading. Paired hormone levels (eg, $T_4$ and TSH) or a similar matching of hormone with another parameter (eg, iodine levels and $T_4$) can lead to the appropriate diagnosis (Table 10-1). Symptoms of hormonal ($T_4$ or $T_3$) excess may

## TABLE 10.1 ● ● ●

### Nomogram: Hormones and Thyroid Status

| Paired Hormone Analysis | Serum $T_4$—Low | Serum $T_4$—Medium | Serum $T_4$—High |
|---|---|---|---|
| TSH—high | Hypothyroidism: 1° thyroid gland failure<br>Iodine deficiency<br>Adrenal insufficiency | | Hyperthyroidism:<br>TSH-secreting tumor (2°), or<br>↑ TRF (3°) |
| TSH—medium | Hypothyroidism: from<br>2° pituitary failure or<br>3° hypothalamic failure | Normal thyroid | Pregnancy |
| TSH—low | | Hyperthyroidism: autonomous 1° secretion from thyroid (eg, Graves' disease, goiter, nodules, or autoimmune thyroiditis) | |

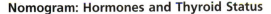

1°, primary; 2°, secondary; 3°, tertiary; $T_4$, thyroxine; TSH, thyroid-stimulating hormone; ↑, increased.

require a suppression test, and symptoms of hormone deficiency may require a stimulation test (TRH stimulation test) to clarify the 1°, 2°, or 3° causes. After an abnormality or hormonal imbalance is identified, additional studies, including nuclear scans, ultrasound (US), x-rays, computed tomography (CT) scans, or magnetic resonance imaging (MRI), may be used to identify the specific location and extent of a nodule or tumor and to select appropriate treatment. Endocrinopathies should be evaluated in light of all clinical, physical, and laboratory data available.

### Thyroid Storm

When hyperthyroid patients are subjected to concurrent illness or stress such as infection, traumatic accident, or heart attack, a medical emergency termed a *thyroid storm* can be triggered. The symptoms are more severe than with thyrotoxicosis and include fever (often above 100.4°F), nausea and vomiting, tachycardia, congestive heart failure (CHF), anxiety, and psychosis. The resulting massive release of thyroid hormones has a fatality rate of 20% to 50% and requires hospitalization and aggressive treatment with high doses of propylthiouracil (PTU), propranolol to treat cardiac arrhythmia, and hydrocortisone to block conversion of $T_4$ to $T_3$. Supportive measures emphasize reducing fever and body temperature, treating any underlying infection, removing any exogenous sources of iodine, and replacing losses of body fluids and glucose (Nathan, 1999).

## Hyperthyroidism

### Incidence and Symptoms

Hyperthyroidism occurs in about 19 per 1000 women and 1.6 per 1000 men in North America (Burman, 1995). The incidence increases in postmenopausal women and elderly men.

Symptoms of hyperthyroidism include restlessness, anxiety, emotional lability, decreased ability to concentrate long term, diminished exercise tolerance because of proximal muscle weakness, heat intolerance with typical warm and moist skin, slight hand tremor, excessive perspiration, increased appetite or tendency for easy weight loss, and ankle edema. Augmented gut motility may lead to increased bowel movements. Patient complaints include cardiopulmonary symptoms (racing heart rate), eye changes (exophthalmos, vision loss), thyroid enlargement (homogeneous or nodular), and problems with personal relationships (increased temper and irritability) (Tables 10-2 and 10-3).

Older patients may respond differently to hyperthyroidism than younger patients and are harder to diagnose. Higher frequencies of tachycardia, atrial fibrillation, fatigue, lethargy, and weight loss with lower frequencies of heat intolerance, tremor, nervousness, and sweating are seen in patients older than 70 years compared with patients younger than 50 years. However, over 35% of thyrotoxicosis cases occur in patients older than 60 (Trivalle et al., 1996).

*Exophthalmos* can occur in one or both eyes and with or without hyperthyroidism, although it usually is linked to elevated levels of TSH secretion. These eye disorders appear to be autoimmune diseases but are not linked to TSH antibody (Figs. 10-3 and 10-4). Exophthalmos responds to corticoid treatment but not to hypophysectomy (Wilson, 1998).

**Clinical Alert**: Hyperthyroidism may cause potassium wasting and loss of muscle tone, leading to periodic paralysis (Burman, 1995); this can be aggravated by exogenous insulin administration, a high carbohydrate diet, alcohol consumption, or strenuous physical activity. Hyperthyroidism may be caused or aggravated by drugs rich in iodine, intravenous contrast media (eg, used in CT scans), excessive use of cough syrup with expectorants (which contain iodine), and antiarrhythmic drugs (eg, amiodarone).

### Physiologic Basis of Treatment for Hyperthyroidism

It is essential to differentiate whether the problem involves the thyroid gland (1°), pituitary tumors (2°), hypothalamic lesions (3°), or other factors (ie, autoimmune, exogenous medicines). Table 10-3 describes the clinical and laboratory differential diagnosis involving hyperthyroidism. Initial treatment of primary hyperthyroidism is to remove or decrease the hypertrophied tissue, either by surgical or medical approaches. Oral medications include thionamide agents (eg, methimazole, carbimazole, or PTU). Inflammatory disease of the thyroid gland or subacute thyroiditis (nonsuppurative thyroiditis, granulomatous thyroiditis, or DeQuervain's disease) is the most common cause of pain and tenderness of the thyroid gland (Lazarus, 1996). Its onset can be abrupt, with or without pain over the thyroid gland, radiating to the jaw, throat, and ears. It often is correlated with a history of fever, sore throat, and myalgia related to recent upper respiratory infection (see the web site of the American Autoimmune Related Disease Association at *http://www.aarda.org*).

## TABLE 10.2

### Signs and Symptoms of Hyperthyroidism

| System | Symptoms Exhibited* |
|---|---|
| Cardiovascular and heart | Palpitations, tachycardia (>90 beats/min), mitral valve prolapse, atrial fibrillation (28% in patients >60 y), increased angina, CHF, shortness of breath, dyspnea on exertion, resistance to digitalis |
| Eyes | Exophthalmos (bilateral or unilateral) and lid retraction, chemosis (conjunctiva edema), ophthalmoplegia (grittiness, blurred, photophobia, diplopia, increased eye pressure), vision loss, limited movement |
| Gastrointestinal | Hyperphagia, hyperdefecation, elevated liver function tests, $\uparrow$ ALT, $\uparrow$ Alk phosphatase |
| General | Nervousness, insomnia, fatigue, heat intolerance, increased appetite but weight loss, anorexia in 33% of elderly, tremulousness, $\uparrow$ sweating, rapid speech |
| Hematologic | Normochromic, normocytic anemia; lymphocytosis; leukopenia ($\downarrow$ neutrophils); requirement $\downarrow$ for anticoagulants (Coumadin) |
| Metabolic | Hypercalcemia, potassium wasting, increased alkaline phosphatase |
| Neurologic | Nervousness, apprehension, emotional lability, fever, delirium, coma, choreoathetosis |
| Neuromuscular | Fine tremors, hyperkinesia, loss of muscle tone, periodic paralysis (possibly from hypokalemia), proximal muscle weakness, seizures, myopathy (males > females) |
| Osseous | Increased ionized $Ca^{2+}$, increased excretion $Ca^{2+}$ and phosphorus, osteoporosis, osteomalacia, osteitis fibrosa |
| Reproductive | Irregular menses (eventually cease altogether), infertility, $\uparrow$ risk miscarriage, $\uparrow$ conversion androgens to estrogens, gynecomastia in men |
| Respiratory | Exertional dyspnea, $\uparrow$ hypercapnic ventilatory drive, $\uparrow$ coexisting asthma |
| Skin | Warm and moist, onycholysis, pretibial myxedema, urticaria, pruritus, vitiligo, palmar erythema, fine hair, hair loss, inability to hold a wave (permanent) |

Alk, alkaline; ALT, alkaline transferase; $Ca^{2+}$, calcium; CHF, congestive heart failure; $\uparrow$, increased; $\downarrow$, decreased.
*Not all symptoms are present in any one patient.
(Adapted from Burman, K.D. [1995]. Hyperthyroidism. In K.L. Becker [Ed.], *Principles and practice of endocrinology metabolism* [2nd ed., pp. 341–346]. Philadelphia: J.B. Lippincott; Larsen, P.R., Davies, T.F., & Hay, I.D. [1998]. The thyroid gland. In J.D. Wilson [Ed.], *Williams textbook of endocrinology* [9th ed., pp 389–516]. Philadelphia: W.B. Saunders; and McPhee, S. & Bauer, D.C. [1997]. Thyroid disease. In S. McPhee [Ed.], *Pathophysiology of disease* [pp. 47–487]. Englewood Cliffs, NJ: Prentice-Hall.)

### Graves' Disease

Graves' disease (called Basedow's disease in Europe) is the most common cause of hyperthyroidism. Graves' disease is an autoimmune disease often characterized by a cyclic course, elevated TSH receptor (stimulating) antibody, diffuse symmetric goiter, thyrotoxicosis, infiltrative orbitopathy, and dermopathy (Table 10-4). Graves' disease occurs in 2.7% of women and 0.27% of men and is exacerbated by physical or emotional stress, with long periods of euthyroidism occurring in over 25%

of patients (when medications can be withdrawn). Treatment initially is offered with antithyroid drugs (inexpensive and more controllable). These include PTU or methimazole (MMI, Tapazole). These antithyroid drugs work by blocking hormone synthesis, blocking iodination and iodotyrosine coupling, and inhibiting the conversion of $T_4$ to $T_3$. Coexisting autoimmune diseases include insulin-dependent diabetes mellitus, hepatitis, pernicious anemia (3%), gastric parietal cell antibody disease, myasthenia gravis (1% to 2%), lupus erythematosis, and rheumatoid arthritis (Larsen et al., 1999).

## TABLE 10.3

**Clinical and Laboratory Differential Diagnosis of Hyperthyroidism**

| Clinical Diagnosis | Symptoms Exhibited |
| --- | --- |
| Goiter, toxic multinodular | Eye (no exophthalmos), inhomogeneous scan, Plummer's disease, enlarged thyroid, difficulty swallowing |
| Graves' disease, autoimmune | Increased iodine uptake, eye (exophthalmos), thyroid autoantibodies (TSHR-Ab) |
| Interleukin-2 or interferon use | Thyroiditis, hyperthyroidism, or hypothyroidism |
| Nodule, toxic | Eye (normal without exophthalmos), usually $T_3$ toxicosis, size >3 cm, age <20 or >60 y |
| Postpartum thyroiditis | Palpitations, rapid weight loss, mood changes, anxiety, transient |
| Thyroiditis, subacute | Fever, tender neck, iodine uptake low, transient |
| Thyroiditis, chronic | Nongoitrous (atrophic), or goitrous (Hashimoto's thyroiditis), +/− autoimmune (95% of diffuse goiter patients are +auto-Ab) |
| Thyrotoxicosis | ↓ Serum TSH, ↑ $fT_4$, ↑ BMR, ↓ serum cholesterol |
| Thyroid storm | Extreme thyrotoxicosis, fever (>100.4°F), nausea, normal catecholamines (epinephrine or norepinephrine), vomiting, tachycardia, CHF, anxiety, confusion, psychosis. High fatality rate |
| TSH-secreting tumor | (+/−) eye signs, CNS signs, increased TSH alpha subunit in serum |

Auto-Ab, autoantibodies; BMR, basal metabolic rate; CHF, congestive heart failure; CNS, central nervous system; $T_3$, triiodothyronine; $T_4$, thyroxine; $fT_4$, free thyroxine; TSH, thyrotropin; TSHR-Ab, thyrotropin receptor antibody; ↑, increased; ↓, decreased.
(Adapted from Burman, K.D. [1995]. Hyperthyroidism. In K.L. Becker [Ed.], *Principles and practice of endocrinology metabolism* [2nd ed., pp. 341–346]. Philadelphia: J.B. Lippincott; Nathan, M.N. [1999]. Diseases of the thyroid and parathyroid glands. In J.K. Singleton, et al. [Eds.], *Primary care* [pp 237–257]. Philadelphia: Lippincott Williams & Wilkins; and McPhee, S. & Bauer, D.C. [1997]. Thyroid disease. In S. McPhee (Ed.), *Pathophysiology of disease* [pp. 470–487].. Englewood Cliffs, NJ: Prentice-Hall.)

Treatment, whether chemical (PTU, carbimazole), surgical, or irradiation, can be adjusted to (1) gradually decrease the symptoms; or (2) aggressively ablate the entire gland, induce a hypothyroid state, and work the patient back to a euthyroid state with replacement thyroid hormones (see Figs. 10-5 and 10-6). Propranolol can be used for symptomatic relief of the autonomic nervous system, and verapamil sometimes is used to control tachycardia.

Diagnostic tests for autoimmune disease can involve a wide variety of thyroid antigens, including thyroglobulin (the storage protein for thyroid hormone), microsomes (mitochondria, lysosomes), thyroid peroxidase, TSH (thyroid-stimulating antibody), or TSH receptor antibody (see Table 10-4).

***Clinical Alert:*** Mild side effects of antithyroid medication include itchy skin and rashes, which can be improved with antihistamines; however, more serious side effect such as hepatitis, fever, agranulocytosis (occurring in 0.3% patients), or leukopenia require immediate cessation of medication and sometimes hospitalization.

Ablative radioactive iodine treatment (causing permanent destruction) is used as a second line of treatment and usually results in hypothyroidism and lifetime requirements for replacement thyroid hormone. Surgical ablation of the thyroid is more expensive than radioiodine but is indicated for pregnant women, patients with large obstructive goiters (compressive symptoms), those intolerant of antithyroid medications, and those believed to have a malignancy. Surgical complications may include vocal cord paralysis and hypoparathyroidism because these structures are buried within the thyroid tissue and are difficult to avoid surgically. Recurrence rate of hyperthyroidism (from remaining remnants) within 5 years of surgery is about 3% to 8% (Torring, 1996).

*Subacute thyroiditis* is a hyperthyroid condition in which stored hormone is released initially in excess and is treated primarily with pain and symptom relief. Anti-inflammatory drugs (salicylate or prednisone) usually resolve the neck pain within 72 hours. Anaplastic thyroid cancer drugs can be added if pain persists. Beta-antagonists (propranolol) can be used to treat palpitations or anxiety. Since there is little increase in thyroid synthesis, PTU and MMI are not clinically valuable (Lazarus, 1995). Postpartum thyroiditis

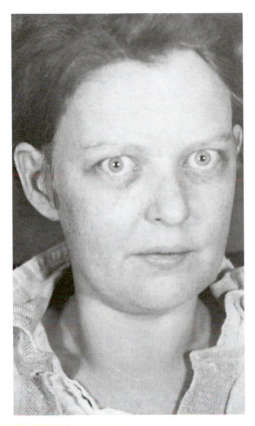

**FIGURE 10.3** ● A woman with Graves' disease. Note the exophthalmos and enlarged thyroid gland.

(PPT), with an incidence of approximately 6% to 9%, can be screened by measuring antithyroid microsomal antibody (MC-Ab) or thyroid peroxidase antibody (TPO-Ab) during or after pregnancy. It has been noted that 20% to 25% of women with PPT will develop permanent hypothyroidism within 5 to 10 years of parturition (Amino et al., 1999).

*Autoimmune thyroiditis*, or *Hashimoto's thyroiditis*, is a result of Graves' hyperthyroid state where the thyroid becomes lymphocytic and goitrous as a result of the autoimmune attack and the patient eventually becomes hypothyroid.

## Hypothyroidism

Hypothyroidism in the adult, or adult myxedema, can be precipitated at multiple levels. Table 10-5 lists the signs and symptoms of hypothyroidism (Fig. 10-7). Decreased thyroid hormone production resulting in hypothyroidism can be caused by thyroid disease (primary hypothyroidism) or by diseases of the pituitary or hypothalamus (secondary or tertiary hypothyroidism). Primary hypothyroidism can be caused by autoimmune destruction of follicular cells (thyroiditis), surgery, or unrelated immune processes (idiopathic). Chronic thyroiditis can occur in an atrophic (nongoitrous, lymphocytic) form or in a goitrous form (Hashimoto's thyroiditis), which shows eosinophilic (Hürthle cells) and fibrotic changes.

Hypothyroidism in children results in truncal obesity, short stature, decreased metabolic rate, and mental sluggishness. Hypothyroidism is more frequent in women than in men, with an incidence of about 2% in women and 0.2% in men between the ages of 20 and 50 years. Postmenopausal women show an incidence of up to 30% to 40% (positive for anti-microsomal antibodies, especially TPO-Ab), with 3% to 4% of all medically

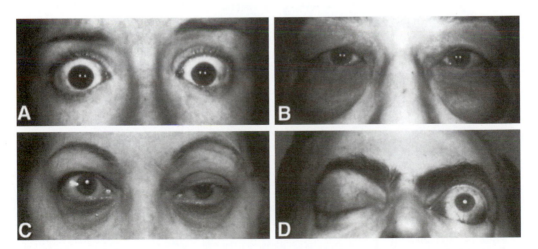

**FIGURE 10.4** ● Clinical presentations of Graves' ophthalmopathy. **(A)** Retraction of both eyelids. **(B)** Severe periorbital edema. **(C)** Predominantly unilateral involvement. **(D)** Spontaneous subluxation of a severely proptotic left eye.

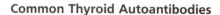

## TABLE 10.4　　● ● ●

### Common Thyroid Autoantibodies

| Antigen | Antibody (IgG type) | Notes |
|---|---|---|
| TSH receptor | TSHR-Ab* | These Abs may mimic TSH, that is, either stimulating or blocking Ab. Association with Graves' disease (~95%) |
| TG　　　or | TG-Ab | Lymphocytic infiltration of thyroid: autoimmune thyroiditis (100%), |
| Thyroid peroxidase (formerly microsomal Ab) | TPO-Ab | Hashimoto's thyroiditis or Graves' disease (50%–80%), IDDM (40%) |

Abs, antibodies; IDDM, insulin-dependent diabetes mellitus; TG, thyroglobulin; TG-Ab, thyroglobulin antibody; TPO-Ab, thyroid peroxidase antibody; TSH, thyroid-stimulating hormone; TSHR-Ab, thyrotropin receptor antibody.
*TSHR-Ab (stimulating) also is known as long-acting thyroid stimulator or thyroid-stimulating immunoglobulin, an IgG.

examined patients showing subclinical hypothyroidism (where TSH is elevated less than three times the upper level of normal, but $T_3$ and $T_4$ are in the low-normal range). Some researchers suggest that these patients are working harder to keep their thyroid levels normal and that its production drops during stress situations, so that the person may become overtly hypothyroid within the next 4 to 5 years. The antiarrhythmic agent amiodarone is an iodinated pharmaceutical used to treat refractory cardiac arrhythmia ranging from paroxysmal atrial fibrillation to life-threatening tachycardia, arrhythmia, CHF, and cardiomyopathy. Structurally, it is similar to $T_4$ and is known to block iodination steps, inhibit conversion of $T_4$ to $T_3$, and

to antagonize $T_3$ activity directly, resulting in abnormal thyroid test results and overt hypothyroidism in some patients (Iudica-Souza & Burch, 1999).

*Clinical Alert:* Up to 28% of patients with Down's syndrome develop autoimmune thyroid disease. Trisomy 21 (Down's syndrome) and several other endocrinopathies are genetically linked to autoimmune disease. For example, the incidence of chronic autoimmune thyroiditis is increased in patients with Addison's disease, polyglandular autoimmune syndrome type II, or Turner's syndrome (Dayan & Daniels, 1996).

*Euthyroid sick syndrome,* or nonthyroidal illness, is a hypothyroid state with normal TSH val-

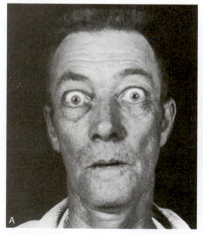
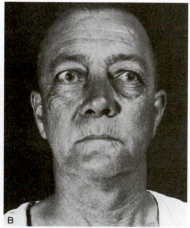

**FIGURE 10.5** ● Patient with Graves' disease treated with antithyroid drug. **(A)** Appearance before therapy. **(B)** Four months after commencement of therapy. Note the markedly decreased stare. Eventually, radioactive iodine treatment was required for permanent cure.

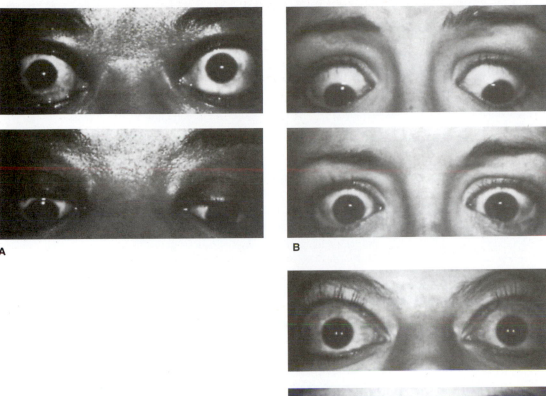

**FIGURE 10.6** ● Results of orbital surgery in patients with Graves' ophthalmopathy. **(A)** Transantral orbital decompression before *(top)* and after *(bottom)*. **(B)** Extraocular muscle surgery before *(top)* and after *(bottom)*. **(C)** Scleral graft insertion to correct eyelid malposition before *(top)* and after *(bottom)*. (Courtesy of Drs. LW DeSanto, J Dyer, and R Waller. Photographs **A** and **C** are from Gorman CA. The presentation and management of endocrine ophthalmopathy. *Clin Endocrinol Metab* 1978;7:67.)

ues, normal $T_4$, low $T_3$, but high $rT_3$ values. It occurs under a variety of aggravated circumstances, including medication with amiodarone, systemic illness, malnutrition, and trauma (Larsen et al., 1998).

*Myxedema coma* is a clinical diagnosis that usually develops gradually among older patients who have concomitant illness, take sedating drugs, or live in cold climates, or it can occur abruptly in cases of infection, gastrointestinal (GI) bleeding, or respiratory disease. Table 10-6 shows patterns of test results seen in the differential diagnosis of various hypothyroid conditions. Physical examination shows overt hypothyroidism, mental stupor, dry skin, lowered body temperature, bradycardia, CHF, or delayed tendon reflexes. A poorer outcome (20% mortality) is associated with body temperature less than 93°F, bradycardia of less than 44 beats per minute, sepsis, myocardial infarction (MI), or hypotension (Jordan, 1995).

*Clinical Alert:* Cabbage, broccoli, cress, and other cruciferous vegetables are natural goitrogens and can induce hypothyroidism when consumed in large amounts by people with a propensity to thyroid nodular disease. The incidence of hypothyroidism in people on lithium treatment is 50% or greater.

## Autoimmune Thyroiditis

Autoimmune diseases occur when the immune system mistakes normal tissue (self) for a foreign invader (nonself) and attempts to destroy it. Autoantibodies are found in the serum of patients with both hyperthyroidism and hypothyroidism because the body tries to resist the initial immune assault by increasing stimulation to the gland under attack. The attacking antibodies destroy thyroid cells but in the process cause excessive release of stored thyroid hormones, resulting initially in hyperthyroid symptoms. As the attack

## TABLE 10.5

### Signs and Symptoms of Hypothyroidism

| Affected System | Symptoms Affected |
|---|---|
| Cardiovascular | Bradycardia, mild hypertension, pericardial effusion |
| Eyes and ears | Edematous upper eye lids, periorbital puffiness, puffy facial expression, hearing loss |
| Gastrointestinal | Nausea, constipation, enlarged tongue (obstructive sleep apnea), ascites |
| General | ↓ levels of $T_3$ and $T_4$, hypothermia, +/− low TSH, anorexia but with ↑ weight gain, lethargy, longer demand for rest (>9 h sleep/night), ↑ obstructive sleep apnea, cold intolerance, fatigue, slow speech, hoarseness |
| Hematologic | Requirement ↑ for anticoagulants (Coumadin); ↑ pernicious anemia; folate deficiency and menorrhagia contribute to microcytic, hypochromic anemia |
| Metabolic | Weight gain, edema in body cavities such as pericardial sac; ↑ creatine phosphokinase, liver enzymes, cholesterol, and triglycerides; ↓ $Na^+$ concentration because of water retention |
| Neurologic | Hoarseness, slow mentation, depression, memory impairment |
| Neuromuscular | Muscle weakness and cramps, slow return of a muscle to neutral position after a tendon jerk, muscle stiffness |
| Respiratory | Pulmonary hypertension (10–20%) is caused by edema, ↑ obstructive sleep apnea |
| Reproductive | Both ↓ testosterone and ↓ estrogens, irregular menses, longer and heavier menstrual bleeding, ↓ fertility, impotence, ↓ libido and oligospermia in men |
| Skin | Cold, rough, dry skin; cold intolerant; loss of hair; coarse, brittle hair; brittle nails; periorbital swelling; facial pallor/swelling; yellow skin (carotenemia); nonpitting edema; myxedema (general and pretibial); arthralgia; infiltrating dermopathy; ↓ sweating; ↑ bruisability; short lateral $1/3$ of eye brows |

$Na^+$, sodium; $T_3$, triiodothyronine; $T_4$, thyroxine; TSH, thyrotropin; ↓, decreased; ↑, increased.
(Adapted from Burman, K.D. [1995]. Hyperthyroidism. In K.L. Becker [Ed.], *Principles and practice of endocrinology metabolism* [2nd ed., pp. 331–346]. Philadelphia: J.B. Lippincott; Larsen, P.R., Davies, T.F., & Hay, I.D. [1998], The thyroid gland. In J.D. Wilson [Ed.], *Williams textbook of endocrinology* [9th ed., pp 389–516]. Philadelphia: W.B. Saunders; and Nathan, M.N. [1999]. Diseases of the thyroid and parathyroid glands. In J.K. Singleton, et al. [Eds.], *Primary care* [pp 237–257]. Philadelphia: Lippincott Williams & Wilkins.)

progresses and more tissue is destroyed, the gland begins to fail, and the patient reverts to hypothyroidism.

### Physiologic Basis for Treatment for Hypothyroidism

*Replacement hormone treatment* for hypothyroidism includes $T_4$, also called L-thyroxine or levothyroxine (Synthroid, approximately 1.7 µg/kg); $T_3$, also called liothyronine (Cytomel, 25–100 mcg/d) and Liotrix ($T_4/T_3$ mixed, approximately 120/30 mcg/d). Older or sedentary patients require approximately half the usual dose. The goal is to reach a replacement dose that results in a normal range for TSH levels. Because the thyroid hormones control metabolic processes and heat production, the body require-

ments change dramatically during various times of the year (winter versus summer), based on physical exertion patterns (eg, taking up a new sport, summer camp for children, working in the garden), and dosages should be adjusted accordingly. Side effects from overmedication include cardiac arrhythmia, angina, and CHF (Toft, 1994). Table 10-7 lists other exogenous factors that can influence the action of replacement thyroid hormone.

*Clinical Alert:* Care should be taken when drawing blood for monitoring thyroid replacement to obtain peak (within approximately 2 hours after taking the next dose) or trough (nadir approximately 2 hours before next dose) values as requested and to carefully note time of the last treatment (refer to Table 10-8 for the half-life of hormones).

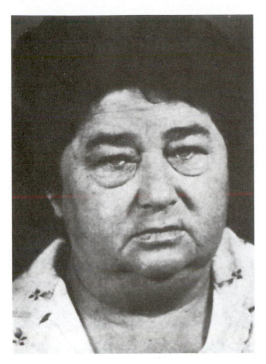

**FIGURE 10.7** ● Patient with myxedema. (Courtesy of Dr. Herbert Langford.) (From Guyton A. & Hall, J. [1996]. *Medical physiology* [9th ed., p. 955.] Philadelphia: W.B. Saunders. Reprinted by permission.)

## Diagnostic Laboratory Tests

Serum concentrations of a variety of hormones can be measured by immunoassay. A laboratory request for a $T_7$ is a combination of three different results: a total $T_3$, a $T_3RUp$, and a calculated free $T_4$. Direct assays of total $T_4$ and free $T_4$ are available and are slightly more specific.

*Clinical Alert*: An elevated total $T_4$ should be combined with a test for TSH before diagnosing hyperthyroidism because pregnancy or menopausal hormone replacement treatment (HRT) with conjugated estrogens will increase the TBG level.

### Radionuclide Imaging Studies

Patients with hyperthyroidism given a tracer dose of radioactive iodine ($^{131}I$) show an increased 24-hour thyroid uptake, which can differentiate between Graves' disease and thyroiditis. Thyroid scans, which allow imaging of the gland, are performed with iodine ($^{123}I$) or pertechnetate (technetium, $^{99}Tc$). The distribution of radionuclide within the gland is homogeneous in Graves' disease but nodular in toxic adenomas or toxic multinodular goiters (Hay & Morris, 1996). Cold nodules (areas of decreased uptake) should be evaluated for thyroid carcinoma in nonfunctioning tissue. Hypothyroid tissue and thyroiditis tissue

may generate no scans or may look patchy (Lazarus, 1996).

*Clinical Alert*: Pregnancy should be deferred for at least 3 months after any radioactive iodine treatment or scan.

### Diagnostic Imaging Tools

Patients with Graves' disease can go into remission for the hyperthyroid symptoms, but continuing problems with unilateral eye movement or eye proptosis may represent a diagnostic dilemma. Ultrasound of a palpable neck thyroid mass is quick, noninvasive (no iodine-containing contrast media), and cost effective. Scanning with CT (x-ray) or MRI offers better resolution in detecting normal tissue from goiter tissue and can be used to measure the thickening of the eye muscles, which is found in more than 50% of euthyroid patients with Graves' disease.

## CALCIUM METABOLISM AND ENDOCRINOPATHIES

Of the total body $Ca^{2+}$, 99% resides in bone; 85% of the body's phosphate and 50% of all magnesium in the body is found in the mineral phase of bone. Blood levels of $Ca^{2+}$ are critical for the functioning of many different tissues (including nerves and muscle) and for the occurrence of different body functions (such as coagulation and endocrine secretory). It must be maintained within the critical window of approximately 7 to 10.5 mg/dL. To accomplish this, several metabolic systems are used to influence blood $Ca^{2+}$ values. The kidneys control secretion of $Ca^{2+}$, the GI tract controls absorption of new $Ca^{2+}$, osteoblast cells remove $Ca^{2+}$ from blood by storing it in bone, and osteoclast cells return $Ca^{2+}$ to the blood by resorbing stored $Ca^{2+}$ from bone. Each system has special requirements and feedback controls.

Total calcium in the blood includes both the free (biologically active) and protein (primarily albumin)-bound components. A variety of factors can change the protein binding: albumin concentrations, the ratio of free to bound (including alkalosis), elevated free fatty acids, lipid infusions, and hepatic diseases. Consequently, direct free or ionized calcium ($iCa^{2+}$) should be measured in the setting of acute illness or severe hypoalbuminemia (Bringhurst & Demay, 1998).

### Parathyroid Control of Bone

The four parathyroid glands are located two on either side of the trachea with one superior and inferior embedded in the thyroid gland (Fig. 10-8). Each of these parathyroid glands is approximately

## TABLE 10.6

### Clinical Diagnosis of Hypothyroid Endocrinopathy

| Clinical Diagnosis | Symptoms Identified | Laboratory Results |
|---|---|---|
| 1° Hypothyroidism (95% of cases) | Infiltrative disease (amyloid, scleroderma), antoimmune thyroiditis, exogenous destruction ($^{131}$I, thyroidectomy, PTU) | ↑TSH, ↑TRH, ↑PRL, ↓fT$_4$, ↓T$_4$ →T$_3$, ↑TRH, ↑PRL, ↑Sed rate |
| Defective thyroid hormone synthesis | Iodine deficiency or drugs that block synthesis (lithium, iodine excess, propylthiouracil/PTU, amiodarone) | ↓Serum iodine, ↑TSH, ↑TRH, ↑PRL, ↓fT$_4$, ↓T$_4$ |
| 2° deficiency (~5% of cases) | Anterior pituitary tumor (macroadenoma), ischemia | ↓TSH, ↑TRH, ↓fT$_4$, ↓T$_4$ |
| 3° deficiency | Hypothalamic lesions, trauma of the pituitary stalk (car accident, concussion) | ↓TRH, ↓TSH, ↓fT$_4$, ↓T$_4$ |
| Thyroiditis, subacute | Silent destruction of thyroid tissue; transient, viral, or postpartum fever; tender neck; low iodine uptake; postpartum incidence ~9% (up to 85% in women with iodine-deficient diets) | ↑TSH, ↑TRH, ↑PRL, ↓fT$_4$, ↓T$_4$ |
| Thyroiditis, chronic | Nongoitrous (atrophic, +HLA-DR3) or goitrous (Hashimoto's thyroiditis, +HLA-DR5), +/− autoimmune (95% +autoantibodies in diffuse goiter patients) | ↑TSH, ↑TRH, ↑PRL, ↓fT$_4$, ↓T$_4$, ↑thyroid Ab, ↑Sed rate |
| Cretinism (childhood myxedema) | Childhood hypothyroidism, failure to thrive, developmental delay, low IQ | ↑TSH, ↑TRH, ↑PRL, ↓fT$_4$, ↓T$_4$, ↑thyroid Ab, ↑Sed rate |
| Myxedema coma | Concomitant illness, drugs, bradycardia, congestive heart failure, hypothermia, ↑creatine phosphokinase, pale, seizures, hypoglycemia, mortality >20% | ↓T4, ↑TSH |

Ab, antibody; fT$_4$, free thyroxine; HLA, human leukocyte antigen; $^{131}$I, radioactive iodine; PRL, progesterone-releasing hormone; PTU, propylthiouracil; Sed, sedimentation; T$_3$, triiodothyronine; T$_4$, thyroxine; TRH, thyrotropin-releasing hormone; TSH, thyrotropin; I°, primary; 2°, secondary; 3°, tertiary; ↑, increased; ↓, decreased; →, converted to.
(Adapted from Burman, K.D. [1995]. Hyperthyroidism. In K.L. Becker [Ed.], *Principles and practice of endocrinology metabolism* [2nd ed., pp 341-346]. Philadelphia: J.B. Lippincott; Jordan, R.M. [1995]. Myxedema coma, pathophysiology, therapy, and factors affecting prognosis. *Medical Clinics of North America*, 79 [1], 185—194; and Nathan, M.N. [1999]. Diseases of the thyroid and parathyroid glands. In J.K. Singleton, et al. [Eds.], *Primary care* [pp 237—257]. Philadelphia: Lippincott Williams & Wilkins,

3 × 6 mm long and weighs about 30 to 50 mg. Each gland is composed of chief cells, which secrete PTH in response to decreasing free or iCa$^{2+}$, plus oxyphil cells and fat cells. PTH is synthesized and stored as a large protein and is cleaved to a smaller protein just before release. Its main target tissues are the bone, gut, and kidneys, where it increases blood levels of calcium and decreases blood phosphorus. Normal bone is constantly undergoing remodeling, with breakdown and rebuilding. PTH specifically stimulates the osteoclast cells (demineralization) and inhibits the osteoblast cells (mineralization) in bone, with the net effect of increasing bone breakdown and put-

ting Ca$^{2+}$ back into the circulation. *Calcitonin* also is synthesized in the thyroid gland in C cells, which are parafollicular and are not located in the parathyroid glands. Increased levels of calcitonin inhibit osteoclast activity and diminish bone resorption. Thus, PTH and calcitonin are opposing or yin-yang controls for Ca$^{2+}$ homeostasis. Replacement of calcitonin is accomplished by treating with Miacalcin nasal spray (Rich, 1999). Hyperplasia of C cells leads to the tumor found in familial medullary carcinoma of the thyroid (Larsen et al., 1998).

GI absorption of calcium is dependent on vitamin D$_3$. However, the body must convert the pre-

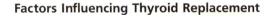

## TABLE 10.7

### Factors Influencing Thyroid Replacement

| | Exogenous Factor | Effect on Thyroid |
|---|---|---|
| Diet: nutrition | Low dietary iodine, fasting, malnutrition | Decreased thyroid synthesis |
| | Excessive iodine, or lithium | Blocked conversion of $T_4$ to $T_3$, decreased thyroid |
| Drugs | Estrogens, clofibrate, opiates | ↑ Total $T_4$ |
| | Androgen, glucocorticoid, danazol | ↓ Total $T_4$ |
| | Salicylates, diphenylhydantoin, furosemide, sulfonylureas, diazepam, heparin | Inhibits binding to carrier molecules (TBG) |
| | Sulfonylureas, interleukin-2 | Inhibits thyroid function |
| | Glucocorticoid, ipodate, propranolol, amiodarone, propylthiouracil | ↓ Conversion $T_4 \rightarrow T_3$ |
| | Dopamine antagonists, cimetidine, iodine, lithium | ↑ TSH |
| | Dopamine agonists, somatostatin, glucocorticoids | ↓ TSH |
| | Cholestyramine, colestipol, soybean flour, iron, sucralfate, cimetidine, aluminum-containing antacids | ↓ Gastrointestinal absorption of replacement thyroid hormone |
| | Antiseizure medications (phenytoin, phenobarbital, carbamazepine), cigarette smoking | ↑ Hepatic metabolism (turnover) of thyroxine, ↓ $T_4$ |
| Pathology | Hepatic, renal dysfunction, systemic illness, trauma, postoperation, iodine imaging agents | ↓ TBG, ↓ conversion $T_4 \rightarrow T_3$ or $rT_3$ |

$rT_4$, reverse thyroxine; $T_3$, triiodothyronine; $T_4$, thyroxine; TBG, thyroxine-binding globulin; TSH, thyrotropin; ↑, increased; ↓, decreased; →, converted to.
(Adapted from Larsen, P.R., Davies, T.F., & Hay, I.D. [1998]. The thyroid gland. In J.D. Wilson [Ed.], *Williams textbook of endocrinology* (9th ed., pp 389–516). Philadelphia: W.B. Saunders; and Nathan, M.N. [1999]. Diseases of the thyroid and parathyroid glands. In J.K. Singleton, et al. [Eds.], *Primary care* [pp 237–257]. Philadelphia: Lippincott Williams & Wilkins.)

cursor vitamin $D_3$ (cholecalciferol) by (1) exposing the skin to sunlight, (2) hydroxylating it in the liver, and (3) hydroxylating it a second time in the kidney to obtain the active form called 1,25 dihydroxyvitamin $D_3$ (calciferol) (Fig. 10-9). If any of these steps are missing or malfunctioning (low dietary vitamin $D_3$, no sun, kidney failure, cirrhosis of the liver), then calciferol will be low and the ability to absorb dietary $Ca^{2+}$ will be limited. There are over 30 different forms of rickets resulting in deficient levels of vitamin $D_3$ or $Ca^{2+}$ (Becker, 1990). If the hydroxylation steps are missing, it is necessary to replace with calciferol and *not* with cholecalciferol (vitamin $D_3$) to have bioactive hormone (Kettyle & Arky, 1999).

Kidney tubules control the reabsorption of $Ca^{2+}$ and the excretion of phosphate ions at the postglomerular filtration level. Increasing release of PTH will induce increasing reabsorption of urinary $Ca^{2+}$ in response to falling blood levels of $iCa^{2+}$.

Disorders of calcium and phosphate metabolism can be life-threatening problems that require prompt attention and careful diagnosis. Hypercalcemia can indicate bone destruction from metastatic disease, PTH excess, or tumor secretion of PTH-like proteins. Initial treatment is hydration for the patient with analysis of the serum $Ca^{2+}$, phosphate, and alkaline phosphatase levels (Table 10-9). Hypocalcemia frequently is associated with

## TABLE 10.8

**Laboratory Diagnostic Tests**

| | Serum Hormone Levels | | | | |
|---|---|---|---|---|---|
| | TSH (mU/L) | T₃RUp (%) | Free T₄ (ng/dL) | Total T₃ (ng/dL) | Total T₄ (μg/dL) |
| Normal Values* (Half-life) | 0.3–5.0 (30 min) | 25–35 | 0.8–2.3 | 80–200 (0.75 d) | 5–12 (7.0 d) |
| *Clinical Diagnosis* | | | | | |
| Primary hypothyroidism | High 15–1000 | Low | Low | +/− | Low |
| Secondary or tertiary hypothyroidism | Low | Low | Low | Low | Low |
| Subclinical hypothyroidism (few symptoms) | ~5–15, < 3 × normal | Low | Normal | Normal | Low |
| Euthyroid sick syndrome | High (early)/ normal (late) | | Normal/high | Low | Normal/high |
| Myxedema coma | High | Low | Low | Low | Low |
| Thyrotoxicosis or Graves' disease | Low < 0.1 | High | High | High | High |
| Primary hyperthyroidism: thyroid nodules (autonomous) | Low | High | High | High | High |
| Pregnancy (normal), hydatidiform mole | 0.2–0.5 | Low | Normal | Normal | High |
| Subclinical hyperthyroidism | Low 0.1–0.3 | Normal | Normal | Normal | Normal |

T₃, triiodothyronine; T₄, thyroxine; T₃RUp, T₃ resin uptake; TSH, thyrotropin.
*May vary slightly between laboratories.
(Adapted from Becker, K.L. [1990]. Interrelationships between hormones and the body. In K.L. Becker [Ed.], *Principles and practice of endocrinology and metabolism* [pp. 1474–1624]. Philadelphia: J.B. Lippincott; Burman, K.D. [1995]. Hyperthyroidism. In K.L. Becker [Ed.], *Principles and practice of endocrinology and metabolism* [2nd ed., pp. 331–346]. Philadelphia: J.B. Lippincott; Larsen, P.R., Davies, T.F., & Hay, I.D. [1998]. The thyroid gland. In J.D. Wilson [Ed.], *Williams textbook of endocrinology* [9th ed., pp 389–516]. Philadelphia: W.B. Saunders; and Nathan, M.N. [1999]. Diseases of the thyroid and parathyroid glands In J.K. Singleton, et al. [Eds.], *Primary care* [pp 237–257]. Philadelphia: Lippincott Williams & Wilkins.)

renal failure, decreased PTH, insensitivity to PTH, magnesium depletion, or vitamin D deficiency. Because of the multiple controls used for calcium, blood levels do not show significant changes in osteoporosis patients until the disease is quite advanced.

## Hyperparathyroidism

Hyperparathyroidism increases with age, and hypercalcemia is seen in 1/500 women and 1/2000 men older than 40 years of age, resulting in a variety of bone diseases. Symptoms of hyperparathyroidism include hypercalcemia and hypophosphatemia, decreased bone mineral density (BMD), decreased pulmonary function, chest deformity and kyphosis, periosteal bone erosion, and azotemia. Of patients with hyperparathyroidism, 20% are found to have kidney stones. Hyperparathyroidism frequently is found in association with multiple endocrine neoplasm syndrome (Silverberg & Bilezikian, 1996). Of the cases of primary hyperparathyroidism, 80% are caused by the development of a tumor (adenoma) in a single parathyroid gland. All four parathyroid glands are enlarged (hyperplasia) in 20% of the cases of primary hyperparathyroidism.

Imaging studies by bone densitometry, US, or ⁹⁹ᵐTc-sestamibi scanning in hyperparathyroidism show accelerated loss of cortical bone (eg, fore-

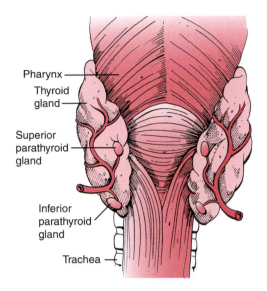

**FIGURE 10.8** ● Location of the four parathyroid bodies.

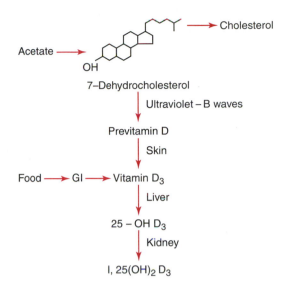

**FIGURE 10.9** ● Biochemical pathway through which activated vitamin $D_3$ is formed. Ultraviolet light is needed for skin synthesis of vitamin $D_3$, which is then converted by the liver into 25-OH $D_3$. Kidney cells then synthesize active $1,25(OH)_2 D_3$.

arm) but not trabecular or cancellous bone (eg, vertebrae are affected first in osteoporosis). These studies can be used to locate adenomas or ectopic rests of parathyroid tissue, such as those in the mediastinum (Sofferman, 1996). Symptoms of severe hyperparathyroidism include conjunctival calcification, hypertension (50%), GI symptoms (anorexia, nausea, vomiting, constipation, or abdominal pain), peptic ulcer, and pancreatitis. Laboratory analysis in primary hyperparathyroidism is characterized by high serum intact PTH, serum total $Ca^{2+}$ of 10.5 to 12.5 mg/dL, reduced serum albumin (seen in patients with anorexia or

cancer), elevated $iCa^{2+}$, elevated alkaline phosphatase, elevated 1,25 dihydroxyvitamin D, and elevated sedimentation rate.

*Clinical Alert*: Severe hypercalcemia ($Ca^{2+}$ above 15 mg/dL), which is called hypercalcemic crisis, can cause arrhythmia, coma, and death. It is sometimes triggered in hyperparathyroid patients during an acute illness, excessive dehydration, or extended immobilization (Bringhurst & Demay, 1998).

## TABLE 10.9 ● ● ●

### Calcium and Phosphate Concentrations Versus Diagnosis

| Serum $Ca^{2+}$ | Serum Phosphate | Serum Alkaline Phosphate | Notes |
|---|---|---|---|
| ↑ | ↑ | N | Vitamin D intoxication |
| ↑ | ↓ | ↑ or N | Hyperparathyroidism |
| ↑ | ↑ or N | ↑ | Metastatic bone disease |
| ↓ | ↑ | ↑ or N | Kidney failure (↑ BUN and creatinine) |
| ↓ | ↑ | N | Hypoparathyroidism |
| ↓ | ↓ | ↑ | Vitamin D deficiency |

BUN, blood urea nitrogen; N, normal; ↑, increased; ↓, decreased.
(From Kettyle, W.M. & Arky, R.A. [1998]. The thyroid. In *Endocrine pathophysiology* [pp 71–98]. Philadelphia: Lippincott Williams & Wilkins.)

## Hypoparathyroidism

Hypoparathyroidism can result from surgical intervention, irradiation of the neck region, or autoimmune destruction. Hypoparathyroidism frequently is associated with other autoimmune disorders (polyglandular autoimmune syndrome) such as Addison's disease (adrenal insufficiency), thymic hypoplasia (DiGeorge's syndrome), and thyroid disease. Hypoparathyroidism is characterized by decreased PTH, decreased $iCa^{2+}$ and total serum $Ca^{2+}$, and high phosphorus levels. Symptoms include paresthesia of the extremities and the circumoral area, and cramping of back and leg muscles, which is exacerbated by hyperventilation and alkalosis. Some patients exhibit subcapsular cataracts, tetany, convulsions, and laryngospasm (Streeten & Levine, 1995). Electrocardiographic abnormalities mimic acute MI or conduction abnormalities with prolonged Q-T intervals.

*Clinical Alert*: Signs of latent tetany include Chvostek's sign elicited by tapping over the facial nerve, which results in twitching of the upper lip on that side. Trousseau's sign can be elicited in patients with falling calcium levels by inflating a blood pressure cuff on the upper arm to 150 mm Hg for 3 minutes (Streeten & Levine, 1995).

First-line treatment includes calcium supplementation in mild cases. In severe hypoparathyroidism, patients are treated with calcitriol (1,25 dihydroxyvitamin $D_3$) or ergocalciferol.

*Osteoporosis* is a silent bone disease that usually is asymptomatic until well advanced and a fracture occurs. It affects more than 25 million Americans, 80% of whom are women. Fifty percent of women and 20% of men older than 65 years of age will have an osteoporotic fracture during their lifetimes. Men older than 50 years have a higher risk of experiencing an osteoporotic fracture than of developing prostate cancer (Rich, 1999). The three most frequently seen problems are (1) vertebral crush fractures, resulting in chronic back, rib, or abdominal pain; kyphosis; poor body image; and curtailed daily activities; (2) Colles' wrist fractures (distal radius); and (3) hip fractures, where 19% of patients require long-term or permanent nursing care, 25% are fatalities within the first year after the fracture (from pneumonia, deep vein thrombosis, or pulmonary embolism), and only 20% return to completely normal functioning (see the web site on bone diseases at *http://www.osteo.org*, or *http://www.nof.org*).

Osteoporosis is classified as type I (postmenopausal, affecting cancellous bone), type II (age associated; seen in both sexes older than 70 years with loss of cancellous and cortical bone) or idiopathic (seen in men and women before the age of 50 years). Secondary osteoporosis is a result of underlying causes such as malignancy (multiple myeloma), chronic liver or renal disease, Cushing's syndrome, hyperthyroidism, hyperparathyroidism, hypogonadism, athletic amenorrhea, anorexia, systemic mastocytosis, rheumatoid arthritis, osteogenesis imperfecta, and hyperprolactinemia. Drugs known to induce or aggravate osteoporosis include glucocorticoids, thyroid hormone, anticonvulsants and antiepileptics, heparin, cyclosporine, lithium, chemotherapy drugs, diuretics, gonadotropin-releasing hormone agonists, and aluminum-containing antacids (Rich, 1999). Lifestyle factors inducing osteoporosis include increased alcohol consumption, increased caffeine consumption, increased protein intake, smoking, excessive exercise, and immobilization or sedentary lifestyle (Harper & Weber, 1998).

*Paget's disease* (*osteitis deformans*) is a form of bone pathophysiology occurring in 1.5% to 8.0% of the population (increased incidence in people older than 50 years of age). It is characterized by deformation and hardening of bone, which may be initiated by a slow virus infection. Diagnosis is made by x-ray and the presence of increased serum alkaline phosphatase. Symptoms include bowing of limbs, kyphosis, pain and deformity, deafness, blindness, and enlargement of the head. It usually is treated with calcitonin and biphosphonate medication.

Diagnostic tests for osteoporosis rely on decreased BMD expressed as the standard deviation from the mean for young adults between the ages of 30 to 40 years. There is a 1.5-fold increase in fracture risk in association with each drop of 1 standard deviation of BMD (Table 10-10). Each drop of 1 standard deviation of BMD also is asso-

---

**TABLE 10.10**

### Osteoporosis Classification of Bone Mineral Density

| BMD (+/− SD)* | Diagnosis |
| --- | --- |
| −1 to −2.5 | Osteopenia |
| −2.5 and more | Osteoporosis |
| −2.5 + history of nonviolent fractures | Severe osteoporosis |

*Standard deviations below young adult mean.
BMD, bone mineral density; SD, standard deviation.
(From Rich, E.R. [1999]. Osteoporosis. In J.K. Singleton, et al. [Eds.], *Primary care* [pp 549–558]. Philadelphia: Lippincott Williams & Wilkins.)

ciated with a 70% increase in death from stroke (Browner et al., 1993).

## Physiologic Basis of Treatment for Osteoporosis

Treatment options for osteoporosis require ruling out any endocrinopathy or metastatic component. Review and adjust any possible medication over-doses, since the dosage requirement frequently decreases with age. Many dietary treatment modalities are designed to increase bone mass, avoid additional bone loss, and prevent fractures. For instance, the recommended dietary intake of calcium ranges from 900 to 1600 mg/day based on age, sex, and lifestyle. Calcium supplementation is available in many forms; however, one of the most important considerations according to nutritionists is to take a calcium-magnesium (ratio of approximately 3:2) combination because calcium without magnesium is not absorbed by the digestive tract. Lactose and vitamin $D_3$ both enhance the absorption of calcium, whereas fats, fiber, and oxalates decrease absorption. Vitamin $D_3$ supplementation can be used for people with inadequate exposure to sunlight but 1,25 dihydroxyvitamin $D_3$ is necessary for people with inadequate liver or kidney function. Sodium-fluoride, using a slow-release sodium-fluoride combined with calcium version, has been shown to increase spine and hip density and reduce vertebral fractures (Pak et al., 1995).

*Clinical Note:* Rolaids tablets (antacids) are formulated with calcium carbonate and magnesium (500 mg $Ca^{2+}$/tablet), are inexpensive and chewable, and can double as appetite suppressants. Tums antacid tablets are an excellent source for calcium but *do not* contain magnesium.

*Pharmaceutical* options for osteoporosis treatment can approach the problem from many angles:

1. Antiresorptive agents include sex steroids such as testosterone or estrogen replacement hormones. The newer selective estrogen receptor modulators, such as raloxifene (Evista), increase BMD in the total body, lower spine, and hip but do not decrease hot flashes or help vaginal dryness, as does estrogen replacement (see the web site regarding raloxifene being approved by the Food and Drug Association at *http://pharminfo.com/drugpr/evista2_pr.html*). Testosterone replacement for elderly men or men with hypogonadism also helps to increase BMD and is available as intramuscular injection every 2 to 4 weeks or as transdermal scrotal patches applied every 24 hours. Dehydroepiandrosterone (DHEA) supplementation has been reported to increase BMD (Labrie et al., 1997). Antiresorptive agents also include biphosphonates such as the third-generation alendronate (Fosamax), which increases bone density at all skeletal sites and reduces vertebral fractures.

2. Replacement hormone treatment with calcitonin in the form of the intranasal medicine, Miacalcin, inhibits osteoclast activity and diminishes bone resorption. However, it has a short half-life and is less effective compared with treatment with steroids or alendronate.

3. The drug paricalcitol (Zemplar) which has been approved for use as a vitamin $D_3$ analog (acting like calcitriol) for renal failure patients.

Primary care providers should encourage appropriate forms of exercise for osteoporotic patients. Exercise for osteoporosis patients, in conjunction with appropriate replacement hormone support, is a key component to rehabilitation and prevention. Strength training (weight-bearing activity) maintains the vascular system, increases bone density, increases muscle mass, and improves flexibility, balance, and agility. High-impact exercise such as jogging or jumping rope should be limited or approached with caution.

The following case study exemplifies the pathophysiologic processes in "hyperparathyroidism." It illustrates the importance of reviewing all history and clinical data because there may be more than one etiology or compounding factor.

---

### ● Case Study 10.1

Janet Mulvihill is a 57-year-old automobile sales clerk who decided to forgo menopausal hormone replacement and take extra calcium with vitamin supplementation as an alternative. The patient presents with intense pain in right flank, radiating into her groin, and is passing bright red urine. Present condition had an acute onset after playing three sets of tennis in the hot sun.

*(Case study continued on page 194)*

## History

### Past Medical History

| | |
|---|---|
| Allergies | Mildew, mold, house dust (dust mites) |
| Illnesses | UTI (uncomplicated), 2× in 5 y |
| Surgery | T&A at age 6 |
| Habits | Nonsmoker, tennis player |
| Prescriptions | None; OTC: calcium, Vit $D_3$, vitamins, bone-building supplements |

### Family History

| | |
|---|---|
| Father | Deceased, age 52, heart attack |
| Mother | 82 y, nursing home (Alzheimer's, osteoporosis) |
| Siblings | None |
| Children | Two children, two grandchildren: all healthy |

## Review of Systems

| | |
|---|---|
| General | Feels well, poor posture, appears slumped |
| Skin | Negative |
| HEENT | Negative |
| CR | Negative |
| GI | Heartburn, occasional recent constipation |
| UG | See past medical history |
| Musculoskeletal | Occasional knee pain and swelling |
| Neurologic | Negative |
| Psychiatric | Stressed over caring for mother and her condition |

## Physical Examination

Healthy-appearing white female

| System | Findings |
|---|---|
| Vital signs | T–98.4°F, P–88, BP–150/98, Height 5'4", Weight 145 lb |
| Skin | Normal |
| HEENT | Normal |
| Neck | Thyroid palpable |
| Chest | Clear to auscultation and percussion |
| Heart | Normal |
| Abdomen | Normal |
| Gyn | Postmenopausal |
| Extremities | Normal |
| Neurologic | Normal |

## Laboratory Studies

| Test | Janet Mulvihill | Normal Range |
|---|---|---|
| WBC | 6600/mm³ | 4300–10500/mm³ |
| HCT | 41% | 37–48% (female) |
| Calcium | 11.3 mg/dL ↑ | 8.5–10.5 mg/dL |
| Phosphate | 1.5 mg/dL ↓ | 3–4.5 mg/dL |
| Alkaline phosphatase | 210 U/L | 30–120 U/L |
| PTH | 145 pg/mL ↑ ↑ | 10–65 pg/mL |

*(Case study continued on next page)*

| Albumin | 4.7 g/dL | 3.5–5.5 g/dL |
|---|---|---|
| Urinalysis | | |
| Color | Amber, cloudy | Yellow, clear |
| Specific gravity | 1.012 | 1.001–1.020 |
| Blood | +4 | Negative |
| Glucose | Negative | Negative |
| Ketones | Negative | Negative |
| Nitrite | Negative | Negative |
| Microscopic | TNTC red cells | <4/high-power field |

## Impression

1. Kidney stones and hematuria
2. R/O UTI
3. R/O 1° and 2° causes for elevated calcium and decreased phosphate

## Discussion

Hematuria with colicky flank pain radiating into the groin strongly suggests a kidney stone and should be evaluated with imaging study (either IVP, US or CT scan) to locate obstruction. Severe dehydration during tennis exercise in hot weather encourages crystals to precipitate, and the stretching movement would have further damaged the kidney tubules. Levels of calcium greater than 13 mg/dL are considered a medical emergency that can lead to cardiac arrest. Acute treatment includes rehydrating (diluting blood calcium), increasing levels of sodium and glucocorticoids to stimulate increased calcium excretion in the kidney, and giving calcitonin or bisphosphonate drugs (etidronate, alendronate, pamidronate) to further block bone demineralization.

An IVP/x-ray confirmed the presence of a right kidney stone. Patient was given narcotics for pain control and a diuretic to facilitate passage of the stones. Sampling of her next urine void revealed two small pieces of brown, irregular, hard materials, which were analyzed later to be calcium oxalate stones.

Mildly elevated blood calcium with low blood phosphate points to an unregulated (autonomous) excess of PTH. Measurement of serum PTH confirmed the diagnosis of hyperparathyroidism. The elevated alkaline phosphatase enzyme suggests high osteoclast activity in response to elevated PTH. The elevated PTH induced an increase in circulating calcitriol (1,25 dihydroxy Vit $D_3$), which further increased the absorption of calcium from the gut. In addition, the patient admitted to taking three times the recommended dose for her "bone building" supplement (containing Vit $D_3$) along with two other OTC medications containing Vit $D_3$. Vitamin $D_3$ toxicosis itself can cause elevated blood calcium.

Mild, relatively asymptomatic hyperparathyroidism can exist for many years, resulting from diffuse hyperplasia (9% of cases), a single adenoma (90%), or malignancy (<1%). Two months after passing the kidney stone, the patient underwent exploratory neck surgery to remove a single adenoma from the right thyroid gland with no involvement of the other parathyroid glands found. Postoperatively, her calcium, phosphate, and PTH levels returned to normal, and she now is taking only a single dose of supplemental Vit $D_3$.

CR, cardiorespiratory; CT, computed tomography; GI, gastrointestinal; Gyn, gynecologic; HCT, hematocrit; HEENT, head, eyes, ears, nose, and throat; IVP, intravenous pyelogram; Neuro, neurologic; OTC, over the counter; PTH, parathyroid hormone; R/O, rule out; T&A, tonsillectomy and adenoidectomy; TNTC, too numerous to count; UG, urinary–genital; US, ultrasound; UTI, urinary tract infection; Vit, vitamin; WBC, white blood cell; 1°, primary; 2°, secondary; ↑, increased; ↓, decreased; ↑↑, markedly increased.

## ADRENAL CORTEX PATHOPHYSIOLOGY

The *hypothalamic-pituitary-adrenal* (HPA) axis is regulated by two hypothalamic peptides, cortisol-releasing hormone (CRH) and arginine vasopressin, through feedback to opioid receptors in the brain. These hypothalamic (3°) peptides regulate secretion of corticotropin (ACTH) (2°) from the anterior pituitary. When ACTH is released into the bloodstream, it is carried to the adrenal cortex, where three families of steroid hormones are produced (Figure 10-10).

1. *Glucocorticoids* (cortisol, prednisone) from the glomerulosa zone are 21-carbon steroids that control multiple metabolic functions. These include hepatic glucose production (gluconeogenesis), liver glycogen storage, permissive functions for other hormones (glucagon, epinephrine, growth hormone), and increased lipolysis in adipose cells.

2. *Mineralocorticoids* (aldosterone) from the fasciculata zone regulate electrolyte transport across epithelial surfaces principally in the kidney, colon, and salivary glands. Increased aldosterone promotes sodium retention and potassium excretion in its major target tissues. Feedback regulation is through the renin-angiotension system.

3. *Adrenal androgens* (DHEA, testosterone, dihydrotestosterone) and *estrogens* (19- and 18-carbon steroids, respectively) are synthesized in the reticularis layer of the adrenal cortex and supplement the gonadal production of sex steroids.

All of these steroids are synthesized and released into the blood. Because they are fairly insoluble in water, they are bound to carrier molecules such as sex hormone-binding globulin (SHBG), albumin, or corticosteroid-binding globulin for transport to their target tissues. The role of these transport proteins is to solubilize, protect from degradation, and ensure uniform distribution of these steroids (Orth & Kovacs, 1998).

Glucocorticoids are metabolized (inactivated) by either the liver (increased blood levels in cirrhosis of the liver and CHF) or the kidneys, where cortisol is converted to the inactive cortisone before excretion. Glucocorticoids have specific cytoplasmic and nuclear receptors in most tissues of the body. Each of these tissues responds to glucocorticoid stimulation in its own specific fashion. For instance, increased cortisol redistributes fat from peripheral sites (where increased cortisol breaks down lipids) to supraclavicular regions, in particular, the body trunk, where it stimulates fat deposition. Increased corticoids also inhibit the immune system, regulate mood swings, change sleep patterns, and induce lung maturation (surfactants).

*Adrenal cortex insufficiency* can result primar-ily from destruction (Addison's disease) of the gland by surgical intervention, by vascular occlusion, or autoimmune causes (see the web site for the National Adrenal Disease Foundation at *http://www.medhelp.org/nadf/*). The hallmark of primary adrenal failure is increased ACTH levels denoted frequently by increased whole-body pigmentation clues. It also can result from a deficiency of ACTH (2°, pituitary deficiency) or deficiency of corticotropin-releasing factor (3°, hypothalamus deficiency) (Table 10-11). The incidence of primary disease is only 40 to 110/million adults, but it has a high morbidity and mortality rate. Tertiary abnormalities are the most common cause of adrenal cortex deficiency. In 2° (ACTH) or 3° (CRH)

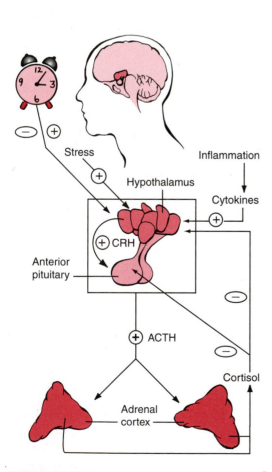

**FIGURE 10.10** ● Control of adrenal cortical function.

## TABLE 10.11

### Clinical Diagnosis of Panhypoadrenal Cortex: Addison's Disease

| Clinical Diagnosis | Symptoms Identified | Laboratory Results |
|---|---|---|
| Addison's disease: autoimmune 1° failure | Hypotension, fatigue, anorexia, weight loss, GI (nausea, vomiting), salt craving, postural dizziness, anemia, eosinophilia, increased pigmentation | ↑ CRF, ↑ ACTH, ↓ cortisol, ↓ FUC, ↓ androgenic steroids |
| Addison's disease: pituitary (2°) or hypothalamus (3°) failure | All the above without hyperpigmentation | ↓ CRF or ↓ ACTH, ↓ cortisol, ↓ FUC, ↓ androgenic steroids |

ACTH, corticotropin; CRF, corticotropin-releasing factor; FUC, free urinary cortisol; GI, gastrointestinal; ↑, increased; ↓, decreased; 1°, primary; 2°, secondary; 3°, tertiary.
(From Orth, D.N. & Kovacs, W.J. [1998]. The adrenal cortex. In J.B. Wilson [Ed.], *Williams textbook of endocrinology* (9th ed., pp. 517–664). Philadelphia: W.B. Saunders.)

deficiency, all three layers of the adrenal cortex are affected, and the initial clinical presentation is hypoglycemia. More than 50% of patients with primary autoimmune adrenal cortex insufficiencies have other associated endocrinopathies, which is referred to as polyglandular autoimmune type I or II.

Several other endocrine pathophysiologies are related to this HPA axis, including Cushing's syndrome, congenital adrenal hypertrophy (CAH) (infant or adult onset), obesity, major depression, posttraumatic stress syndrome, alcoholism, and chronic fatigue syndrome (Nye, 1999).

*Hypercortisolism* is called Cushing's disease (CD) (Table 10-12). Cushing's disease exhibits hypercortisolism of either ACTH dependent (2°) or independent (1° tumor or hyperplasia) origin.

## TABLE 10.12

### Clinical and Laboratory Differential Diagnosis of Hyperadrenal Cortex

| Clinical Diagnosis | Symptoms Identified | Laboratory Results |
|---|---|---|
| **Cushing's disease: ACTH independent** (adrenal adenoma, carcinoma, nodular adrenal hyperplasia) | Upper body and truncal obesity | ↓ CRF, ↓ /N ACTH, ↑ cortisol, ↑ FUC |
| **Cushing's disease: ACTH dependent** (pituitary tumor) | Upper body and truncal obesity, hyperpigmentation | ↑ CRF or ↑ ACTH, ↑ cortisol, ↑ FUC |
| **Pseudo-Cushing's disease** | Visceral obesity, alcoholism, neuropsychiatric medicines, PCOD, infertility | |
| **Ectopic ACTH secretion** | Lung tumor (nodules), +/− hyperpigmentation | ↓ CRF, ↑ ACTH, ↑ cortisol |
| **Hypertension** | ↑ BP, hypokalemia | ↑ Aldosterone |
| **Hirsutism and masculinization** | ↑ Androgenization | ↑ Androgens |
| **Adult CAH** | Upper body and truncal obesity, hyperpigmentation | ↑ ACTH, N/ ↓ cortisol, ↑ androgens, +/− ↓ aldosterone |

ACTH, corticotropin; BP, blood pressure; CAH, congenital adrenal hyperplasia; CRF, corticotropin-releasing factor; FUC, free urinary cortisol; PCOD, polycystic ovarian disease; N, normal; ↓, decreased; ↑, increased.

Symptoms of CD include weight gain, increased upper body and truncal obesity, increased cortisol, increased free urinary cortisol, and decreased leptin secretion. Hyperpigmentation (ie, skin, nail beds, mucosal lining of mouth) is correlated with elevated ACTH levels (Figure 10-11).

*Adult-onset congenital adrenal hyperplasia* (adult CAH) has all of the symptoms of inadequate production of glucocorticoids (cortisol). The classic CAH patient is identified with a genetic deficiency as an infant. Adult CAH syndrome occurs gradually in later life because of a partial enzyme block involving a deficiency in any 1 of about 20 different adrenal enzymes. For instance, a 21-hydroxylase enzyme deficiency requires greater secretion of ACTH to maintain cortisol, which induces a buildup of cortisol precursor steroids, including 17α-hydoxyprogesterone (17-OHP) and androgens. Similarly, a deficiency in 11-β-hydroxylase enzyme forces higher secretion of ACTH to maintain cortisol, resulting in a fall in the mineralocorticoid aldosterone and an increase in the precursor 11-desoxycorticosterone (11-DOC) (Nye et al., 1999). The classic symptoms of adult CAH include truncal obesity, elevated 17-OHP with or without elevated renin (from decreased aldosterone), hypertension (from elevated 11-DOC), hirsutism or virilization (in-creased androgens and

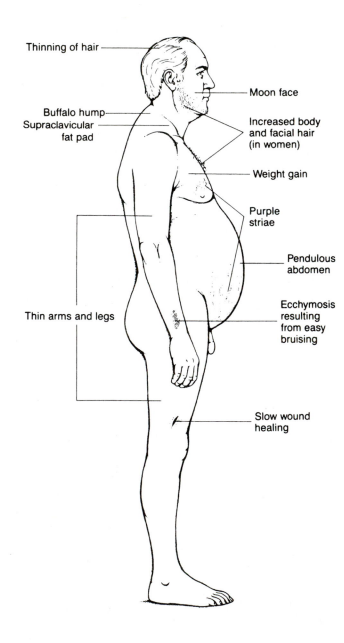

**FIGURE 10.11**  ●  The major clinical manifestations of Cushing's syndrome. (Smeltzer, S.C. & Bare, B.G. *Brunner and Suddarth's Textbook of Medical-Surgical Nursing.* [7th ed.]. Philadelphia: J.B. Lippincott, 1992.)

DHEA), polycystic ovarian disease (PCOD), and oligomenorrhea (Orth & Kovacs, 1998).

Patients with PCOD show irregular cycles; androgynism; hirsutism; alopecia; an increased incidence of endometrial cancer, insulin resistance (insulin levels above 28 mIU/L), diabetes before 30 years of age, and hypertension; and a decrease in SHBGs (Nestler, 1998). Even mild adult CAH can result in sinus and pulmonary infections, orthostatic syncope, severe acne, oligomenorrhea, and infertility (PCOD).

Treatment of nonclassic, or adult, CAH requires identifying the elevated precursor buildup and giving glucocorticoid replacement (usually hydrocortisone or dexamethasone) therapy (Deaton et al., 1999), with fludrocortisone for patients deficient in aldosterone. Two recent FDA-approved medications, metformin (Glucophage) and Avondia, are called insulin sensitizers. These are used for type 2 diabetics, have been shown to induce weight loss, decrease CAH, and decrease PCOD symptoms (Nestler, 1998; Glueck et al., 1999).

### ● Case Study 10.2

The following case study exemplifies the pathophysiologic processes in adult-onset CAH and polycystic ovarian disease. It illustrates the importance of reviewing all history and clinical data because more than one etiology or compounding factor may be present.

Beverly Bointon is a 31-year-old woman who has been amenorrheic for 6 months. She always has had irregular periods with intervals between 3 and 12+ weeks, and bleeding patterns lasting 2 to 7 days. Recently, she noticed increasing facial and body hair. Despite exercising 2 to 3 times/week, she is 30 to 40 lb overweight.

### History

#### Past Medical History

| | |
|---|---|
| Allergies | Mildew, mold, house dust (dust mites) |
| Illnesses | None |
| Surgery | T&A at age 10 |
| Habits | Nonsmoker |
| Prescriptions | None; OTC: diet pills |

#### Family History

| | |
|---|---|
| Father | Overweight, hypertensive |
| Mother | Overweight, acne problem |
| Siblings | Three brothers, one sister |
| Children | None |

### Review of Systems

| | |
|---|---|
| General | Well nourished; oily complexion |
| Skin | Moderate facial sideburns and hair on upper lip. Periareolar and presternal hair. Striae |
| HEENT | Negative, no thyroid enlargement |
| CR | Negative |
| GI | Obese abdomen |
| UG | Negative |
| Musculoskeletal | Normal extremities |
| Pelvic | Normal external genitalia and uterus |
| Psychiatric | Somewhat lethargic or depressed |

*(Case study continued on page 200)*

## Physical Examination

Healthy appearing white woman

| System | Findings |
| --- | --- |
| Vital signs | T –98.6°F, P–72, BP–115/75, Height 5'4", Weight 210 lb |
| Skin | Moderately increased facial sideburns |
| HEENT | Normal |
| Neck | Normal |
| Chest | Clear to auscultation and percussion |
| Heart | Normal |
| Abdomen | No organomegaly |
| Gyn | Some ovarian enlargement, oligomenorrhea |
| Extremities | Normal |
| Urinalysis | Normal |

## Laboratory Studies

| Test | Beverly Bointon | Normal Range |
| --- | --- | --- |
| WBC | 9000/mm$^3$ | 4300–10,500/mm$^3$ |
| HCT | 48% | 37–48% (female) |
| Glucose, fasting | 118 mg/dL ↑ | 70–110 mg/dL, fasting |
| Phosphate | 3.5 mg/dL | 3.0–4.5 mg/dL |
| Cortisol | Normal | |
| HCG | <10 mIU/mL | <10 mIU/mL (negative) |
| LH/FSH ratio | >4.2 ↑ | <2.5 = normal |
| Testosterone, total | 82 ng/dL | 20–90 ng/dL |
| Testosterone, free | 1.9 ng/dL ↑ | 0.1–1.3 ng/dL, (female) |
| DHEA-sulfate | 642 µg/dL ↑ | 80–443 µg/dL |

## Impression

1. Patient is not pregnant with normal cortisol levels. R/O Cushing's disease with the dexamethasone suppression test, 17-OHP levels, and ACTH
2. Androgen excess. R/O adrenal or ovarian tumors. Do US to confirm PCOD
3. Evaluate blood insulin levels and peripheral insulin resistance to R/O diabetes

## Discussion

The features of polycystic ovary syndrome include hyperandrogenism (biochemical and anatomical), oligomenorrhea, and cystic ovaries, with an LH/FSH ratio (during the follicular stage) of >2.5 and elevated 17-OHP.

*Infertility patients* with CAH and PCOD historically have been unresponsive to the normal treatments with clomiphene, gonadotropins, or pulsatile GnRH to trigger ovulation. Surgical ovarian wedge resection has had a moderate degree of success for restoring normal menstrual cycles.

*Treatment* with a 10-day course of medroxyprogesterone acetate will allow withdrawal bleeding, but oligomenorrhea usually returns. Regular use of oral contraceptives will provide contraception as well as regular menstrual bleeding and should decrease androgenization. Cortisol supplementation should be considered if ACTH levels suggest CAH. Insulin-sensitivity medications such as metformin and troglidizone have been successful in inducing weight loss as well as increasing the probability of successful conception for infertility patients (Kettyle & Arky, 1998).

ACTH, corticotropin; CAH, congenital adrenal hypertrophy; CR, cardiorespiratory; DHEA, dehydroepiandrosterone; FSH, follicle-stimulating hormone; GI, gastrointestinal; GnRH, gonadotropin-releasing hormone; Gyn, gynecologic; HCG, human chorionic gonadotropin; HCT, hematocrit; HEENT, head, eyes, ears, nose, and throat; LH, luteinizing hormone; 17-OHP, 17-hydroxyprogesterone; PCOD, polycystic ovarian disease; R/O, rule out; T&A, tonsillectomy and adenoidectomy; UG, urinary–genital; US, ultrasound; WBC, white blood cell; ↑, increased.

## INSOMNIA AND NEUROENDOCRINOPATHIES

The pineal gland is a neuroendocrine gland located in the roof of the third ventricle in the brain that begins to regress in size at about 7 years of age. Two primary neurohormones are found in the adult pineal: serotonin and melatonin. The pineal is controlled by the suprachiasmatic nucleus (SCN) in the hypothalamus, which is the primary center for circadian rhythms in the body. The enzymes that convert the precursor neurohormone serotonin to melatonin are inhibited by light. During the day, neural (autonomic nervous system) pathways from the eye's retina to the hypothalamus depress the SCN and thus decrease enzyme activity in the pineal. At night, these enzymes increase their activity, and thus, the production of melatonin increases. Normal melatonin plasma values range from 0.17 to 0.43 nmol/L, with the highest values occurring at approximately 4 AM and the nadir at approximately 8 PM (Becker, 1990). Insomnia patients treated with melatonin have shown shorter times required to fall asleep and increased duration of rapid eye movement sleep (Fig. 10-12).

Replacing melatonin has been shown to be effective in inducing sleep and resetting circadian rhythms when used to overcome jet lag. Excessive production of melatonin causes a delay in the onset of puberty. Phototherapy using bright fluorescent lamps (mimicking the inhibitory effect of sunlight) has been shown to decrease the high melatonin levels found in "winter depression," or seasonal affective disorder. Side effects of excessive melatonin (natural or replacement) are daytime drowsiness and inability to concentrate.

Insomnia occurs in approximately 10% of adults. These patients show one or more of the following difficulties: falling asleep, maintaining sleep, waking up too early, or experiencing nonrefreshing sleep. In persons older than 65 years, 50% or more report at least one chronic sleep complaint (Neubauer, 1999). Daytime consequences are fatigue, lack of energy, difficulty concentrating, and irritability. Depression is a major contributor to insomnia; however, patients with other pathologies such as hyperthyroidism, hypothyroidism, and fibromyalgia (closely related to chronic fatigue syndrome) also exhibit insomnia (see the web site on fibromyalgia at *http://www.fmnetnews. com/pages/basics.html*). Treatment should correlate with analysis of causative factors (Table 10-13). Behavioral and sleep hygiene factors, hypnotic medications, and menopausal status should be evaluated.

Postmenopausal insomnia is characterized by multiple cycles of hot flashes (hyperthermia and night sweats) occurring between about 1 AM and 6 AM. These result from the autonomic nervous system's response to decreased estrogen feedback. Insomnia is further aggravated by increased nocturia (multiple trips to the bathroom per night), which disrupts sleep. This can be partly caused by excessive fluid intake in the evening or by the decrease in both androgens and estrogens in menopause contributing to urinary incontinence (Bachmann, 1999).

HRT has been discussed in another section, but several generalizations are mentioned here.

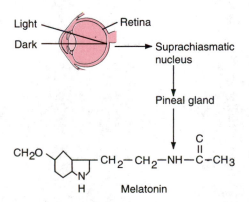

**FIGURE 10.12** ● Light stimulates the pineal gland to produce melatonin.

### ● Internet References

1. *Drugstore.com*
   Lists prescription drugs by name, doses available, usage, and side effects

2. *Medscape.com*
   Search by disease name, pathophysiology

3. *Biomednet.com*
   Contains more than 170 biologic and medical journals with abstracts and some full articles

4. *Mdconsult.com*
   Over 45 full medical texts available (some charges, free at most large libraries)

5. *NursingCenter.com*
   Nursing references, journals, and chatroom

6. *Pdr.net/nurse*
   Free access to Physician's Desk Reference

7. *Pharminfo.com*
   Lists prescription drugs by generic or trade name and gives information on usage and side effects

## TABLE 10.13

### Causes of Insomnia and Possible Treatments

| Extenuating Factors | Treatment Approaches |
| --- | --- |
| Sleep hygiene and emotional factors: (1) caffeine, nicotine, diet pills, stimulants; (2) depression, serotonin | Review sleep hygiene practices, ↓ dietary or smoking stimulants, try antidepressants or antihistamines |
| Sleep apnea: obstructive or central | Question sleep partner, do sleep study, R/O hypoxia and hypothyroidism |
| Restless leg syndrome, periodic limb movement (nocturnal myoclonus) | Try replacement $K^+$, $Mg^+$, or $Fe^+$ pills, low-dose antiparkinson (levodopa), R/O hyperthyroidism |
| UTI or vaginal infections, low grade | R/O infections (which disturb sleep), pinworms, and vaginitis |
| Vasomotor hot flashes (postmenopausal), increased nocturia | Increase HRT (+ androgens) to aid urethral sphincter muscle integrity and ↓ hot flashes |
| Fibromyalgia with ↓ serotonin, ↑ pain, ↑ trigger points, ↑ depression | Antidepressant (eg, fluoxetine [Prozac]), which ↑ serotonin |

$Fe^+$, iron; HRT, hormone replacement therapy; $K^+$, potassium; $Mg^+$, magnesium; R/O, rule out; UTI, urinary tract infection; ↓, decreased; ↑, increased.

Decreased hormone levels and hot flashes occur in women between the ages of 45 and 65 years and in men between 65 and 85 years. The following are guidelines for HRT:

1. Use natural estrogens, not synthetic estrogens, when possible.
2. Use natural progesterone, not synthetic progestins (such as medroxyprogesterone acetate), so that the progesterone can be used as precursor for synthesis in other essential steroid pathways.
3. Monitor androgen levels in both men and women and use low-dose androgen replacement when appropriate. These androgen levels are important in supporting the muscular integrity and development (bladder sphincter muscle), and they curtail excessive autoimmune processes.

## REFERENCES

Amino, N., Tada, H., Hidaka, Y., Crapo, L.M., & Stagnaro-Green, A. (1999). Screening for postpartum thyroiditis. *Journal of Clinical Endocrinology and Metabolism, 84* (6), 1813–1821.

Bachmann, G.A. (1999). Role of androgens in the menopause: Vasomotor flushes in menopausal women. *American Journal of Obstetrics and Gynecology, 180* (3), S302–S306.

Becker, K.L. (1990). Interrelationships between hormones and the body. In K.L. Becker (Ed.), *Principles and practice of endocrinology and metabolism* (pp. 1474–1624). Philadelphia: J.B. Lippincott.

Bornstein, S.R. & Chrousos, G.P. (1999). Adrenocorticotropin (ACTH) and non-ACTH–mediated regulation of the adrenal cortex: Neural and immune inputs. *Journal of Clinical Endocrinology and Metabolism, 84* (5), 1729–1736.

Braverman, L.E. (1996). Thyroid diseases. In L.E. Braverman & R.D. Utiger (Eds.), *Werner and Ingbar's The Thyroid: A fundamental and clinical text* (7th ed., pp. 522–889). Philadelphia: Lippincott-Raven.

Bringhurst, F.R. & Demay, M.B. (1998). Hormones and disorders of mineral metabolism. In J.D. Wilson (Ed.), *Williams Textbook of Endocrinology* (9th ed., pp. 1155–1199). Philadelphia: W.B. Saunders.

Browner, W.S., Pressman, A.R., Nevitt, M.C., Cauley, J.A., & Cummings, S.R. (1993). Association between low bone density and stroke in elderly women: The study of osteoporotic fractures. *Stroke, 24* (7), 940–946.

Burman, K.D. (1995). Hyperthyroidism. In K.L. Becker (Ed.), *Principles and practice of endocrinology and metabolism* (2nd ed., pp. 331–346). Philadelphia: J.B. Lippincott.

Cauffield, J.S. & Forbes, H.J. (1999). Dietary supplements used in the treatment of depression, anxiety, and sleep disorders. *Primary Care Practice, 3* (3), 290–298.

Dayan, C.M. & Daniels, G.H. (1996). Chronic autoimmune thyroiditis. *New England Journal of Medicine, 335* (2), 99–107.

Deaton, M.A., Glorioso, J.E., & McLean, D.B. (1999). Congenital adrenal hyperplasia: Not really a zebra. *American Family Physician, 59* (5), 1190–1196.

Downs, R.W. & Levine, M.A. (1995). Hypoparathyroidism and other causes of hypocalcemia. In K.L. Becker (Ed.), *Principles and practice of endocrinology and metabolism* (2nd ed., pp. 447–456). Philadelphia: J.B. Lippincott.

Eddy, M. & Walbroehl, G.S. (1999). Insomnia. *American Family Physician, 59* (7), 1911–1925.

Fox, S.I. (Ed.). (1999). Endocrine glands: Secretion and action of hormones. In *Human physiology* (6th ed., pp. 284–323). Boston: WCB/McGraw-Hill.

Glueck, C.J., Wang, P., Fontaine, R., Tracy, T., & Sieve-Smith, L. (1999). Metformin-induced resumption of normal menses in 39 of 43 (91%) previously amenorrheic women with polycystic ovary syndrome. *Metabolism, 48,* 1–10.

Hall, R., Evered, D., & Greene, R. (1979). *A colour atlas of endocrinology.* London, England: Wolfe Medical Publications.

Harper, K.D. & Weber, T.J. (1998). Secondary osteoporosis: Diagnostic considerations. *Endocrinology and Metabolism Clinics, 27* (2), 325–348.

Hay, I.D. & Morris, J.C. (1996). Toxic adenoma and toxic multinodular goiter. In L.E. Braverman & R.D. Utiger (Eds.), *Werner and Ingbar's The Thyroid: A fundamental and clinical text* (7th ed., pp. 890–986). Philadelphia: Lippincott-Raven.

Invitti, C., Giraldi, F.P., DeMartin, M., & Cavagnini, F. (1999). Diagnosis and management of Cushing's syndrome: Results of an Italian multicentre study. *Journal of Clinical Endocrinology and Metabolism, 84,* 440–448.

Iudica-Souza, C. & Burch, H.B. (1999). Amiodarone induced thyroid dysfunction. *The Endocrinologist, 9,* 216–227.

Jordan, R.M. (1995). Myxedema coma. Pathophysiology, therapy and factors affecting prognosis. *Medical Clinics of North America, 9* (1): 185–194.

Kamal, A. & Brocklehurst, J.C. (1992). *Color atlas of geriatric medicine* (2nd ed., pp. 80–122). St. Louis: C.V. Mosby.

Kettyle, W.M. & Arky, R.A. (Eds.) (1998). The thyroid. In *Endocrine pathophysiology* (pp. 71–98). Philadelphia: Lippincott-Raven.

Labrie, F., Diamond, P., Cusan, L., Gomez, J., Belanger, A., & Candas, B. (1997). Effect of 12-month dehydroepi-androsterone replacement therapy on bone, vagina, and endometrium in postmenopausal women. *Journal of Clinical Endocrinology and Metabolism, 82* (10), 3498–3503.

Larsen, P.R., Davies, T.F., & Hay, I.D. (1998). The thyroid gland. In J.D. Wilson (Ed.), *Williams textbook of endocrinology* (9th ed., pp 389–516). Philadelphia: W.B. Saunders.

Lazarus, J.H. (1996). Silent thyroiditis and subacute thyroiditis. In L.E. Braverman & R.D. Utiger (Eds.), *Werner and Ingbar's The thyroid: A fundamental and clinical text* (7th ed.). Philadelphia: J.B. Lippincott.

McPhee, S. & Bauer, D.C. (1997). Thyroid disease. In S. McPhee (Ed.), *Pathophysiology of disease* (pp. 470–487). Englewood Cliffs, NJ: Prentice-Hall.

Nathan, M.N. (1999). Diseases of the thyroid and parathyroid glands In J.K. Singleton, et al. (Eds.), *Primary Care* (pp 237–257). Philadelphia: Lippincott Williams & Wilkins.

Nestler, J.E. (1998). Effects of metformin on spontaneous and clomiphene-induced ovulation in the polycystic ovary syndrome. *New England Journal of Medicine, 338,* 1876–1880.

Neubauer, D.N. (1999). Sleep problems in the elderly. *American Family Physician, 59* (9), 2551–2559.

Nye, E.J., Hockings, G.I., Grice, J.E., Strakosch, C.R., Torpy, D.J., & Jackson, R.V. (1999). The use of naloxone for investigating disorders of the hypothalamic-pituitary-adrenal axis. *The Endocrinologist, 9* (3), 161–182.

Orth, D.N. & Kovacs, W.J. (1998). The adrenal cortex. In J.B. Wilson (Ed.), *Williams textbook of endocrinology* (9th ed., pp. 517–664). Philadelphia: W.B. Saunders.

Pak, Y.C., Kakhaee, K., Adams-Hunt, B., Piziak, V., Petersen, R.D., & Poindexter, J.R. (1995). Treatment of postmenopausal osteoporosis with slow-release sodium fluoride. *Annals of Internal Medicine, 123* (6), 401–408.

Papanicolaou, D.A. & Chrousos, G.P. (1999). The endocrine system: Cushing's syndrome. In R.E. Rakel (Ed.), *Conn's current therapy* (51st ed., pp. 632–656).

Raisz, L.G., Kream, B.E., & Lorenzo, I.A. (1998). Metabolic bone disease. In J.D. Wilson (Ed.), *Williams textbook of endocrinology* (9th ed., pp. 1211–1239). Philadelphia: W.B. Saunders.

Reed, L. & Pangaro, L.N. (1995). Physiology of the thyroid gland. Part I: Synthesis and release, iodine metabolism binding and transport. In K.L. Becker (Ed.), *Principles and practice of endocrinology and metabolism* (2nd ed., pp 285–291). Philadelphia: J.B. Lippincott.

Rich, E.R. (1999). Osteoporosis. In J.K. Singleton, et al. (Eds.), *Primary Care* (pp 549–558). Philadelphia: Lippincott Williams & Wilkins.

Silverberg, S.J. & Bilezikian, J.P. (1996). Extensive personal experience: Evaluation and management of primary hyperparathyroidism. *Journal of Clinical Endocrinology and Metabolism, 81* (6), 2036–2040.

Singleton, J.K., Sandowski, S.A., Green-Hernandez, C., Horvath, T.V., Digregorio, R.V., & Holzemer, S.P. (Eds.) (1999). *Primary care.* Philadelphia: Lippincott Williams & Wilkins.

Sofferman, R.A. (1996). Preoperative technetium-Tc99m-sestamibi imaging: Paving the way to minimal-access parathyroid surgery. *Archives of Otolaryngology Head and Neck Surgery, 122,* 369–374.

Toft, A.D. (1994). Thyroxine therapy. *New England Journal of Medicine, 331* (3): 174–180.

Torring, O. (1996). Graves' hyperthyroidism: Treatment with antithyroid drugs, surgery or radioiodine. A prospective, randomized study. *Journal of Clinical Endocrinology and Metabolism, 81,* 2986–2993.

Trivalle, C., Doucet, J., Chassagne, P., Landrin, I., Kadri, N., Menard, J., & Bercoff, E. (1996). Differences in the signs and symptoms of hyperthyroidism in older and younger patients. *Journal of the American Geriatrics Society, 44* (1), 50–64.

Walsh, J.K., et al. (1999). National Heart Lung and Blood Institute: Insomnia: Assessment and management in primary care. *American Family Physician, 59* (11), 3029–3038.

# Diabetes

Ronda Hart

In the United States, diabetes mellitus is the seventh leading cause of death, estimated to affect 16 million people, 5.4 million of whom are undiagnosed and at increased risk for serious complications (Satcher, 1998). If deaths caused by the cardiovascular complications of diabetes were to be attributed to diabetes, then diabetes mellitus becomes the fourth leading cause of death in the United States (Davidson, 1998). Recognition of diabetes, especially type 2 diabetes, in time to prevent complications is a major goal for providers dealing with this disease. Most people are unaware that they have diabetes or that it has serious consequences. If primary care providers are to prevent diabetic morbidity and mortality, they must become adept at screening, diagnosing, and treating this disease.

Diabetes affects 6% to 7% of the total population, affecting different ethnic and age groups unequally. There is a 6% disease prevalence in whites, 10% prevalence in African and Asian Americans, 15% prevalence in Hispanics, and up to a 50% prevalence in Native Americans (Davidson, 1998; Satcher, 1998). In the ever-growing population of individuals older than 65 years, an estimated 20% are affected, with half remaining undiagnosed (Butler et al., 1998; Davidson, 1998). Knowing such statistics can help primary care providers to focus their efforts on at-risk individuals.

Diabetes consumes an enormous number of health care resources. Providers spend a great deal of time and effort delivering direct patient care, and treating the complications of diabetes consumes large amounts of allocated health care funds. One third of the cases of end-stage renal disease (ESRD) result from diabetic nephropathy. In 1997, the cost of providing renal replacement therapy averaged about $12 billion per year

(Kobrin & Aradhye, 1997). In 1995, more than half of all lower-extremity amputations occurred as a complication of diabetes, at a cost of nearly $600 million annually (Satcher, 1998). In all, 15% of the health care dollar is care is spent on treating diabetes, with most spent on treating preventable diabetic complications (Davidson, 1998). With a strong practice focus on disease prevention and patient education, primary care providers can significantly impact these numbers. A thorough understanding of the disease process assists the practitioner in diagnosing and treating diabetes and enables the practitioner to provide accurate client education.

## PHYSIOLOGY OF FUEL METABOLISM

Diabetes is a disease of altered fuel metabolism, which produces hyperglycemia. The physiology of fuel metabolism provides a foundation from which to begin an examination of the pathophysiology of diabetes mellitus and the physiologic basis for treatment of the disease. All body tissues use glucose for fuel, with the brain using approximately 25% of the total. The brain cannot store glucose, so a constant source must be available to maintain nervous system function. To assure this constant source, blood glucose levels must remain in the 60- to 120-mg/dL range, with several hormones responsible for maintaining this steady state. The endocrine pancreas secretes insulin from the β cells, glucagon from the α cells, and somatostatin from the δ cells in response to changes in blood glucose, amino acid, ketone bodies, and fatty acid levels. Catecholamines and glucocorticoid hormones also play an important role in fuel metabolism and homeostasis. These influences are illustrated in Table 11-1.

## TABLE 11.1

### Hormonal Action in Fuel Metabolism

**Glucagon**

Glucose

  Promotes the breakdown of glycogen into glucose phosphate

  Increases gluconeogenesis

Fat

  Enhances lipolysis in adipose tissue, freeing glycerol

  Activates adipose cell lipase

  Enhances lipolysis in adipose tissue, freeing fatty acids

Protein

  Increases breakdown of protein into amino acids

  Increases transport of amino acids into hepatic cells

  Increases conversion of amino acids into glucose precursors

**Insulin**

Glucose

  Increases glucose transport into skeletal muscle and adipose tissue

  Increases glycogen synthesis

  Increases gluconeogenesis

Fat

  Increases glucose transport into fat cells

  Increases fatty acid transport into adipose cells

  Increases triglyceride synthesis

  Inhibits adipose cell lipase

  Activates lipoprotein lipase in capillary walls

Protein

  Increases active transport of amino acids into cells

  Increases protein synthesis

  Decreases protein breakdown by enhancing the use of glucose and fatty acids for fuel

**Epinephrine**

  Mobilizes glycogen stores

  Decreases movement of glucose into cells

  Inhibits insulin release

  Mobilizes fatty acids from adipose tissue

## Insulin

Diabetes is a disease primarily involving insulin. This hormone is made in stages by the β cells. First, *preproinsulin* is formed into a *proinsulin* molecule composed of 81 amino acids, which is the precursor of insulin. The β cells then process the proinsulin to insulin by removal of a C-peptide structure, leaving behind the 51-amino acid structure of insulin (Fig. 11-1). The C peptide is biologically inactive, but it is produced in amounts equal to insulin and is measurable in the blood. Measurement of C peptide levels are a good indicator of β-cell function. A healthy pancreas can release 40 to 50 units of insulin daily, with several hundred units available in storage in secretory granules, which is released if blood glucose rises.

Glucose enters the β cells through a glucose transporter (GLUT 2), which has a low glucose affinity, allowing for gradient glucose uptake into the cell. The enzyme *glucokinase* regulates the first step of glucose metabolism by catalyzing the phosphorylation of glucose into glucose 6-phosphate. This metabolism of glucose, not necessarily the presence of glucose itself, is thought to be the trigger for insulin release, with glucokinase functioning as a "glucose sensor" (McPhee et al., 1997). Changes in cell electrophysiology, triggered by glucose metabolism, result in the release of insulin from cytoplasmic granules (McPhee et al., 1997). Insulin then enters the bloodstream and binds to insulin receptors on the membranes of liver, muscle, and fat cells. In these insulin-sensitive cells, insulin promotes glucose uptake into cells, encourages fuel storage (anabolism), and prevents the breakdown of stored fuel (catabolism).

### Liver Activity

In the liver, increased insulin secretion suppresses the breakdown of stored glycogen (glycogenolysis), suppresses the formation of new glucose (gluconeogenesis), and increases the synthesis of glycogen. Insulin also stimulates glycolysis (metabolism of glucose to pyruvate), which provides the precursors for the formation of fatty acids. Insulin also discourages the production of ketones.

### Muscle and Fat

In muscle and fat cells, insulin encourages glucose uptake by causing a shift of another insulin-sensitive glucose transporter, GLUT 4, to the surface of the cells (Fig. 11-2). In muscle, insulin encourages the storage of glucose by promoting glycogen synthesis and inhibiting glycogen catabolism. Insulin also promotes protein synthesis in muscle cells. Uptake of glucose by muscle accounts for approximately 85% of glucose disposition (McPhee et al., 1997).

Insulin increases the production of very low-density lipoproteins by the liver. These lipoproteins deliver triglycerides to fat tissue for storage,

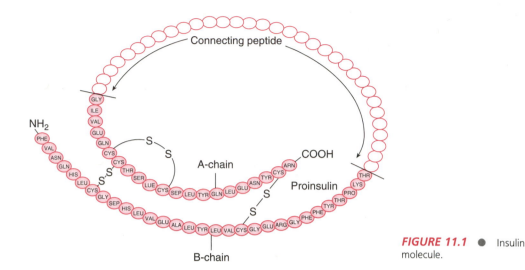

**FIGURE 11.1** ● Insulin molecule.

thus promoting fat storage. Lipoprotein lipase, a membrane-bound enzyme that breaks down triglycerides into fatty acids for uptake by fat cells, also is stimulated by insulin. Glucose taken into fat cells by the GLUT 4 transporter also aids in fat storage by increasing intracellular levels of fatty acid substrates produced from glucose. These eventually are stored as triglycerides. Insulin inhibits hormone-sensitive lipase, an enzyme that breaks down stored fat into fatty acids.

### Glucagon

The α cells of the pancreas produce two major hormones, glucagon and glucagon-like peptide-1 (7-36). Glucagon opposes the action of insulin, whereas glucagon-like peptide-1 (7-36) stimulates insulin synthesis and secretion. Glucagon release is inhibited by glucose through an unknown feedback mechanism. Another β-cell product, γ-aminobutyric acid, also is thought to inhibit glucagon release (McPhee et al., 1997). Glucagon

has important actions on a host of other processes (see Table 11-1). Glucagon binds to glucagon receptors on the surface of hepatocytes, which, through a cascade of reactions, stimulates enzymes responsible for glucagon's effect on metabolism.

### Somatostatin

Somatostatin, produced by the δ cells of the pancreas, is stimulated by the ingestion of every type of food substance. Somatostatin is thought to inhibit both insulin and glucagon release through paracrine effects by binding to somatostatin receptors on the α and β cells. This action may modulate and regulate excessive insulin and glucagon release in response to a meal. Somatostatin also decreases gastrointestinal activity after eating, extending the amount of time available for food absorption.

### Catecholamines and Glucocorticoid Hormones

The catecholamines epinephrine and norepinephrine maintain and increase blood glucose levels in times of stress by inhibiting the release of insulin from the β cells, increasing lipase activity, and promoting glycogenolysis in the skeletal muscles and liver. This action promotes local muscle glucose bioavailability without directly increasing blood glucose and also conserves blood glucose for use by the brain and nervous system.

The glucocorticoid hormones, released from the adrenal cortex, are crucial for maintaining

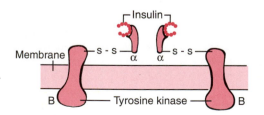

**FIGURE 11.2** ● Insulin receptor. When insulin binds to α subunits, a conformational change occurs which activates tyrosine kinase on β subunits. This activates a sequence of events which allows glucoside to be transported across the membrane.

blood glucose levels, especially between meals or during periods of fasting. These hormones increase gluconeogenesis in the liver and decrease the uptake of glucose by muscle and fat. They also stimulate protein catabolism and inhibit protein synthesis. Cortisol accounts for most glucocorticoid activity, with the hypothalamus and the anterior pituitary gland regulating its release. Cortisol levels are elevated during the early morning hours in individuals with regular sleep patterns, as well as during periods of anxiety or stress. Cortisol also appears to have permissive action, enhancing the effects of catecholamines.

## CLINICAL PRESENTATION

### Signs and Symptoms

Diabetes mellitus is not a single disease but instead is a complex syndrome characterized by *hyperglycemia* resulting from altered carbohydrate, fat, and protein metabolism. This altered metabolism is secondary to insulin insufficiency, insufficient insulin activity, or both, and to increases in the counter-regulatory hormones that oppose the action of insulin. Because of the sequelae of altered fuel metabolism, diabetes is characterized by vascular and neurologic changes throughout the body.

Absence of insulin or ineffective insulin activity prevents glucose from entering muscle and fat cells. As the blood glucose level approaches 180 mg/dL, the ability of the kidney to reabsorb glucose (the tubular maxima) is surpassed, and glucose is excreted into the urine (glucosuria). Because it is an osmotic diuretic, glucose causes the osmosis of large amounts of water into the tubules, causing frequent urination in large quantities (polyuria), notably at night (nocturia). Dehydration, hunger (from calorie loss), and fatigue follow. The classic symptoms of diabetes mellitus ensue: *polyuria, polydipsia,* and *polyphagia.*

To overcome the lack of glucose, the body begins breaking down protein stores, leading to a negative nitrogen balance. In the continued absolute absence or ineffectiveness of insulin, fat stores are mobilized into free fatty acids (FFAs). In the liver, excess amounts of fatty acids cannot enter into the Krebs cycle and instead condense into acetoacetic acid and beta hydroxybutyrate, called ketone bodies, which are acidic. To buffer these acids, the body excretes acidic urine and buffers the blood acidity with bicarbonate and buffer base reserves. However, continued production and buffering of ketones causes a drop in plasma pH, acidosis, and eventually death if left untreated.

### Diagnostic Criteria

New criteria for diagnosing diabetes were presented at the 57th Annual Meeting of the American Diabetes Association (ADA) (ADA, 1997). The ADA expert panel stated that diabetes may be diagnosed by any one of the following three methods, followed by a confirming test on a different day:

1. A fasting plasma glucose (FPG) level of ≥ 126 mg/dL or higher (after no caloric intake for at least 8 hours). This no longer must be confirmed with an oral glucose tolerance test (OGTT).
2. A casual plasma glucose (taken at any time of the day without regard to time of last meal) of ≥ 200 mg/dL, combined with the classic signs and symptoms of diabetes.
3. An OGTT value of ≥ 200 mg/dL in the 2-hour sample.

The ADA expert committee prefers the FPG and recommends its universal use for the testing and diagnosis of diabetes. It is easy to administer, acceptable to patients, and lower in cost when compared with the OGTT.

A new state also was defined at the annual ADA meeting. The committee defined the upper limit of normal for the FPG test as 110 mg/dL and recognized two states of impaired glucose metabolism that are considered risk factors for developing diabetes:

1. *Impaired fasting glucose*: a new category in which FPG is ≥ 110 mg/dL but < 126 mg/dL.
2. *Impaired glucose tolerance* (IGT): an existing category in which results of the OGTT are ≥ 140 mg/dL but < 200 mg/dL at the 2-hour sample.

### Classification and Etiology

At the same ADA annual meeting, revised nomenclature for the two chief categories of diabetes was recommended to clarify diagnosis (ADA, 1997). The term *type 1 diabetes* replaced insulin-dependent diabetes mellitus (IDDM), juvenile-onset diabetes, or type I diabetes. The term *type 2 diabetes* replaced non–insulin-dependent diabetes mellitus, adult-onset diabetes, or type II diabetes. The older terminology was misleading because the nomenclature did not accurately reflect the underlying disease process. Also, treatment methods often confused the issue (ie, type II diabetics receiving insulin therapy often were incorrectly labeled as type I or insulin-dependent diabetics).

## Type 1 Diabetes

Type 1 diabetes is typified by autoimmune destruction of the β cells of the pancreas. It can be subdivided into two types: type 1A, immune-mediated diabetes, and type 1B, idiopathic diabetes. Type 1 diabetes affects 10% to 20% of those with diabetes in the United States and Europe, with most having type 1A diabetes. Commonly developing in childhood or the teenage years, it can occur at any age. The presence of blood ketones, hyperglycemia, and an absolute absence of endogenous insulin characterize type 1 diabetes. All individuals with type 1 diabetes require exogenous insulin to control hyperglycemia and to prevent ketosis.

## Type 1A Diabetes

Several theories exist regarding the etiology of type 1A diabetes. One is that type 1A diabetes results from genetic predisposition coupled with an environmental trigger that stimulates β-cell autoimmune destruction.

### Autoimmune Disease and Genetic Predisposition

The failure of the body to distinguish self-antigens from foreign antigens is the fundamental cause of autoimmune disease. This ability to recognize self is dependent on cell surface glycoprotein molecules called the major histocompatibility complex (MHC). In humans, the MHC proteins are termed the human leukocyte antigens (HLAs) and are designated by both letters (A to D) and numbers (eg, HLA-A1, HLA-DR3). Genes on chromosome 6 code for these molecules. Individuals inherit a chromosome from each parent, and with each chromosome inherit a HLA gene. They therefore end up with two HLA units known as HLA haplotypes. Each HLA haplotype is inherited intact from the parent; thus, the offspring shares a HLA haplotype with each parent. A susceptibility to type 1 diabetes has been linked to HLA-DR3 and HLA-DR4 (Honeyman et al., 1995). Individuals appear to inherit an abnormal immune response affecting the β cells when they inherit these haplotypes. It is thought that antibodies are directed against and initiate an immune response to the β-cell antigens. In fact, inheritance of specific HLA types has been associated with a 50-fold higher rate of type 1 diabetes

(Fantus et al., 1997). Type 1 diabetes–associated autoantibodies are classified as islet cell antibodies (ICAs) and insulin autoantibodies (IAAs). In newly diagnosed individuals, ICAs are present in most individuals, whereas IAAs are present half of the time. These antibodies are detectable years before the disease becomes apparent and are predictive of the disease eventually developing. When neither antibody is present, the risk of developing type 1 diabetes is essentially zero. In individuals who have both antibodies and diagnosed first-degree relatives, the risk of developing disease escalates to 70% (McPhee et al., 1997). Antibodies to glutamic acid decarboxylase (GAD), an islet cell antigen, also have been identified and may be more predictive of type 1 diabetes than either ICAs or IAAs.

Identification of these autoantigens has led to the hope that tolerance can be induced in individuals, thereby preventing the development of type 1 diabetes. In a trial by the National Institutes of Health (NIH) titled Diabetes Prevention Trial-Type 1, individuals having high ICA titers, poor insulin response, and first-degree relatives diagnosed with type 1 diabetes are being treated with oral or parenteral administration of insulin. It is hoped that administration of these initiators of the autoimmune response will induce tolerance and prevent or delay diabetes (Fantus et al., 1997; NIH, 1996). In a similar trial (Canadian-European Nicotinamide Diabetes Intervention Trial), nicotinamide administration has shown to be an effective preventative in at-risk children (Fantus et al., 1997). In animal studies, oral administration of insulin and GAD has provided protection against the development of type 1 diabetes.

However, some HLA types have been associated with resistance to type 1 diabetes, and identical twin studies show a concordance rate of less than 33% (Fantus et al., 1997). This indicates that genetic susceptibility alone cannot explain the autoimmune response.

### Environmental Triggers

A prevalent theory regarding genetic-environmental interaction is one of "molecular mimicry" (Fantus et al., 1997). It is believed that an environmental antigen found in microbial or food proteins stimulates an autoimmune response in some individuals because of structural similarities to islet cell proteins. For example, a coxsackie viral protein has been found to share homology with an islet cell antibody (GAD) and may induce β-cell destruction (McPhee et al., 1997). Other viruses also may trigger immune response and progression to type 1 diabetes, but the mechanism is unknown.

It is possible that, rather then molecular mimicry, islet damage results from bystander damage from the inflammation, tissue damage, and the release of sequestered islet antigen, which then stimulates resting autoreactive T cells (Horwitz et al., 1998). Based on a positive correlation between increased numbers of bank voles (small rodents) and the number of new cases of type 1 diabetes, a Swedish study has hypothesized that type 1 diabetes is caused or triggered by an infectious agent carried by the voles. Isolates of three viruses resembling picornaviruses (which include the polio and coxsackie viruses) have been identified and are presumed to be the causative agents (Niklasson et al., 1998).

Food triggers also are implicated as causative agents. There has been much debate over the idea that exposure to cow's milk protein at an early age (younger than 6 months) may be associated with an increased risk for developing type 1 diabetes. In countries with early and high consumption of cow's milk, there is a high incidence of type 1 diabetes. In children with type 1 diabetes, there have been reports of increased anti-bovine serum albumin (Fantus et al., 1997). In Finland, a clinical trial has been initiated to study 5000 newborns who have first-degree relatives diagnosed with type 1 diabetes and who also have HLA genetic predisposition. Known as the Trial to Reduce IDDM in the Genetically at Risk, it is a double-blind study to determine if early avoidance of cow's milk reduces the incidence of type 1 diabetes.

In the Diabetes Autoimmunity Study of the Young, US researchers found no positive correlation between early exposure to cow's milk and increased risk of β-cell antibodies associated with the development of type 1 diabetes (Norris et al., 1996). Animal studies yield the same results (Schatz & Maclaren, 1996).

## Type 1B Diabetes

Type 1B idiopathic diabetes describes cases of β-cell destruction that are not of an autoimmune origin. This type of diabetes is fairly uncommon and is seen predominantly in individuals of African or Asian origin. Need for use of exogenous insulin is not constant with this classification.

## Type 2 Diabetes

Type 2 diabetes is characterized by insulin resistance and a relative lack of insulin production as opposed to the total lack of insulin production seen in type 1 diabetics. It also is characterized by increased hepatic glucose production. Type 2 diabetes occurs in 80% to 90% of those with diabetes, usually affecting those older than 40 years (Satcher, 1998). It is generally distinguished by the absence of ketosis in a hyperglycemic state, secondary to the body's ability to produce insulin, even in small quantities. Individuals with type 2 diabetes may be able to control their hyperglycemia with diet and lifestyle modification or oral drug therapy, never needing exogenous insulin to achieve glycemic control. However, these same individuals eventually may require exogenous insulin to control their hyperglycemia. These people are, nevertheless, considered to have type 2 diabetes. Several theories abound regarding the cause of type 2 diabetes.

### Impaired Insulin Secretion/Hyperinsulinemia

β-cell dysfunction, with consequent impaired insulin secretion, has been proposed as a key contributing factor to the pathogenesis of type 2 diabetes. In a study of first-degree relatives of type 2 diabetics, those who had IGT also were found to have marked β-cell dysfunction, which continued to worsen as glucose tolerance worsened (Fernandez-Castaner et al., 1996). β-cell dysfunction also was exhibited in first-degree relatives with normal glucose tolerance or in those with advancing age. Paired with the insulin-resistance commonly found in type 2 diabetes, it is proposed that the β cells become "exhausted" in an attempt to constantly overcome the insulin requirements of hyperglycemia (Fernandez-Castaner et al., 1996).

β-cell dysfunction also may be caused by a decrease in the number of functioning β cells, by abnormal function of the β cells, or by a combination of the two. Amyloid deposits are associated with β-cell destruction and normally increase in number with advancing age. Fatty amyloid deposits in the pancreas are associated with the elevated serum lipid levels frequently seen in diabetes and are thought to play a role in the development of β-cell dysfunction with increasing length of disease (Kahn et al., 1999). A gene product known as islet amyloid polypeptide, or amylin, has been isolated in these amyloid deposits, and amyloid fibrils may fill the β cells, replacing functional cytoplasm with amyloid deposits. A decrease in weight and number of β cells also can occur, but the cause is unknown.

Hyperinsulinemia, a β-cell defect, has been suggested in the pathogenesis of type 2 diabetes. Increased production of insulin, with elevated serum insulin levels, down-regulates the number of insulin receptors, leading to eventual β-cell exhaustion. In addition, failure of the pancreas to release insulin in an initial response to a glucose load (impaired first-phase insulin release) could lead to hyperglycemia and hyperinsulinemia, with resultant β-cell exhaustion. Other β-cell dysfunctions thought to contribute to the pathology of type 2 diabetes include altered patterns of pulsatile insulin release (Reusch, 1993) and an increased exhaustion of proinsulin levels (Fernandez-Castaner et al., 1996; Reusch, 1993).

## Insulin Resistance/Reduced Insulin Binding

Insulin resistance is thought to contribute significantly to the pathogenesis and progression of type 2 diabetes. Insulin resistance is defined as "a blunted response of the body to normal or even supranormal insulin concentrations. That is, for a given amount of insulin, the body will store less glucose and fat." (Reusch, 1993, p. 188). The expected physiologic response to insulin resistance would be hyperglycemia, with the β cells producing increasingly larger amounts of insulin to compensate (hyperinsulinemia). In those with type 2 diabetes, the insulin demand is not met, and the subsequent hyperglycemia increases insulin resistance. It is theorized that the insulin resistance triggers hyperinsulinemia to the point of β-cell exhaustion in a continuous, vicious cycle.

Obesity (especially central or android obesity) has been highly associated with insulin resistance. Obesity is "a state of insulin resistance" with hyperinsulinemia as an "adaptive response" to insulin resistance (Muscelli et al., 1998). Individuals with severe obesity have a 10-fold increase in risk for developing type 2 diabetes. In addition, fat cells produce cytokines such as tumor necrosis factor-α (TNF-α), which impair insulin action (Reusch, 1993). TNF-α is thought to exert its effects by inducing insulin resistance in skeletal muscle tissue, thus inhibiting insulin action through paracrine effects on muscle tissue, or by release of factors such as FFAs, which inhibit insulin action on muscle (Boden, 1997). A study of obesity reveals that obese individuals exhibit hyperinsulinemia, insulin resistance, and insulin hypersecretion compared with a nonobese control group (Muscelli et al., 1998). However, individuals who had an early onset of obesity and longer duration of obesity had better insulin sensitivity and secretion than did individuals who had recently become obese. This is inconsistent with many theories that propose insulin resistance as a mechanism to protect from weight gain. These findings suggest that increased insulin sensitivity might be useful in predicting obesity and resistance to developing type 2 diabetes (Muscelli et al., 1998).

Insulin resistance also can result from poor insulin delivery to the tissues. Because insulin normally is a vasodilator (through nitric oxide–dependent vasodilation), insulin-resistant individuals can have decreased skeletal muscle and capillary blood flow (Salonen et al., 1998). If this occurs, delivery of insulin to insulin-sensitive tissue is decreased (Reusch, 1993). Similarly, insulin resistance may be linked to higher whole-blood viscosity, which reduces the blood flow and, therefore, delivery of both insulin and glucose to skeletal muscle. Higher blood viscosity has been associated with increased serum triglycerides and total cholesterol, as well as decreased high-density lipoprotein concentrations found in type 2 diabetes (Hoieggen et al., 1998).

There are other proposed mechanisms for insulin resistance. Approximately 41% of hypertensive patients exhibit insulin resistance and hyperinsulinemia (Laviades et al., 1998). Many studies suggest that both normotensive and hypertensive individuals who exhibit salt sensitivity also exhibit insulin resistance (Galletti et al., 1997; Sharma et al., 1991, 1993; Ferrannini et al., 1987; Capaldo et al., 1991; DeFronzo & Ferrannini, 1991); however, other studies refute this (Egan et al., 1994; Lind et al., 1992). One study found that insulin-like growth factor 1 (IGF-1), which participates in glucose metabolism and is similar to proinsulin, may contribute to the development of hypertension and insulin resistance. Administration of IGF-1 to hypertensive, insulin-resistant patients decreases plasma glucose levels and insulin concentrations. IGF-1 also may play a role in glycemic control by inhibiting secretion of glucagon (Laviades et al., 1998).

Alterations in GLUT 4, the insulin-sensitive glucose transporter that assists in transporting glucose across the cell membrane, are being studied as a cause for insulin resistance. In type 2 diabetes, there may be faulty gene coding for the GLUT 4 transporter, or there may be decreased quantities of GLUT 4 in skeletal muscle (Reusch, 1993). Similarly, alterations in cell surface receptors are being studied. To become active, insulin first must bind and interact with cell surface receptors, which stimulate the enzyme tyrosine kinase (TK) to begin a cascade reaction that results in insulin's effects. Genetic mutations can cause diminished TK activity (Elbein, 1997). In addition, hyperglycemia or hyperinsulinemia can cause faulty binding and activation of the cell surface receptors (Reusch, 1993).

### Failure to Suppress Endogenous Glucose Production

One of the primary effects of insulin is to suppress endogenous production of glucose. Traditionally thought to exert its effect directly on the liver through portal circulation, insulin also is believed to indirectly affect glucose production by extrahepatic suppression of adipocyte lipolysis (which releases FFAs) (Mittelman et al., 1998). Glucagon release, stimulated by hypoglycemia and the ingestion of amino acids, stimulates the release of insulin, which then suppresses glucagon's stimulation of endogenous glucose production. In type 2 diabetes, there is an impaired suppression of glucose production by the liver.

In type 2 diabetes, FFAs fail to stimulate insulin secretion, which results in hepatic overproduction of glucose and underutilization of this glucose (Boden, 1997). Increased plasma levels of FFAs produce peripheral and hepatic insulin resistance and promotion of gluconeogenesis. In obesity, FFAs are elevated, being released from intramuscular fat deposits, especially intraabdominal fat deposits. FFAs are thought to inhibit insulin-stimulated glucose uptake by (1) inhibiting glucose transport or phosphorylation, (2) decreasing glycogen synthase activity, (3) interfering with GLUT 4 gene expression in muscle and fat tissue, and (4) altering insulin receptor binding through alterations in the lipid layer of the plasma membrane in which insulin receptors are located (Boden, 1997).

### Stress Response

Psychological stress is a factor that has been identified as having a significant negative impact on diabetic control (Jablon et al., 1997; Aikens et al., 1997). Life stress generally is associated with an increase in sympathetic nervous system (SNS) outflow and activation of the hypothalamic-pituitary-adrenocorticoid (HPA) axis (Pennisi, 1997). In a study of chronic and acute stress, researchers found that individuals who were subjected to chronic stress showed greater increases in circulating levels of both epinephrine and cortisol when exposed to an acute stressor than did control subjects. In addition, the cortisol levels of the chronic stress group never returned to prestress levels during the study. Cortisol not only elevates blood glucose, but it enhances the effects of epinephrine. Elevated epinephrine levels can decrease insulin-stimulated utilization of glucose (Hoieggen et al., 1998).

A similar study sought to determine if biologic stressors, both acute and chronic, could condition individual biologic responses in ways that alter vulnerability to disease, including type 2 diabetes. The biologic stress responses examined included the neural and endocrine adaptations of the central nervous system (CNS) that maintain homeostasis, particularly catecholamine release and stimulation of the HPA axis (Pike et al., 1997). Research suggests a link between stress and the development of central or android obesity, which already has been linked with type 2 diabetes. Cortisol, which is elevated during stress, influences the accumulation of adipose tissue, especially deep abdominal fat. Adipose tissue contains glucocorticoid receptors that help to regulate fat deposits. Individuals with central obesity, also measured as a high waist-to-hip ratio (WHR), secreted higher levels of cortisol during stress than individuals with a low WHR. This suggests that abdominal obesity might be evidence of an underlying process that conditions the individual's biologic response, as opposed to a direct risk factor for disease development (Kelly et al., 1997).

### Genetics

Type 2 diabetes is strongly inherited. A positive history of type 2 diabetes in first-degree relatives doubles an individual's risk for diabetes, and a child of two diabetic parents has an 80% lifetime risk of developing the disease (Elbein, 1997). The fact that type 2 diabetes is so prevalent among specific ethnic groups also suggests a strong genetic link. For example, the Pima Indians of Arizona have approximately a 50% disease prevalence rate, with 90% who exhibit IGT developing diabetes within 10 years (Elbein, 1997; Noble, 1996). Results of genetic research in the Pima Indians suggests several genomic regions with possible links to glucose metabolism.

By studying the pathophysiologic process of type 2 diabetes, several theories in support of genetic inheritance of type 2 diabetes have been proposed. Many laboratories are using genetic tools to search for type 2 susceptibility genetic loci in humans. In the realm of insulin action, areas of study include insulin-sulfonylurea receptors, muscle and liver glycogen synthase, GLUT 4, Ras-like protein associated with diabetes, multiple loci associated with lipid metabolism, and insulin receptor substrate-1. With regard to insulin secretion, areas of study include glucose sensing (glucose kinase, GLUT 2), insulin gene transcription factors (MODY 1, MODY 3), glucagon and glucagon-like peptide receptor, and amylin (Elbein, 1997). Because type 2 diabetes does not follow simple Mendelian inheritance, identifying a genetic basis for the disease is difficult (Pratley et al., 1998; Turner et al., 1997).

### Autoantibodies

Antibodies to islet cells (ICAs) and to glutamic acid decarboxylase (GADAs), already known to play a major role in the development of type 1 diabetes, are being investigated as causative agents in the development of type two diabetes. ICAs and GADAs also appear in a subset of younger adults with type 2 diabetes. At the time of diagnosis, these younger, nonobese patients have higher levels of ICAs and GADAs than do older patients. ICA and GADA levels continually decline with increasing age. The younger patients typically have a clinical presentation similar to that of type 1 diabetes. However, initially, these patients can be treated successfully with oral diabetic agents. They slowly progress to a point of insulin dependence and are thought to have an evolving form of type 1 diabetes, or latent autoimmune diabetes in adults. Testing for GADA and ICA antibodies in newly diagnosed, young diabetics might help to determine proper disease classification, which sometimes can be difficult. High levels of ICAs and GADAs are thought to be predictive of future insulin dependence (Turner et al., 1997).

### Secondary Causes of Hyperglycemia

Any condition that causes an impairment of insulin secretion or faulty insulin uptake can result in hyperglycemia. Several disease states and common medications induce hyperglycemia (Table 11-2). Hyperglycemia usually is reversible once the offending drug is discontinued or the underlying disease process is corrected.

## COMPLICATIONS

### Acute Complications

#### Diabetic Ketoacidosis

Diabetic ketoacidosis (DKA) is a common and serious complication of diabetes mellitus, with average mortality rates of 3% to 10% (Davidson, 1998). DKA develops when there is a deficiency of insulin, which is needed to use available glucose stores. Because the glucose cannot be used,

| TABLE 11.2  |
| :--- |
| **Drugs Commonly Associated With Hyperglycemia** |

*Hormones*
  Glucocorticoids
  Estrogens and oral contraceptives
  Thyroid replacement hormones
*Antihypertensives*
  Beta blockers
  Loop diuretics
  Prazosin
  Clonidine
  Diazoxide
*Miscellaneous*
  Phenytoin
  Levodopa
  Sympathomimetics and catecholamines
  Phenothiazine
  Lithium
  Tricyclic antidepressants
  Niacin
  Isoniazid
  Indomethacin

plasma glucose levels rise and counterregulatory hormones are stimulated. Catecholamines, cortisol, and glucagon increase hepatic glucose production, decrease utilization of glucose, and stimulate lipolysis, which provides fatty acids for use by the CNS. As lipolysis continues in the face of insulin deficiency, ketone by-products build and are excreted in the urine along with sodium bicarbonate. Continued ketone production can overcome the acid-buffering ability of the kidneys. If plasma pH continues to fall, deep and rapid respirations (Kussmaul breathing) occur to lower $P_{CO_2}$ and compensate for metabolic acidosis. Acetone, a product of ketosis, is blown off during these respirations and gives the person with DKA the characteristic fruity-smelling breath. Severe hyperglycemia can occur, resulting in diuresis and eventual cellular dehydration. This diuresis depletes sodium stores and results in low plasma sodium levels. Total potassium also is depleted, but acidosis and hyperglycemia drive intracellular potassium into the extracellular space, resulting in normal or even elevated serum potassium levels.

DKA strikes patients with type 1 diabetes, although those with type 2 occasionally manifest this complication. Severe stress, infection, surgery, myocardial infarction (MI), and interruption of insulin administration can be precipitating factors. DKA can occur at the onset of type 1 diabetes, and the need for treatment of its signs and symptoms frequently is how the diagnosis of type 1 diabetes is first made. Polyuria, dehydration and thirst, anorexia, nausea and vomiting, Kussmaul respirations, abdominal pain, postural hypotension, tachycardia, and CNS depression are typical presenting symptoms. Treatment includes administration of intravenous (IV) fluids for replacement of lost fluid volume, electrolyte replacement therapy, and continuous infusion of insulin to control hyperglycemia and halt lipolysis. As hyperglycemia is corrected, extracellular potassium begins to shift back into the cell, causing dangerously low levels of potassium and a potential for cardiac arrhythmias. Treatment is best conducted in an acute-care setting.

### *Hyperglycemic Hyperosmolar Nonketotic Syndrome*

Hyperglycemic hyperosmolar nonketotic syndrome (HHNKS) also is a serious complication of diabetes mellitus, with mortality rates of 10% to 20% (with older reports suggesting a mortality rate as high as 30% to 50%) (Davidson, 1998). There is no universally accepted pathophysiologic mechanism to explain the difference between DKA and HHNKS. It is thought that the amount of insulin necessary to inhibit lipolysis is much smaller than that needed to accommodate glucose transport. Individuals with type 2 diabetes who retain even minimal insulin production develop HHNKS as opposed to DKA. Those who exhibit extreme insulin resistance are more prone to developing HHNKS. Patients generally present for medical treatment later in the course of HHNKS, when plasma glucose levels reach as high as 800 to 2400 mg/dL (McPhee et al., 1997). Glucosuria, polyuria, and extreme depletion of intravascular volume result from the grossly elevated blood glucose levels. Electrolyte changes are similar to those of DKA.

Development of HHNKS can be insidious and may be the first presenting symptom that leads to a diagnosis of diabetes. There is usually a precipitating cause such as infection, MI, or cerebrovascular accident (CVA). Drugs that cause insulin resistance also may be implicated. The presenting signs and symptoms are similar to those in DKA. In addition, HHNKS also presents with significant neurologic changes, especially changes in responsiveness and sensorium. Other neurologic manifestations include hemiparesis, aphasia, positive Babinski reflex, seizure, and coma. These signs and symptoms frequently are mistaken for a stroke, especially in the elderly.

Treatment of HHNKS is similar to that of DKA. However, the dehydration of HHNKS is more severe and requires massive IV hydration. Care must be taken during IV replacement therapy that cerebral edema does not occur. Potassium replacement also is crucial, with replacement of potassium stores taking several days to a week. This condition also requires treatment in an acute-care setting.

## Chronic Complications

The diagnosis of diabetes carries with it a host of chronic complications with serious health implications. With improvements in therapy, many of those with diabetes are living longer lives but, unfortunately, are experiencing the long-term complications of the disease.

Macrovascular and microvascular disease, as well as neuropathies, are potential sequelae.

### Macrovascular Disease

Known risk factors for coronary artery disease (CAD) include smoking, hypertension, hyperlipidemia, obesity, positive family history of CAD, increasing age (men, 45 years and older; women, 55 years and older without hormone replacement therapy [HRT]), any state of hypercoagulability, and diabetes mellitus (Davidson, 1998; Schernthaner, 1996). Diabetes acts synergistically with any of these risk factors, but diabetes mellitus is considered an independent risk factor, even when associated with none of the other factors. Macrovascular disease is especially prominent in type 2 diabetes, causing 75% to 80% of deaths for these patients (American Heart Association, 1998; Davidson, 1998). In the general population, women are less affected with CAD than men, but CAD affects men and women with diabetes equally (Schernthaner, 1996). Men with type 2 diabetes have a twofold risk of developing CAD; women, a fourfold increase (especially true in women who forgo HRT). Both diabetic men and women have a twofold increased risk of CVA (Davidson, 1998). MI, angina, and sudden death occur twice as often in the diabetic population, especially in those 65 to 75 years of age (Schern-thaner, 1996). There also is an increased frequency of silent ischemia (no pain with MI), increased risk of MI, and higher mortality rate after MI in the diabetic population.

Diabetes is an independent risk factor because of both the numerous physiologic changes that contribute to the development of this disease and the physiologic changes that occur as a consequence of the disease. Diabetes increases the risk for atherosclerosis because of (1) an increase in lipid levels and an alteration in the lipoprotein composition, which makes the lipoproteins more atherogenic; (2) a relative procoagulant state with increased clotting factors, increased tissue plasminogen activator, and platelet aggregation; (3) changes in the vessel walls secondary to hyperinsulinemia or exogenous insulin administration; (4) deposition of advanced glycosylation end products (AGEs); and (5) a high prevalence of hypertension (type 1 after nephropathy, type 2 present at diagnosis) (McPhee et al., 1997; Schernthaner, 1996). Glycosylated proteins (AGEs) cause a change in vascular and neural tissue and may cause impaired release of the vasodilator nitric oxide, contributing to CAD (Noble, 1996; Schernthaner, 1996).

The prevalence of atherosclerosis in diabetes is greatly increased over the general population (McPhee et al., 1997). One study hypothesizes that cytomegalovirus (CMV) may be a causative agent in CAD and atherosclerosis. CMV can replicate in human smooth muscle cell and remain dormant there after a primary infection. Because there is impaired immune response in diabetes mellitus, it is thought that the virus can reactivate, damage vessel walls, and initiate atherosclerosis (Visseren et al., 1997). CMV antibodies detectable in diabetic patients with atherosclerosis are higher than in diabetic patients without atherosclerosis. This is especially true in women who become more susceptible to atherosclerosis than male diabetics or the nondiabetic population in general (Visseren et al., 1997).

Insulin resistance syndrome (*syndrome X*, see earlier section, Insulin Resistance/Reduced Insulin Binding) increases the risk of CAD secondary to increased central obesity and increased WHR (ratios > 0.85 to 0.90 in women and > 1.0 in men) (Davidson, 1998; McPhee et al., 1997; Meigs et al., 1998; Salonen et al., 1998). Hyperinsulinemia also can induce sodium retention and the development of hypertension, leading to CAD (Muscelli et al., 1998). As glucose tolerance decreases, the risk for CAD increases (Meigs et al., 1998). The risk also rises with increasing length of disease. A recent study found no clear threshold where increasing risk levels begin, indicating that there is no cut point where risk starts and stops (Meigs et al.,1998). Studies such as this prompted change in ADA guidelines, which lowered the plasma glucose levels for diagnosing diabetes.

## Microvascular Disease

Microvascular complications are thought to be related to elevated glucose levels, thickening of the capillary basement wall membranes by AGEs, and accumulated sugar alcohol through the polyol pathway.

### *Nephropathy*

The first clinical abnormality evident in nephropathy is the presence of microalbuminuria (urinary excretion of 30 to 300 mg albumin/24 hours). The earliest pathophysiologic change characteristic of nephropathy is the thickening of the glomerular basement membrane, thought to be secondary to hyperglycemia and hypertension. Elevated glucose levels cause a decreased glomerular filtration of macromolecules and increased intraglomerular pressure. Filtration in the kidney is regulated by the glomerular basement membrane permeability and glomerular pressure (a combination of glomerular capillary hydrostatic pressure and the opposing forces of the glomerular capillary colloid osmotic pressure and Bowman's capsule hydrostatic pressure). Glomeruli are further damaged by the formation of AGEs and increasing intraglomerular hypertension. Histologic changes include renal hypertrophy, capillary basement membrane thickening, and diffuse glomerulosclerosis. Nodular glomerulosclerosis (Kimmelstiel-Wilson disease) occurs in 10% to 35% of diabetics. Development of these lesions in the glomerular capillaries of the kidneys allows proteins to escape because of changes in the basement membrane (Noble, 1996). Structural changes are similar in types 1 and 2, although there may be more glomerulosclerosis in type 2 (Aiello, 1998).

Type 1 patients generally remain asymptomatic for about 10 years after diagnosis. Type 1 progression is slow, with a time frame of about 30 years. Type 2 patients usually are diagnosed farther along in the disease process, and many already are at stage 3 on diagnosis. However, not all diabetics develop nephropathy. Diabetic nephropathy occurs in family clusters, suggesting a family predisposition. Risk factors for developing nephropathy include having genetic or family risk factors, kidney or glomerular enlargement, poor glycemic control (the risk of microalbuminuria rises abruptly if $HbA_{1c}$ is above 8.1%), and systemic hypertension. Hypertension in type 1 diabetes worsens as kidney function declines, is a strong predictor of clinically overt nephropathy, and is predated by hyperglycemia (Equiluz-Bruck et al., 1996). Hypertension may predate hyperglycemia in type 2 diabetes and is associated with an increased albumin excretion rate. Continuous proteinuria heralds a life expectancy of less than 10 years. However, 10-year mortality in diabetics with overt nephropathy is three to four times lower if hypertension is effectively treated.

The five clinical stages of nephropathy are as follows (McPhee et al., 1997):

*Stage 1 (diagnosis)*: There is a 30% to 40% increase in glomerular filtration rate (GFR) above normal. This does not reverse immediately with institution of hyperglycemic therapy but eventually may return to normal. It is associated with enlarged kidneys and increased intraglomerular pressure, possibly secondary to hypertension. This is seen in most type 1 diabetics at diagnosis.

*Stage 2 (2 years)*: Albumin excretion is normal ($<$ 20 μg/min or 30 mg/24 hours). There may be an initial decline in renal function at this stage.

*Stage 3 (7 to 15 years; incipient diabetic nephropathy)*: There is microalbuminuria at rest (30 to 300 mg/24 hours). Those with less microalbuminuria have increased or normal GFR. Those with significant microalbuminuria show significant decrease in GFR. Blood pressure begins to elevate.

*Stage 4 (overt diabetic nephropathy)*: Stage 4 is characterized by clinical proteinuria (a urinary level detectable by simple tests such as urine dipstick). There is microalbuminuria ($\geq$ 300 mg/24 hours). Urinary protein is τ 0.5 g/24 hours. GFR declines slowly as the disease progresses. Rate of GFR fall varies between patients, but the decreased GFR is consistent within each patient. Retinopathy is common at this stage. As nephropathy worsens, hypertension worsens. Aggressive treatment of hypertension slows the rate of disease progression. Once destruction of the nephrons has occurred, improved glycemic control has little effect.

*Stage 5 (ESRD)*: Renal replacement therapy is required.

### Retinopathy

Retinopathy appears to be a response to retinal ischemia secondary to blood vessel changes and red blood cell aggregation, and develops more quickly in type 2 than type 1 diabetes. Diabetes can affect the lens, vitreous fluid, and retina. The lens changes shape with high glucose levels and causes blurring (glucose levels equalize between the lens and the aqueous humor, leading to shifts in water and an altered lens shape). Hyperglycemia in the aqueous humor draws fluid out of the lens and causes nearsightedness (myopia) (Davidson, 1998). It can take weeks to months of good glycemic control for vision to return to baseline. There is an increased risk for diabetics to develop cataracts and optic neuropathies, and at a younger age. There is background retinopathy in 20% of type 2 diabetics at the time of disease diagnosis. Diabetic retinopathy risk increases with the duration of the disease. In those with type 1 diabetes of longer than 30 years' duration, there is a greater than 90% prevalence of retinopathy. Renal disease manifested by proteinuria and elevated blood urea nitrogen and serum creatinine is highly correlated with the presence of retinopathy.

The stages of diabetic retinopathy are as follows (McPhee et al., 1997; Noble, 1996):

- *Nonproliferative* (also known as background retinopathy): Microaneurysms, splinter hemorrhages, venous tortuosity, macular edema, hard exudates
- *Preproliferative*: Areas of capillary nonperfusion, increased retinal hemorrhage, aneurysms, cotton-wool spots, intraretinal microvascular abnormalities
- *Proliferative*: Proliferation of neovascular vessels; vitreous hemorrhage; increased risk of retinal detachment; neovascularization of the iris, which leads to glaucoma

### Neuropathies

Diabetic neuropathy, the most common cause of neuropathy in the West, is thought to result from genetic, metabolic, and environmental interaction. The earliest changes in the nervous system are in the distal portions of the neurons, with the unmyelinated nerve fibers affected initially. These changes can occur in the spinal cord, the posterior root ganglia, and the peripheral nerves, with both motor and sensory nerves affected. The neuropathies can occur at any time during disease progression and may be reversible. Good glycemic control can prevent or reverse their progression. However, some neuropathies occur initially during periods of good control, leaving the mechanism of neuropathic change in question.

### Peripheral Neuropathies

Peripheral neuropathies probably are the most common form of neuropathies, with prevalence increasing with duration of disease. At the time of diagnosis, 20% of type 2 patients have peripheral neuropathy, with the overall prevalence in the diabetic population at 25% to 35% (Davidson, 1998). "Peripheral neuropathy is a generalized, sensorimotor polyneuropathy of gradual onset that is usually progressive" (Davidson, 1998, p. 298). Patients typically present with painful burning and tingling in the feet and lower extremities. Physical examination frequently reveals loss of tendon reflexes and decreased sensation to vibration and touch. With disease progression, there is increased risk for other complications. Impairment of motor and sensory function can lead to falls, burns, and injury to the feet. There is frequently atrophy of the structures of the feet, causing areas of increased pressure and deformity of joints and bone. Callous formation leading to ulceration, infection, and amputation frequently goes unnoticed because of sensory impairment. Diabetes is the largest contributor to nontraumatic lower extremity amputations in the United States.

One suggested cause of neuropathy is through the polyol pathway (Wunderlich et al., 1999). In this pathway, glucose in changed first to sorbitol then to fructose in a rate-limited reaction. In conditions of hyperglycemia, conversion of glucose to sorbitol exceeds conversion of sorbitol to fructose. These elevated sorbitol levels are hypothesized to cause the damage of peripheral neuropathy. Another theory behind peripheral neuropathy is that vessel ischemia leads to a thickening of the vessel walls that supply the nerves.

### Autonomic Neuropathy

Autonomic neuropathy affects more patients with type 1 diabetes than type 2, but frequently is found in both groups (McPhee et al., 1997). Appearing clinically later in the course of the disease than peripheral neuropathy, autonomic neuropathy affects both the SNS and the parasympathetic nervous system (PNS). The cardiovascular, gastrointestinal, and genitourinary systems are affected most often, with the PNS affected earlier and more heavily than the SNS (Davidson, 1998; McPhee, et al., 1997). Clinical manifestations of both autonomic and peripheral neuropathy are seen in Table 11-3.

## PHYSIOLOGIC BASIS FOR TREATMENT

The treatment objectives for diabetes mellitus must be designed with the knowledge that diabetes is a disease unique to the individual patient. There is no "best" method for treating the disease, there are only guidelines that must be adapted to suit the needs of each patient. The first step in developing

---

### TABLE 11.3

**Neuropathic Complications of Diabetes Mellitus**

***Peripheral***

Sensory

    Paresthesia, hyperesthesia, burning

    Usually bilateral and symmetric

    Loss of vibratory sense

    Decreased sense of touch

    Loss of tendon reflex

Motor

    Muscle weakness and atrophy

    Joint destruction

***Autonomic***

Cardiovascular

    Resting tachycardia, exercise intolerance, postural hypotension

Gastrointestinal

    Gastroparesis, nausea and vomiting, anorexia, reflux, constipation and/or diarrhea

Genitourinary

    Bladder dysfunction, overflow incontinence, urinary retention, impotence (> 50%), retrograde ejaculation

Sudomotor

    Anhidrosis, hyperhidrosis, gustatory sweating

Cranial nerves

    Cranial nerve III affected, pain, diplopia, ptosis

Hypoglycemic

    Type 1, no glucagon and occasionally no catecholamine response

Unawareness

    Type 2, retain glucagon response, can occur with sulfonylurea agents

---

appropriate therapy is classifying the type of diabetes. Although therapy differs between types 1 and 2, the goals are similar (Table 11-4). Treatment is multipronged, with patients from both disease types requiring lifestyle modification and administration of antidiabetic agents.

### Lifestyle Modification

#### Diet

Treatment of type 1 diabetes involves diet and exercise coordinated with insulin therapy. Diet is

## TABLE 11.4

### Treatment Objectives

Maintain blood glucose levels as near to normal as possible, with individual targets set for each patient

Maintain target Hb $A_{1c}$

| | |
|---|---|
| Pre-meal | 80–120 mg/dL |
| Post-meal (2 h) | 100–180 mg/dL |
| Bedtime glucose | 100–140 mg/dL |
| Hg $A_{1c}$ | < 7% without episodes of severe hypoglycemia |

Achieve optimal lipid levels

Provide adequate calories to maintain/attain goal weight; maintain normal growth and development in adolescents

Prevent acute and/or multiple episodes of hypoglycemia

Prevent long-term complications

Educate the patients to take charge of their condition

Enjoy a normal life

---

important in normalizing blood glucose levels in those with type 1 diabetes. Timing of meals in relation to exogenous insulin administration is crucial to prevent hypoglycemia and wide fluctuations in glucose levels. The recommended method of therapy is to adjust insulin administration to the individual's existing daily pattern of food intake. Trying to change daily meal patterns to fit into a prescribed insulin regime is difficult and often results in poor compliance. Therapy can be conventional (less than three daily injections) or intensive (three or more daily injections or continuous infusion pump), depending on the motivation of the patient and the willingness of the practitioner to work with the patient in developing this type plan. In addition, adherence to a strict ADA diet is no longer recommended. Nutritional planning is based on individual goals and nutritional needs, with clients planning meals around a dietary exchange system or carbohydrate counting (Kalergis et al., 1998). At the initiation of therapy, patients are encouraged to eat consistently throughout the day, with three meals and two to three snacks to prevent hypoglycemia. As patients become more attuned to their own physiologic responses to diet and insulin therapy, they can begin to adjust both to better fit their needs.

Nutritional therapy for type 2 diabetes involves achieving optimal glycemic control with a diet, which also helps to improve the lipid profile and control hypertension. Weight loss, which usually is indicated in type 2, also should be addressed during nutritional planning. A reasonable, realistic weight loss goal should be set. It does not necessarily include reaching ideal body weight (which may be unachievable), since a loss of as little as 10 to 15 lb can contribute significantly to glycemic control by reducing insulin resistance (Davidson, 1998; Noble, 1996). Perhaps the hardest part of nutritional therapy is creating a diet with which clients are able to comply. Great consideration should be given to a client's dietary preference when creating nutritional guidelines. A diet that cannot be followed sets the client up for failure and potential noncompliance with all aspects of therapy. Excellent guidelines for dietary change can be obtained from the ADA (*http://www.diabetes.org*), the American Heart Association (*http://www.americanheart.org*), and the American Dietetic Association (*http://www.eatright.org*). As in meal planning for type 1 diabetics, the diet is centered on carbohydrate counting. Meals should be spread into five to six small meals daily to control large glycemic fluctuations, diminish hunger, and alleviate gastrointestinal distress secondary to diabetic gastroparesis.

### Exercise

Exercise can play a significant role in the diabetic patient. It is important for cardiovascular fitness, flexibility, and maintenance of muscle strength and endurance as the disease progresses. However, exercise influences those with type 1 diabetes differently from those with type 2. In individuals with type 1 diabetes, insulin levels fall and counterregulatory hormones rise during exercise. The increased skeletal muscle uptake of glucose is matched by a rise in glucose production. Response to exercise varies depending on the physical condition of the individual, level of exercise intensity, the degree of glycemic control achieved, and the levels of insulin and glucose at the start of exercise (Davidson, 1998). In addition, injected insulin may be taken up more quickly during exercise than in a resting state. In a well-controlled individual, the risk of hypoglycemia is heightened by exercise. Not only can acute hypoglycemia occur, but delayed effects also can be seen for several hours after exercise. The cause is unknown but may be related to increased glucose uptake by the skeletal muscles as they replenish glycogen stores (Davidson, 1998). The type 1 patient must be aware of the potential for delayed hypoglycemia and adjust insulin administration, carbohydrate intake, or both to compensate. In a poorly controlled individual, exercise may further elevate glucose levels and lead to ketosis if insufficient insulin is available to control the rise of counterregulatory hormones. Self-monitoring of glucose levels both before and after exercise is essential.

Exercise in the type 2 patient is a mainstay of therapy. Exercise increases insulin sensitivity, decreases insulin requirements, enhances glucose uptake, lowers cholesterol and triglyceride levels, and promotes weight loss (Gautier et al., 1995; Laine et al., 1998; Mayer-Davis et al., 1998). Exercise also may have antithrombotic effects by decreasing plasma fibrinogen (Gautier et al., 1995). The potential for exercise-induced hypoglycemia also exists in type 2 patients, especially those on insulin or sulfonylurea therapy. Exercise should be performed after a meal or snack, with self-monitoring of glucose levels performed before and after exercise.

There are potential adverse effects of exercise for both types of diabetic patients. No exercise program should be initiated without a thorough physical examination to detect underlying cardiac disease. Intense exercise may exacerbate ischemic cardiac disease and cause silent MI or sudden death. Those with underlying proliferative retinopathy increase their risk of vitreous hemorrhage and retinal detachment, and those with neuropathy increase their risk of lower extremity injury (Gautier et al., 1995; Noble, 1996). Exercise programs should begin slowly, working up to periods of 20 to 45 minutes 3 days a week. To enhance weight loss, exercise frequency should be increased to at least 5 days a week.

## Stress Reduction

Because stress has been implicated as a causative agent in poor glycemic control, it has been hypothesized that stress reduction should have significant clinical implications for diabetes. Several research studies, using methods such as biofeedback and progressive relaxation training to improve glycemia, yield conflicting results (Aikens et al., 1997; Jablon et al., 1997; Lammers et al., 1984; Rosenbaum, 1983). There is insufficient evidence to conclude that stress reduction will help clients improve glycemic control.

## Antidiabetic Agents

The agents used to treat diabetes can be broadly classified into oral antidiabetic agents and insulin. Oral agents, which are further subdivided into classes based on mechanism of action, are effec-

tive only in treating type 2 diabetes (Burge et al., 1998; Romano et al., 1997; Schwartz et al., 1998). Insulin is required to treat type 1 diabetics and type 2 patients unresponsive to other treatment.

### Oral Medications

Oral medication is added to the treatment of type 2 diabetics who are unable to achieve glycemic control with dietary change, exercise, and weight loss. The treatment proceeds in a stepwise approach, based on responsiveness to therapy (Fig. 11-3). At each step, increasing dosages of drug can be given for improved response (using caution not to induce severe or multiple episodes of hypoglycemia with the sulfonylureas) (Burge et al., 1998). Sufficient time should be allowed at each step to achieve maximum response. FPG should be measured every 1 to 2 weeks (with medication dosage adjusted as necessary), and $HbA_{1c}$ should be measured every 2 to 3 months until glycemic goals are met (see Table 11-4). It is tempting to advance quickly to the next step or to initiate insulin therapy if goals are not met immediately. However, insulin

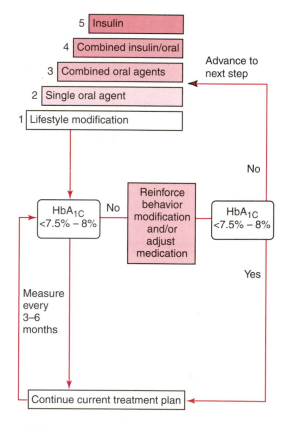

**FIGURE 11.3** ● Stepwise approach to management of type 2 diabetes.

therapy can have several drawbacks. If the client is responding to diet, exercise, and oral therapy with continued reductions in FPG and HbA$_{1c}$, then the practitioner should continue to monitor the client and proceed with this method of treatment until the patient fails to respond to therapy. Advancing to the next step is appropriate at this point.

## Insulin

Insulin is required to treat type 1 diabetes and is used as an adjunct to oral therapy in type 2 diabetes. Several types of insulin are available, with different onsets and durations of action (Herfindal & Gourley, 1996; Noble et al., 1998). Also, there are several different methods for dosing insulin. Conventional therapy requires less than three injections of insulin daily but produces worse glycemic control. Intensive treatment requires three or more injections daily, greatly improves glycemic control, and increases the risk of acute hypoglycemia. Because there is no "perfect" insulin regimen, treatment must be tailored to the individual's lifestyle and eating behaviors.

## Adjunctive Therapy

Because of the multisystem effects that diabetes exerts on the patient, the practitioner often ends up treating the sequelae of the disease as well as the disease itself. Studies indicate that treating hypertension with angiotensin converting enzyme (ACE) inhibitors provides renoprotective effects and slows progression of nephropathy (Aiello, 1998; Allen et al., 1997). Angiotensin II receptor antagonists, a new class of antihypertensive drugs, have not been studied sufficiently to determine their renoprotective effects. ACE inhibitors also may inhibit structural vascular change after long-term use (Bijlstra et al., 1995). Using beta blockers to treat hypertension may be contraindicated because of their ability to mask autonomic symptoms of impending hypoglycemia. Beta blockers also tend to worsen glycemic control, dyslipidemia, and peripheral vascular disease. Treatment of painful neuropathies with tricyclic antidepressants and topical creams that deplete substance P has been shown to be useful.

Clinical trials are under way to study aminoguanidine and its effect on AGEs, as well as the effect of aldose reductase inhibitors (which decrease sorbitol levels) on the prevention of neuropathies and CAD. A comprehensive review of the literature, as well as the standards of care set forth by the ADA, should guide the practitioner in treating the complications and comorbid conditions of diabetes.

## BENEFITS AND COMPLICATIONS OF THERAPY

With the publication of results from the Diabetes Control and Complications Trial (DCCT) in 1993, the need for good control of blood glucose levels became apparent. Results of the trial of 1441 volunteers with type 1 diabetes established that intensive therapy and maintenance of blood glucose levels as near to normal as possible delayed the onset of retinopathy, neuropathy, and nephropathy. Risk for developing retinopathy decreased by 76%, and progression of disease slowed by 54%. Microalbuminuria occurrence decreased by 39%, and albuminuria decreased by 54%. The risk of developing neuropathy dropped by 60% (The Diabetes Control and Complications Trial Research Group [DCCTRG], 1993). It also indicated, but did not prove, that macrovascular complications were decreased with tight control (Bantle, 1996a; DCCTRG, 1993; Karl & Riddle, 1996). DCCT researchers recommend intensive therapy for most type 1 patients.

The Japanese Kumamoto Study sought to determine if intensive treatment in type 2 patients would yield results similar to the DCCT. Although the study was much smaller (110 patients), the results matched those of the DCCT. Development of retinopathy was reduced by 69%, and nephropathy by 70% (Karl & Riddle, 1996). This suggests that good glycemic control should greatly reduce the risks of microvascular disease in type 2 patients (Bantle, 1996a). Results of the United Kingdom Prospective Diabetes Study, started in 1977 and recently concluded, also indicate that intensive therapy significantly improves health care status of type 2 diabetics, supporting the results of the DCCT and Kumamoto studies (Nathan, 1998).

The major side effects experienced by type 1 diabetics treated with intensive insulin regimens are weight gain (cause unknown) and severe hypoglycemia (Table 11-5) (Bantle, 1996b; Karl & Riddle, 1996). Side effects of oral hypoglycemic agents vary and generally are tolerable. The major side effect experienced by patients with type 2 diabetes treated with intensive insulin therapy is an increase in mild, not severe, hypoglycemia. The possibility also exists that insulin treatment increases the risk of cardiac disease (Niskanen, 1996). Insulin also can stimulate renal sodium retention and fluid overload, putting patients with compromised cardiac function at risk (DiGregorio, 1998).

## TABLE 11.5

### Signs and Symptoms of Hypoglycemia*

| Adrenergic | Central Nervous System Symptoms |
|---|---|
| Heart palpitations | Headache |
| Increased heart rate | Dullness |
| Perspiration | Confusion |
| Nervousness | Irritability |
| Tingling around the mouth | Hostility |
| Hunger | Mood swings |
| Weakness (this response frequently lost in type 1 diabetics; also masked by beta blockers) | Visual disturbances |
| | Drowsiness |
| | Lethargy (may be unable to help self at this point) |

*Treatment Guidelines*

1. Always check blood sugar first, if able.

2. Treat immediately with 15–20 g of carbohydrate (4 glucose tablets, ½ can sweetened cola, 1 cup juice, 4 tsp sugar in water, tube of icing gel, or 2 cups of skim milk.) Food with high fat content is absorbed more slowly so will not correct hypoglycemia quickly (Bantle, 1996b).

Individuals with severe hypoglycemic reactions should carry a Glucagon Emergency Kit.

3. In an acute-care setting, if patient is unconscious and cannot swallow, IV administration of $D_{50}W$ should be given, or 1 g of IM glucagon (Cydulka, 1997).

4. Recheck blood glucose in 15–20 min. If levels are not > 80, repeat the treatment. If patient does not plan to eat soon, patient also should eat a small snack.

$D_{50}W$, 50% dextrose in water; IM, intramuscular; IV, intravenous.
*Sudden drop in blood levels may cause more signs and symptoms than a slow fall.

## IMPLICATIONS FOR PRIMARY CARE PRACTICE

The ADA has set forth standards of practice to assist the provider in delivering quality care and education to the client with diabetes. Guidelines for taking an accurate history and performing a thorough physical examination are well defined (ADA, 1998). These standards are not intended to replace more extensive evaluation by specialists when indicated. The standards of diabetes care seek to provide the health care professional with a means to set treatment goals, assess quality of treatment, and determine the need for referral. It also provides persons with diabetes a way to assess the quality of care that they receive and to compare their progress with standard goals (ADA, 1998). Setting specific goals of therapy includes forming individualized targets of glycemic control, taking into account the patient's ability to understand and complete the prescribed regimen, and weighing benefit of therapy against risk. To achieve the goal of intensive therapy set forth in the DCCT and the Kumamoto studies, clients must be willing to perform frequent self-monitoring of blood glucose, to properly administer their own medication (or have a family member willing to learn to do so), and actively participate in managing their own disease. Figure 11-4 presents a stepped care treatment plan for type 2 diabetes.

## SUMMARY

There is no question that diabetes is a serious health threat. With a sixfold increase in the number of cases in the last 40 years and with the number of cases of diabetes expected to double by 2008, it is imperative that both the public and the health care professional become aware of the ramifications of this disease. Goals of all primary health care providers must include timely screening of at-risk individuals as well as prompt diagnosis and early intervention for individuals with diabetes mellitus. As nurse practitioners and other non-

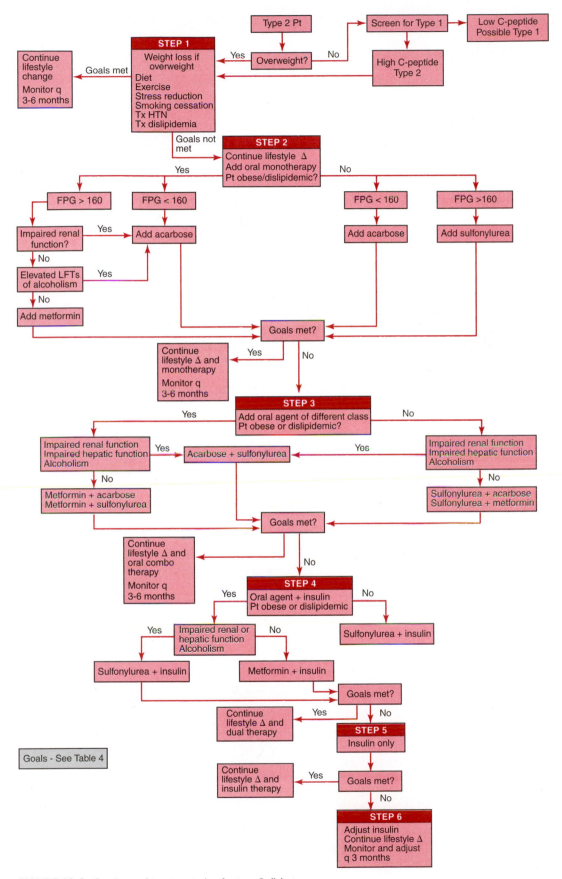

**FIGURE 11.4** ● Stepped treatment plan for type 2 diabetes.

physician providers continue to enter new arenas of primary care, they must be well prepared to encounter patients with this disease. Diabetes appears to be both preventable and predictable, and proper detection and management has been proven to decrease the sequelae of this disease. Building on a strong history of disease prevention and health promotion, primary care providers can change the direction that diabetes appears to be taking.

● **Case Study 11.1**

### Presentation

A 54-year-old Hispanic man presents to the primary care clinic with a 6-month history of worsening fatigue, hunger, and thirst. He also complains of polyuria with frequent episodes of nocturia, which are worsening his fatigue. He has gained approximately 35 lb in the last 2 years but has lost about 5 lb in the last week. He denies other medical conditions. His last physical examination was 3 years ago.

### History

#### Past Medical History

| | |
|---|---|
| Allergies | NKDA |
| Current medications | Occasional OTC NSAIDs for headache |
| | No prescription medications |
| Surgeries | Appendectomy, age 22. Tonsillectomy, age 8 |
| Injury/Trauma | Unremarkable |
| Childhood illness | Chicken pox, age 5 |
| Immunizations current | (No hx influenza, pneumonia, or Hep B vaccines) |

#### Social History

| | |
|---|---|
| Married | 31-y, monogamous relationship, 2 children |
| Tobacco | ½–1 ppd × 30 y |
| Alcohol | None |
| Social drugs | None |
| Caffeine | Several cups of coffee and tea daily |
| Exercise | Infrequent, sedentary job |
| Employment | Loan officer at a local bank × 15 y, source of stress |

#### Family History

| | |
|---|---|
| Mother | 77 y, HTN, DM type 2, MI @ 63 y |
| Father | 79 y, HTN |
| PGM | Died @ 45 of MI, hx of HTN, DM type 2 |
| Sister | 52 y, hyperlipidemia, DM @ 47 y |

#### 24-Hour Dietary Recall

Breakfast: 2 cups coffee, Danish
Lunch: Cheeseburger, chips, tea
Snack: Candy bar
Dinner: Steak, potato with butter and sour cream, salad with ranch dressing,
    roll and butter
Snack: Ice cream
Drinks tea and coffee all day long, constant thirst

*(Case study continued on next page)*

### Review of Systems

| | |
|---|---|
| General | Wt gain 35 lb in 2 y. Lost 5 lb in last wk |
| Skin | No problems. Denies trouble with healing. No hx rash, pruritus, lesions |
| HEENT | Denies visual change or disturbance (last exam 10 y ago). Does not wear corrective lenses. Denies dizziness. Has occasional stress headache. Denies difficulty swallowing, hoarseness, or sore throat. No hx thyroid disease |
| Lungs | Denies SOB at rest or on exertion. No PND. No hx asthma, pneumonia, or bronchitis |
| CV | Denies chest pain or palpitations at rest or on exertion. No hx MRG. No prior ECG |
| GI | No N&V. C/O increased hunger and thirst. Occasional constipation |
| GU | Denies dysuria, retention, hesitancy in starting a stream. C/O increased frequency and volume of urine × 6 months. Denies impotence |
| MS | Denies pain, tenderness, swelling of joints. Occasional low back pain from overexertion |
| Neurologic | Denies numbness, tingling, blackouts, seizures |

### Differential Diagnosis

1. Hypothyroidism
2. Anemia
3. BPH
4. Diabetes insipidus
5. Diabetes mellitus

### Physical Examination

| System | Findings |
|---|---|
| Vital signs | T–98.4°F, P–92, R–20<br>BP–176/94 sitting, 148/82 standing<br>Height 5'11", Weight 208 lb |
| General | Alert and oriented. In no acute distress<br>Mild/moderately obese |
| HEENT | Normocephalic. Vision 20/40 OU uncorrected. Cranial nerves intact. Funduscopic exam w/o hemorrhage or AV nicking. Optic disc margins well defined. Neck supple, no thyromegaly. No bruit, no palpable nodes. TMs intact, hearing normal at conversational levels. Throat clear, tonsils 1+ |
| Lungs | CTA bilat. Breath sounds equal |
| Cardiac | HRRR. No MRG |
| Abdomen | Nontender. No masses. No HSM. BS × 4 quad |
| GU | Circumcised man. No penile discharge. Testes nontender, no masses. No herniation |
| Rectal | Prostate nonenlarged, firm. No nodules |
| Extremities | Pulses 1+ bilateral lower, 2+ bilateral upper. No pedal edema. Skin warm, dry, and intact. Several calluses. Sensation intact |

*(Case study continued on page 224)*

## Laboratory Studies

| Test | Result |
|------|--------|
| CBC | WNL |
| Hg $A_{1c}$ | 10% |
| Urine | 2+ glucose, ketone negative |
| UA | Negative |
| Chem | FPG 251, otherwise WNL |
| Lipid profile | Cholesterol 345, triglycerides 317 |
| | HDL 24  LDL 174 |
| Thyroid profile | WNL |
| PSA | Pending |
| Baseline ECG | Normal sinus rhythm |

## Impression

1. Diabetes mellitus type 2
2. Obesity
3. Probable hypertension
4. Dyslipidemia

*Diagnosis of type 2 diabetes mellitus can be based on several key factors:*

Elevated FPG
Elevated Hg $A_{1c}$
Positive family history
Classic signs and symptoms of polyuria, polyphagia, polydipsia
History of weight gain
Negative ketones
Associated symptoms of HTN and dislipidemia

## Immediate Plan

1. Initiate patient education today regarding the risk factors, disease process, treatment options, and consequences of type 2 diabetes.
2. Agree on lifestyle and dietary modifications that the patient can implement until his next examination. Encourage weight loss, exercise, and healthy diet. Mention smoking and consequences of CAD, encourage cessation if patient is receptive. (When confronted with a new diagnosis such as this, a patient may not be able to make multiple lifestyle changes all at once. If not receptive to smoking cessation today, then approach it at each subsequent visit.)
3. Refer to a diabetes educator if available. This patient will need to learn to monitor his own glucose levels, plan an appropriate diet, and learn about his disease so that he can become an active participant in his own care.
4. Recheck in 2 weeks. If glycemic control is not improved, begin stepped therapy with oral agents. If significant improvement is noted, continue lifestyle and diet modifications and recheck in 2 more weeks.
5. Follow-up examinations should be agreed on. Follow ADA clinical guidelines.
6. Refer to an ophthalmologist for a dilated exam.
7. Institute treatment for hyperlipidemia per the AHA guidelines.
8. Continue to monitor blood pressure and institute therapy if indicated.
9. Encourage influenza, pneumonia, and Hep B vaccinations.

ADA, American Diabetes Association; AHA, American Heart Association; AV, arterial-venous; BP, blood pressure; BS, bowel sounds; BPH, benign prostatic hypertrophy; CAD, coronary artery disease; CBC, complete blood count; Chem, chemistry; C/O, complains of; CTA, clear to auscultation; DM, diabetes mellitus; ECG, electrocardiogram; FPG, fasting plasma glucose; GU, genitourinary; HDL, high-density lipoprotein; HEENT, head, eyes, ears, nose, and throat; Hep, hepatitis; HRRR, heart rate and rhythm regular; HSM, hepatosplenomegaly; HTN, hypertension; hx, history; LDL, low-density lipoproteins; MI, myocardial infarction; MRG, murmur, rub, or gallop; NKDA, no known drug allergy; NSAIDs, nonsteroidal anti-inflammatory drugs; OTC, over the counter; PGM, paternal grandmother; PND, paroxysmal nocturnal dyspnea; PSA, prostate-specific antigen; quad, quadrants; SOB, shortness of breath; TMs, tympanic membranes; WNL, within normal limits; w/o, without; UA, urinalysis.

A 21-year-old white female presents to the clinic with a 3-month history of worsening fatigue, hunger, and thirst. She also C/O all symptoms steadily worsening over the last 2 weeks. She has lost about 8 lb in the last week despite a ravenous appetite. Her last physical examination was approximately 18 months ago. She denies other medical conditions.

## History

### Past Medical History

| | |
|---|---|
| Allergies | Penicillin |
| Current medications | Low-dose oral birth control pills × 3 y |
| | Daily multivitamin. No prescription medications |
| Surgeries | None |
| Injury/Trauma | Fractured left ulna, age 7 y |
| Childhood illness | Mumps age 2 |
| Immunizations | Current (No hx influenza or pneumonia, +Hep B vaccines) |
| Pregnancy | G0,P0,A0 |

### Social History

| | |
|---|---|
| Single | Sexually active in a monogamous relationship |
| Tobacco | Denies |
| Alcohol | 1–2 beers/wk |
| Social drugs | Denies |
| Caffeine | Infrequently |
| Exercise | Runs 2–3 miles 3 × wk. Walks/lifts weights opposite running days |
| Employment | College senior: works part time in the bookstore 15–20 h/wk |

### Family History

| | |
|---|---|
| Mother | 46 y, no current medical conditions |
| Father | 47 y, HTN |
| PGM | 69 y, Graves' disease @ age 45, rheumatoid arthritis |
| MGM | 70 y, HTN, osteoarthritis |

### 24-Hour Dietary Recall

Breakfast: Orange juice, bagel, nonfat cream cheese
Lunch: Salad, dressing, crackers, apple, water
Snack: 4 chocolate chip cookies and milk
Dinner: Baked potato, tuna steak, salad, dressing, diet cola
Snack: Cheese sticks

## Review of Systems

| | |
|---|---|
| General | Weight loss 8 lb in 1 week. Generally fatigued |
| Skin | No problems. Denies trouble with healing. No hx rash, pruritus, or lesions |
| HEENT | Denies visual change or disturbance (last exam 1 y ago). Wears corrective lenses. Denies dizziness. Denies headache. Denies difficulty swallowing, hoarseness, or sore throat. No hx thyroid disease |

(Case study continued on page 226)

| Lungs | Denies SOB at rest or on exertion. No PND. No hx asthma, pneumonia, or bronchitis. Infrequent colds |
| Cardiac | Denies chest pain or palpitations at rest or on exertion. No hx MRG. No prior ECG |
| GI | No N&V. C/O increased hunger and thirst. Occasional diarrhea |
| GU | Denies dysuria, retention, hesitancy in starting a stream. C/O increased frequency and volume of urine × 3 months, worsening over the last 2 wk |
| MS | Denies pain, tenderness, swelling of joints |
| Neurologic | Denies numbness, tingling, blackouts, seizures |

### Differential Diagnosis

1. Hyperthyroidism
2. Anemia
3. Urinary tract infection
4. Diabetes insipidus
5. Diabetes mellitus

### Physical Examination

| System | Findings |
| --- | --- |
| Vital signs | T–98.8°F, P–68, R–16, BP-110/74 sitting, 106/68 standing Height 5'8", Weight 107 lb |
| General | Alert and oriented. In no acute distress. Thin but well-nourished female in NAD |
| HEENT | Normocephalic. Vision 20/20 OU corrected. Cranial nerves intact. Funduscopic exam without hemorrhage or AV nicking. Optic disc margins well defined. Neck supple, no thyromegaly, no bruit, no palpable nodes. TMs intact, hearing normal at conversational levels. Throat clear, tonsils 1+ |
| Lungs | CTA bilat. Breath sounds equal |
| Cardiac | HRRR. No MRG |
| Abdomen | Thin, nontender. No masses. No HSM. BS × 4 quad |
| GU | Deferred |
| Extremities | Pulses 2+ bilateral lower and upper. No pedal edema. Skin warm, dry, and intact. Sensation intact |

### Laboratory Studies

| Test | Result |
| --- | --- |
| CBC | WNL |
| $HbA_{1c}$ | 14% |
| Urine | 3+ glucose, ketone positive |
| UA | Negative |
| Chem | FPG 411, $HCO_3$ 19 mEq/L, pH 7.29 |
| Lipid profile | Cholesterol 179, triglycerides 115 HDL 45   LDL 110 |
| Thyroid profile | WNL |

*(Case study continued on next page)*

### Impression

Diabetes mellitus type 1

*Diagnosis of type 1 diabetes mellitus can be based on several key factors*

Elevated FPG
Elevated $HbA_{1c}$
Classic signs and symptoms of polyuria, polyphagia, polydipsia
History of weight loss
Positive ketones
Metabolic acidosis ($HCO_3$ 19, pH 7.29)

### Immediate Plan

1. Initiate patient education today regarding the risk factors, disease process, treatment options, and consequences of type 1 diabetes.
2. Initiate insulin therapy.
3. Agree on lifestyle and dietary modifications that the patient can implement until her next examination.
4. This patient will need to learn to monitor her own glucose levels, plan an appropriate diet, and learn about her disease so that she can become an active participant in her own care. Depending on the client's level of motivation and ability to learn, she could be treated on an outpatient basis. However, this client would be a good candidate for hospitalization. She can use hospital resources for education and training while she is receiving medical care.
5. After stabilization/hospitalization, this client will need frequent education and monitoring. Provide her with as much time as she needs, make frequent office appointments, and find community resources for her.
6. Follow-up examinations should be agreed on. Follow ADA clinical guidelines.

ADA, American Diabetic Association; AV, arterial-venous; BP, blood pressure; CBC, complete blood count; C/O, complains of; CTA, clear to auscultation; ECG, electrocardiogram; FPG, fasting plasma glucose; GI, gastrointestinal; GU, genitourinary; $HCO_3$, bicarbonate; HDL, high-density lipoprotein; HEENT, head, eyes, ears, nose, and throat; Hep, hepatitis; HSM, hepatosplenomegaly; HRRR, heart rate and rhythm regular; HTN, hypertension; Hx, history; LDL, low-density lipoprotein; MGM, maternal grandmother; MRG, murmur, rub, or gallop; MS, musculoskeletal; NAD, no apparent distress; N&V, nausea and vomiting; P, pulse; PGM, paternal grandmother; PND, paroxysmal nocturnal dyspnea; quad, quadrants; R, respiration; SOB, shortness of breath; T, temperature; TMs, tympanic membranes; UA, urinalysis; WNL, within normal limits.

---

### ● Professional Resources

The following is a list of resources for primary care providers and their patients that may prove useful in dealing with the management of diabetes.

Organizations:

American Diabetes Association
National Office
1660 Duke Street
Alexandria, VA 22314
(800) 232-3472
*http://www.diabetes.org/ada/Info.html*

American Dietetic Association
216 W. Jackson Blvd.
Chicago, IL 60606-6995
(800) 877-1600
*http://www.eatright.org*

*(continued)*

American Heart Association
7272 Greenville Ave.
Dallas, TX 75231
1 (800) AHA-USA1
*http://www.americanheart.org/contact.html*

Canadian Diabetes Association
National Office
15 Toronto St. Ste. #800
Toronto, ON
M5C 2E3
*http://www.diabetes.ca*

Centers for Disease Control and Prevention
1600 Clifton Rd., NE
Atlanta, GA 30333
(404) 639-3311
*http://www.cdc.gov*

CDC's Diabetes and Public Health Resource
*http://www.cdc.gov/nccdphp/ddt/ddthome.htm*

Diabetes Australia-NSW
GPO Box 9824
Sydney NSW 2001
*http://www.diabetes-australia.com.au*

Diabetes Australia House
26 Arundel Street
Glebe NSW 2037
02 9552 9900
*http://www.talent.com.au/diabetes/diabeteswelcome*

The Diabetes Center of the Albert Einstein
College of Medicine
Yeshiva University in New York
Jack D. Weiler Hospital
1825 Eastchester Road
Bronx, NY 10461
*http://medicine.aecom.yu.edu/diabetes/DC.htm*

Federation of European Nurses in Diabetes
(FEND)
*http://www.fend.org*

International Diabetes Federation
1 rue Defacqz
B-1000 Brussels
Belgium
32-2/538 55 11
Fax: 32-2/538 51 14
*http://www.idf org*

Joslin Diabetes Center
Room 616
One Joslin Place
Boston, MA 02215
(617) 735-1932
*http://dnacore.joslab.harvard.edu/core/contact.html*

Juvenile Diabetes Foundation International
120 Wall Street
New York, NY 10005-4001
(212) 785-9500
(800) JDF-CURE
*http://www.jdf.org*

National Diabetes Information Clearinghouse
1 Information Way
Bethesda, MD 20892-3560
E-mail:ndicC~irfo.niddk.m.h.gov
*http://www.niddk.nih.gov/health/diabetes/ndic.htm*

National Institute of Diabetes and Digestive
and Kidney Diseases
*http:/Iwww.niddk.nih.gov*

National Institutes of Health
Bethesda, MD 20892
http://www.nih.gov

● **Journals:**

American Diabetes Association
*Diabetes* and *Diabetes Care*
*http://journal.diabetes.org*

Canadian Diabetes Association
*Diabetes Dialogue*
http://www.diabetes.ca/cda/ddsum.htm

*Journal of the American Medical Association*
Directory of Specialty Journals
*http://www.ama~assn.org/public/journals/jama/ jamahome.htm*

*The New England Journal of Medicine*
10 Shattuck Street
Boston, MA 02115-6094
(617) 734-9800
*http://www.nejm.org/content/index.asp*

● **World Wide Web:**

CliniWeb—An index and table of contents to
clinical information
Oregon Health Sciences University
*http://www.ohsu.edu/cliniweb/search.html*

## REFERENCES

Aiello, J.H. (1998). Preventing diabetic nephropathy: The role of primary care. *The Nurse Practitioner, 23* (2), 12–31.

Aikens, J.E., Kiolbasa, T.A., & Sobel, R. (1997). Psychological predictors of glycemic change with relaxation training in non-insulin-dependent diabetes mellitus. *Psychotherapy and Psychosomatics, 66* (6), 302–306.

Allen, T.J., Cao, Z., Youssef, S., Hulthen, U.L., & Cooper, M.E. (1997). Role of angiotensin II and bradykinin in experimental diabetic nephropathy. *Diabetes, 46* (10), 1612–1618.

American Diabetes Association. (1997). 57th Annual meeting and scientific sessions June 21–24, 1997. *Clinician Reviews, 7* (8), 162–165, 168–170.

American Diabetes Association. (1998). Clinical practice recommendations 1998. *Diabetes Care, 21* (Suppl. 1).

American Heart Association. (1998). *Diabetes mellitus statistics.* Available at: http://207.211.141.25/Heart_and_Stroke_A_Z_Guide/diabs.html.

Bantle, J.P. (1996a). Diabetes mellitus: Guide to implementing intensive therapy. *Consultant, 36* (11), 2353–2362.

Bantle, J.P. (1996b). How to recognize and manage hypoglycemia in diabetes. *Consultant, 36* (11), 2363–2364.

Bijlstra, P.J., Smits, P., Lutterman, J.A., & Thien, T. (1995). Effect of long-term angiotensin-converting enzyme inhibition on endothelial function in patients with the insulin resistance syndrome. *Journal of Cardiovascular Pharmacology, 25* (4), 658–664.

Boden, G. (1997). Perspectives in diabetes: Role of fatty acids in the pathogenesis of insulin resistance and NIDDM. *Diabetes, 46* (1), 3–10.

Burge, M.R., Schmitz-Fiorentino, K., Fischette, C., Qualls, C.R, & Schade, D.S. (1998). A prospective trial of risk factors for sulfonylurea-induced hypoglycemia in type 2 diabetes mellitus. *Journal of the American Medical Association, 279* (2), 137–143.

Butler, R.N., Rubenstein, A.H., Gracia, A.G., & Zweig, S.C. (1998). Type 2 diabetes: Causes, complications, and new screening recommendations. *Geriatrics, 53* (3 Pt. 1), 47–54.

Capaldo, B., Lembo, G., Napoli, R., Rendina, V., Albano, G., Sacca, L., & Trimarco, B. (1991). Skeletal muscle is a primary site of insulin resistance in hypertension. *Metabolism, 40* (12), 1320–1322.

Cydulka, R.K. (1997). Thwarting the glucose-related crisis. *Emergency Medicine, 29* (6), 18–29.

Davidson, M.B. (1998). *Diabetes mellitus: Diagnosis and treatment* (4th ed.). Philadelphia: W.B. Saunders.

DeFronzo, R.A. & Ferrannini, E. (1991). Insulin resistance: A multifaceted syndrome responsible for NIDDM obesity, hypertension, dyslipidemia, and atherosclerotic cardiovascular disease. *Diabetes Care, 14* (3), 173–194.

The Diabetes Control and Complications Trial Research Group. (1993). The effect of intensive treatment of diabetes on the development and progression of long-term complications in insulin-dependent diabetes mellitus. *The New England Journal of Medicine, 329* (14), 977–986.

DiGregorio, R.V. (1998). Managing heart failure in diabetic patients. *U.S. Pharmacist,* June, 101–112.

Egan, B.M., Stepniakowski, K., & Nazzaro, P. (1994). Insulin levels are similar in obese salt-sensitive and salt-resistant hypertensive subjects. *Hypertension, 23* (Suppl.), 11–17.

Elbein, S.C. (1997). Obesity: Common symptom of diverse gene-based metabolic dysregulations. *American Society for Nutritional Sciences* (Suppl.), 1891S–1896S.

Equiluz-Bruck, S., Schnack, C., Kopp, H.P., & Schernthaner, G. (1996). Nondipping of nocturnal blood pressure is related to urinary albumin excretion rate in patients with type 2 diabetes mellitus. *The American Journal of Hypertension, 9* (11), 1139–1143.

Fantus, I.G., Delovitch, T.L., & Dupre, J. (1997). Prevention of diabetes mellitus: Goal for the twenty-first century: Part II. *Canadian Journal of Diabetes Care, 21* (4), 14–20.

Fernandez-Castaner, M., Blarnes, J., Camps, I., Ripolles, J., Gomez, N., & Soler, J. (1996). Beta-cell dysfunction in first-degree relatives of patients with non-insulin dependent diabetes mellitus. *Diabetic Medicine, 13* (11), 953–959.

Ferrannini, E., Buzzigoli, G., Bonadonna, R., Giorico, M.A., Oleggini, M., Graziadei, L., Pedrinelli, R., Brandi, L., & Bevilacqua, S. (1987). Insulin resistance in essential hypertension. *The New England Journal of Medicine, 317* (6), 350–357.

Galletti, F., Strazzullo, P., Ferrara, I., Annuzzi, G., Rivellese, A.A., Galto, S., & Mancini, M. (1997). NaCl sensitivity of essential hypertensive patients is related to insulin resistance. *Journal of Hypertension, 15* (12 Pt. 1), 1485–1491.

Gautier, J.F., Scheen, A., & Lefebvre, P.J. (1995). Exercise in the management of non-insulin-dependent (type 2) diabetes mellitus. *International Journal of Obesity, 1995, 19* (Suppl. 4), S58–S61.

Hendey, G.W. (1998). Screening for ketones: Do use the dip test. *Emergency Medicine, 28* (2), 129–130.

Herfindal, E.T. & Gourley, D.R. (Eds.). (1996). *Textbook of therapeutics: Drug and disease management* (6th ed.). Baltimore: Williams & Wilkins.

Hoieggen, A., Fossum, E., Moan, A., Enger, E., & Kjeldsen, S.E. (1998). Whole-blood viscosity and the insulin-resistance syndrome. *Journal of Hypertension, 16* (2), 203–210.

Honeyman, M.C., Harrison, L.C., Drummond, B., Colman, P.G., & Tait, B.D. Analysis of families at risk for insulin-dependent diabetes mellitus reveals that HLA antigens influence progression to clinical disease. *Molecular Medicine 1* (5), 576–582.

Horwitz, M.S., Bradley, L.M., Harbertson, J., Krahl T., Lee, J., & Sarvetnick, N. (1998). Diabetes induced by coxsackie virus: Initiation by bystander damage and not molecular mimicry. *Nature and Medicine 4* (7), 781–785.

Jablon, S.L., Naliboff, B.D., Gilmore, S.L., & Rosenthal, M.J. (1997). Effects of relaxation training on glucose tolerance and diabetic control in type II diabetes. *Applied Psychophysiology and Biofeedback, 22* (3), 155–169.

Kahn, S.E., Andrikopoulos, S., & Verchere, C.B. (1999). Islet amyloid: A long-recognized but underappreciated pathological feature of type 2 diabetes. *Diabetes, 48* (2), 241–253.

Kalergis, M., Pacaud, D., & Yale, J.F. (1998). Attempts to control the glycemic response to carbohydrate in diabetes mellitus: Overviews and practical implications. *Canadian Journal of Diabetes Care, 22* (1), 20–29.

Karl, D.M. & Riddle, M.C. (1996). Diabetes mellitus: Lessons from the DCCT and how to implement them. *Consultant, 36* (8), 1670–1681.

Kelly, S., Hertzman, C., & Daniels, M. (1997). Searching for the biological pathways between stress and health. *Annual Review of Public Health, 18,* 437–462.

Kobrin, S. & Aradhye, S. (1997). Preventing progression and complications of renal disease. *Hospital Medicine, 33* (11), 11–12, 17–18, 20, 29–31, 35–36, 39–40.

Laine, H., Knuuti, M.J., Ruotsalainen, U., Raitakari, M., Iida, H., Kaponen, J., Kirvela, O., Haaparanta, M., Yki-Jarvinen, H., & Nuutila, P. (1998). Insulin resistance in essential hypertension is characterized by impaired insulin stimulation of blood flow in skeletal muscle. *Journal of Hypertension, 16* (2), 211–219.

Lammers, C.A., Naliboff, B.M., & Straatmeyer, A.J. (1984). The effects of progressive relaxation on stress and diabetic control. *Behavioral Research and Therapy, 22* (6), 641–650.

Laviades, C., Gil, M.J., Monreal, I., Gonzalez, A., & Diez, J. (1998). Tissue availability of insulin-like growth factor I is inversely related to insulin resistance in essential hypertension: Effects of angiotensin converting enzyme inhibition. *Journal of Hypertension, 16* (6), 863–870.

Lind, L., Lithel, H., Gustaffson, I.B., Pollare, T., & Ljungal, S. (1992). Metabolic cardiovascular risk factors and sodium sensitivity in hypertensive subjects. *American Journal of Hypertension, 5* (8), 502–505.

Mayer-Davis, E.J., D'Agostino, R., Karter, A.J., Haffner, S.J., Rewers, M.J., Saad, M., & Bergman, R.N. (1998). Intensity and amount of physical activity in relation to insulin sensitivity. *Journal of the American Medical Association, 279* (9), 669–674.

McPhee, S.J., Lingappa, V.R., Ganong, W.F., & Lange, J.D. (Eds.). (1997). *Pathophysiology of disease: An introduction to clinical medicine* (2nd ed.). Stamford, CT: Appleton & Lange.

Meigs, J.B., Nathan, D.M., Wilson, P.W.F., Cupples, L.A., & Singer, D.E. (1998). Metabolic risk factors worsen continuously across the spectrum of nondiabetic glucose tolerance: The Framingham Offspring Study. *Annals of Internal Medicine, 128* (7), 524–533.

Mittelman, S.D., Fu, Y., Rebrin, K., Steil, G., & Bergman, R.N. (1998). Indirect effect of insulin to suppress endogenous glucose production is dominant, even with hyperglucagonemia. *Journal of Clinical Investigation, 100* (12), 3121–3130.

Muscelli, E., Camastra, S., Gastaldelli, A., Natali, A., Masoni, A., Pecori, N., & Ferrannini, E. (1998). Influence of duration of obesity on the insulin resistance of obese non-diabetic patients. *International Journal of Obesity, 22* (3), 262–267.

Nathan, D.M. (1998). Some answers, more controversy, from the UKPDS. *The Lancet, 352* (9131), 832–833.

National Institutes of Health. (1996, Sept. 10) News release.

Niklasson, B., Hornfeldt, B., & Lundman, B. (1998). Could myocarditis, insulin-dependent diabetes mellitus, and Guillain-Barré syndrome be caused by one or more infectious agents carried by rodents? *Emerging Infectious Diseases, 4* (2), 187–193.

Niskanen, L. (1996). Insulin treatment in elderly patients with non-insulin-dependent diabetes mellitus: A double-edged sword? *Drugs and Aging, 8* (3), 183–192.

Noble, J. (Ed.). (1996). *Textbook of primary care medicine* (2nd ed.). New York: Mosby.

Noble, S.L., Johnston, E., & Walton, B. (1998). Insulin lispro: A fast-acting insulin analog. *American Family Physician, 57* (2), 279–286.

Norris, J.M., Beaty, B., Klingensmith, G., Yu, L., Hoffman, M., Chase, H.P., Erlich, H.A., Hamman, R.F., Eisenbarth, G.S., & Rewers, M. (1996). Lack of association between early exposure to cow's milk protein and beta-cell autoimmunity. *Journal of the American Medical Association, 276* (8), 609–614.

Pennisi, E. (1997). Tracing molecules that make the brain-body connection. *Science, 275* (5302), 930–931.

Pike, J.L., Smith, T.L., Hauger, R.L., Nicassio, P.M., Patterson, T.L., McClintock, J., Costlow, C., & Irwin, M.R. (1997). Chronic life stress alters sympathetic, neuroendocrine, and immune reponsivity to an acute psychological stressor in humans. *Psychosomatic Medicine, 59* (4), 447–457.

Pratley, R.E, Thompson, D.B, Prochazka, M., Baier, L., Mott, D., Ravussin, E., Sakul, H., Ehm, M.G., Burns, D.K., Foroud, T., Garvey, W.T., Hanson, R.L., Knowler, W.C., Bennett, P.H., & Bogardus, C. (1998). An autosomal genomic scan for loci linked to prediabetic phenotypes in Pima Indians. *The Journal of Clinical Investigation, 101* (8), 1757–1764.

Reusch, JE. (1993). Focus on insulin resistance in type 2 diabetes: Therapeutic implications. *The Diabetes Educator, 24* (2), 188–193.

Romano, G., Patti, L., Innelli, F., DiMarino, L., Annuzzi, G., Iavicoli, M., Coronel, G.A., Riccardi, G., & Rivellese, A.A. (1997). Insulin and sulfonylurea therapy in NIDDM patients: Are the effects on lipoprotein metabolism different even with similar blood glucose control? *Diabetes, 46* (10), 1601–1606.

Rosenbaum, L. (1983). Biofeedback-assisted stress management for insulin-treated diabetes mellitus. *Biofeedback and Self-Regulation, 8* (4), 519–532.

Salonen, J.T., Lakka, T.A., Lakka, H., Valkonen, V., Everson, S.A., & Kaplan, G.A. (1998). Hyperinsulinism is associated with the incidence of hypertension and dyslipidemia in middle-aged men. *Diabetes, 47* (2), 270–275.

Satcher, D. (1998). *Diabetes: A serious public health problem*. Atlanta: Centers for Disease Control and Prevention. Available on-line at: http://www.cdc.gov/nccdphp/ddt/glance/html.

Schatz, D.A. & Maclaren, N.K. (1996). Cow's milk and insulin-dependent diabetes mellitus: Innocent until proven guilty. *Journal of the American Medical Association, 276* (8), 647–648.

Schernthaner, G. (1996). Cardiovascular mortality and morbidity in type-2 diabetes mellitus. *Diabetes Research and Clinical Practice, 31* (Suppl.), S3–S13.

Schwartz, S., Raskin, P., Fonseca, V., & Graveline, J.F. (1998). Effect of troglitazone in insulin-treated patients with type II diabetes mellitus. *The New England Journal of Medicine, 338* (13), 861–866.

Sharma, A.M., Ruland, K., Spies, K.P., & Distler, A. (1991). Salt sensitivity in young normotensive subjects is associated with a hyperinsulinemic response to oral glucose. *Journal of Hypertension, 9* (4), 329–335.

Sharma, A.M., Schorr, U., & Distler, A. (1993). Insulin resistance in young salt-sensitive normotensive subjects. *Hypertension, 21* (3), 273–279.

Turner, R., Stratton, I., Horton, V., Manley, S., Zimmet, P., Mackay, I.R., Shattock, M., Bottazzo, G.F., & Holman, R. (1997). UKPDS 25: Autoantibodies to islet-cell cytoplasm and glutamic acid decarboxylase for prediction of insulin requirements in type 2 diabetes. *The Lancet, 350* (9087), 1288–1293.

Wunderlich, R.P., Peters, E.J., Bosma, J., & Armstrong, D.G. (1998). Pathophysiology and treatment of painful diabetic neuropathy of the lower extremity. *Southern Medical Journal 91* (10), 894–898.

# Common Breast Disorders

Margaret Pierce

It has been estimated that one of two American women will consult a health care provider about a breast disorder at some time in her life. Most of these women will not have a malignancy, but breast cancer is the most feared diagnosis by women according to a recent Gallup poll, and it is the second leading cause of cancer death in women. Once the diagnosis of breast cancer is ruled out, providers may consider the woman's concern unimportant, perhaps because of a lack of understanding of nonmalignant breast problems. The primary care provider must be able to accurately assess a breast problem, determine referral needs, and, often, provide treatment and follow-up for nonmalignant breast problems. This chapter focuses on common nonmalignant breast problems. It is divided into common presenting "complaints," with potential pathologies for each complaint addressed. The pathology of breast cancer will also be discussed.

Most breast problems present as palpable masses, inflammatory lesions, nipple discharge, or suspicious mammogram findings. In a study in which women were evaluated for a breast concern, 30% were found to have no breast disease, 40% had fibrocystic changes, and another 7% had fibroadenoma. Approximately 10% were diagnosed with breast cancer, and the remainder had a variety of nonmalignant pathologies.

## ANATOMY AND NORMAL BREAST PHYSIOLOGY

The breasts are basically a collection of lobes and ducts surrounded by layers of fat and fibrous connective tissue lying under the skin and on the pectorales muscle and fascia. The ligaments of Cooper anchor the breast to this muscle. A small portion of breast tissue extends into the axilla, forming the tail of Spence (Fig. 12-1). The ducts and periductal tissue respond to hormonal stimulation, accounting for changes in size and function through the life span and through the menstrual cycle, pregnancy, and lactation.

Each lobe of the breast is drained by a specific duct, which joins with other ducts to form lactiferous sinuses; these sinuses enlarge and open on the surface of the nipple. The nipple and areola are covered by more darkly pigmented skin and contain bands of smooth muscle. The nipples become erect when these muscles contract. In a nonpregnant state, the nipples usually are sealed with a keratin plug.

The breasts are found along two lines, the milk lines. Accessory, or supernumary, breast tissue can develop anywhere along these milk lines, and, rarely, pathologic conditions associated with the breast may occur in them.

The breasts are essentially identical in both the male and female until puberty, when hormones from the pituitary gland and ovaries stimulate development in girls. With the onset of menarche, breast development increases rapidly and significantly. The five stages of development, Tanner stages, are pictured in Figure 12-2. They begin with stage 1, elevation of the nipple in the preadolescent stage, and move to stage 2, the appearance of breast buds, enlargement of the areola, and slight raising of the nipple. Stage 3 is characterized by growth of both the areola and breast tissue, with little distinction between the elevation of these structures. In stage 4, the areola and nipple again become more distinct, forming a small second mound on the breast. Stage 5 represents the mature female breast with the areola flattened again and only the nipple projecting above the

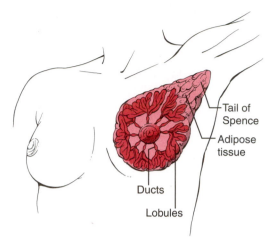

**FIGURE 12.1** ● The glandular anatomy of the breast, including the tail of Spence.

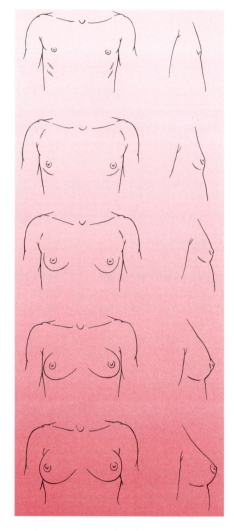

**FIGURE 12.2** ● Tanner's stages of breast development. (From Mitchell, G.W. & Bassett, G.W. [1990] *The female breast and its disorders.* Baltimore: Williams & Wilkins.)

breast. This development occurs primarily because of the influence of estrogen and progesterone, but additional hypothalamic-pituitary-ovarian hormones are believed to be important in this process.

During pregnancy, the breasts enlarge and develop more prominent vasculature, and the areola and nipple usually become more deeply pigmented. Lactogen and prolactin influence this development early in pregnancy. Microscopically, fat and connective tissue decrease as glandular hyperplasia occurs. Existing lobules enlarge, and new lobules form in preparation for lactation.

## COMMON BREAST COMPLAINTS

### Breast Pain (Mastalgia)

Breast pain is a common complaint of women, especially in the reproductive years. It is the most common concern brought to the attention of the health care provider, one that is often accompanied by a high level of fear (Blackwell & Grotting, 1997). Many women present with a triad of symptoms of pain, tenderness, and nodularity. Cyclic discomfort and nodularity are so common that most practitioners, and many women, consider them "normal" and do not seek any care for these symptoms. Some, however, have had their concerns dismissed as "nothing to worry about" when the symptoms were debilitating. Differentiating normal cyclic changes from pathologic conditions is critical, and management of the nonpathologic cyclic mastalgia can enhance health and well-being for many women.

### Cyclic Mastalgia

Mastalgia is classified as cyclic, noncyclic, and nonbreast in origin. Cyclic mastalgia is experienced so commonly that often it is considered physiologic. It occurs most frequently among women in their 30s and 40s. Women typically report a sense of fullness, heaviness, tenderness, or heightened awareness of the breasts, which may extend into the axilla or even upper arms, for 3 to 7 days before menses and which disappears, or at least diminishes, with the onset of menstrual flow. For some women, however, these symptoms occur for most, or even all, of the menstrual cycle.

The terminal ducts of breast lobules undergo changes during the regular menstrual cycle. During the luteal phase, after ovulation, mitotic activity in the ducts increases, epithelium becomes vacuolated, and the intralobular stroma becomes edematous (Rubin & Farber, 1994). Women perceive these changes as increasing heaviness, fullness, and tenderness premenstrually. As estrogen and progesterone levels decrease with the onset of menses, there is an increase in cell death and regression of the ducts. Most women with mastalgia report diminished symptoms at this time, hence the term *cyclic mastalgia*. No consistently abnormal estrogen or progesterone levels have been found in women experiencing cyclic mastalgia. However, the fact that hormonal disruption from drugs, surgery, or menopause often results in reduction of symptoms suggests a relationship between hormones and mastalgia. An elevated release of prolactin and thyrotropin-releasing hormone was noted in women with cyclic breast pain (Gately et al., 1992). Fatty acid and lipid levels also have been though to have a potential relationship with cyclic mastalgia. Theoretically, altered levels of fatty acids in the plasma would affect hormone receptors. Several studies show that women with cyclic mastalgia are more likely than controls to have low levels of gamma linolenic acid and its metabolites, which are important in maintaining the integrity of cell membranes.

### Noncyclic Mastalgia

Noncyclic mastalgia tends to occur in women who are in their 40s or older, with symptoms spontaneously resolving in approximately 50% of patients. This pain may be constant, or intermittent and irregular. It usually is unilateral; often is in the upper outer quadrant, radiating to the axilla or arm; and usually is associated with nodularity. This pain is not related to the menstrual cycle and may be localized to a "trigger spot." Women often describe it as an ache, throbbing, or burning sensation. In postmenopausal women, this presentation should lead to a careful evaluation for malignancy. Early lobular carcinoma has been associated with a presenting complaint of breast pain (Preece, 1990). Breast pain typically is not associated with malignancy, and its presence as a symptom of early breast cancer is not uniformly acknowledged. However, research suggests that lobular carcinoma may be more likely to cause pain. Therefore, it is important for the health care provider to consider this diagnosis in any woman presenting with breast pain.

It is critical for the clinician to consider multiple etiologies when evaluating a woman with noncyclic mastalgia. Nonbreast etiologies should be considered, and an appropriate history and physical examination should be performed. Although a detailed discussion is beyond the scope of this chapter, the clinician should consider the following possible diagnoses: musculoskeletal etiologies such as costochondritis or Tietze's syndrome, cervical radiculopathy, myocardial infarction or coronary artery disease, hiatal hernia, myalgia, neuralgia, pleurisy, cholecystitis, cervical rib anomaly, psychological pathologies, and tuberculosis. After a mastectomy, women may experience phantom pain in this region, which understandably causes fear of cancer recurrence. Once these etiologies have been ruled out, mammary etiologies should be considered and evaluated.

### General Management Principles

The management approaches of cyclic and noncyclic mastalgia are similar. Once a malignant or infectious etiology is ruled out, cyclic breast pain may be managed in a variety of ways. Often, the patient with cyclic mastalgia also has some degree of nodularity and may be diagnosed as having "fibrocystic disease" or "fibrocystic changes." These terms are considered to be inaccurate and confusing by most health professionals. (Breast nodules or lumps are discussed in another section of this chapter.) The overall management of cyclic and noncyclic mastalgia is the same. Therapy can be divided into nonhormonal and hormonal approaches.

## PHYSIOLOGIC BASIS OF TREATMENT

### Nonhormonal Approaches

For many women, understanding the normal physiologic process causing breast pain, coupled with reassurance that there is no malignancy, infection, or other identifiable pathology, is enough to relieve pain significantly. However, for others, reassurance does not alleviate symptoms sufficiently, and other approaches are necessary. A breast pain calendar is useful to determine if there is a hormonal relationship. The calendar includes dates of menses, treatments used, and a pain-rating scale for each day. Patterns are identified easily using this tool. If pharmacologic interventions are used, responses to treatment also can be evaluated.

The importance of a properly fitting brassiere often is overlooked when managing breast pain. Support of the ligaments of the breast, especially for large-breasted women, relieves pain for many. The role of diet and exercise has not been confirmed in large studies, but several reports recommend increased physical activity as one approach to managing mastalgia. Aerobic exercise has been demonstrated to increase endorphins, thereby decreasing chronic pain. Weight loss may decrease estrogen levels, which may play a significant role in cyclic breast pain.

Varieties of treatments have been advocated in the literature, many of them without significant scientific basis. Diuretics have been prescribed based on the belief that breast pain results from premenstrual fluid and sodium retention. This approach is not effective and may increase discomfort by causing rebound edema. Caffeine abstention and consumption of vitamins A, B₆, and E have been recommended, but none of these have been shown to have more that a placebo effect in controlled trials.

Nonsteroidal anti-inflammatory drugs (NSAIDs) have been shown to relieve pain for many women, often negating the need for other interventions. The prostaglandin-inhibiting effects of NSAIDs may not only decrease pain, but also may play a role in reducing engorgement of ducts. Evening primrose oil has a high concentration of linoleic acid, which also may affect prostaglandin metabolism, thereby decreasing cyclic mastalgia. It is apparently nontoxic and may be an attractive therapeutic intervention for women who want to avoid hormonal therapies.

### Hormonal Therapies

Oral contraceptives both increase and decrease breast pain. Breast pain is a common side effect of hormonal therapy, especially during the first months. However, these agents are successful in relieving cyclic mastalgia. Also, many women report an increase in symptoms when they discontinue oral contraceptives. The basis of this approach is the association of mastalgia with changes in estrogen levels during the menstrual cycle. However, because the true etiology of cyclic mastalgia still is poorly understood, it remains unclear whether this approach has a solid scientific rationale.

Bromocriptine, a dopamine agonist, stimulates dopamine release from the posterior pituitary, which inhibits prolactin release. Some clinicians believe that prolactin is a cause of cyclic breast pain based on its role in lactation. Although this drug relieves breast pain, it also has significant side effects, including postural hypotension and decreased fertility, making it an option to be used with caution.

Danazol is an androgen variant that decreases secretion of follicle-stimulating hormone (FSH) and luteinizing hormone, inhibiting ovulation, corpus luteum development, and menstruation. It has been found to decrease breast pain, but because it suppresses menstruation, many clinicians use it only for 3 to 4 months at a time. In women with cystic changes, danazol does decrease cyst size. Hot flashes, irritability, and masculinizing effects make it another drug to be used with caution.

Tamoxifen, an antiestrogen that has been used primarily to treat breast cancer, blocks estrogen receptor sites, thereby counteracting the effects of estrogen on cells. It is reported to be effective in reducing breast pain, but some clinicians are reluctant to prescribe it, possibly because of its association with cancer therapy.

## NODULARITY

The appropriate terminology to use when describing palpable lumps in the breast has been a matter of debate in the medical community. The terms "fibrocystic disease" and "fibrocystic changes" are controversial. Many clinicians and researchers observe that these terms are used to describe conditions ranging from swelling and pain to nipple discharge, and that they sometimes are used to describe normal developmental changes in breast tissues. Although there is not a complete consensus, it is useful to divide these changes into three categories: nonproliferative lesions, proliferative lesions without atypia, and atypical hyperplasia, as recommended by The College of American Pathologists as a clinically and histologically relevant taxonomy (Cancer Committee of the American College of Pathologists, 1986).

## NONPROLIFERATIVE CHANGES

In premenopausal women, the normal breast is somewhat nodular, especially in the upper outer quadrant and the inframammary ridge. Nodules that change in size with the menstrual cycle are normal findings, albeit sometimes associated with mastalgia (cyclic mastalgia is discussed in an earlier section of this chapter). Fibrocystic changes account for 70% of palpable breast masses. These commonly include cysts, fibrosis, ductal ectasia, mastitis, fibroadenomas, metaplasia, squamous or papillary apocrine changes, mild epithelial hyperplasia, and mild sclerosing adenosis.

Cysts may develop in one breast but are more likely bilateral and often multiple. Lobules and ducts may be dilated by the cyst, producing a poorly defined thickening or discrete palpable lumps: clusters of microcysts, which have a pallet-like or "shotty" texture to palpation. On mammogram, microcalcifications often are noted because of the calcification of secretions within the cyst. Surgically removed benign cysts typically are dark brown or blue because of the accumulation of turbid fluid within the cyst; however, this is not discernible on physical examination.

When cysts spontaneously rupture, the inflammatory response results in scarring and fibrosis, making the area firm. Cystic lesions in post-menopausal women are more worrisome than those found in premenopausal women. The health care provider must consider the likelihood of cyst formation caused by malignant obstruction of a duct or lobule, most likely making surgical biopsy necessary. In a premenopausal woman, a discrete macrocyst may be aspirated, usually causing it to resolve. If it recurs, the possibility of malignancy is greater, and biopsy is needed.

Apocrine change, or metaplasia, refers to cellular changes in the ductal epithelium resulting in larger cells that are more characteristic of apocrine sweat glands. Although clinically these lesions usually are rubbery and smooth, it is difficult to discern the difference, and biopsy usually is necessary. Even the pathology specimen may be difficult to evaluate. Large lesions may appear grossly malignant. Whereas these benign lesions are more common than malignant lesions, in the premenopausal woman they require careful evaluation and usually are surgically removed for microscopic evaluation (Blackwell & Grotting, 1996; Rubin & Farber, 1994; Cotran et al., 1999).

## DUCT ECTASIA

Duct ectasia is a condition usually diagnosed in premenopausal women. It occurs when one or more terminal collecting ducts beneath the nipple become distended with cellular debris, macrophages, and fat. Women typically present with a complaint of spontaneous, pasty, thick discharge from the nipple, which varies from straw colored to green or black. The discharge does not contain blood in duct ectasia. It often occurs bilaterally, and with progression, the duct walls atrophy and may become necrotic. The inflammatory response intensifies as ductal erosion allows extrusion of lipids into the underlying stroma, resulting in a palpable, round, fixed nodule; occasional skin retraction and dimpling; and pain, redness, and tenderness—resembling signs of a malignancy. Surgical removal of the affected ducts and surrounding tissue then is required (Cotran et al., 1999; Handle, 1990; Marchant, 1997).

## FIBROADENOMA

Fibroadenoma is the most common benign breast neoplasm, usually occurring in women aged 20 to 35 years but also found in adolescents and elderly women. They are more common in African-American than white women. These lesions often are detected clinically in pregnant women, when they grow more rapidly. Clinically, they are round, well circumscribed, rubbery, and movable. They may be small and nonproliferative or large and rapidly growing. Although usually a single lesion, they can present as multiple nodules, and they may be painful. Women usually describe them as feeling like a "marble." Nipple discharge or skin changes are not present. They are not associated with an increased risk of malignancy but usually are surgically removed for biopsy. Microscopically, fibroadenomas consist of fibrous connective tissue and ducts and may include areas of hyperplastic epithelial cells. In adolescent girls, fibroadenomas usually are detected near menarche, when the adenomas tend to grow rapidly (Powell & Stelling, 1994; Rubin & Farber, 1994).

## PROLIFERATIVE LESIONS WITHOUT ATYPIA

According to Hansen and Morrow (1998), proliferative lesions without atypia are associated with a slightly increased risk (1.5 to 2.0 times the relative risk) of breast cancer. Atypical cellular changes increase the risk of malignancy substantially (4.0 to 5.0 times the relative risk), and women with atypical hyperplasia should be examined every 6 months and should have an annual mammogram.

The common proliferative lesions without atypia are noted in Table 12-1.

### Moderate or Florid Hyperplasia

Normally in the breast, two layers of epithelial cells line the ducts. An increased number of layers of cells lining the ducts, hyperplasia, may result from increased mitotic activity of the epithelial cells but is believed to be caused by diminished apoptosis. With increasing mitotic activity, the risk of malignant transformation increases. On clinical examination, it is not possible to determine

## TABLE 12.1

**Benign Breast Disease and Relative Risk for Subsequent Invasive Breast Cancer**

| Classification | Relative Risk |
|---|---|
| Nonproliferative lesions | 1 (no increase in risk) |
| Cyst, micro or macro          Fibrosis | |
| Duct ectasia          Mastitis | |
| Fibroadenoma          Metaplasia, squamous or apocrine | |
| Papillary apocrine changes          Mild epithelial hyperplasia | |
| Mild sclerosing adenosis | |
| Proliferative lesions | 1.5–2.0 (slight increase in risk) |
| Moderate or florid hyperplasia | |
| Intraductal papilloma | |
| Florid sclerosing adenosis | |
| Proliferative lesions with atypia | 4.0–5.0 (moderate increase in risk) |
| Atypical hyperplasia, lobular or ductal | |
| Carcinoma in situ | 8.0–10.0 (high risk) |
| Ductal carcinoma in situ | |
| Lobular carcinoma in situ | |

(From Hansen, N & Morrow, M. [1998]. Breast disease. *Medical Clinics of North America, 82,* [2]. 203–222.)

whether a palpable mass is benign or malignant. Mammography, fine-needle aspiration and, possibly, surgical biopsy are needed to determine the type of lesion. The risk of malignancy is believed to be directly related to the degree of atypia.

### Papillomas

Sometimes, the epithelial hyperplasia cells form finger-like projections (papillomas) in the ducts. These usually are found in the small peripheral ducts and may be described in a pathology report as "papillomatosis" when several lesions are present. When present in the large lactiferous ducts beneath the nipple, there may be serous or bloody nipple discharge. A solitary intraductal papilla is not associated with an increased risk of malignancy (Rubin & Farber, 1994; O'Grady et al., 1995), despite the frightening occurrence of nipple discharge. However, any palpable lump beneath the nipple should be evaluated by an expert in breast diseases, since the subareolar area is the second most common location for malignancy.

### Atypical Hyperplasia

Whether found in the lobes or the ducts, hyperplasia associated with atypical cells significantly increases the risk of malignancy.

### Fat Necrosis

Fat necrosis can occur spontaneously, but usually patients provide a history of trauma, prior surgery, or radiation therapy. The patient presents with pain, tenderness, and swelling that usually is well localized and and confined to one breast. Mammography often is not helpful because the area of fat necrosis may look like a malignant lesion or a calcified spot. The initial response to the trauma usually is bleeding, followed by necrosis of fat cells. Macrophages and neutrophils infiltrate the area, resulting in an acute inflammatory response. Later, debris such as blood pigments and calcium salts may accumulate, scar tissue develops, and the lesion may become encapsulated. Usually, symptoms resolve in a few weeks, but referral for further evaluation is essential if the lesion does not disappear within this time.

### Ruptured Cyst

Trauma to the breast of a woman with known cystic changes may result in the rupture of one or more cysts. Common causes are motor vehicle accident and mammogram. The cyst's contents stimulate inflammation, swelling, and tenderness.

Careful history usually verifies this etiology, and symptoms resolve within a few weeks.

## NIPPLE SECRETION

Discharge from the nipple in a nonlactating woman is the third most common symptom of those seeking care for breast problems. Until the 1950s, it was thought to be a sign of malignancy. Because more women are performing breast self-examination, it is reported more frequently, and it is now understood that a variety of nonmalignant etiologies exist. Fluid can be expressed from the breasts of more than 50% of white and African-American women and from approximately 40% of Asian-American women (O'Grady et al., 1995). For more than 80% of women, this represents a normal finding and a physiologic response to manipulation; however, it is associated with malignancy nearly half of the time in women older than 60 years of age. Discharge may be associated with nipple or ductal pathology or may result from neuroendocrine or drug effects. Most clinicians agree that spontaneous, persistent, nonlactational discharge from the nipple ducts requires careful evaluation.

Nipple discharge is categorized as spontaneous or provoked, or by the characteristics of the discharge. Generally, provoked discharge is less worrisome than spontaneous. For this discussion, milky, opalescent, and bloody or serous discharge are differentiated.

### Milky Discharge

Milky nipple discharge is thin, nonsticky, and clear to white. This type of discharge most often is the physiologic lactation seen in the postpartum period. Suckling stimulates further milk secretion. It also can occur after ovulation and is considered to be physiologic. Nonlactational milky discharge most likely is caused by mechanical stimulation, medications, or increased prolactin levels. The mature female breast is a secretary organ, normally producing milky fluid in small amounts. Keratin plugs in the nipples typically prevent these secretions from exiting the breast, and they are absorbed into the blood and lymphatics, but these keratin plugs may be softened or moved by heat, friction, or manipulation, allowing fluid to exude from the breast. Mechanical stimulation such as sucking, fondling, vigorous breast examination, trauma, surgery, or even irritation during vigorous exercise may result in stimulation of the afferent nerves of the thorax and reflex stimulation of the breast tissue. Lung tumors and herpetic lesions also have been reported as a possible source of afferent nerve stimulation. Small amounts of discharge are not unusual in these circumstances.

Unexplained, spontaneous, bilateral milky discharge not associated with lactation is galactorrhea. It mostly results from the hormonal alterations associated with menarche or early menopause, thyroid disorders, pituitary tumors, or drugs. Thyrotropin-releasing hormone stimulates prolactin release, and in the presence of hypothyroidism, hyperprolactinemia occurs, which stimulates lactation. In the presence of a pituitary adenoma, prolactin levels may be significantly higher than normal. Normally, prolactin levels are stable throughout the menstrual cycle, so elevated levels require evaluation of thyroid and pituitary function.

Several drugs have been associated with galactorrhea. Marijuana and opiates increase prolactin levels; tricyclics and some antihypertensives deplete dopamine and the $H_2$ blockers; and phenothiazines and antigastroplegics antagonize dopamine action, increasing serum prolactin levels. Oral contraceptives stimulate breast tissue, leading to increased prolactin levels. Management of galactorrhea in these cases entails discontinuing the medication involved, and if possible, substituting another drug.

### Opalescent Discharge

Opalescent discharge may be clear, yellow, green-brown, or black. It most often results from duct ectasia or cysts. It does not contain blood and usually is described as thick, pasty, or cheesy. It is rarely associated with malignancy.

### Bloody or Serous Discharge

Bloody or serous discharge may be red, pink, brown, or clear. The chance of malignancy is greatest with this finding, but it usually has a benign etiology. Bloody discharge may occur during pregnancy and lactation, probably because of increased vascularity within the ducts. If it persists after delivery, it is considered to be more significant and should be evaluated carefully. The most common diagnosis is papilloma, where a bloody or serous discharge occurs. Duct ectasia also may present with bloody discharge. Approximately 10% of women presenting with bloody nipple discharge have a carcinoma. Meticulous evaluation is critical for anyone with this symptom.

## INFECTION

Mastitis is an infection of the breast with fever and localized erythema, tenderness, heat, and induration. Frequently, malaise and nausea and vomiting are associated symptoms. Mastitis usually is associated with lactation, occurring most often in the first few weeks postpartum, or when there is a significant decrease in frequency of breast-feeding. Mastitis is caused by obstruction of the ductal system, usually by milk, and concomitant exposure to bacteria, often secondary to nipple and areola irritation. Granulomatous mastitis is uncommon but has been associated with mycobacteria infections or silicone injections for augmentation. Fungi also have caused this condition. The usual organisms involved are *Staphylococcus aureus* or *Staphylococcus epidermis*, although it can be caused by other organisms such as streptococci or Gram-negative rods. Ten percent of women with mastitis develop an abscess. With appropriate antibiotic therapy, 80% to 90% of women with mastitis can be cured without abscess complications. The risk of this complication is reduced by having the woman continue to breast-feed or by mechanically emptying the breast on a regular schedule.

Mastitis in a nonlactating woman is more serious, requiring prompt evaluation for inflammatory carcinoma. It also may be caused by a subareolar abscess from squamous metaplasia of ductal epithelial cells. With this condition, cellular debris builds up, and because of keratin plugs of the lactiferous ducts, inflammation and infection may develop. The offending bacteria usually are *S. aureus*. Smoking is a major risk factor for this condition, and treatment should involve smoking cessation intervention. Surgical excision of the involved duct also may be required for resolution.

## CONGENITAL ANOMALIES

Most abnormalities of size or shape of the breast are a result of hormonal influences during fetal development. Testosterone inhibits breast development. When levels of this hormone are too high or estrogen levels are low, the breasts do not fully develop. Some of these anomalies are noted at birth, whereas others do not become apparent until puberty.

Asymmetry usually is recognized at menarche, when one breast develops more rapidly than the other. By the time a woman reaches adulthood, the degree of asymmetry usually is slight. Marked asymmetry has been linked to inhibited glandular development and often results in lactation failure in the postpartum period. Musculoskeletal anomalies such as pectus excavatum or pectus carinatum may give the appearance of asymmetry. Poland's syndrome of the pectoralis major muscle is associated with hypoplasia or, possibly, total absence of the nipple or of the entire breast.

Supernumary or accessory nipples occur when there is failure of regression of the milk line during fetal development. These nipples usually are rudimentary, looking more like a nevus than a nipple, and can occur anywhere along the milk line from the axilla to the groin. These areas of breast tissue may undergo hypertrophy during pregnancy and rarely produce milk. Malignancy and other breast pathology in these tissues are rare.

Hyperplasia of the breasts usually results from development of excessive fat or connective tissue and is not associated with increased risk for breast disease. Surgical reduction is recommended when musculoskeletal or psychological well-being is significantly affected.

Complete absence of the breast (amastia) or of the nipple (athelia) is rare, occurring as a result of failure of embryonic differentiation of breast tissue. This usually is a unilateral finding, and cosmetic surgery is the only treatment. Failure of maturation of breast tissue at adolescence may indicate ovarian failure, requiring evaluation for etiologies. On successful resolution of ovarian dysfunction, breast tissue development will occur.

Premature breast development, occurring before 8 years of age without precocious puberty, is believed to be caused by elevated FSH concentrations, which stimulate ovarian production of estradiol, resulting in breast tissue proliferation. This may result from endocrine tumors, exogenous sources of estrogen, or true precocious puberty. The underlying etiology must be determined and rectified, with surgical revision sometimes necessary for cosmetic care.

## GYNECOMASTIA

Proliferation of breast tissue in the male, gynecomastia, is common, especially during puberty or in older men. The most common etiology is a low androgen-to-estrogen ratio, which resolves with maturation in the adolescent. In older men, the incidence of gynecomastia increases with age; however, reported prevalence varies widely because of a lack of standard criteria for the condition. Nevertheless, possible etiologies must be investigated in any male patient with this condition.

Male breast glandular tissue is responsive to the same hormonal influences as the female breast. Estrogen stimulation results in proliferation of both the connective tissue and the ducts. Hyperplasia of the ductal epithelium results in palpable, rubbery, or slightly firm tissue, which is easily differentiated from increased adipose tissue. Excessive estrogen effects can result from drugs containing estrogen or estrogen-like substances, liver disease, hormone-secreting tumors, or inadequate production of testosterone. Drugs associated with gynecomastia include alcohol, marijuana, opioids, anabolic steroids, digitalis, calcium channel blockers, $H_2$ receptor blockers, and psychoactive agents. Hepatic and renal dysfunction results in an altered ability to metabolize and excrete estrogen, thereby increasing the circulation of estrogen-like substances. Testicular or adrenal tumors may secrete estrogen, and paraneoplastic syndromes associated with production of estrogen from malignancies of the lung and liver have been reported (Rubin & Farber, 1994). Altered metabolism rates associated with thyroid dysfunction also have been reported

as a possible etiology of gynecomastia. Inadequate secretion of testosterone is associated with Klinefelter's syndrome, castration, and orchitis. Table 12-2 shows the association of drugs with gynecomastia.

### Physiologic Basis of Management

Careful history and physical examination, including a history of drug ingestion, must be completed with the possible etiologies in mind. Transient pubertal gynecomastia is the most common cause, followed by drug-induced and idiopathic gynecomastia. Resolution of the hormone imbalance leads to involution and regression of breast tissue in most cases when it is a recent development. Long-standing gynecomastia may not resolve even with treatment. However, breast pain and tenderness usually diminish over time. Spontaneous regression also has been reported in many male patients. Hormonal therapy with testosterone, antiestrogens, or both has been used, with reports of varying degrees of successful regression of glandular breast tissue.

## TABLE 12.2

**Drugs Associated With Gynecomastia**

| *Hormones* | *Cancer Chemotherapeutic Agents* | *Psychoactive Agents* |
|---|---|---|
| Androgens and anabolic steroids* | Alkylating agents* | Diazepam |
| Chorionic gonadotropin* | *Cardiovascular Drugs* | Haloperidol |
| Estrogens and estrogen agonists* | Amiodarone | Phenothiazine |
| *Antiandrogens or Inhibitors of Androgen Synthesis* | Captopril | Tricyclic antidepressants |
| Cyproterone* | Digitoxin* | *Drugs of Abuse* |
| Flutamide* | Diltiazem | Alcohol |
| *Antibiotics* | Enalapril | Amphetamines |
| Isoniazid | Methyldopa | Heroin |
| Ketoconazole* | Nifedipine | Marijuana |
| *Antiulcer Medications* | Reserpine | *Other* |
| Cimetidine* | Spironolactone* | Phenytoin |
| Ranitidine | Verapamil | Penicillamine |
| Omeprazole | | |

*A strong relation has been established. Other relations have been proposed on the basis of epidemiologic studies or challenge–rechallenge studies of individual patients or small groups of patients (Braunstein, G.D. [1993]. Gynecomastia. *New England Journal of Medicine, 328,* 490). (From Harris, J.R., Lippman, M.C., Morrow, M., & Hellman, S. [Eds.] [1996]. *Diseases of the breast.* Philadelphia: Lippincott-Raven.)

## BREAST CANCER

Breast cancer is the most common malignancy and the second leading cause of cancer death in women in the United States. The American Cancer Society estimated that 182,200 American women would be diagnosed and 40,800 women would die of this disease in 2000 (American Cancer Society, 2000). Lifetime risk of developing breast cancer is one in eight women, with the risk increasing with age. Many risk factors for breast cancer have been identified, but most women diagnosed with breast cancer have only the risk factors of sex and age. The following box indicates the risk factors for breast cancer.

Approximately, 1% of breast cancer occurs in men. Ninety-five percent of breast cancers are found in women aged 40 years and older, and only 5% to 10% of them have a family history of it (American Cancer Society, 2000). Whereas white women have a higher incidence of breast cancer, African-American women have a higher mortality rate, possibly because of an increased rate of later stage diagnosis and because estrogen-receptor negative tumors are more commonly diagnosed in that group. Worldwide, breast cancer mortality is highest in Western, industrialized nations and lowest in developing countries and Asia. Biobehavioral differences among population groups appear to reinforce previously identified risk factors. Age at birth of first child is one example. It has been

recognized for over a century that breast cancer occurs more frequently in women who were never pregnant or were pregnant for the first time after 30 years of age. Both of these phenomena are more common in industrialized nations, which have a high rate of breast cancer, than in developing countries. Dietary fat is another correlate with breast cancer occurring in certain populations. However, its relationship to the development of breast cancer has been questioned based on several reports. Attention has moved to the significance of the ratio of monosaturated to polyunsaturated fat in the diet.

Family history continues to be the most recognized risk factor after sex and age. Maternal family history appears to be more significant, but genetic alterations also have been documented from paternal lineage. Several genetic mutations are linked to breast cancer. The BRCA1 gene is linked especially to premenopausal breast cancer but also appears to be associated with post-menopausal occurrence and to an increased risk for cancers of the ovary, prostate, and colon. The BRCA2 gene has been associated with a similar risk of development of breast cancer but with a poorer prognosis. These genes have been associated with approximately 10% of breast cancer cases. There is a relationship between the BRCA genes and a high incidence of p53 tumor suppressor gene mutations. An important role is played by p53 in growth suppression and normal apoptosis of damaged cells. Mutations in this gene may allow abnormal cells to proliferate unchecked and inhibit DNA repair (Smith et al., 1999). This is thought to be the effect of the gene product of p53, which normally prevents cells from moving into the G1 phase of the cell cycle. Damaged cells or cells with mutations thus would have time to repair such damage and then either proceed into mitosis or undergo apoptosis. This effect is illustrated in Figure 12-3. Mutations of p53 then would result in mutated and damaged cells dividing and producing clones of like cells.

The her-2/*neu* oncogene also is found in breast cancers with a poorer prognosis. Its role in breast cancer development continues to be explored (Hansen & Morrow, 1998; Youngkin & Davis, 1998). This gene appears to play a role in normal cell growth as well as the development of malignancy. It codes for a membrane-related protein. When bound with other growth factors, this protein initiates a reaction that signals the nucleus to begin cell division. In approximately 25% of women with breast cancer, overproduction of this protein may stimulate both increased cell division and tumor growth. This protein also may alter es-

---

● **Risk Factors for Breast Cancer**

Female

Age older than 40 years

Prior history of breast cancer

Early menarche, before age 12

Late menopause, after age 55

Late first pregnancy, after age 30

Family history of breast cancer, especially maternal

BRCA1 or BRCA2 gene

Nulliparity

Daily alcohol consumption

Atypical lobular hyperplasia

Lobular carcinoma in situ

Ionizing radiation exposure

Obesity

(Love, 1995; Powell & Stelling, 1994; Harris et al., 1996)

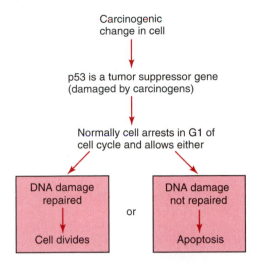

Carcinogenic
change in cell

p53 is a tumor suppressor gene
(damaged by carcinogens)

Normally cell arrests in G1 of
cell cycle and allows either

DNA damage
repaired

or

DNA damage
not repaired

Cell divides

Apoptosis

**FIGURE 12.3** ● With decreased amounts of p53, a carcinogenically damaged cell does not arrest in G1 and may go on to proliferate into cancer cells.

trogen receptor activity on cell membranes, making these tumors more resistant to antiestrogen therapies. Overexpression of the her-2/*neu* oncogene is associated with poor prognosis in breast cancer. Its presence and relative amount can be assayed in tumor tissue, and monoclonal antibody therapy has demonstrated effectiveness in limiting the expression of the protein as a component of anticancer therapy (Slamon et al., 1989).

## PATHOLOGY OF BREAST CANCER

Cellular changes are believed to occur over time, progressing to malignancy. The first change is a proliferation of cells resulting in hyperplasia. Genetic changes appear next, with the development of clones of cells with an atypical structure. On the pathology report, "atypical hyperplasia" would be the common conclusion. Progression leads to the recognition of genetic changes such as those noted earlier, loss of cellular adhesion, angiogenesis, growth factor abnormalities, and further aberrations in cell structure. These changes are seen in both noninvasive and invasive breast cancers.

Malignancy is more common in the left breast than the right and more often located in the upper outer quadrant followed by the subareolar region. Reasons for this pattern of occurrence are unclear. Lymph node metastasis is the most common route of spread. The development of sentinel-node biopsy promises to increase the accuracy of identifying or ruling out progression of disease beyond the breast.

Most authorities agree that breast cancers should be categorized as noninvasive (in situ) or invasive.

### Noninvasive Carcinomas

Lobular carcinoma in situ (LCIS) often is an incidental finding in a biopsy done for another reason. It is a proliferation of cells within a terminal duct but does not invade the underlying cell lining and does not usually alter the size of the duct. It does not form a palpable mass and rarely forms calcifications. Women with LCIS have an increased risk of developing invasive carcinoma, although not necessarily in the same breast.

Ductal carcinoma in situ (DCIS) has become one of the most common malignancies found on mammogram. Although these cells can spread along ducts involving relatively large areas, they usually do not invade the underlying basement membrane of the duct and rarely metastasize. They can, however, distort the shape and size of the ducts, creating a palpable mass. Five structural subtypes have been noted: comedo carcinoma, cribriform, papillary, micropapillary, and solid. Many specimens contain mixed cellularity. Comedo DCIS is characterized by the presence of necrotic (comedones-like) tissue surrounded by sheets of large cells with pleomorphic nuclei. Inflammation and calcification of debris may render the area palpable. Microscopic invasion into the lining of the duct or other breast tissue is most common with this type. Cribriform DCIS is described as having a sievelike pattern with relatively small uniform cells. Mitotic activity is relatively low, and necrosis may be present but is limited. Micropapillary DCIS looks like stalks of cells projecting into the lumen with low levels of mitosis. These may be called well-differentiated DCIS. Papillary DCIS differs from micropapillary DCIS in that it has a microvascular core and usually lacks a myoepithelial layer of cells. In solid DCIS, ductal spaces are filled with tumor cells that often vary in size but exhibit necrosis on papillary forms.

Paget's disease is considered a variant of ductal carcinoma. It is not clear whether the Paget cell arises from the breast or the epidermis, but the patient typically reports a history of erosion or "eczema" of the nipple with the common complaint of itching and increased sensitivity. The disease likely involves the nipple and areola first, and later the ductal cancer develops. Paget cells are large, clear, mucin-containing cells found in the epidermis. Approximately half of women presenting with Paget's disease have a palpable mass. Anyone presenting with a history of nipple excoriation should undergo a biopsy for Paget's disease.

### Invasive Carcinomas

Ductal carcinoma, or infiltrating ductal carcinoma, represents approximately 75% of invasive breast cancers. These tumors invade and sometimes replace normal cells within the breast. Cell size and differentiation varies, and mixtures of cell architecture may be seen. These tumors form hard, painless, often-fixed nodules of varying size. Because they often are fixed, retraction and dimpling (peau d'orange) of the overlying skin is common. When poorly differentiated, they usually are estrogen-receptor negative, and, conversely, well-differentiated tumors tend to be estrogen-receptor positive.

Invasive lobular carcinomas comprise approximately 10% of invasive cancers. Patients typically present with an upper outer quadrant lesion that often is indistinct and may be described as a thickening rather than a mass. A unique feature of this type is that it often is multicentric and more often bilateral than other types. The cells tend to be in a single layer, loosely lining breast tissues. This lack of cell adhesion helps to explain the lack of a distinct mass and the possibility of early micrometastasis. Well-differentiated tumors usually are hormone-receptor positive, but central nervous system and bone marrow metastases are more common with this cell type than others.

Tubular carcinomas usually are well differentiated and have an excellent prognosis when detected early. Axillary metastases occur late. The cells and tumor architecture closely resemble normal breast ductules. Most women present with a palpable lump that usually is mobile, without skin retraction. It usually forms one tumor, but boundaries often are irregular, and multifocal lesions have been reported. These tumors tend to be estrogen-receptor and progesterone-receptor positive.

Colloid, or mucinous, carcinoma represents only 1% to 2% of breast cancer and usually occurs in older women. It tends to be relatively slow growing and usually is a soft, almost gelatinous mass. Microscopically, there are large areas of mucin with small foci of tumor cells. Most are estrogen-receptor positive.

Medullary carcinoma occurs in younger women more than other types of breast cancer. These tumors are soft and usually well defined. Cells usually are highly proliferative, poorly differentiated, and estrogen-receptor negative. However, they metastasize less often than other types of breast cancer. The cells appear to grow in closely packed sheets, indicating that cell adhesion is preserved.

Papillary invasive carcinomas are rare, accounting for less than 1% of breast malignancies. These tumors usually are well circumscribed, soft to firm, and sometimes lobulated. Papillary fronds are found on microscopic examination. Because these tend to be low-grade lesions, they must be carefully analyzed to distinguish them from benign papillomas.

## PHYSIOLOGIC BASIS OF TREATMENT

The careful microscopic analysis of a breast lesion is the only way to determine absolutely whether a malignancy is present. History, including identification of risk factors and physical examination, is critical in determining the need for referral for mammography or surgical biopsy. When a diagnosis of breast cancer is confirmed, the cellular characteristics and stage of disease directly influence treatment decisions. The biopsy specimen is examined, cell type is identified, and several special studies are used to identify estrogen receptor and progesterone receptor status, her-2/*neu* oncogene presence, and lymphocyte infiltration of the tumor. The hormone receptor studies are important because it is widely accepted that the growth of estrogen-receptor or progesterone-receptor positive tumors can be altered by hormonal approaches. The drug tamoxifen is classified as an antiestrogen that competes with estradiol at cellular receptor sites in breast, uterine, and vaginal tissues. By binding to the estrogen receptor sites on breast cancer cells, it inhibits tumor growth in estrogen-receptor positive tumors.

Staging of breast cancer involves measuring the primary tumor, both clinically and pathologically, and determining if lymph node or distant metastasis has occurred. Based on these findings, the appropriate surgical, radiation therapy, or chemotherapy regimen can be determined. Although it is beyond the scope of this chapter to discuss specific treatment, the primary care provider should recognize that for most women with invasive breast cancer, a course of adjuvant chemotherapy will be recommended, even in early disease, because of the risk of early micrometastasis.

### CLINICAL VIGNETTE 12.1

A 36-year-old female presents with the complaint of breast pain that has been increasing over the last few months. Initially, she perceived the discomfort 3 to 4 days before her menses each month but now states that the pain is constant. She has been taking ibuprofen with some relief but is worried that the pain is a sign of cancer.

History and physical examination reveal that the pain is bilateral and present daily. It increases during the week before her menses and is quantified as a "6" on a 0 to 10 scale when at its worst. She describes the pain as a sense of heavy achiness and states that she cannot tolerate anyone touching her breasts during this time. The pain occasionally wakens her from sleep. She reports no palpable mass or nipple discharge and denies any weight change or change in activity level. She participates in an aerobics class twice a week. She has no family history of breast cancer or other breast disease. She has a 10-year-old son and a 7-year-old daughter. She performs breast self-examination sporadically but has an annual clinical breast examination. She never has had a mammogram. A coworker, aged 37, recently was diagnosed with breast cancer.

Physical examination reveals an anxious white female, 5 feet, 5 inches tall weighing 125 pounds. Systematic breast examination reveals no masses, no skin changes, and no nipple discharge. The client appears to be uncomfortable during the breast examination. The remainder of the physical examination is normal.

This client should have a mammogram and repeat clinical examination. If both are normal, she should keep a breast pain calendar for 1 to 2 months, recording her pain, any medications taken, and days of menstruation. Her brassiere also should be evaluated for proper fit. Reassurance of normalcy could only be given after such evaluation. Possible pharmacologic management could be considered.

---

Breast cancer in men is treated with the same therapeutic interventions as in women. Unfortunately, male breast cancer frequently is diagnosed late because of the lack of awareness of both men and their health care providers of the importance of assessing the male breast during a physical examination.

## SUMMARY

Breast changes range from expected physiologic responses to life-threatening pathologies. The continuum from benign to malignant changes sometimes is confusing to the health care provider and anxiety-provoking for the patient. All male and female patients presenting with a concern about breast health should be evaluated with a careful history and physical examination, and any suspicious pathology should be evaluated by an expert in breast care. Most concerns will not be malignant, and many resolve without definitive treatment, but only careful evaluation will differentiate the pathologic conditions.

### CLINICAL VIGNETTE 12.2

Ms. S. is a 24-year-old African-American female who presents with a painless lump in the upper outer quadrant of her left breast. She states that she just noticed it when bathing last week. Her mother insisted that she have it evaluated. She has never been pregnant, began menstruation at age 14, and has no family history of breast cancer.

Physical examination reveals a 2-cm palpable, firm, nodular, but movable mass in the left breast, upper outer quadrant. No skin changes are noted, and the axillary exam is negative. The remainder of the physical examination is normal, including evaluation of the right breast.

Despite her young age and negative family history, this patient should be referred for further evaluation of the mass with mammogram and possibly biopsy. Although unusual, breast cancer can and does occur in young women.

---

## CLINICAL VIGNETTE 12.3

Mr. A., a 59-year-old white male, presents with a complaint of a small lump just below his nipple and occasional spontaneous serous discharge. He has noted the discharge on his shirt three times in the last month and is concerned that he has an infection. He denies any fever, pain, malaise, or lymphadenitis. Physical examination reveals a 1-cm, smooth, movable subareolar mass in the right breast. Gentle squeezing of the nipple produces a few drops of serous fluid that tests negative for red blood cells.

This patient should be immediately referred to a breast care expert for evaluation. Breast cancer does occur in men, and its presentation, although similar to that of a woman, often is not recognized as requiring further diagnostic evaluation. This presentation is suggestive of a malignancy until proven otherwise.

## REFERENCES

American Cancer Society. (2000). *Cancer facts and figures.* Atlanta: American Cancer Society.

Arnold, G.J. & Neiheisel, M.B. (1997). A comprehensive approach to evaluating nipple discharge. *The Nurse Practitioner, 22* (7), 96–111.

Bedinghaus, J.M. (1997). Care of the breast and support of breast feeding. *Primary Care, 24* (1), 147–160.

Blackwell, R.E. & Grotting, J.C. (1996). *Diagnosis and management of breast disease.* Cambridge, MA: Blackwell Science.

Cady, B., Steele, G.D., Morrow, M., Gardner, B., Smith, B.L., Lee, N.C., Lawson, H.W., & Winchester, D.P. (1998). Evaluation of common breast problems: Guidance for primary care providers. *CA: A Cancer Journal for Clinicians, 48* (1), 49–63.

Cancer Committee of the American College of Pathologists. (1986). Is fibrocystic disease of the breast precancerous? *Archives of Pathology and Laboratory Medicine, 110,* 173.

Cotran, R.S., Kumar, V., & Collins, T. (1999). *Robbins pathologic basis of disease* (6th ed.). Philadelphia: W.B. Saunders.

Davies, E.L., Gateley, C.A., Miers, M., & Mansel, R.E. (1998). The long-term course of mastalgia. *Journal of the Royal Society of Medicine, 91,* 462–464.

Donegen, W.L. (1992). Evaluation of a palpable breast mass. *New England Journal of Medicine, 327,* 937.

Gateley, C., Miers, M., Mansel, R., & Hughes, L. (1992). Drug treatment for mastalgia: 17 years' experience in the Cardiff mastalgic clinic. *Journal of the Royal Society of Medicine, 85,* 12–15.

Goehring, C. & Morabia, A. (1997). Epidemiology of benign breast disease, with special attention to histologic types. *Epidemiologic Reviews, 19* (2), 310–327.

Goodwin, D.J., Miller, A., Delguidice, M.E., & Ritchie, K. (1997). Breast health and associated premenstrual symptoms in women with severe cyclic mastopathy. *American Journal of Obstretrics and Gynecology, 176* (5), 998–1005.

Hansen, N. & Morrow, M. (1998). Breast disease. *Medical Clinics of North America, 82* (2), 203–222.

Harris, J.R., Lippman, M.E., Morrow, M., & Hellman, S. (Eds.). (1996). *Diseases of the breast.* Philadelphia: Lippincott-Raven Publishers.

Hindle, W.H. (1990). *Breast disease for gynecologists.* Norwalk, CT: Appleton & Lange.

Holland, P. & Gately, C. (1994). Drug therapy of mastalgia: What are the options? *Drugs, 48,* (5), 709–716.

Kumar, S., Mansel, R.E., Scanlon, M.E., Hughes, L.E., Edwards, G.A., Woodhead, J.S., & Newcombe, R.G. (1984). Altered responses of prolactin leutinizing hormone and follicle stimulating hormone secretion to thyrotrophin releasing hormone/gonadotrophin releasing hormone stimulation in cyclical mastalgia. *British Journal of Surgery, 71* (11), 870–873.

Love, S.M. (1995). *Dr. Susan Love's breast book* (2nd ed.). Reading, MA: Addison–Wesley.

Maddox, P.R. & Mansel, R. (1989). Management of breast pain and nodularity. *World Journal of Surgery, 13,* 699–705.

Mansel, R. (1992). Benign breast disease. *The Practitioner, 236,* 833–837.

Marchant, D.J. (1997). *Breast disease.* Philadelphia: W.B. Saunders.

McCool, W.F., Stone–Condry, M., & Bradford, H.M. (1998). Breast health care. *Journal of Nurse–Midwifery, 43* (6), 406–430.

McDermott, M.M., Dolan, N.C., & Rademaker, A. (1996). Effect of breast–tissue characteristics on the outcome of clinical breast examination training. *Academic Medicine, 71* (5), 505–507.

Mitchell, G.W. & Bassett, L.W. (Eds.) (1990). *The female breast and its disorders.* Baltimore: Williams & Wilkins.

Mudan, S.S., Ibrahim, A.E., Wise, M., & Perry, P.M. (1998). Nipple discharge in a teenager. *Journal of the Royal Society of Medicine, 91,* 490–491.

O'Grady, L.F., Lindfors, K.K., Howell, L.P., & Rippon, M.B. (1995). *A practical approach to breast disease.* Boston: Little, Brown & Company.

Perna, W.C. (1996). Mastalgia: Diagnosis and treatment. *Journal of the American Academy of Nurse Practitioners, 8* (12), 579–584.

Powell, D.E. & Stelling, C.B. (1994). *The diagnosis and detection of breast disease.* St. Louis: Mosby.

Preece, P. (1990). Mastaglia. In J.A. Smallwood & I. Taylor (Eds.), *Benign breast disease.* Baltimore: Urban & Schwarzenburg.

Rode, S., Favre, C., & Thivolet, C. (1998). Diabetic mastopathy. *Diabetes Care, 21* (2), 322.

Rubin, E. & Farber, J.L. (Eds.) (1994). *Pathology* (2nd ed.). Philadelphia: J.B. Lippincott.

Scott, J.R., Disaia, D.J., Hammond, C.B., & Spellacy, W.N. (Eds.) (1994). *Danforth's obstetrics and gynecology* (7th ed.). Philadelphia: J.B. Lippincott.

Smith, P.D., Crossland, S., Parker, G., Osin, P. Brooks, L., Waller, J., Philip, E., Crompton, M.R., Gusterson, B.A., Allday, M. J., & Crook, T. (1999). Novel p53 mutants selected in BRCA associated tumours which dissociate transformation suppression form other wild-type p53 functions. *Oncogene, 18* (15), 2451–2459.

Smallwood, J.A. & Taylor, I. (Eds.) (1990). *Benign breast disease.* Baltimore: Urban & Schwarzenberg.

Thompson, W.D. (1994). Genetic epidemiology of breast cancer. *Cancer, 74* (Suppl. 1), 279–287.

Youngkin, E.Q. & Davis, M.S. (1998). *Women's health: A primary care clinical guide* (2nd ed.). Norwalk, CT: Appleton & Lange.

# Arthritis

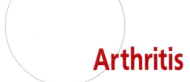

Karen Lasater

Maureen Groer

P rimary care providers treat many patients who complain of some type of joint pain. However, patients often report arthritic symptoms only in the review of systems, since they consider arthritis to be a natural consequence of aging and, therefore, not a cause for medical concern. Others clearly experience major pain and disability from arthritis, some so significantly that their quality of life becomes seriously threatened. Of all chronic diseases that affect the quality of life, especially of older persons, arthritis is, by far, the leading contender.

The practitioner must be able to distinguish and diagnose the major forms of human arthritis to appropriately refer patients with infectious or rheumatoid arthritis (RA) and medically manage most of those with osteoarthritis (OA). It also is important to recognize the arthritic patients who need surgical referral.

Practitioners should evaluate patients with arthritis symptoms for their general health and the presence of any systemic disease, to determine if the disease is monoarticular or polyarticular, and if there are signs of inflammation (redness, warmth, swelling) in the involved joints. The location and characteristics of the pain and stiffness also are critical diagnostic factors, as is be seen in the case study in this chapter.

The most common arthritis observed in primary care is OA (16 million in the United States). However, patients can be misdiagnosed with primary OA and treated improperly when an underlying disease process, such as an endocrinopathy, or an inflammatory disease, such as RA, is the true etiology.

Table 13-1 lists the common presentations of arthritis, depending on inflammatory signs and symptoms and number of joints involved, that the practitioner will observe in ambulatory care practice.

## OSTEOARTHRITIS

Ninety percent of people older than 50 years of age have, on x-ray, some evidence of OA, but only a third of these individuals have symptoms. OA is thus a ubiquitous disease with a range of severity. It is the most common joint disease and has affected the human skeleton since prehistoric times. Its incidence increases with age, but it does not result merely from normal aging processes of cartilage. Other factors associated with OA include chronic microtrauma to the joint structures, genetic factors, and obesity. Men are more commonly affected than women before the age of 50, but thereafter the incidence is approximately equal. Typically OA affects one or only a few joints such as the knees, hips, spine, and hands. The pain and stiffness are aggravated by activity and alleviated by rest.

The following definition of OA has been proposed by the American College of Rheumatology (ACR): "a heterogeneous group of conditions that lead to joint symptoms and signs which are associated with defective integrity of articular cartilage, in addition to related changes in the underlying bone at the joint margins." (Altman et al., 1996, p 1039).

## TABLE 13.1

### Common Types of Arthritis

| Noninflammatory Monoarticular Arthritis | Inflammatory Monoarticular Arthritis | Noninflammatory Polyarticular Arthritis | Inflammatory Polyarticular Arthritis |
|---|---|---|---|
| Trauma | Crystalline | Osteoarthritis | Rheumatoid arthritis |
| Metabolic diseases | Infections | Metabolic diseases | Psoriatic arthritis |
| Hyperparathyroidism | Inflammatory diseases (most are polyarticular; see last column) | Hyperparathyroidism | Seronegative arthritis |
| Acromegaly | Reiter's syndrome | Acromegaly | Ankylosing spondylitis |
| Paget's disease | Sarcoid | Paget's disease | Serum sickness |
| Thyroid disorders | | Thyroid disorders | Vasculitis |
| Infiltrative disease | | Infiltrative diseases | |
| Amyloid | | Hemochromatosis | |
| Foreign body | | Amyloid | |
| Tumor | | | |
| Mechanical derangement | | | |
| Meniscal tears | | | |
| Aseptic necrosis | | | |
| Neuropathic | | | |

(From Silverman J. [1997] Evaluation of joint pain. In L. Dornbrand, A. Hoole, & R. Fletcher [Eds.], *Manual of clinical problems in adult ambulatory care.* On *MAXX: Maximum access in diagnosis and therapy. The electronic library of medicine* [CD-Rom]. Lippincott-Raven.)

## PATHOPHYSIOLOGIC CHANGES IN OSTEOARTHRITIS

Osteoarthritis is a progressive degenerative disease of diarthrodial joints causing pain, stiffness, and limited range of motion (Uphold & Graham, 1998). Historically, OA has been viewed as resulting from acute or chronic injury or repetitive use ("wear and tear") (Brandt et al., 1998a). Prevailing research, however, suggests that this former theory of pathogenesis of OA is too limited. Current thoughts on the pathologic process propose OA as a disease with multiple etiologies driven by local and systemic mechanisms, resulting in pathologic changes in and around the joint (Cooper & Dennison, 1998). Architectural and cellular changes lead to limited joint function and eventual joint destruction (Pritzker, 1998). This disease process affects the articular cartilage, subchondral bone, and synovial membranes. The cartilage is degraded, the bone hypertrophies and thickens, and the synovial membranes inflame (Pelletier et al., 1998).

A classification of OA has been established to organize the different presentations and etiologies of OA. In *primary* or idiopathic OA, no underlying etiologies have been identified. It presents either as localized or generalized, depending on the number of involved joints. There are multiple etiologies involved in *secondary* OA, including metabolic and endocrine diseases (Kraus, 1997). However, trauma is the most common cause of secondary OA.

The precise mechanisms that initiate the OA disease process are unknown. The progression, severity, and outcomes vary widely with each etiology; however, the signs and symptoms of OA can be generalized to each of the different etiologies (O'Reilly & Doherty, 1998). A full list of contributing risk factors for OA are found in Table 13-2.

## CLINICAL PRESENTATION: SIGNS AND SYMPTOMS

The common clinical presentation of OA is that of an insidious onset of joint pain related to activity, with joint stiffness occurring after periods of inactivity. Morning stiffness rarely exceeds 15 minutes

## TABLE 13.2  ● ● ●

### Classification of Osteoarthritis

*Primary*
*Localized*
  Hands
    Heberden's and Bouchard's nodes (nodal)
    Erosive interphalangeal arthritis (nonnodal)
    Carpal—first metacarpal
  Feet
    Hallux valgus
    Hallus rigidus
    Contracted toes (hammer/cockup toes)
    Talonavicular
  Hip
    Eccentric (superior)
    Concentric (axial, medial)
    Diffuse (Coxae senilis)
  Spine
    Apophyseal joints
    Intervertebral joints (disc)
    Spondylosis (osteophytes)
    Ligamentous (hyperostosis, Forestier's disease, diffuse idiopathic skeletal hyperostosis)
    Glenohumeral
    Acromioclavicular
    Tibiotalar
    Sacroiliac
    Temporomandibular
*Generalized*
  Includes 3 or more areas listed above

*Secondary*
  *Trauma*
    Acute
    Chronic (occupational, sports)
*Congenital or developmental*
Localized
  Legg-Calvé-Perthes syndrome
  Diseases
  Congenital hip dislocation
  Slipped epiphysis

Mechanical
  Unequal lower extremity length
Factors
  Valgus/varus deformity
  Hypermobility syndromes
*Metabolic*
  Ochronosis (alkaptonuria)
  Hemochromatosis
  Wilson's disease
  Gaucher's disease
*Endocrine*
  Acromegaly
  Hyperparathyroidism
  Diabetes mellitus
  Obesity
  Hypothyroidism
*Calcium deposition diseases*
  Calcium pyrophosphate dihydrate deposition
  Apatite arthropathy
*Other bone and joint diseases*
  Localized
    Fracture
    Avascular necrosis
    Infection
    Gout
  Diffuse
    Rheumatoid (inflammatory) arthritis
    Paget's disease
    Osteopetrosis
    Osteochondritis
*Neuropathic (Charcot joint)*
*Endemic*
  Kashin-Bek disease
  Mseleni disease
*Miscellaneous*
  Caisson disease
  Hemoglobinopathies

(From Brandt, K.D., [1996]. Diagnosis and non-surgical management of osteoarthritis. Professional Communications, McNeil Consumer Products, Caddo, Oklahoma.)

and resolves with movement. Stiffness may be worse when the weather becomes cold and humid. The pain often is described as deep, aching, and poorly localized. Other symptoms of OA include restrictions in the range of motion of the affected joints and collapse of the joint on weight bearing. Joints typically affected by this disease are seen in Figure 13-1. The hands, fingers, knees, cervical and lumbar vertebrae, and hips are the most commonly involved. OA usually affects one to two joints at a time, and the disease does not produce systemic symptoms. Considering the multiple etiologies of OA, the duration and progression, the pattern of joint involvement, and the severity of the disease are unpredictable; however, the long-term clinical outcomes, regardless of the different etiologies, are similar (O'Reilly & Doherty, 1998). The clinical signs of OA for the practitioner to evaluate are listed in Table 13-3.

These signs are variable, depending on the progression of the disease and the joints affected. Tenderness at or around the joint and muscle wasting are signs usually found in the late stages of the disease. Crepitus, a crunching feeling or sound (like Rice Krispies), during range of motion is a result

## TABLE 13.3

### Signs of Osteoarthritis

Tenderness on palpation (may involve widely separated areas of the joint)

Pain on passive motion

Crepitus (crunching or grinding sounds heard on joint motion)

Joint enlargement (spur formation, synovitis, prolonged disease)

Limitation of motion (joint surface incongruity, muscle spasm, fibrotic changes, contracture, osteophytes, joint mice)

Deformity, subluxation (cartilage degeneration, subchondral bone collapse, bone cysts, bony growth, muscle atrophy, rarely ankylosis)

Modified from Moskowitz, R. (1992). Osteoarthritis: Symptoms and signs. In R. Moskowitz, D. Howell, V. Goldberg, & H. Markin (Eds.), *Diagnosis and medical/surgical management* (p. 257). Philadelphia: W.B. Saunders.

of irregularly shaped bony surfaces and cartilage breakdown. Joint deformities, such as Heberden's and Bouchard's nodes of the interphalangeal joints, are caused by loss of cartilage, bone remodeling and loss, and osteophyte formation (O'Reilly & Doherty, 1998) (Fig. 13-2). A common sign of OA is decreased range of motion and loss of joint function resulting from proliferation of bony prominences, spurs, and osteophytes on the joint surfaces.

### Normal Joint Function

Understanding normal joint function and cartilage physiology is essential before the cellular and gross anatomic changes that occur in OA can be appreciated. Bullough (1992) describes the characteristics required for proper joint functioning as follows:

1. The freedom of the opposed articular surfaces to move painlessly over each other within the required range of motion
2. A proper distribution of load across joint tissues that might otherwise be damaged by overloading, or that fail to be maintained because of habitual underloading (disuse)
3. The maintenance of stability during use

These three characteristics are dependent on the structural development and integrity of the joint anatomy, as well as the cellular components

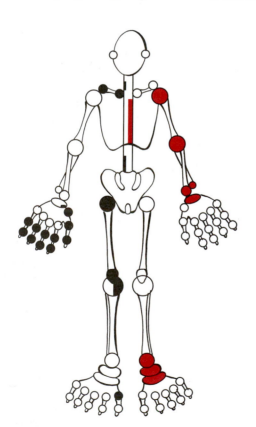

**FIGURE 13.1**  ●  Common sites for osteoarthritis are in black and spared sites are red.

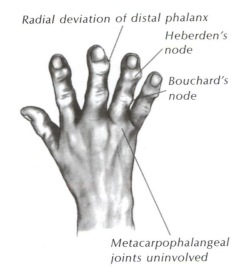

Radial deviation of distal phalanx

Heberden's node

Bouchard's node

Metacarpophalangeal joints uninvolved

**FIGURE 13.2** ● Characteristics of the hand in osteoarthritis. (From Bates, B. [1995]. *A guide to physical examination and history taking*. Philadelphia: J.B. Lippincott.)

within the joint tissues. The basic anatomy of a typical diarthrodial joint is illustrated in Figure 13-3. Normal joint structure is compared with a joint affected by OA. The design or shape of the articular surfaces of the joint must be flawlessly matched for unimpeded movement and full range of motion. Ligaments, tendons, and muscles offer the essential stability, support, and strength to the joint, whereas the neurologic innervation of the joint allows for sensory input and proprioception. Both muscular support and neurologic input are essential for normal joint

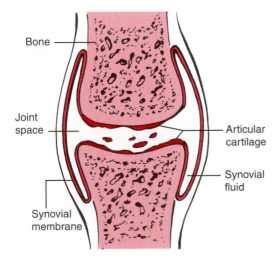

Bone

Joint space

Articular cartilage

Synovial fluid

Synovial membrane

**FIGURE 13.3** ● Normal joint and osteoarthritis damage (in red).

functioning and coordination (Bullough, 1992). Alterations in any of these components can lead to the development of OA through joint misalignment, unequal load bearing through alterations in muscular and ligament support, injury, and pathologic alterations in the characteristics of the tissues of the joint.

## Physiology of Joint Tissues

A series of feedback mechanisms regulate the physiologic processes involved in the maintenance and remodeling of subchondral bone and cartilage. These mechanisms must be maintained in a state of equilibrium so that the joint can stay functional (Bullough, 1992).

### Subchondral Bone

The subchondral bone is composed of subarticular tissues and contains both calcified cartilage and cortical bone (Burr, 1998) (see Fig. 13-3). This bone is vascular; however, in healthy tissues, vessels do not impinge on calcified cartilage. Therefore, cartilage is totally dependent on the synovial fluid bathing it for nutrition, waste removal, and oxygenation. The bony tissue underlying joint cartilage is dynamic tissue, and changes in subchondral bone may alter the morphology of the joint. Bone is constantly remodeled in healthy humans, and factors that change the load forces on bone play a direct role in these changes. Bone is broken down by osteoclasts and new bones formed by osteoblasts in a state of dynamic equilibrium. Calcification of the new bone matrix is the process that changes the density and strength of the newly remodeled bone. Remodeling also affects the Haversian systems and the trabeculae within the bone—a process described by Wolff's law (1986). This law states that the density and composition of the bone respond to the applied environmental forces. An extreme example of the necessity for weight and gravity to act on the bone is seen in immobilized patients. Without loads being placed on bone, the skeletal tissue atrophies, weakens, and decalcifies.

The calcified cartilage and noncalcified cartilage at the ends of bone are constantly interacting at the *tidemark*, or *calcified front* (Fig. 13-4). At the tidemark, a balance exists between deposition and inhibition of mineral deposition within the cartilage. The subchondral bone absorbs the calcified cartilage at a rate similar to that of the calcified cartilage invading the noncalcified cartilage, so that an equilibrium between bone and cartilage is maintained. Thus, the calcified cartilage provides an intermediate layer between the subchondral

NORMAL

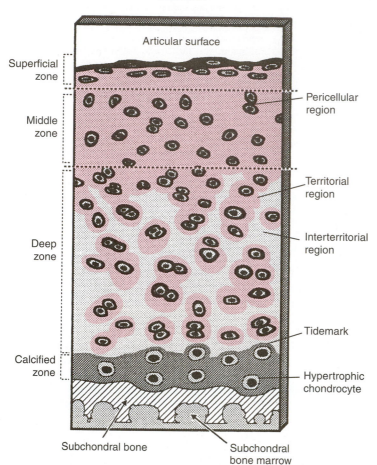

**FIGURE 13.4**  ●  Regional organization of adult cartilage. (From Poole, R. [1997] Cartilage in health and disease. In W. Koopman [Ed.], *Arthritis and allied conditions.* Baltimore: Williams & Wilkins.)

bone and the noncalcified cartilage, protecting the joint from stress (Burr, 1998).

## Cartilage

Articular cartilage is a solid material composed primarily of extracellular matrix surrounded by water (Mow & Setton, 1998). The major cell type of cartilage is the chondrocyte, although other cells such as lymphocytes may be found. Chondrocytes regulate and repair the extracellular matrix, which is composed primarily of type II collagen, proteoglycans or *aggrecan*, and water (Jacobson, 1996). The chondrocytes synthesize and degrade the extracellular matrix for the joint tissue to remain healthy and functional (Sandy & Lark, 1998). The amounts and ratio of the cellular and extracellular components are variable, depending on the joint involved and the depth within the cartilage itself. Collagen in joint cartilage is tightly packed and has a high tensile strength to transfer the load across the joint

(Bullough, 1992). Collagen provides tensile strength through its unique design, whereas the proteoglycans provide stiffness (Hollander et al., 1994).

Proteoglycans are negatively charged glycosaminoglycans that attract water molecules (Brandt & Fife, 1986). They exist as aggregates and are attached to hyaluronic acid. Water provides the cartilage with elastic properties, thus preventing excessive compression (Bullough, 1992). Water binds with the negative charges of the glycosaminoglycans, and as the joint compresses and pressure is applied to the cartilage, the bond between the two is broken, forcing the water to detach from its binding site. As the pressure is relieved, the water again attaches to its binding site. Nutrients and oxygen are supplied to cartilage through synovial fluid as the joint moves in this way (Kraus, 1997).

The extracellular components comprising the matrix, proteoglycans, collagen, and hyaluronic acid are regulated by the chondrocytes, and a balance exists between degradation and repair. In OA, both the type II collagen fibers and proteoglycan molecules are broken down excessively. The chondrocyte itself seems responsible for this destruction of the matrix of cartilage. In adults, long bone growth has been completed, so collagen activity normally shows limited remodeling, but the proteoglycans are in constant flux. Various proteinases, produced by chondrocytes, are responsible for degradation of the cartilage matrix. Metalloproteinases (MMPs) released by chondrocytes degrade the cartilage tissues and include collagenase (MMP1), galatinases (MMP2 and MMP9), and stromelysin (MMP3) (Sandy et al., 1998). Collagenase destroys collagen, whereas galatinase and stromelysin digest the proteoglycans. Active MMPs are sensitive to tissue inhibitors of MMPs (TIMPs), which also are secreted by synovial cells and chondrocytes (Woessner & Gunja-Smith, 1991). In healthy cartilage, there is a balance between the inhibitory properties of the TIMPs and the degradation of the MMPs, but in OA, there is an upregulation of the genes that code for MMPs in chondrocytes. Excessive proteinase production therefore may be at the heart of the pathophysiologic mechanisms that produce OA. Cytokines

are thought to be major factors that stimulate the genetic switching, so that excessive proteinases are produced by chondrocytes activated by catabolic cytokines. Inflammatory changes in the synovium, debris in the synovial fluid, and hyperplasia of synovial cells promote macrophage infiltration into the joint. Macrophages and chondrocytes release prostaglandin $E_2$ (PGE$_2$) and other proinflammatory cytokines such as interleukin-1β (IL-1β) and tumor necrosis factor-alpha (TNF-α). This pathologic process is illustrated in Figure 13-5.

Whereas the MMPs break down cartilage, other chondrocyte factors promote cartilage growth. Several important growth factors have been identified in the remodeling process of the cartilage matrix. Transforming growth factor-beta is thought to be responsible for the proliferation of aging chondrocytes, for increases in the synthesis of the extracellular matrix, and for slowing the proinflammatory effects of IL-1 (Ling & Bathon, 1998). Insulin-like growth factor also has been found to play a significant role in the production of collagen and proteoglycans by stimulating the chondrocytes (Dore et al., 1994). Both the proteinases and the growth factor substances must remain in homeostasis with one another for the joint's equilibrium to be maintained.

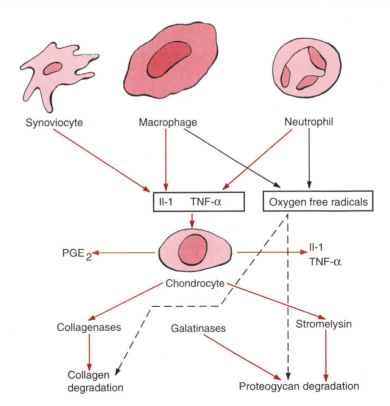

**FIGURE 13.5** ● The cytokines interleukin-1 and tumor necrosis factor-alpha stimulate protease release and cartilage breakdown.

## Factors That Influence Osteoarthritis

### Genetic Influences

A role for genetics is postulated in OA, and forms of the disease clearly are familial. For example, an early onset, severe OA occurs in 100% of the carriers of a mutation in the gene that codes for type II collagen (the Arg519-Cys mutation) (Bleasel et al., 1999). Another study from the Baltimore Longitudinal Study on Aging found an association between an aggrecan gene polymorphic allele and OA of the hands in elderly men (Horton et al., 1998). A genetic association was found between the presence of OA on x-ray with specific genotypes of the insulin-like growth factor I gene (Muelenbelt et al., 1998). How genetic risk is transmitted is not known, but statistical models of the data from the Framingham Heart study suggest that a recessive gene with a Mendelian pattern of inheritance is plausible. The model requires not only recessive genetic transmission, but also a multifactorial component that may be related to other genes or to environmental factors (Felsen et al., 1998). As in other genetic diseases, data from twin studies are available for OA; based on these studies, the contribution of familial risk to OA occurrence is thought to be on the order of 50% to 65% (Cicuttini & Spector, 1997).

### Obesity

Being overweight is a risk factor for OA of the knees, particularly in women, but not for other common joints such as the hip. As demonstrated in the Framingham Heart Study, being overweight as a young adult significantly increased risk of OA within the following 36 years, and losing as little as 5 kg reduced these odds by half (Hahn & Edwards, 1998). However, obesity is not believed to cause the disease, but to potentiate its expression and increase its severity. Weight loss does not alter the degree of disease present, but it reduces the load on damaged joints, thus alleviating some of the pain and disability.

### *Joint Shape and Trauma*

A popular notion is that repetitive activity of a joint will increase its risk for developing OA. Certainly there is evidence that misalignment or instability of joint surfaces and some joint injuries (eg, anterior cruciate ligament tears) ultimately may lead to OA over the years. There also are certain occupational groups that, because of the repetitive work or stress on joints, have increased risk for OA. However, there is little evidence to suggest that engaging in recreational sports over a lifetime, including sports such as marathon running, causes OA (Hahn & Edwards, 1998). For many OA patients, the strengthening of muscle groups and lubrication of joints through exercise has a positive effect.

## PATHOLOGIC CHANGES IN OSTEOARTHRITIS

Osteoarthritis is a disease in which the equilibrium between natural synthesis and degradation processes of the extracellular matrix is disrupted (Dore et al., 1994). This disruption leads to the degradation of the extracellular matrix and is followed by alterations in the subchondral bone and inflammation of the synovial membrane. Early in the disease, there is a softening of the articular cartilage. The disease then progresses to a structural breakdown of cartilage, consisting of fibrillation and fissuring, focal and diffuse erosions of the cartilage surface, and thinning and denudation of cartilage. The subchondral bone undergoes sclerosis, cyst formation, thickening, and reactive bone formation, producing spurs and osteophytes. Occasionally there also is synovial membrane inflammation.

The initiator of the disruption in OA is unknown. As the disease progresses, genetic abnormalities occur within the synovial cells, osteophyte cells, and chondrocytes, specifically, trisomies of chromosomes 5 and 7 (Broberg et al., 1997). Multiple biochemical abnormalities also are found in these cells, but the links between genetic changes and molecular perturbations are just being discovered.

Alterations in equilibrium between synthesis and degradation of collagen and proteoglycans occur throughout the disease process. There is excessive degradation of the matrix components, which overcomes cartilage synthesis, causing the depletion of the proteoglycans and a weakened collagenous net (Ling & Bathon, 1998). Collagen proteinases are in high concentrations, overwhelming their counterparts, the TIMPs, leading to collagen resorption. When stromelysin cleaves the proteoglycans, more water binding sites become available and the cartilage swells (Kraus, 1997). The swelling of the cartilage leads to softening and the development of cracks and fissures within the cartilage matrix. As these mechanical defects form, debris from the cartilage matrix is released into the synovial fluid and then may initiate inflammatory changes. The natural response to the progressive damage is for chondrocytes to proliferate and increase the production of proteoglycans. This attempt produces an abnormal matrix and immature chondrocytes (Kraus, 1997). Throughout the disease process, degradation overpowers these reparative efforts (Ling & Bathon, 1998). This process is illustrated in Figure 13-6.

As the cartilage is damaged and thinned, increased pressures and loads are forced onto the subchondral bone. This bone then remodels to accommodate these loads. To repair and restore joint functioning, the osteoblasts and osteoclasts resorb and create new subchondral bone tissue. The formation of new bony tissue is greater than the resorption, leading to bone thickening. In the areas where the bone-cartilage border is thin, bony outgrowths occur (Pritzker, 1998).

## PATHOPHYSIOLOGY OF THE SIGNS AND SYMPTOMS

Pain usually is the major presenting symptoms of OA. It is caused by structural changes within the joint, microfractures of the bone, and intra-articular hypertension resulting from swelling, synovial hypertrophy, and accompanying synovitis (O'Reilly & Doherty, 1998). Joint stiffness resulting from a mild inflammatory process usually occurs in the morning and lasts less than 30 minutes.

Crepitus, limited range of motion, and deformity can result from osteophyte formation, bone remodeling, and cartilage loss. Whereas the osteophytes' function is to support and stabilize the joint, they also are a source of pain, crepitus, and decreased range of motion (Kraus, 1997). Along with crepitus, there is joint deformity. Tenderness, increased warmth, and effusions are not commonly seen in OA; however, associated inflammatory conditions such as bursitis can lead to them (Jacobson, 1996).

### Diagnosing Osteoarthritis

The diagnosis of OA is based on both subjective and objective data collection. No diagnostic tests

OSTEOARTHRITIS
(Grades 2–6)

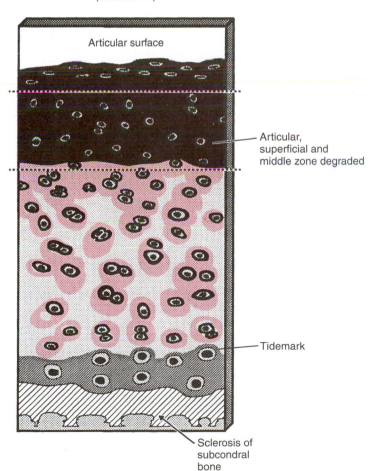

**FIGURE 13.6** ● Early cartilage damage in osteoarthritis. (From Poole, R. [1997]. Cartilage in health and disease. In W. Koopman [Ed.], *Arthritis and allied conditions.* Baltimore: Williams & Wilkins.)

Articular surface

Articular, superficial and middle zone degraded

Tidemark

Sclerosis of subcondral bone

can diagnose OA. Numerous test results, such as erythrocyte sedimentation rate, complete blood count, serum calcium and phosphate levels, chemistry profile, and uric acid level, are normal in OA, but these tests are ordered to rule out other disease processes in the presence of suggestive subjective or clinical findings (O'Reilly & Doherty, 1998). X-rays may reveal joint deformity, osteophytes, and joint narrowing, which are important in determining the progression of the disease (Uphold & Graham, 1998). Radiographic findings do not correlate with onset or severity of symptoms and therefore should be used only to compare progression of the disease (O'Reilly & Doherty, 1998).

## PHYSIOLOGIC BASIS FOR MANAGEMENT OF OSTEOARTHRITIS

The goals in the management of OA include patient education, minimizing pain, maximizing joint functioning, and reducing joint limitation (Brandt et al., 1998b). The therapeutic modalities chosen for the patients depend on the joints involved. The management of OA involves pharmacologic, nonpharmacologic, and surgical interventions. Patient education is important in any disease process. It allows patients to understand the prognosis, disease severity and progression, and any limitations that they will have.

Pharmacologic therapies include analgesic and anti-inflammatory medications. Acetaminophen is the analgesic of choice (Uphold & Graham, 1998). Nonsteroidal anti-inflammatory drugs (NSAIDs) are widely used for their analgesic and anti-inflammatory effects on secondary inflammations (Jacobson, 1996). Topical capsaicin relieves the pain through altering the levels of substance P, a neurotransmitter used in the pain pathways. Systemic steroids have not been effective in the treatment of OA; however, intra-articular corticosteroid injections have been shown to be effective by altering the inflammatory response (Brandt, 1996). People who have repeated cortisone injections into a joint ultimately progress to greater pathophysiologic joint alterations, however, because these drugs eventually increase connective tissue breakdown and muscle weakening around the joint.

A new, natural approach to OA has become popular in Europe and the United States. The supplements glucosamine and chondroitin have been widely touted as relieving the symptoms of OA. The theory behind the action of these agents is that they supply substrates for collagen and proteoglycan production in damaged OA cartilage. Clinical trials are under way to determine the true efficacy of these substances, but many patients with OA have discovered these "joint replacement" agents and are using them with varying degrees of relief.

Some of the nonpharmacologic therapies are exercise, heat and cold application, and ultrasound. Exercise is one of the most important therapeutic modalities for treatment of OA. Exercise has been shown to increase general fitness, range of motion, muscle strength, and neuromuscular control over proprioception. Brandt, Lohmander, and Doherty (1998b) report that persons in poor physical condition describe more pain with OA. Weight loss decreases load bearing on the joint tissues (bone and cartilage), thus allowing for ease of movement. Deep heat with ultrasound increases muscle relaxation and the tendons' ability to stretch (Kraus, 1997). Topical application of ice decreases secondary inflammation and increases the pain threshold (Brandt, 1996). Physical therapy offers concentrated nonpharmacologic therapies in a structured setting, which enhances patient compliance (Brandt et al., 1998b).

# OTHER FORMS OF ARTHRITIS

The primary care provider usually does not manage patients with inflammatory or infectious arthritis. However, the signs and symptoms of these other forms must be differentiated from OA, and if discovered in a patient in the clinic, appropriate referral to an infectious disease physician or rheumatologist is necessary.

# INFECTIOUS ARTHRITIS

Infectious disease agents can cause joint involvement through several pathophysiologic mechanisms. Bacterial sepsis can develop in a joint that has been surgically opened or traumatized. Microorganisms also spread to joints through hematogenous routes. Bacteria, viruses, mycobacteria, fungi, and parasites all are known to cause infectious arthritis. Infectious arthritis may be divided into gonococcal and nongonococcal causes, and 50% of septic arthritis in young, sexually active people is caused by the gonococcus. Infectious arthritis usually involves one joint and presents with fever. Arthritis resulting from hematogenous spread (eg, hepatitis B) may be polyarticular. The differentiating factors from OA are

● **Case Study 13.1**

A 55-year-old white female presents at a primary care clinic with a chief complaint of a painful and stiff left knee. She states that her knee has been hurting for several years but has progressively gotten worse over the last month. The pain is interfering with her daily activities of walking and gardening. It usually is worse in the evenings and at night. Stiffness occurs at rest and on awakening and improves with movement and use. Stair climbing has become progressively more painful. She denies any recent falls, trauma, or injury to her knees. She has been participating in more gardening activities recently. In the past, she has taken two OTC ibuprofen, 200 mg each, intermittently for the pain with minimal relief. She never sought medical care for knee pain. She denies any problems with other joints. No inflammation, loss of range of motion, redness, numbness or tingling in her lower extremities.

## History

### Past Medical History

| | |
|---|---|
| Current medication | Captopril 25 mg BID, multivitamin daily |
| Surgeries | Cesarean section × 2 (1969, 1971) |
| Injury/Trauma | History of left patellar subluxation in 1985 after a snow skiing accident, required no surgical intervention. No other injuries, fractures or trauma |

### Social History

| | |
|---|---|
| Retired nurse | Happily married for 30 years. G2,P2,AO |
| Tobacco | Denies |
| Alcohol | Denies |
| Social drugs | Denies |
| Exercise | Walks in neighborhood 2–3 times/week for 20 minutes. Enjoys gardening |

### Family History

| | |
|---|---|
| Mother | 82 y, hypertension |
| Father | 86 y |
| Brother | 54 y |
| Sister | 59 y |
| | No diabetes, cancer, or rheumatologic problems |

## Review of Systems

| | |
|---|---|
| General | No recent weight changes, fever, weakness, or fatigue |
| HEENT | No changes in visual acuity. Has worn glasses for 25 years for near-sightedness. No ear or eye pain, nasal drainage or congestion. Denies sinus pressure, sore throat or neck stiffness |
| Lungs | Denies SOB, cough, orthopnea, or PND |
| Cardiac | Denies palpitations, chest pain, peripheral edema, discoloration of extremities, blood clots, Raynaud's phenomenon, or varicosities |
| GI | No change in appetite; no abdominal pain, nausea, vomiting; no change in bowels. No history of GI bleeds, ulcers, or reflux |

*(Case study continued on page 256)*

| | |
|---|---|
| GU | Denies dysuria, retention or frequency. Menopausal for 5 years. No vaginal irritation or discharge |
| MS | No previous diagnosis of arthritis. Denies any weakness, inflammation or redness of joints. Left knee with pain and stiffness for several years, progressively worsening over the last month. Interfering with walking and gardening. No limited range of motion or deformity. History of left patellar subluxation in 1985 after a snow skiing accident, required no surgical intervention. No back or ankle injuries. No history of gout |
| Endocrine | Denies changes in hair or nails. No constipation, cold/heat intolerance, sweats, or fatigue |
| Neurologic | Denies numbness, tingling in extremities. No history of back or neck injuries |

## Differential Diagnosis

1. Osteoarthritis
2. Gout
3. Rheumatoid arthritis
4. Soft tissue injuries: bursitis, tendinitis

## Physical Examination

| System | Findings |
|---|---|
| General | 55-year-old white female in NAD. Alert and oriented × 3 |
| Vital Signs | T–98.3°F, R–20, P–88<br>BP–120/87<br>Height 5′4″, Weight 175 lb |
| HEENT | Eyes—PERRLA. TMs pearly gray. Canals clear. No maxillary or frontal sinus tenderness. Posterior pharynx without redness or inflammation. No lymphoid patches or exudes noted |
| Neck | Supple without lymphadenopathy, thyroid enlargement, or carotid bruits. No JVD |
| Lungs | Clear with good bilateral air exchange. Respirations even and unlabored |
| CV | $S_1$ and $S_2$ noted. No murmurs or extra heart sounds. No peripheral edema noted. Pedal, radial, and post-tibia pulses at 2+. No varicosities noted |
| Abdomen | Obese, soft, nontender. Bowel sounds × 4 quad. No organomegaly noted |
| GU | Deferred |
| MS | No joint deformity noted. Decreased ROM with full extension and flexion of the left knee. Pain elicited with palpation of the left knee, medial and lateral joint lines, and with passive/active ROM. Crepitus in left knee with ROM. No inflammation, redness, or warmth noted in any joints. No ligament laxity or muscle weakness noted. Negative drawer, Lachman, and McMurray's test. Gait—patient favoring left leg |
| Neurologic | Cranial nerves intact. DTRs 2+ bilaterally |

*(Case study continued on next page)*

### Diagnostic Testing

No laboratory testing is indicated
X-ray: narrowing joint space in the left knee with osteophyte formation

### Assessment

Osteoarthritis

### Plan

1. Analgesics for relief of pain.
2. Ice 3 × a day for 20 minutes and after strenuous physical activity. Decreases secondary inflammation
3. Exercise: increase walking regimen to at least 30 minutes, 5 times a week. Improves fitness level and helps weight loss
4. Provide strengthening exercises for the quadriceps. Gives more support to the knee joint, protecting it from further damage
5. Plan: follow-up in 4 weeks, sooner if needed. If without improvement at this time, refer to physical therapy

BID, twice daily; CV, cardiovascular; DTRs, deep tendon reflexes; GI, gastrointestinal; GU, genitourinary; HEENT, head, eyes, ears, nose, and throat; JVD, joint and vascular disease; MS, musculoskeletal; NAD, no apparent distress; Neuro, neurologic; OTC, over the counter; PERRLA, pupils equal, round, regular to light accommodation; PND, paroxysmal nocturnal dyspnea; quad, quadrants; ROM, range of motion; SOB, shortness of breath; TMs, tympanic membranes.

that patients may be young or immunocompromised and may present with acute-onset illness; signs of acute inflammation usually are apparent. Patients also may present with a postinfectious polyarthritis. Examples of this include Lyme disease, rheumatic fever, and Reiter's syndrome. The following clinical vignette illustrates this type of polyarthritis.

# GOUTY ARTHRITIS

Arthritis can result from the deposition of crystals in joints, and the most common type in humans is caused by gout. Crystals of uric acid deposit in joints and initiate a cascade of inflammatory events, resulting in swelling, heat, redness, and throbbing pain in the affected joint. The general incidence is 2 of 1000, with a higher prevalence in men. Risk increases also in patients with obesity, diabetes mellitus, renal disease, and sickle cell anemia. Certain drugs that interrupt normal purine metabolism also increase uric acid levels, leading to gouty arthritis. There is a strong hereditary tendency to develop gout, and attacks of the disease can be caused by excessive alcohol ingestion or heavy, rich meals.

## PURINE METABOLISM

Purines are one of the building blocks of DNA. The purine base adenine is a compound in adenosine triphosphate, which is used in all cells for energy. When purines are broken down in cells, the end product is, in humans, uric acid. Humans are the only species unable to further degrade uric acid to a more soluble and easily excreted compound, allantoin, because humans lack the enzyme uric acid oxidase. Normal metabolism leads to a load of uric acid of 600 mg/day, which must be excreted by the kidneys (Morris, 1998). When the uric acid levels in the blood and tissue fluids exceed the limit of solubility of the compound, then needle-like crystals—about the size of an erythrocyte—of monosodium urate precipitate. The precipitation of crystals in synovial fluid leads to gout when levels of uric acid are greater than 6.8 mg/100 mL (Morris, 1998), making the patient hyperuricemic. Depending on the chronicity of the disease (usually longer than 10 years) and serum levels of uric acid (greater than 10 mg/100 mL), uric acid can deposit in many structures in the body. These nodular deposits of uric acid are called tophi and are found in the skin, on bone and tendons, on the ear, in the kidney, and in

## CLINICAL VIGNETTE 13.1

A 40-year-old female patient presents to the primary care clinic with complaints of low-grade fever, fatigue, and arthralgia. During the review of systems, the nurse practitioner notes that the patient reports having a rash about a month ago but otherwise felt well. Now she reports extreme malaise, fatigue, pain, and swelling in her left knee and right elbow.

On physical examination, her vitals signs are noted to be elevated, with a fever of 101°F and tachycardia: 92. A red macular rash is noted in her groin area and on her abdomen. She also is found to have asymmetric paresthesia in her feet and legs. The only joints involved are the right elbow, which is painful on range of motion and feels slightly warm and swollen, and her left knee joint, which has an effusion and is warm to touch. She has limitation of full range of motion in this joint and reports pain on palpation and with movement. Her gait favors this leg.

The history in this patient was unremarkable except that she mentioned casually that she had been on vacation about 6 weeks previously on Martha's Vineyard in Massachusetts and remembers being bitten by a small, barely visible tick.

The patient presents history and physical findings strongly suggestive of Lyme disease, which is the most common tick-borne illness in the United States. The organism is the spirochete *Borrelia burgdorferi,* which is carried in the ticks (*Ixodes dammini*) that infest deer, and most cases have occurred in New England and New York. The incubation period is 7 to 10 days and is followed by mild constitutional symptoms and a rash (erythema migrans). The disease involves multiple other structures in the next weeks to months such as the skin, peripheral nervous system, heart, and joints. Joint involvement is typically asymmetrical and involves one to a few joints, and often the arthritis is migratory, moving from one joint to another. Low-grade fever, malaise, and fatigue are typical symptoms in the early disease. Any of these systems can develop chronic disease if the organisms are not eradicated. Arthritis is one of the most common long-term sequelae in untreated patients. Diagnosis of Lyme disease is made definitively by serologic tests (immunofluorescence assay, enzyme-linked immunosorbent assay, Western blot), and the disease is treated in the early stages by antibiotic therapy. Resolution of arthritis symptoms varies in response to antibiotics.

---

joints. They have been known to be large enough to simulate soft tissue tumors.

## HISTORY OF THE DISEASE

People can develop hyperuricemia slowly and over many years, or may not have any symptoms. However, it is believed that during this time, small tophaceous accumulations are developing in many tissues, including joints. Gout is divided into four stages: asymptomatic, acute, intercritical, and chronic. The asymptomatic stage can last 10 years, and the occurrence of an acute attack depends largely on the level of uric acid during the asymptomatic period. It is not uncommon for males to have their first attack during adolescence, whereas females may not have their first attack until after menopause.

The acute attack of gout usually is an episode of extreme monoarticular joint pain, and although any joint could theoretically be involved, half of the patients with gout have their first attack in the first metatarsophalangeal joint. The big toe

appears red, hot, swollen, and throbs, often with excruciating pain. Patients experience an extreme sensitivity to touch, and even bedsheets may be intolerable (Sacks, 1998). The more distal the joint is from the heart, the lower the temperature of the fluids in the joint, and the big toe is the most distal joint, with a temperature of 27°C. As body temperature drops, uric acid's solubility decreases, thus increasing the likelihood of precipitation into monosodium urate crystals (Morris, 1998).

Subsequent attacks may be in the big toe or other distal joints (ankle, wrist, finger, and elbow). Particularly susceptible are joints already damaged by OA. Most patients have a subsequent attack after the first attack within a year.

Chronic gouty arthritis develops in patients who are untreated and involves the continuous deposition of urate with chronic inflammation ensuing; production of tophi, which may calcify and alter joint morphology; and, in some cases, production of a thick, white effusion of urate known as urate milk.

# INFLAMMATORY PATHOPHYSIOLOGY OF GOUTY ARTHRITIS

Gout can occur when levels of uric acid accumulate either because of impaired excretion or overproduction of uric acid. The inability to excrete uric acid seems to be the most common form of the disease. Another cause is overexpression of the gene that codes for the enzyme phosphoribosylpyrophosphate synthetase. This is an X-linked disorder characterized by overproduction of purine nucleotides and uric acid (Ahmed et al., 1999).

The initiators of inflammation in gouty arthritis are the monosodium urate crystals, which are foreign body–like irritants in the synovial fluid. Aspiration of joint fluid and identification of the crystals definitively diagnoses gout. Like other inflammatory conditions, acute gouty arthritis involves a network of cytokines that promote inflammation. Monocyte chemoattractant proteins released by synovial cells promote macrophage infiltration into the joint fluid. A wave of other proinflammatory cytokines also appear to be released from the synovial cells and include IL-1β, IL-8 and TNF-α, which are released into the synovial fluid in response to monosodium urate crystal precipitation. IL-8 is a powerful neutrophil chemoattractant agent and IL-1 and TNF-α are major proinflammatory cytokines. Infiltrating leukocytes then produce a second wave of cytokines, including IL-8, IL-1, and IL-1 receptor antagonist (Matsukawaw et al., 1998). Cytokines then initiate further inflammatory changes, as discussed in Chapter 2.

# PHYSIOLOGIC BASIS OF TREATMENT

High doses of colchicine historically have been the treatment of choice for the inflammation associated with acute gouty attacks, although their mechanism of action is unknown. Colchicine may interrupt leukocyte function and thus suppress inflammation. NSAIDs have proven equally or more effective and less toxic than colchicine in the treatment of acute gout attacks.

Long-term therapy for patients with uric acid levels greater than 7 mg/100 mL usually is necessary, although some patients may achieve low enough uric acid levels by lifestyle modification alone, which should be encouraged. Weight loss is helpful, and the choice of diet is critical to preventing gouty attacks, requiring an avoidance of high-purine foods and alcohol. Also, the use of concurrent medications for other conditions that increase uric acid may be modified. Choosing medication for gout depends on whether the disease is caused by impaired renal excretion or excessive purine metabolism and urate production. The practitioner can determine the proper choice through creatinine clearance and 24-hour uric acid excretion levels. Allopurinol is used when hyperuricemia is present with decreased renal function or with high uric acid levels in the urine. Allopurinol is a xanthine oxidase inhibitor. For patients who do not overexcrete uric acid, a uricosuric agent such as probenecid often is used. This drug increases uric acid excretion (Sack, 1997).

# RHEUMATOID ARTHRITIS

Rheumatoid arthritis is the most common inflammatory joint disease afflicting humans, with an incidence of 0.8% across all worldwide populations. It is a disease only of humans; no natural animal models exist. The highest prevalence is in women, and the average age at onset is in the late 40s to early 50s. The cause of RA is unknown, although genetic, environmental, hormonal, immune, and aging factors probably interact to cause this disease. Most authorities consider RA to have an underlying autoimmune etiology. Certain anatomic and physiologic characteristics of cartilage and synovium perpetuate immunologic destruction of joints in this disease.

## SPECIAL PROPERTIES OF JOINTS

Recall that articular cartilage is avascular, depending on the synovial fluid for nutrition. Because there is not constant exchange between cartilage and blood, antigens may persist in cartilage for a longer time than in other tissues. The cells of cartilage, mainly chondrocytes, are functionally autonomous, producing a variety of cytokines and chemokines. On the other hand, the synovium is highly vascular and contains type A synoviocytes, which are derived from monocytes that migrate from the blood. These cells carry antigens and even microorganisms into the joints, act as antigen-presenting cells (APCs), and secrete a variety of immune-modulating cytokines (Albani & Carson, 1997). Cartilage, as was discussed in the section on OA, is subject to potential injury, and as cartilage ages, it is less capable of repair. These anatomic and physiologic properties make joints ideal sites for potentially extensive immunologic responses.

# ETIOLOGIC FACTORS IN RHEUMATOID ARTHRITIS

## Genetic Factors

Several hereditary factors influence both the occurrence and severity of RA. It has been known for 30 years that the human leukocyte antigen (HLA) class II antigens might be involved in the genetically inherited influences in RA. The haplotypes HLA-DR4 and HLA-DR1 increase the severity of the disease. Other HLA haplotypes have been implicated in influencing disease expression and incidence. A five-amino acid sequence, known as the *rheumatoid (or shared) epitope*, is found as a common sequences among all suspected HLA haplotypes.

The extent of concordance between identical twins for RA is only about 15% (Albani & Carson, 1997), but the immune systems even of monozygotic twins are different, based on their personal immunologic history. Environmental factors clearly are important in disease expression in RA.

## Infectious Agents

No known microbes have been found to have a positive association with RA. However, the amino acid sequence of the rheumatoid epitope on human cells has been discovered to be identical to sequences on certain Epstein-Barr virus proteins and other Gram-negative microorganism-induced heat shock proteins. This is the basis for theories of cross-reactivity, in which the human immune response to the microorganisms is beneficial, but because of shared epitopes, there may be immunologic attack on self-antigens.

## Hormonal Factors

Because RA is more prevalent in women (3:1 ratio), as are most of the autoimmune diseases, the female hormones are thought to be involved in susceptibility, or, conversely, male hormones might be involved in protection. RA is considered to be a $T_H1$ disease, which means that the T-helper subset involved mostly in cellular immune responses and delayed hypersensitivity reactions is thought to be aberrant. Proinflammatory cytokines released by $T_H1$ cells may produce some of the inflammatory changes seen in the joints of RA. RA is well known to essentially disappear or become less severe during pregnancy, when estrogen and progesterone are high, and to exacerbate during the postpartum period, particularly if the mother breast-feeds. The hormones estrogen, progesterone, and prolactin may be key factors in the regulation of these subpopulations of T-helper cells. However, the picture is not simple, since RA appears with a peak incidence in the menopausal years when estrogen levels are falling, and there may be some protection for women on estrogen replacement therapy.

## Autoimmunity

The most ubiquitous and well-known autoimmune factor discovered in RA is *rheumatoid factor* (RF). Serum levels of RF are elevated in RA. RFs are IgM, IgA, and IgG antibodies against the Fc region of IgG. Evidence indicates that the RFs are produced by antigenically stimulated circulating B cells, with the marker CD5+ on their surface (Youinou et al., 1990). These types of B cells can increase remarkably in patients with RA. It is thought that the production of autoantibodies against a patient's own immunoglobulins causes complexing and cross-linking of antibodies, potentially leading to inflammation in the synovium.

# PATHOPHYSIOLOGIC MECHANISMS IN RHEUMATOID ARTHRITIS

There are some similarities between the disruption in cartilage homeostasis that has been described as occurring in OA and observed in RA. Critical differences include the degree of immunologically mediated inflammation and the amount of erosive damage that occurs in RA. Also, RA is considered to be a systemic inflammatory disease, which can affect multiple structures. For example, granulomatous, subcutaneous rheumatoid nodules can occur in many different tissues, lung lesions have been observed, and vasculitis occasionally is found.

In early RA, there is synovial cell proliferation, endothelial changes in the blood vessels, and infiltration of lymphocytes and neutrophils into the joint, producing a highly cellular joint effusion. Later, further lymphocytic infiltration and chronic, granulomatous necrotic changes in the joints produce cartilaginous and subchondral bone destruction, largely through the invasive *pannus*, an erosive granulomatous tissue. The pannus is unique to RA compared with OA. This granulation tissue is filled with fibroblasts and inflammatory cells and destroys the articular cartilage first, and then destroys subsequent layers of cartilage down to and including the subchondral bone. Often, there also is damage to the joint ligaments and tendons (Jasin, 1997), leading to deformity and instability. The effects of RA on cartilage and bone are illustrated in Figure 13-7.

RHEUMATOID ARTHRITIS
(Early Changes)

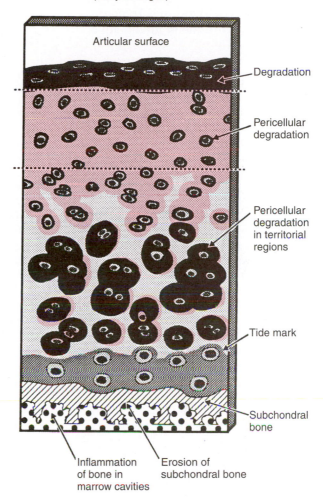

Articular surface

— Degradation

— Pericellular
degradation

— Pericellular
degradation
in territorial
regions

— Tide mark

— Subchondral
bone

Inflammation
of bone in
marrow cavities

Erosion of
subchondral bone

**FIGURE 13.7** ● Early cartilage and bone changes in rheumatoid arthritis. (From Poole, R. [1997]. Cartilage in health and disease. In W. Koopman [Ed.], *Arthritis and allied conditions.* Baltimore: Williams & Wilkins.)

As in OA, the cytokines, with their paracrine and autocrine effects, play important roles in the pathophysiologic disruptions in the affected joints. The most critical cytokines are IL-1 and TNF-α. The initiating event in RA probably results from autoimmunologic reactivity to components of cartilage. Collagen degradation and exposure of hidden collagen epitopes may be the critical first step. How collagen breakdown is stimulated initially is unknown, but it could be through inflammatory, immune, or infectious events. The collagen fragments then are presented by APCs such as B cells, macrophages, and synovial cells, which process and present the antigen to T cells. These APCs release IL-1 or TNF-α when they are immunologically activated by antigen. The T-activated helper cells then stimulate B cells to release immunoglobulins, which react to the fragments of type II collagen, causing immune precipitation of complexes

into the joint. This further aggravates the inflammatory processes. Additionally, high levels of RF are found in the joint fluid in RA, and these complex with IgG, leading to further immune complex formation and deposition.

IL-1 and TNF-α have several important effects on cartilage and bone (Table 13-4). The proinflammatory cytokines act at various levels on cartilage and bone. They produce a synovitis, which causes synovial cells to proliferate and transform into macrophage-like cells, which act as APCs and release cytokines. They cause vascular endothelial expression of adhesin and selectin molecules, causing neutrophils to migrate into the joint. Proteases, IL-1, and TNF-α produced by these neutrophils then act on the articular surface of cartilage. They also stimulate chondrocytes to release proteases that degrade cartilage and matrix. Finally, they stimulate osteoclast activity, causing

## TABLE 13.4 ● ● ●

### Effects of Interleukin-1 and Tumor Necrosis Factor-Alpha in Rheumatoid Arthritis

Proinflammatory

Induces T-cell clonal expansion

Induces chondrocytes to secrete proteases, prostaglandin $E_2$, nitric oxide, oxygen free radicals, proinflammatory cytokines

Inhibits collagen synthesis

Stimulates osteoclasts to increase bone resorption

Stimulates endothelial cells to express adhesion receptors

Induces neutrophil degranulation and superoxide synthesis

bone resorption. All of these effects are important in producing the joint damage seen in RA. Additionally, levels of these cytokines rise in the blood in the patient with active RA and can cause periarticular disease, sickness behavior effects, and other systemic problems.

## CLINICAL PRESENTATION

Although primary care providers usually refer patients with RA to appropriate specialists, they will have patients with RA in their practices. This is a chronic disease that deeply affects people's lives, and sensitivity to patients' limitations and pain are important for providers who care for their primary disease or for providers who manage other minor illnesses that might bring them to the ambulatory care clinic. The primary care practitioner should understand not only the pathophysiologic basis of this disease, but also the clinical presentation. This helps the provider to judge the stage and severity of the disease, and the possibility that disease symptomatology or medication is masking symptoms of other illnesses. Practitioners using a holistic approach to patients with RA must be aware of the stressful nature of this illness, the potential role of stress in exacerbation, and must be able to help patients to manage and alleviate stress in their lives.

The clinical presentation of the patient with RA depends on disease severity and chronicity. The

1987 criteria of the ACR are used to diagnose this disease (Arnett, et al., 1998). They are as follows:

- Morning stiffness for at least 1 hour in three or more joints
- Arthritis (defined as soft tissue swelling or fluid) of three or more joints
- Arthritis of hand joints
- Rheumatoid nodules
- RF-positive serum
- Typical radiographic changes in the hand and wrist
- Symmetrical arthritis

If patients meet all of these criteria, they are diagnosed as having *classic* RA; if they meet five of the seven, they are diagnosed with *definite* RA; and patients who meet three criteria are diagnosed with *probable* RA. Some patients have an initial diagnosis of RA based on symptoms and are symptom-free when reexamined 3 to 5 years later. However, most patients who are diagnosed with RA in a rheumatology setting show progression over time to increasingly severe disease (Pincus & Callahan, 1993). In-long term studies of patients with RA, progressive and severe morbidity generally is seen in terms of joint space narrowing, pannus formation, and functional status declines. The first two are measured radiographically, whereas the latter is measured by questionnaires that inventory activities of daily living, grip strength, morning stiffness, and work disability (Pincus & Callahan, 1993).

The primary care provider should be aware there is evidence that patients with RA have an increased mortality rate. Although the cause of death may not be RA, the general physical weakening, systemic and local immune changes, and social and stress effects all may contribute to decreased resistance to a variety of diseases, leading to early death.

The major findings on history and physical examination in the RA patient include joint pain both at rest and on motion, tenderness to palpation, morning stiffness, joint swelling, and deformity. The fingers are involved most often, and over time, characteristic deformities develop (boutonniere deformity, swan neck deformity). The joints involved in RA are metacarpophalangeal joints compared with the more distal finger joints of OA. Other joints include the wrists, elbows, shoulders, and, rarely, the sternoclavicular and manubriosternal joints of the chest wall. The knees are commonly affected in RA, as are the metatarsophalangeal joints. Many patients also develop arthritis of the cricoarytenoid joint, which can cause sever dysphagia and hoarseness. Another common site

---

## CLINICAL VIGNETTE 13.2

Mrs. Carla Spellman, a 53-year-old female, comes to the clinic with a chief complaint of sore throat. She is well known to the clinic as a patient recently diagnosed with rheumatoid arthritis. She was referred to a rheumatologist and has been on Celebrex twice daily for the last 3 months, with some relief of her pain and stiffness. She has bilateral joint involvement of her hands, knees, and cervical spine.

Today she asks for antibiotic treatment for her sore throat, since "it feels like a strep throat." Physical examination reveals that Mrs. Spellman has lost about 10 lbs since her last visit and has mild anemia (Hct: 32%, Hgb: 10). Her vital signs are within normal limits. Mrs. Spellman's involved joints are swollen and slightly warm to the touch and moderately painful on range of motion. She feels that she is somewhat better than when first diagnosed, but she states, "I didn't know that this was going to go on and on! When am I going to get better?"

She is noted to have a small subcutaneous nodule on her right olecranon process. She has swollen, red turbinates, clear nasal discharge, and mildly injected throat with 2+ tonsils. No exudate is seen. She has no cervical adenopa-

thy, and has a negative strep test. Results from the rest of her physical examination are unremarkable. During the course of the examination she begins to cry and states that she feels "very stressed about having this disease," and that she "doesn't know how she can cope."

Social history indicates that she lives with her husband, who is employed as a banker, and that she is on long-term disability from her job as an insurance agent. Her children are grown and live out of state. She has not been able to engage in any physical activity since diagnosis. Previously her social life revolved around her tennis club activities.

Plan: Mrs. Spellman's current symptoms are caused by a mild viral rhinitis with postnasal drip. It is likely that she came to the clinic with this symptom because she needed to talk to a professional about her illness, pain, and disability. She needs advice and teaching about her disease, connection with information resources such as World Wide Web addresses, a peer support group, and help in thinking about new recreational and social outlets. Because she has lost weight and is anemic, dietary assessment needs to be done, and a stool for guaiac analyzed. Her viral rhinitis requires only symptomatic treatment.

---

of involvement is the cervical spine, which occurs in most patients with long-term disease.

Extra-articular manifestations include rheumatoid nodules, pericarditis, pleuritis, and vasculitis.

## PHYSIOLOGIC BASIS OF TREATMENT

Therapy for the patient with RA is to symptomatically treat the inflammation of this disease. The first-line approach is to use salicylates or NSAIDs. These drugs then become the background therapy (Weinblatt, 1997). The second-line drugs are directed at the pathophysiologic basis of the disease and include numerous drugs that act in different ways to modify the disease. Included in this list are antimalarials, sulfasalazine, methotrexate, gold salts, cyclophosphamide, cyclosporine, and corticosteroids. Sometimes, these second-line drugs are used in combination (Weinblatt, 1997). Their general mechanism of action is to suppress the immune system. A new type of drug with promis-

ing results blocks TNF-α's proinflammatory effects.

One of the most powerful nonpharmacologic tools that a practitioner can use in patients with chronic illness is that of *written disclosure*. Numerous studies indicate that for all types of chronic problems, from depression to RA, keeping a daily written diary, or using other methods for writing down events and emotions, is beneficial. In a study of patients with RA or asthma (see Chapter 8), clinically relevant improvements in both types of patients were observed after 4 months of writing about stressful events compared with the control condition, in which subjects wrote about neutral events (Smyth et al., 1999). Other studies of the effects of daily hassles on symptoms in patients with RA show a significant relationship between stress and flares of the disease (Zautra et al., 1997).

Teaching patients about their disease may help them to understand symptoms and manage their lives more effectively. Practitioners can suggest that patients with RA keep up with the latest knowledge about their disease by using the World Wide Web. One site that is useful for all patients with arthritis is *http://www. arthritis.org*, which is the home page of the Arthritis Foundation.

## REFERENCES

Altman, R., Asch, E., Bloch, D., et al. (1996). The American College of Rheumatology criteria for the classification and reporting of osteoarthritis of the knee. *Arthritis and Rheumatism, 29,* 1039–1049.

Ahmed, M., Taylor, W., Smith, P., & Becker, M. (1999). Accelerated transcription of PRPS1 in X-linked overactivity of normal human phosphoribosylpyrophosphate synthetase. *Journal of Biological Chemistry, 274* (11), 7482–7488.

Albani, S. & Carson, D. (1997). Etiology and pathogenesis of rheumatoid arthritis. In W. Koopman (Ed.), *Arthritis and allied conditions* (13th ed.). Baltimore: Williams & Wilkins.

Arnett, F., Edworthy, S., Block, D., McShane, D. Fries, J., Cooper, N., Healey, L., Kaplan, S., Liang, M., & Luthra, H. (1988). The American Rheumatism Association 1987 revised criteria for the classification of rheumatoid arthritis. *Arthritis and Rheumatism, 24,* 315–324.

Bleasel, J., Poole, A., Heinegard, D., Saxne, T., Holderbaum, D., Ionescu, M., Jones, P., & Moskowitz, R. (1999). Changes in serum cartilage marker levels indicate altered cartilage metabolism in families with the osteoarthritis-related type II collagen gene COL2A1 mutation. *Arthritis and Rheumatism, 42* (1), 39–45.

Brandt, K. & Fife, R. (1986). Aging in relation to the pathogenesis of osteoarthritis. *Clinics of Rheumatic Diseases, 12* (1), 117–130.

Brandt, K. (1996). *Diagnosis and nonsurgical management of osteoarthritis.* USA: Professional Communications.

Brandt, K., Lohmander, S., & Doherty, M. (1998a). Pathogenesis of osteoarthritis. In K. Brandt, S. Lohmander, & M. Doherty (Eds.), *Osteoarthritis* (pp. 70–73). Oxford: Oxford University Press.

Brandt, K., Lohmander, S., & Doherty, M. (1998b). Management of osteoarthritis. In K. Brandt, S. Lohmander, & M. Doherty (Eds.), *Osteoarthritis* (pp. 251–255). Philadelphia: W.B. Saunders.

Broberg, K., Limon, J., Palsson, E., Lindstrand, A., Toksvig-Larsen, S., Mandahl, N., & Mertens, F. (1997). Clonal chromosome aberrations are present in vivo in synovia and osteophytes from patients with osteoarthritis. *Human Genetics, 101* (3), 295–298.

Bullough, P. (1992). The pathology of osteoarthritis. In R. Moskowitz, D. Howell, V. Goldberg, & H. Markin (Eds.), *Osteoarthritis: Diagnosis and medical/surgical management* (pp. 39–69). Philadelphia: W.B. Saunders.

Burr, D. (1998). Subchondral bone. In K. Brandt, S. Lohmander, & M. Doherty (Eds.), *Osteoarthritis* (pp. 144–156). Oxford: Oxford University Press.

Campbell, J. & Linc, L. (1999). Managing osteoarthritis pain. *Advances for the Nurse Practitioner 7* (4), 57–60.

Cicuttini, F. & Spector, T.D. (1997). What is the evidence that osteoarthritis is genetically determined? *Baillieres Clinical Rheumatology, 11* (4), 657–669.

Cooper, C. & Dennison, E. (1998). The natural history and prognosis of osteoarthritis. In K. Brandt, S. Lohmander, & M. Doherty (Eds.), *Osteoarthritis* (pp. 237–249). Oxford: Oxford University Press.

Dore, S., Pelletier, J., DiBattista, J., Tardif, G., Brazeau, P., & Martel-Pelletier, J. (1994). Human osteoarthritic chondrocytes possess an increased number of insulin-like growth factor 1 binding sites but are unresponsive to its stimulation. *Arthritis and Rheumatism 17* (2), 253–263.

Felson, D.T., Couropmitree, N., Chaisson, C., Hannan, M., Zhang, Y., McAlindon, T.E., LaValley, M., Levy, D., & Myers, R.H. (1998). Evidence for a Mendelian gene in a segregation analysis of generalized radiographic osteoarthritis: The Framingham Study. *Arthritis and Rheumatism, 41,* 1064–1071.

Hahn, P. & Edwards, L. (1998). Osteoarthritis: Presentation, pathogenesis, and pharmacologic therapy. *Clinical Reviews, Summer,* 9–13.

Hollander, A., Heathfield, T., Webber, C., Iwata, Y., Bourne, R., & Poole, R. (1994). Increased damage to type II collagen in osteoarthritic articular cartilage detected by a new immunoassay. *Journal of Clinical Investigation, 93,* 1722–1732.

Horton, W., Jr., Lethbridge-Cejku, M., Hochberg, M., Balakir, R., Precht, P., Plato, C., Tobin, J., Meek, L., & Doege, K. (1998). An association between an aggrecan polymorphic allele and bilateral hand osteoarthritis in elderly white men: Data from the Baltimore Longitudinal Study of Aging (BLSA). *Osteoarthritis Cartilage, 16*(4), 245–251.

Jacobson, E. (1996). Osteoarthritis. In J. Noble (Ed.), *Textbook of primary care medicine* (2nd ed., pp. 1093–1097). St. Louis: Mosby.

Jasin, H. (1997). Mechanisms of tissue damage in rheumatoid arthritis. In W. Koopman, (Ed.), *Arthritis and allied conditions.* Baltimore: Williams & Wilkins.

Kraus, V. (1997). Pathogenesis and treatment of osteoarthritis. *Advances in Rheumatology 81* (1), 85–112.

Ling, S. & Bathon, J. (1998). Osteoarthritis in older adults. *Journal of the American Geriatrics Society, 46* (2), 216–225.

Marieb, E. & Mallatt, J. (1992). *Human anatomy.* Redwood City: California: The Benjamin/Cummings Publishing Company.

Martel-Pelletier, J., DiBattista, J., Lajeunesse, D., & Pelletier, J. (1998). IGF/IGFBP axis in cartilage and bone in osteoarthritis pathogenesis. *Inflammation Research, 47,* 90–100.

Matsukawa, A., Yoshimura, T., Maeda, T., Takahashi, T., Ohkawara, S., & Yoshinaga, M. (1998). Analysis of the cytokine network among tumor necrosis factor alpha, interleukin-1 beta, interleukin-8, and interleukin-1 receptor antagonist in monosodium urate crystal-induced rabbit arthritis. *Laboratory Investigation, 78* (5), 559–569.

Meulenbelt, I., Bijkerk, C., Miedema, H.S., Breedveld, F.C., Hofman, A., Valkenburg, H.A., Pols, H.A., Slagboom, P.E., & van Duijn, C.M. (1998). A genetic association study of the IGF-1 gene and radiological osteoarthritis in a population-based cohort study (the Rotterdam Study). *Annals of Rheumatic Disease, 57* (6), 371–374.

Morris, A. (1998). Gout: An old clinician's approach to an even older arthropathy. *Clinical Reviews, Summer,* 18–22.

Moskowitz, R. (1992). Osteoarthritis: Symptoms and signs. In R. Moskowitz, D. Howell, V. Goldberg, & H. Markin (Eds.), *Osteoarthritis: Diagnosis and medical/surgical management* (pp. 255–261). Philadelphia: W.B. Saunders.

Mow, V. & Setton, L. (1998). Mechanical properties of normal and osteoarthritic articular cartilage. In K. Brandt, S. Lohmander, & M. Doherty (Eds.), *Osteoarthritis* (pp. 108–122). Oxford: Oxford University Press.

O'Reilly, S. & Doherty, M. (1998). Clinical features of osteoarthritis and standard approaches to the diagnosis. In K.

Brandt, S. Lohmander, & M. Doherty (Eds.), *Osteoarthritis* (pp. 197–217). Oxford: Oxford University Press.

Pelletier, J., Martel-Pelletier, J., & Howell, D. (1997). Etiopathogenesis of osteoarthitis. In W. Koopman (Ed.), *Arthritis and allied conditions: A textbook of rheumatology* (13th ed., pp. 1969–1984). Baltimore: Williams & Wilkins.

Pincus, T. & Callahan, L. (1993). What is the natural history of rheumatoid arthritis? *Rheumatic Disease Clinics of North America 19*(1), 123–151.

Pritzker, K. (1998). Pathology of osteoarthritis. In K. Brandt, S. Lohmander, & M. Doherty (Eds.), *Osteoarthritis* (pp. 50–61). Oxford: Oxford University Press.

Sack, K. (1997). Gout, pseudogout, and asymptomatic hyperuricemia. In L. Dornbrand, A. Hoole, & R. Fletcher (Eds.), *Manual of clinical problems in adult ambulatory care. On MAXX; Maximum access to diagnosis and therapy: The electronic library of medicine* (CD-ROM). Philadelphia: Lippincott-Raven.

Sandy, J. & Lark, M. (1998). Proteolytic degradation of normal and osteoarthritic cartilage matrix. In K. Brandt, S. Lohmander, & M. Doherty (Eds.), *Osteoarthritis* (pp. 84–93). Oxford: Oxford University Press.

Smyth, J.M., Stone, A.A., Hurewitz, A., & Kaell, A. (1999). Effects of writing about stressful experiences on symptom reduction in patients with asthma or rheumatoid arthritis:

A randomized trial. *Journal of the American Medical Association, 281* (14), 1304–1309.

Towle, C., Hung, H.H., Bonasser, L., Treadwell, B., & Mangham, D. (1997). Detection of interleukin-1 in the cartilage of patients with osteoarthritis: A possible auto-crine role in pathogenesis. *Osteoarthritis and Cartilage, 5* (5), 293–299.

Uphold, C. & Graham, M. (1998). *Clinical guidelines in family practice* (3rd ed.). Florida: Barmarrae Books.

Weinblatt, M. (1997). Treatment of rheumatoid arthritis. In W. Koopman (Ed.), *Arthritis and allied conditions* (13th ed.). Baltimore: Williams & Wilkins.

Woessner, M. & Gunja-Smith, Z. (1991). Role of metalloproteinases in human osteoarthritis. *Journal of Rheumatology, 96*, 2454–2460.

Wolff, J. (1986). *The law of bone remodeling*. Translated by P. Magret & R. Furlog. New York: Springer-Verlag.

Youinou, P., Mackenzie, L., Katsikis, P., Merdrignac, G., Isenberg, D.A., Tuaillon, N., Lamour, A., Le Goff, P., Jouquan, J., Drogou, A., et al. (1990). The relationship between CD5-expressing B lymphocytes and serologic abnormalities in rheumatoid arthritis patients and their relatives. *Arthritis and Rheumatism, 33* (3), 339–348.

Zautra, A., Hoffman, J., Potter, P., & Matt, K. (1997). Examination of changes in interpersonal stress as a factor in disease exacerbations among women with rheumatoid arthritis. *Annals of Behavioral Medicine, 19*, 279–286.

# Common Cardiovascular Illnesses

Maureen Groer

Cardiovascular diseases (CVDs) are the number one cause of death in the United States. Consequently, primary care providers are caring for people with some type of CVD every day. These individuals may require primary care for many other minor or major health problems, and their CVD then becomes another factor to consider in their treatment plan. They may need primary care preventive strategies to reduce their risk for experiencing major life-threatening events from CVD. Moreover, almost all Americans require assessment of their risk factors, teaching, and wellness-oriented strategies for preventing CVD, since this is such a prevalent disease process.

At the root of many circulatory diseases is the process of *atherogenesis*, the formation of atherosclerotic plaque. Plaque evolution begins in early life and ultimately leads to the formation of occlusive arterial disease. A tremendous amount of research has been directed at understanding the causative factors that influence atherogenesis, and many of the known factors are lifestyle related and preventable. Included in the list of risk factors are familial risk, hypercholesterolemia, hypertension, diabetes mellitus, cigarette smoking, infectious agents (*Chlamydia* and cytomegalovirus), obesity, lack of physical activity, and hyperhomocysteinemia. The cumulative risk increases for the individual as the number of factors increases.

## ATHEROGENESIS

Atherosclerosis is a subtype of arteriosclerosis, a general term meaning thickening or hardening of the arteries. Atherosclerosis causes changes in large arterial walls, particularly in areas of the arterial system associated with increased turbulence or sheer forces (branchings, bifurcations) through the accumulation of atherosclerotic plaque. The development of atherosclerotic plaque begins during early childhood, with the earliest sign of a developing lesion being the *fatty streak*, which is a smooth, subendothelial, raised lesion in the arterial wall. These lesions may diminish in size, remain dormant, or evolve into atherosclerotic plaques. The fatty streak is primary composed of *foam cells*, which are macrophages filled with lipid. The morphology of the fatty streak is illustrated in Figure 14-1. The presence of these activated and phagocytic macrophages suggests that an early pathophysiologic process in atherogenesis may be inflammatory.

An initial insult that begins the process of atherogenesis could be an injury to the endothelial cells that line the lumen of blood vessels. Once damaged, the endothelial cells release a variety of mediators that alter the patency and vasodilatory responsiveness of the vessel. Growth factors from damaged endothelium may promote smooth muscle growth within the vessel wall. The endothelium also expresses factors such as leukocyte adhesion molecules, which cause blood monocytes and neutrophils to adhere and stick to the lumen. The endothelial injury believed to be the primary event may result from a variety of independent and interacting factors. Dyslipidemia—particularly high cholesterol levels with high levels of low-density lipoproteins (LDL) and low levels of high-density lipoproteins (HDL)—diabetes, cigarette smoking, high levels of homocysteine, autoimmune mechanisms, high blood viscosity, and, possibly, certain infectious agents may cause endothelial damage, leading to atherosclerosis.

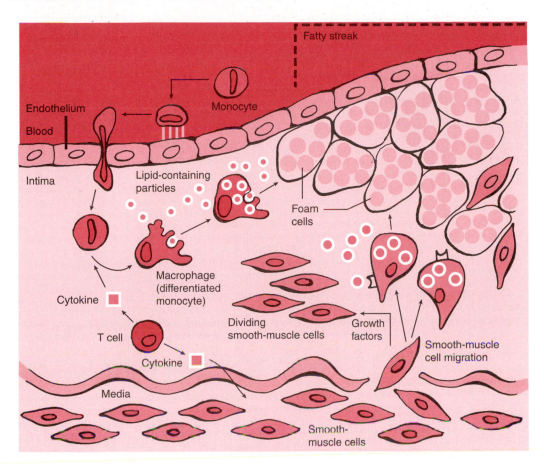

**FIGURE 14.1** ● Morphology of the fatty streak found in the development of atherosclerotic plaque. (Adapted from Hajjar, D. & Nicholson, A. [1995]. Atherosclerosis. *American Scientist, 83*(5), 460.)

A relationship exists between high levels of LDL cholesterol, with the corresponding low levels of HDL cholesterol, and the development of atherosclerotic plaque. When the levels of LDL cholesterol are higher than normal, these lipoproteins are able to damage the vessel wall, which then becomes more permeable. The lipoproteins then enter the vessel wall, where they become oxidized. This is a critical event. The degree of lipid oxidation within vessels is determined partly by the genetic mechanism that increases an individual's risk of CVD. Oxidized lipid within the extracellular matrix of the subendothelial space is actively phagocytosed by macrophages that have migrated to the damaged endothelium. These cells become full of oxidized lipid and convert into foam cells. Conversion of monocytes into macrophages may require T cell cytokines. The fatty streak lesion is filled with macrophages and T cells, and thus appears much like a chronic inflammatory process.

Over time, the fatty streak may progress into a fibrous plaque. Normally, the arterial smooth mus-

cle cells are confined to the tunica media. However, in evolving plaque, smooth muscle cells migrate into the tunica intima in response to cytokines released by endothelium and macrophages. Here, the muscle cells are stimulated to proliferate and secrete collagen, and they may even ingest lipid, much like the macrophages (Hajir & Nicholson, 1995). This process leads to a remodeling of the extracellular matrix in the subendothelial space, causing hardening and thickened and enlarging plaque. This stage of atherogenesis is associated with the development of the fibrous cap, a covering over the lipid core made up of connective tissue fibrils (Koga & Sasaki, 1999) (Fig. 14-2). The lesion now is significant enough to produce thickening of the arterial wall and potential occlusion of the vessel; the next stage of atherogenesis produces extracellular conditions in the subendothelium that may ultimately lead to rupture of the thin, fibrous cap (Newby & Zaltsman, 1999). The atherosclerotic plaque becomes calcified, which mineralizes the plaque, giving it a gritty, hardened texture. Cholesterol crystal forma-

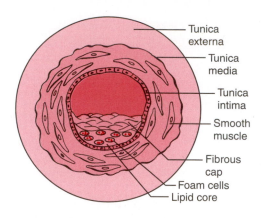

Tunica externa
Tunica media
Tunica intima
Smooth muscle
Fibrous cap
Foam cells
Lipid core

**FIGURE 14.2** ● Late stage atherosclerotic lesion with fibrous cap.

tion and continuing lipid deposition cause the plaque to eventually produce a rigid arterial tube that offers increased resistance to blood flow, produces turbulent flow through the vessel, and occludes the blood supply to the tissue. This plaque is susceptible to rupture and propagates thrombus formation within the vessel. Macrophages and smooth muscle cells produce enzymes such as the metalloproteinases, which weaken the fibrous cap. When the fibrous cap is destroyed, the plaque itself ruptures, which then produces an acute occlusive event (see Fig. 14-2). Whereas the fissuring of the fibrous cap is a critical event leading to an acute thrombotic event, not all atherosclerotic plaques develop to this point. However, these plaques are more likely to produce catastrophic effects. The process of thinning and fissuring of the fibrous cap can undergo regression when rigorous cholesterol-lowering treatments are instituted, thus decreasing the risk of myocardial infarction and stroke in high-risk patients.

## THE ROLE OF LIPIDS

Serum lipids are important factors in the development of atherosclerosis. An elevated level of cholesterol, particularly LDL cholesterol, is a CVD risk factor, along with hypertension, cigarette smoking, obesity, a sedentary lifestyle, and diabetes. All of these factors can be modified by lifestyle change and good health care. Other risk factors such as age, male sex, and family history are not modifiable but help the primary care provider to determine an individual's risk for development of atherosclerosis. Obesity usually is defined as a body mass index (BMI) of 30 or higher. The BMI is a calculation of weight in kilograms divided by the height in meters, squared. A

convenient way to perform this calculation can be found at the web site *http://www.nhlbisupport.com/bmi.*

Primary serum lipid disorders are termed *dyslipidemias* and are classified as types I, IIA, IIB, III, IV, and V. Secondary dyslipidemia may be caused by diseases such as diabetes, liver disease, or hypothyroidism. The primary dyslipidemias have a strong genetic basis, with 1 of 500 persons having either a heterozygous or a homozygous genetic hypercholesterolemia. The most common type is type IV, with an incidence of 1 of 300 in the US.

### Primary Dyslipidemias

Figure 14-3 illustrates the normal lipid pathways after fat is ingested in the diet. After lipids are repackaged as chylomicrons (which are a type of lipoprotein) in intestinal epithelial cells, they enter the circulatory system. Chylomicrons transport triglycerides (TGs) to adipocytes, muscle, and liver cells, which have an abundance of the enzyme lipoprotein lipase (LPL) on their surfaces. LPL acts on chylomicrons to hydrolyze TG molecules into glycerol and fatty acids, and leaves behind a cholesterol-rich chylomicron remnant. The cell takes the fatty acids and makes new TGs for use or storage by the cell, while the liver removes the chylomicron remnant from the blood. Chylomicrons contain the apo B-48, apo A, apo C, and apo E apolipoproteins; they are large compared with other lipoproteins and have a low density. All other lipoproteins are synthesized by the liver or form in the blood as remnants of these lipoproteins. All lipoproteins have apolipoproteins as part of their structures, which regulate the removal of lipoprotein from the plasma by acting as an enzyme activator or as a ligand for certain cell receptors. Several genetic conditions are characterized by abnormalities in apolipoprotein synthesis.

The liver synthesizes very–low-density lipoprotein (VLDL) from lipid and protein, with the apo B-100 apolipoprotein being an essential component. Other apolipoproteins on the VLDL include apo C and apo E. Apo B-100 is a structural protein as well as a ligand for cellular receptors. The size of the VLDL is determined by the amount of TG available, but it has the lowest density (g/mL) of the lipoproteins and is more TG rich than the other lipoproteins. If hypertriglyceridemia is present (as occurs in alcoholism, diabetes, or obesity), more TG may be carried on the VLDL. VLDL can be acted on by cell-bound LPL, again liberating the TG for hydrolysis into glycerol and fatty acid. Once hydrol-

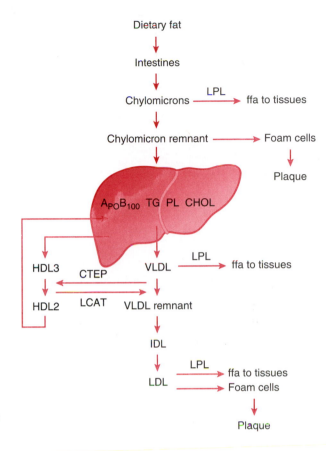

**FIGURE 14.3** ● Normal lipid pathways after fat is ingested in the diet. Ffa, free fatty acids.

ysis has occurred, the VLDL becomes a remnant, the intermediate-density lipoprotein (IDL). The IDL contains cholesterol esters and TGs and is removed by the liver or is subject to further breakdown, forming the remnant LDL. The LDL has the lowest density and the highest cholesterol content of the lipoproteins; it contains only apo B-100, and if present in higher than normal concentrations, it is atherogenic. Normally, 75% of the cholesterol on the LDL is removed by LPL, and remaining cholesterol may be phagocytosed by macrophages, producing the classic foam cell that was described in the fatty streak.

HDLs are formed by the liver and are small, high-density lipoproteins carrying the apo A and apo C apolipoproteins. When formed by the liver, the HDL contains apo A and phospholipid, and the nascent particles then add cholesterol, which is converted to cholesterol esters by the enzyme lecithin cholesterol acetyl transferase, which is activated by apo A-I. HDL-3 is formed in this way, which then adds more cholesterol, forming HDL-2. The cholesterol in the HDL particles can be transferred to LDLs and VLDLs or can be delivered to the liver. The former action requires

another enzyme, cholesterol ester transfer protein (CTEP). The cholesterol thus can be cycled back to the liver. The HDLs transfer cholesterol to the liver and are thought to be anti-atherogenic because they reverse cholesterol transport, protect LDL particles from oxidation, and decrease endothelial expression of cytokine-mediated cell adhesion molecules.

Most of the cholesterol in the body is actually synthesized, with only about 25% having a dietary origin. The synthesis occurs mostly in the liver, where cholesterol is used for production of bile acids and lipoproteins. Excess cholesterol in the liver is excreted through the bile.

Hyperlipidemias are classified in the Fredrickson classification system as types I, IIA, IIB, III, IV, or V. Table 14-1 lists the characteristics of these dyslipidemias.

Elevations in total cholesterol and LDL cholesterol are the most important atherogenic influences. A total cholesterol value of less than 200, a LDL level less than 130, and a TG level less than 200 mg/dL are the desirable fasting values in a normal person. Borderline high TG levels are 200 to 400 mg/dL, high are 400 to 1000 mg/dL, and

## TABLE 14.1

### Hyperlipidemias

| Type | Effect on Lipids | Cause | Symptoms |
| --- | --- | --- | --- |
| I | High levels of chylomicrons causing high triglyceride levels | Deficiency of LPL or apo C-II | Xanthomas<br>Pancreatitis |
| IIA | High level of LDL cholesterol | Inherited: familial hypercholesterolemia from mutated LDL receptor gene | Premature coronary artery disease |
| IIB | Increased VLDL and LDL cholesterol and triglycerides | Inherited: familial combined hyperlipidemia | Premature coronary artery disease |
| III | High levels of IDL cholesterol and triglyceride | Inherited: familial dysbetalipo-proteinemia from decreased ability to remove VLDL remnants | Xanthomas<br>Premature coronary artery disease |
| IV | Hypertriglyceridemia from elevated VLDLs | Inherited or acquired (diabetes, nephrosis, diet, alcohol) | Atherosclerosis<br>Pancreatitis |
| V | Elevated levels of chylomicrons and VLDL; high levels of triglycerides | Familial or acquired over-production of VLDLs and impaired lipolysis | Xanthomas<br>Pancreatitis<br>Atherosclerosis |

IDL, intermediate-density lipoprotein; LDL, low-density lipoprotein; VLDL, very–low-density lipoprotein.

very high levels are above 1000 mg/dL. The mean total cholesterol in the United States is 205 mg/dL. HDL cholesterol, the anti-atherogenic form, has a normal range of 29 to 77 mg/dL, with the optimal level considered to be greater than 50 mg/dL. When the ratio of LDL–HDL is greater than 3.1, the patient is considered to be at high risk for CVD. Most of the total cholesterol is carried on LDLs, and LDL levels are directly related to atherosclerosis risk, so LDLs usually are the target of most therapies. When hyperlipidemia is caused by diet and obesity, weight loss and a reduced calorie and fat intake can reduce LDL and TG levels and increase HDL levels. Several medications may elevate cholesterol levels as a side effect. These include thiazide diuretics, beta blockers, cyclosporine, anabolic steroids, isoretinoin, glucocorticoids, oral contraceptives, and alcohol.

### Stress and Hyperlipidemia

Diagnosis of dyslipidemia is made based on a serum lipid profile, which often is performed after a screening sample of total cholesterol indicates hyperlipidemia. The approach to the patient should consider lipid levels, category of hyperlipidemia, lifestyle, evidence of atherogenic disease, medica-

tions, and stress. A person's level of psychological stress may affect levels of serum lipids. Experiments in which subjects were exposed to laboratory stressors found elevations in lipids related to the degree of stress. LDL and VLDL, TG, and free fatty acids all become elevated with stress (McCann et al., 1995). Positive life events were found to improve the lipid profile in middle-aged men in another study (Helminen et al., 1999). Work stress also has been associated with increased levels of LDLs in a large study of men and women in Sweden (Peter et al., 1998).

Stress may exert its effects on the serum lipid profile through endocrine and metabolic mechanisms. Chronic stress also may be associated with poor diet and unhealthy lifestyle, which could indirectly lead to elevated serum lipids. The effects of chronically elevated glucocorticoids could account, in part, for dyslipidemia. Glucocorticoids antagonize the action of growth hormone and gonadal steroids of fat catabolism, thus promoting adiposity and hyperlipidemia. Syndrome X resembles a cushingoid syndrome in many ways, with hyperglycemia, hyperlipidemia, hyperinsulinemia, hypertension, central adiposity, and coronary artery disease (CAD) all being part of the picture. Chronic stress may therefore be a contributing factor to this clinically high-risk syndrome. Syndrome X is more fully described elsewhere (see Chapter 15).

## Homocysteine

Homocysteine is an amino acid normally present in the plasma. It is produced by the breakdown of methionine. People who have the genetic disease homocystinuria have high rates of CVD. Moderately elevated levels of homocysteine have been identified as a significant risk factor for CVD for those in the highest quartile of homocysteine levels. The normal homocysteine level is between 5 and 15 mmol/L. Higher levels than normal were found in men who had experienced myocardial infarctions in the large Physician's Health Study (Verhoef & Stampfer, 1997). In another study of women, the risk of heart attack was increased 2.3 times for women in the top 10%. There was an inverse relationship between homocysteine and folate (see *http://www.americanheart.org/Whats_News/AHA_News_Releases/974566.htm*). A common gene mutation, present in up to 12.3% of American whites, increases the level of homocysteine and thus the risk for CVD. The mechanisms by which homocysteine perpetuates the atherogenic process are unknown but may involve impaired endothelial function. A Norwegian study found a striking relationship between cardiovascular mortality and serum homocysteine levels when other factors, including lipids, were adjusted. The authors suggest that serum lipids might be involved in the atherosclerotic process, whereas homocysteine may be involved in the thrombotic process (Nygard et al., 1997).

## Microbial Agents

The relationship between microbial infection and atherosclerosis has been a matter of intense speculation since the observation that vascular changes in the atherogenic process involve inflammatory cells, cytokines, and growth factors. A study of Alaskan Native Americans who had died for reasons other than CVD found that the atherosclerotic plaques of these individuals contained immuno-globulins to *Chlamydia pneumoniae*. Seventy-five percent of the Native Americans, who normally have a lower rate of heart disease than nonnative Alaskans, had macrophages that had ingested *C. pneumoniae*. The organism causes pulmonary infection, and there is a high incidence of chronic infection in the Eskimo population. The theoretical mechanism by which chlamydiae may be involved could be through damage to the endothelium,

which then initiates the atherosclerotic process (Davidson et al., 1998).

This relationship between chlamydiae and CVD could be a general model for other microorganisms' effects. Cytomegalovirus (CMV) also has been suggested as a potential etiologic agent in atherosclerosis. Viral antigens and nucleic acid sequences in arterial smooth muscles suggest that CMV may be a latent virus playing a role in atherogenesis.

Animal viral infection is known to damage the arterial wall and produce vascular atherosclerotic lesions. Marek's disease in fowl is well described vis-à-vis this process. The relationship between herpesviruses and CVD has been studied for over 30 years, with recent work suggesting that CMV may be an initiating factor (Melnick, Adam, & DeBakey, 1997). CMV causes an endothelial infection that does not kill the cells, but produces an inflammatory response in the endothelium characterized by attachment and influx of inflammatory cells. This may be an initiating event for the ultimate development of plaque. Another observation is that heart transplants develop atherosclerosis when the immunosuppressed recipient is infected with CMV (Melnick et al., 1997).

## Physiologic Basis of Treatment of Dyslipidemia

Because the large epidemiologic studies that follow populations over time indicate that the strongest CVD risk is a high level of LDL, the treatment for hypercholesterolemia usually is aimed at reducing LDL cholesterol. The first approach is a nonpharmacologic one in which the patient modifies the diet, often dramatically, to reduce intake of saturated fats; loses weight; and increases physical activity. This approach may reduce cholesterol levels significantly, which then reduces the amount of LDLs that, in a high-fat diet, are not sufficiently cleared from the blood and deposit cholesterol in the vascular endothelium. The National Cholesterol Education Program (NCEP) (1993) recommended dietary approach is a step 1 diet in which fat is reduced to 30% of total calories (8% to 10% from saturated fat, no more than 10% from polyunsaturated fats, and no more than 15% from monounsaturated fats). The total caloric intake should either cause weight loss, if needed, or maintain optimal weight. If this approach does not achieve the desired serum cholesterol levels, a step 2 approach then is recommended. This diet is more rigorous, reducing fats to 7% of the total calories. This diet is recommended if the patient already has CAD. Patients using the step 1 or 2 diets are monitored for cholesterol-lowering effects after starting the diet and again at 3 months. Most people who adhere to these diets require a full 6 months for the maximum effect on cholesterol levels to be seen.

Adherence to the NCEP diets often is a problem for people because it requires a true lifestyle change in the way they eat, how they prepare foods, and their restaurant choices. Patients must maintain weight loss, adhere to exercise programs, and follow the dietary changes just described. Because of these difficulties—although research clearly shows that diet, weight loss, and exercise produce significant drops in both total cholesterol and HDL cholesterol—many hyperlipidemic patients eventually require medication. However, people on medication should continue to make appropriate lifestyle accommodations, including reducing fat in their diets.

## Pharmacology Update

Several pharmacologic approaches are used to treat the hyperlipidemic patient. For elevated LDL cholesterol and TG levels greater than 200 mg/dL, the NCEP recommends bile acid sequestrants, either alone or in combination with hydroxymethylglutaryl coenzyme A (HMG-CoA) reductase inhibitors. The bile acid sequestrants act in the bowel by binding bile acids that normally circulate through the enterohepatic circulation back to the liver. By binding bile acids in the intestines, fecal excretion of the cholesterol-containing bile acids is increased. Since cholesterol in the liver is reduced by these drugs, there is increased removal of LDLs and VLDLs from the circulation. The enzyme HMG-CoA reductase may become upregulated when liver cholesterol is decreased, however, and could oppose the actions of the bile acid sequestrants. Therefore, patients may need a HMG-CoA reductase inhibitor added to maintain the lower cholesterol and TG levels. The HMG-CoA reductase inhibitors (*statins*) also may be used as monotherapy. The introduction of these drugs has been a major advance in the treatment of hyperlipidemic patients. Statins affect the synthesis of cholesterol through liver metabolic pathways. Cholesterol synthesis is illustrated in Figure 14-4. Notice that the rate-limiting step in cholesterol synthesis is the conversion of 3 hydroxy-3-methylglutaryl-CoA to mevalonic acid. This step requires the reduced form nicotinamide-adenine dinucleotide phosphate (NADPH) and the enzyme HMG-CoA reductase. As cholesterol is synthesized in this pathway in liver cells, it acts as a feedback inhibitor of the enzyme, thus reducing further cholesterol synthesis. The statins therefore decrease total liver cholesterol synthesis through inhibition of this enzyme.

Another drug that may be used as monotherapy or in combination with other drugs is nicotinic acid. This drug, a B vitamin, affects liver synthesis of VLDLs, consequently decreasing IDLs and LDLs. Nicotinic acid has a well-known effect on the endothelium, causing prostaglandin release, which produces vasodilation, and, clinically, a flushing response in patients after taking the drug.

For patients with high cholesterol levels (200 to 400 mg/dL), fibric acid derivatives are added to the arsenal of pharmacotherapy. The actions are complex and are not completely described, although increasing the activity of LPL is one mechanism of action.

Providers can access information about the various drugs at web sites of pharmaceutical companies. Latest research findings also are available at the web site of the American Heart Association (*http://www.americanheart.org*).

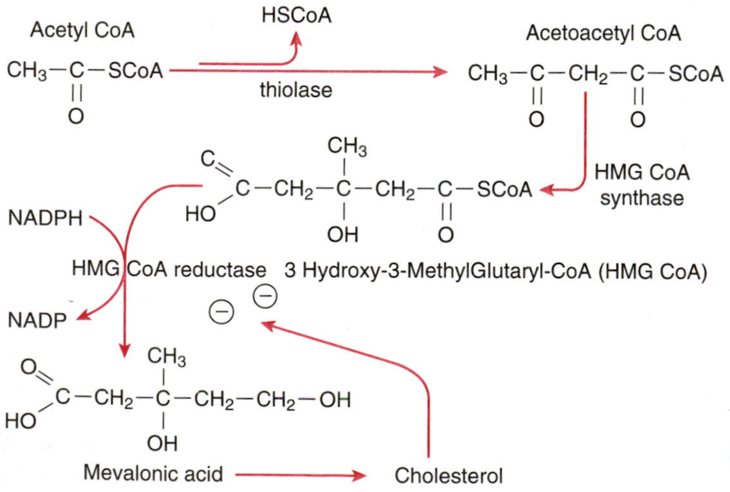

**FIGURE 14.4** • Cholesterol synthesis.

# CORONARY ARTERY DISEASE

This chapter described the pathophysiologic processes that produce atherosclerotic plaque within arterial walls. The fact that this process has a predilection for certain arterial sites is significant. Wherever atherosclerotic plaque forms, two potential clinical effects may occur. One effect is occlusion: the growing plaque occupies space within the arterial wall, causing it to bulge inward into the lumen of the vessel. This defect causes increased resistance to blood flow and stiffening of the artery, both of which restrict the nutrient arterial supply to the tissue and increase the turbulence of blood flow through the affected segment. Second, as the atherosclerotic plaque progresses, thinning of the fibrous cap increases the risk of rupture of plaque into the arterial lumen. This creates a potentially catastrophic event in which platelet activation and thrombus formation at the site of the plaque can lead to complete occlusion of the tissue supplied by the artery, producing profound ischemia.

When the affected vessels are the coronary arteries, the muscle tissue of the myocardium becomes compromised by occlusion and threatened by the potentiality of a thrombotic event. This is the situation in CAD, the most common cause of death for both men and women in the US.

## Epidemiology

Coronary artery disease caused 476,124 deaths in the United States in 1996 (one of every 4.9 deaths). There are about 12,000,000 people with CAD in the United States (slightly more women than men), with 6,000,000 experiencing angina attacks. The racial differences are significant, with prevalence rates of 3.4% for non-Hispanic white men, 2.6% for non-Hispanic black men, and 3.4% for Mexican-American men. For women, the estimated prevalence of angina is 4.1% for non-Hispanic white women, 5.2% for non-Hispanic black women, and 4.6% for Mexican-American women. (*http://www.americanheart.org/Heart_and_Stroke_A_Z_Guide/has.html*).

## Gender Differences

The death rate for CAD in women is six times that for breast cancer, with 233,000 women dying and 625,000 women experiencing myocardial infarctions each year. There are 28 million women in the US who have CVD, half of whom are younger than 65 years of age. A woman's risk of CAD increases dramatically during postmenopause, and they are more likely to develop CAD at an age that is 10 years older than when men develop CAD. Although the death rate for men is higher than for women between the ages of 35 and 55, this difference disappears after 55, and the death rate for women continues to increase, whereas it declines for men after 55 years of age. This is related to both the later development of symptoms and later presentation to the health care provider. Atypical symptoms of CAD are more common in women compared with men, and misdiagnosis, undertesting, and undertreatment all are problems. Women have a greater incidence of symptoms such as abdominal pain, dyspnea nausea, and fatigue (Redberg, 1998). In addition, when a woman experiences chest pain, she often attributes it to noncardiac causes, as does her physician. Unfortunately, women are more likely to have a fatal heart attack than are men.

## Response of the Heart to Atherosclerosis

The presence of atherosclerosis in the coronary arteries produces occlusion, leading to myocardial ischemia. When this is transient, the person is considered to have angina; when it is severe, prolonged, and produces myocardial tissue necrosis, it is considered a myocardial infarction. The response of the heart to chronically compromised circulation is the development of collateral vasculature. This is the growth and dilation of existing small vessels that connect two coronary arteries or two segments of the same artery. The development of collateral circulation in the compromised myocardium allows tissue to receive nutrition and oxygen through alternate flow pathways. The greater the extent of collateralization, the more protected the myocardium is from ischemia. Patients with angina may have one or more coronary arteries occluded. Chronic, stable angina, particularly if it is superimposed by unstable angina, may be associated with three-vessel disease, whereas new-onset anginal pain at rest may represent only single-vessel disease (Gersh et al., 1997).

### Regulation of Myocardial Perfusion and Oxygenation

The heart is extraordinarily dependent on a constant supply of oxygen through perfusion of the myocardium by the coronary arteries. The major proportion of myocardial perfusion occurs during diastole, when the ventricles are relaxed.

Myocardial oxygen consumption is influenced by three mechanical factors: stress on the ventricular wall during systole, heart rate, and contractility of the myocardium. Preload and afterload influence these factors. For example, increased preload from increased end diastolic pressures distends the ventricular wall, reducing perfusion of the myocardium, so decreasing preload reduces the work and energy consumption of the myocardium. The afterload is related to the ventricular wall tension that develops during systolic ejection, which is increased when total peripheral resistance is increased. Reducing the afterload improves the perfusion in the myocardium.

## Angina

Angina pectoris is the term given for myocardial ischemic pain caused by an imbalance between myocardial oxygen demand and coronary blood supply. The ischemia may result from an episode of increased demand (exercise, sexual intercourse) or from decreased blood supply caused by coronary vasoconstriction (stress, cigarette smoking). Anginal pain is variable, with some patients experiencing silent ischemia, and thus no pain, and others describing a crushing, unbearable retrosternal pain. Anginal pain often radiates to the left arm and frequently occurs in the morning hours. Anginal pain is caused by coronary artery atherosclerosis, but the primary care provider needs to rule out other causes of chest pain that can mimic angina. Included in this category are heartburn, cervical radicular pain, and pulmonary embolism.

### Types of Angina

Angina may present as stable or unstable, with unstable angina representing an intermediate state between stable angina and an acute myocardial infarction (AMI). Stable angina is commonly classified according to the Canadian Classification System. Class I angina describes pain evoked by prolonged exertion; class II, by walking more than two blocks; class III, by walking less than two blocks; and class IV, pain experienced on minimal exertion or at rest. Stable angina is more predictable than the unstable form and is relieved by rest and nitroglycerin. Unstable angina occurs even at rest, during sleep, or after meals and is associated with more severe pain, often requiring two sublingual nitroglycerin tablets (2.5 mg each) for relief. Persons with unstable angina are more likely to develop AMI than those with stable angina. Risk of death increases with the number of coronary vessels involved and presence of impaired left ventricular function. In patients with unstable angina, a reduction in coronary blood flow is the initial event, followed by depression of the ST segment on the electrocardiogram, and then, finally, pain (Gersh et al., 1997).

The pathophysiology of unstable angina involves the nature of the atherosclerotic lesions in the affected coronary arteries. Fissuring and rupturing occur in an unstable plaque, causing platelet aggregation and thrombus formation along the vessel. This may lead to AMI and sudden death. The possibility of this type of plaque disruption is related to the size and consistency of the core of the plaque, the thickness of the fibrous cap, and the ongoing inflammatory and repair process that occurs within the plaque (Kristensen et al., 1999). The inflammatory process within the vessel involves both the endothelium and aggregating platelets. Blood levels of inflammatory proteins are increased in unstable angina patients (Caligiuri et al., 1998). Because platelets perpetuate the clotting process, their actions must be inhibited by drugs such as aspirin in patients with unstable angina. Treatment guidelines for unstable angina are found at *http://www.ahcpr.gov*.

Another less common form of angina is variant or Prinzmetal angina that results from vasospasm of the coronary vessels. This may occur in both normal and atherosclerotic coronary arteries, and usually involves a large septal or epicardial vessel (Gersh et al., 1997). Cigarette smoking is a significant risk factor for this variant form of angina. The anginal pain typically occurs at rest, often in the morning, is associated with ST segment *elevation*, and is relieved by nitroglycerin. It most commonly affects women younger than 50 years of age.

---

### ● Case Study 14-1

Dr. Hubert Hillman is a 60-year-old chemistry professor at the local university. He comes to the primary care provider with complaints of chest pain during sexual intercourse, a problem he has noted over the last few weeks. He has pain in his left anterior chest, which disappears with rest.

*(Case study continued on next page)*

## History

### Past Medical History

| | |
|---|---|
| Allergies | NKDA |
| Current medications | No prescription medications |
| Surgeries | Cholescystectomy at 45; hernia repair at 50 |
| Injury/Trauma | None |
| Childhood illness | Had the "usual illnesses," including chicken pox, measles, mumps |

### Social History

Married in a monogamous relationship for 35 years; has three adult children

| | |
|---|---|
| Tobacco | 1ppd × 15 y; has not smoked for 15 y |
| Alcohol | Occasional beer or glass of wine |
| Social drugs | None |
| Caffeine | 2 cups of coffee every morning and several caffeinated beverages during the day |
| Exercise | None |
| Employment | Employed as a professor in the local university. Enjoys his work, which centers mostly on research, with occasional lectures. Is busy preparing manuscripts and grant proposals at this time. Has no thoughts of retirement. Wife is 55 years old and a biology professor. She recently has been diagnosed with hypertension |
| Sleep | States that he sleeps poorly; has been diagnosed with sleep apnea; awakens frequently |

### Family History

| | |
|---|---|
| Mother | Deceased, aneurysm at age 70 |
| Father | Deceased at age 40 of a stroke |
| Sister | 55 years old; no health problems |

### 24-Hour Dietary Recall

| | |
|---|---|
| Breakfast | 2 cups coffee, coffee cake |
| Lunch | Deli sandwich, french fries, Coke |
| Dinner | Salad, steak, mashed potatoes, bread, pie |
| Snack | Fruit, Fritos |

## Review of Systems

| | |
|---|---|
| General | Describes himself as overweight for 30 years. Was diagnosed with hypertension 20 years ago. Currently on ACE inhibitor. Usually remembers to take the medication |
| Skin | No rashes or lesions |
| HEENT | Wears reading glasses; denies nosebleeds, dizziness, sore throats |
| Lungs | No asthma, bronchitis, SOB, pneumonia |
| Cardiac | Has noticed that his heart occasionally "skips a beat." No previous episodes of chest pain. Has noticed chest pain only with intercourse but admits that he does not exercise |
| GU | No dysuria, urgency. No change in urination. No STDs |
| MS | Has arthritis in both knees and a bit in hands |

*(Case study continued on page 276)*

| | |
|---|---|
| Neurologic | Reports occasional light-headedness; no numbness, tingling, fainting, seizures, weakness |

## Physical Examination

| System | Findings |
|---|---|
| Vital Signs | T–97.4°F, P–86, R–14, BP 155/90 Height 5'9", Weight 230 lb |
| General | Alert, friendly, fully oriented. Marked abdominal adiposity, round face; skin warm and dry |
| HEENT | Normocephalic, neck size 16.5", cranial nerves intact. TMs intact. Rinne and Weber negative. Hearing normal. Throat negative. No adenopathy. Thyroid not palpable. No carotid bruits. AV ratio 1:2 in retina (grade 1 hypertensive retinopathy (see Chapter 15, Figure 15-7) |
| Lungs | Clear to auscultation and percussion bilaterally |
| Cardiac | Heart rate regular. $S_3$ is present. No murmurs. Cardiac borders indicate somewhat enlarged heart by percussion |
| Abdomen | Soft, nontender, no masses. BS in all 4 quad. No CVA tenderness. Cholescystectomy incision scar |
| GU | Circumcised. No lesions, discharge. Testicles descended |
| Rectal | Mild prostatic hypertrophy |
| Extremities | Femoral pulses 2+; pedal pulse 1+; radial, brachial pulses 3+. Grip strength good; little hair growth on ankles and feet |
| Neurologic | DTRs 3+ in upper and lower extremities. Romberg negative. Sensations intact |

## Laboratory Results

| Test | Result |
|---|---|
| WBC | 6000 (52% neutrophils, 30% lymphocytes, 6% monocytes, 1% eosinophils, 1% basophils) |
| Chem | BUN 5, creatinine 0.8, total cholesterol 360, LDLs 250, HDLs 30, triglycerides 400, FBS 90, sodium 14 1 mEq/L, potassium 3.0 mEq/L |
| Urine | Small amount sediment, yellow, neg glucose, neg ketones, albumin 1+; pH 5 |
| ECG | Q wave in lead III wider than 1 mm (1 small square) and a Q wave in lead aVF wider than 0.5 mm and Q wave of any size in lead II indicating old inferior myocardial infarction |

## Impression

Previous MI
Hypertension
Dyslipidemia
CAD

*(Case study continued on next page)*

### Discussion

The patient has evidence of long-standing cardiovascular disease. His blood lipids are elevated with high LDLs and triglycerides. He is hypertensive but not adequately controlled. He is significantly obese with a large amount of abdominal fat. He has evidence of PVD because of diminished pedal pulses and lack of hair growth on ankles and feet. Finally, he has evidence of an old MI on ECG, which apparently was a silent attack. His current symptoms of chest pain on exertion and relief with rest are classic anginal attacks, and he has no symptoms of GERD or radiculitis that could cause chest pain. He requires a comprehensive assessment, including angiograms, and needs referral to a cardiologist.

A useful website for patients with CAD and their families is *http://www.med-edu.com/patient/cad/cad-index.html.*

ACE, angiotensin converting enzyme; AV, atrioventricular; BS, bowel sounds; BUN, blood urea nitrogen; CAD, coronary artery disease; CV, cardiovascular; CVA, cardiovascular accident; DTRs, deep tendon reflexes; ECG, electrocardiogram; FBS, fasting blood sugar; GERD, gastroesophageal reflux disease; GU, genitourinary; HDL, high-density lipoprotein; HEENT, head, eyes, ears, nose, and throat; LDL, low-density lipoprotein; MI, myocardial infarction; MS, musculoskeletal; neg, negative; NKDA, no known drug allergy; PVD, peripheral vascular disease; quad, quadrants; SOB, shortness of breath; STDs, sexually transmitted diseases; TMs, tympanic membranes; WBCs, white blood cells.

## PERIPHERAL CARDIOVASCULAR DISEASE

The atherosclerotic processes that result in angina and myocardial infarction also occur in other vessels of the body, where they produce the similar pathophysiologic effects of occlusion, plaque rupture, and ischemia. Any site other than the coronary vessels is considered a peripheral site. Common locations for atherosclerosis are the carotid, iliac, femoral, popliteal, and subclavian arteries. When these arteries are involved, the atherosclerotic process is termed organic peripheral vascular disease (PVD). Another type of PVD is functional, in which there is a nonatherosclerotic vascular occlusive disease such as Raynaud's syndrome.

The incidence of PVD has increased as the percentage of the elderly population also has increased, and a third of patients with PVD have significant CVD. The diabetic patient is up to five times more likely than a nondiabetic patient to develop this disease. Because there is occlusion in major vessels supplying blood to tissue, the symptoms are related to ischemia. In the arms and legs, this translates into poor circulation. Patients complain of coldness, pallor, numbness, and discoloration of the most distal part. Ischemic pain develops as the person exercises, producing the classic symptom of *intermittent claudication*. This is a cramp-like pain that can be felt in the hips, thighs, and calves during any exercise; is relieved by rest; and can be very disabling. Often, affected individuals cannot walk more than a few steps without pain. Because there is poor arterial perfusion, another problem experienced is that of decreased skin integrity and poor healing. The skin may appear shiny, hairless, and dry. Wounds do not heal well and may progress to gangrene if not carefully attended.

Carotid artery involvement can lead to significant and even catastrophic symptoms. Dizziness may occur when the head is turned sharply. The atherosclerotic plaque may fissure and thrombose, or an embolism can develop. Symptoms are that of a stroke, or a transient ischemic attack, if the occlusion is temporary: weakness, numbness, loss of speech, falling, and loss of vision.

A less commonly recognized problem related to atherosclerosis is erectile dysfunction. Lesions in the vessels supplying the penis produce a decrease in arterial flow into the erectile tissue, so that the veins leaving the tissue do not become occluded, as normally occurs, and blood leaves as quickly as it enters, inhibiting the ability of the penis to remain erect. This problem is associated with diabetes, hypertension, cigarette smoking, and hyperlipidemia (McKee, 1999). In younger men, arterial injury may be caused by perineal traumatic injury from bicycling and other activities involving prolonged straddling, leading to decreased arterial flow.

## CONGESTIVE HEART FAILURE

It is not uncommon for primary care providers to manage patients with mild, chronic congestive heart failure (CHF). This is an extremely common cardiovascular disorder, affecting 3 million individuals in the US, many of whom are elderly and on Medicare. The cost of CHF in the US ranges from $10 to 15 billion per year, and the mortality rate is high.

Heart failure is defined as an inability of the heart to pump adequate amounts of blood to meet the perfusion needs of the tissues. The term "congestive" implies that not only is there inadequate perfusion (a *forward* effect), but also venous congestion, leading to either pulmonary or systemic congestion (a *backward* effect). CHF occurs as a result of hypertension, CAD, diabetes, cardiomyopathy, valvular heart disease, and congenital heart defects, all of which ultimately lead to a dilated, damaged, and ineffective heart—the final pathway for CHF. The development of CHF involves neurohumoral and inflammatory responses in the myocardium, exercise intolerance, and pump failure.

### Pathophysiologic Changes in Heart Failure

Recall that cardiac output is the product of stroke volume (SV) and heart rate. Stroke volume is largely determined by the Frank-Starling mechanism, which is the effect of an increased end diastolic volume (EDV) causing an increased strength of contraction and SV. This is because the length-tension relationship in the heart is similar to that in skeletal muscle. As muscle is stretched, it responds with greater tension and thus is able to perform more optimally. The lengthening of the muscle produces an optimized sarcomere length, which results in greater binding of myosin cross-bridges to actin, so that the strength of the contraction improves. However, there is an optimal sarcomere length beyond which further stretching of the muscle fiber produces less and less myosin-actin binding. In the heart, this sarcomere length is 2.2 μm, and at this sarcomere length, stretching of the myocytes by increased EDV results in a stronger ventricular contraction, thus producing a greater SV on systole. The Starling curve for a normal and failing heart is illustrated in Figure 14-5. In heart failure, the Frank-Starling mechanism may be effective only in early disease. As long as the heart responds to increased filling with an increased cardiac output, the heart is said to be compensating for the heart failure. As the EDV increases, associ-

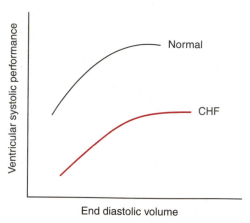

**FIGURE 14.5** ● Starling curve for normal and failing hearts.

ated with increased end diastolic pressure, a failing heart eventually cannot produce an increased SV, and the end systolic volume (ESV) becomes higher than normal. As volumes and pressures increase in the left or right ventricles, the heart stretches even more, and ultimately stretches to a point of dilation. Then the sarcomere length is too great for effective contraction, and the contraction rate is impaired. A dilated heart also is subject to remodeling, which is described later.

### Factors Governing Cardiac Output

The factors that govern cardiac output are preload, afterload, myocardial contractility, and heart rate. Preload is the pressure at the end of diastole and is determined by the EDV.

### Preload

Increasing the EDV is a major compensatory mechanism in heart failure produced through the renin-angiotensin system (RAS). Renal perfusion is reduced as the cardiac output falls, and renal beta receptors are stimulated as the sympathetic nervous system (SNS) is activated, and both effects cause the release of renin by the cells of the juxtaglomerular apparatus. Renin produces activation of angiotensin I, which then produces angiotensin II, causing the adrenal cortex to release the hormone aldosterone. Aldosterone acts on the kidney tubules to increase sodium and water reabsorption. As sodium and water increase in the peripheral circulation, the venous return to the right atrium increases, causing an increased right atrial pressure. A right atrial pressure between 5 and 14 mm Hg can result in improved cardiac performance by increasing preload (EDV) through Starling mechanisms. However, when right atrial pressure rises beyond 14 mm Hg, then the compensatory effect diminishes, and right-sided congestive symptoms appear.

### Afterload

The afterload is the pressure in the aorta, against which the left ventricle pumps its output. Increasing pressure offers resistance to that output and strains the heart. Hypertension is the most common cause of heart failure resulting from increased afterload. Any mechanism that reduces aortic pressure thus reduces the work of the heart and alleviates symptoms of heart failure.

### Myocardial Contractility

Myocardial contractility is a third influence on cardiac output. The myocytes of cardiac muscle are cells that contract by actin-myosin filament sliding when they are stimulated by a wave of depolarization and when calcium and adenosine triphosphate are available to produce a strong contraction. A variety of factors influence the strength of the myocardial contraction. When the heart undergoes inflammatory or ischemic damage, the myocardial cells may be damaged or die and are replaced by white, fibrous connective tissue. The areas of damaged myocardium are not efficient contractile elements, and the strength of the systolic contraction is less than optimal, leading to heart failure.

### Heart Rate

The fourth influence on cardiac output is heart rate. Significant bradycardia can reduce cardiac output so that the metabolic needs of the body are not met. Another way that heart rate and metabolic needs are mismatched is in situations of extremely increased metabolic activity, as might occur in thyrotoxicosis, severe anemia, or fever. The accumulation of metabolites in the peripheral tissues causes massive vasodilation of the supplying arterioles, leading to a great drop in total peripheral resistance through autoregulation. Although cardiac output is high rather than low in this scenario, there is, nevertheless, an inability of the heart to supply the tissue with adequate metabolic fuels and oxygen.

### Systolic and Diastolic Dysfunction

When the heart begins to fail, several compensatory mechanisms are important in restoring cardiac output. However, over time, either systolic, diastolic, or combined dysfunction of the left ventricle occurs. A reduced systolic ejection fraction from the left ventricle is a common measure of left ventricular dysfunction. When ejection fraction is reduced, there is an increased ESV of blood left in the ventricular chamber at the completion of systole. This increased volume and concomitant increased pressure ultimately produces CHF when compensatory mechanisms are no longer able to maintain the SV. Diastolic dysfunction occurs in the absence of left ventricular systolic dysfunction, particularly in the elderly and in people with hypertension. In this situation, the heart may be less elastic and stiffer than normal so that the left ventricular pressure during diastolic filling is increased, leading to congestive symptoms. In reality, many patients with CHF have both diastolic and systolic dysfunction.

Chronic activation of the SNS in CHF initially is a compensatory mechanism because of the inotropic and chronotropic influences of the SNS on the heart. Over time, this may cause progressive deterioration of cardiac function. Desensitization of cardiac beta$_1$-receptor–G protein complex may explain the loss of myocardial contractility in CHF (Fowler et al., 1986). The adrenergic receptors and their G proteins may down-regulate in response to the massively increased degree of sympathetic discharge that occurs in chronic heart failure. An important compensation for the decrease in cardiac output experienced in CHF is SNS activation. With time, however, the failing heart does not respond to adrenergic stimulation by a significant enough increase in ventricular contraction strength, so compensation by the SNS becomes inadequate.

### Remodeling

Remodeling is defined as a change in geometry, volume, mass, and myocellular structure of the cardiac chambers. In the early stage of heart failure, the Frank-Starling forces are important in producing a stretch that achieves an optimal sarcomere length in the myocytes. Hypertrophy is the next phase, which occurs as a response to afterload; wall stress; loss of myocytes through apoptosis or necrosis; and hormonal, chemical, and neurohumoral factors (Sonnenblick & Anversa, 1999). If there is a pressure (systolic) overload, the hypertrophic remodeling involves growth of the myocyte cells, laying down of cells in parallel, and concentric thickening of the ventricular wall (Colucci & Braunwald, 1997). If the hemodynamic stress is a volume (diastolic) overload, the individual myocytes add additional sarcomeres to the length of the fiber, and ventricular dilatation occurs (Colucci & Braunwald, 1997). Remodeling also involves the release of fetal growth factors and cytokines released by cardiac myocytes and other cells, as well as enzymes such as the matrix metalloproteinases, which are involved in extracellular matrix remodeling. The initial response to the stressors on the heart is hypertrophy of the left ventricle to make it a stronger pump, a process that is well described in the athletic heart. In the failing heart, it does improve cardiac output for a period of time, but eventually it, too, fails to provides sufficient compensation for the deteriorating cardiac function. A key factor is thought to be the inadequacy of collateral circulation in the failing heart compared with the athletic heart.

The hypertrophic remodeling is accompanied by continuing myocyte apoptosis. Apoptosis is programmed cell suicide in which cells shrink and deteriorate and the remnants are removed by phagocytosis with little stimulation of an inflammatory response. It is regulated by cellular enzymes, the caspases. Apoptosis is triggered by nuclear or mitochondrial damage and is further stimulated by tumor necrosis factor-alpha (TNF-α). Apoptosis of myocytes appears to occur in heart failure. There are many reasons for this, including normal aging. However, excessive beta-adrenergic blockade, such as occurs in heart failure, accelerates this process and beta-adrenergic blockade inhibits it in experimental animals (Asai et al., 1999). Additional influences include glucose deprivation, nitric oxide, hypoxia, and cytokines. As cells die, they are replaced with connective tissue, and the remaining myocytes experience an increase in workload and demand.

## Inflammatory-like Processes

Along with apoptosis, cellular necrosis with inflammatory-like changes in the myocardium occurs in CHF. The proinflammatory cytokines, IL-1β, IL-6 and TNF-α are produced by the dilated heart and are found in higher than normal serum concentration in patients with heart failure. IL-1 and TNF-α act as myocardial depressants (Cain, et al., 1999). IL-1 and TNF-α are released by cardiac myocytes and regulate the expression of factors that increase matrix degradation in the heart. Cytokines contribute to the evolution of heart failure in several ways: they may cause left ventricular dysfunction, pulmonary edema, cardiomyopathy, reduced peripheral organ perfusion, ventricular remodeling, activation of fetal gene programs, anorexia, and cachexia (Kapadia, 1999).

Circulating TNF-α affects not only cardiac muscle, it also is a powerful cachectic and is at least partly responsible for the severe wasting in CHF patients. As many as 16% of CHF patients have *cardiac cachexia*, a condition characterized by significant loss of lean, fat, and bone tissue (Anker & Rauchhaus, 1999). Cardiac cachexia predicts poor survival in CHF patients.

## Pathophysiologic Effects of Congestive Heart Failure

The cellular and neurohumoral events occurring in heart failure have been described. The clinical implications of these pathophysiologic changes are enormous. The patient with CHF often compensates well for a time through the mechanisms that have been described; namely, RAS and SNS activation. They may be so well compensated that they have no symptoms, or show symptoms only when they stress the cardiovascular system, such as through exercise or during illness. On the other hand, elderly patients in CHF also may have several comorbid conditions that severely limit their abilities to adequately compensate. The symptoms that ultimately appear indicate which compensatory mechanism have begun to fail.

### Left-Sided Heart Failure

Congestive heart failure usually results when the left ventricle has failed. Whereas right-sided failure ultimately often occurs, it does not result from a primary dysfunction in the right ventricle, but rather from the effects of the left ventricle on total cardiac performance. The most common and disturbing symptoms that occur in CHF patients are respiratory distress complaints. The origin of dyspnea, orthopnea, and paroxysmal nocturnal dyspnea is the increasing left ventricular end diastolic pressure, which causes left atrial and, ultimately, pulmonary venule and capillary pressures to increase. The pulmonary capillary pressure normally is balanced by the pulmonary capillary blood osmotic pressure, and the lung parenchyma is kept dry. When the pulmonary capillary hydrostatic pressure begins to exceed the osmotic pressure, excess filtration into the lung tissues and, ultimately, the alveoli, occurs (Fig. 14-6). The patient experiences shortness of breath, first with exercise and then, ultimately, at rest. Alveolar ventilation is impaired because of the boggy tissue and alveolar transudation that prevents gas diffusion. Careful history may elicit orthopnea and also paroxysmal nocturnal dyspnea (PND) as the disease progresses. The pulmonary vascular pressures may rise to levels high enough to cause frank pulmonary edema.

As CHF progresses, the right side of the heart becomes congested as pulmonary vascular pressures increase. The chambers of the right heart hypertrophy to increase the pumping efficacy of the right ventricle, but these chambers ultimately

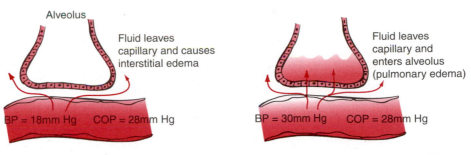

Alveolus

Fluid leaves capillary and causes interstitial edema

BP = 18mm Hg     COP = 28mm Hg

Fluid leaves capillary and enters alveolus (pulmonary edema)

BP = 30mm Hg     COP = 28mm Hg

**FIGURE 14.6** ● Development of pulmonary edema as seen in patient with congestive heart failure.

dilate, becoming less and less effective. Venous blood returning to the right atrium encounters increased pressure and resistance, and so filling is impaired. The venous pressure increases, and the capillaries eventually experience increased hydrostatic pressure (Fig. 14-7). The forces at the capillary level are hydrostatic and osmotic forces, and filtration becomes favored over reabsorption as the venous pressure increases, causing capillary pressure to increase. This results in excess fluid filtration into tissue spaces, causing edema. In the CHF patient, this edema is first noticed in the most distal parts of the body: the feet and ankles. Vascular congestion and edema also occur in the abdominal organs such as the liver and spleen.

If CHF patients have significant systolic dysfunction, they also will experience the effects of poor tissue perfusion. This may be manifested in weakness, fatigue, cachexia, and lack of strength and endurance.

The pathophysiologic changes in the heart and lungs may be assessed through clinical evaluations. Most patients in heart failure have abnormally stiff and noncompliant chambers. This then produces a gallop rhythm, which can be assessed by cardiac auscultation. They also often have cardiomegaly, jugular venous distension, and murmurs. The respiratory effects produce rales and rhonchi. The hepatic venous engorgement leads to hepatomegaly and tenderness to palpation. Tissue edema can advance to severe pitting edema and usually is prominent in the most gravity-dependent parts of the body.

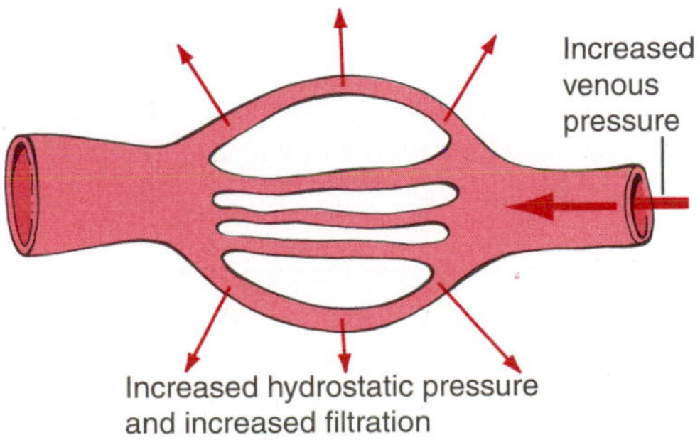

## Cor Pulmonale

Whereas cardiac dysfunction arises from abnormalities in the left ventricle, leading to failure, it is possible for the right ventricle to be the origin of failure. This occurs most often as *cor pulmonale*. The normally low-pressure, high-compliance circuit of the right heart meets with little resistance in the pulmonary vasculature, but in situations in which there is pulmonary hypertension, a strain is placed on the right ventricle. The right ventricle responds to the overload by hypertrophy and dilation. Cor pulmonale occurs either as an acute state or, more commonly, as a chronic condition. Acute cor pulmonale most often is the response of the heart to pulmonary embolism, whereas the chronic right-sided failure appears in patients with chronic obstructive pulmonary disease and, less commonly, in patients with pulmonary vascular diseases. Recall that the vascular autoregulatory response of the pulmonary vessels to hypoxia is vasoconstriction. (This stands in strong contrast to the systemic vessels vasodilation in response to hypoxia.) Chronic states of alveolar hypoxia, whatever the pathogenesis, lead to pulmonary vasoconstriction, which increases resistance to the output from the right ventricle. Disease processes that produce fibrosis and mechanical contributions to resistance are involved.

The architecture of the right ventricle is different from that of the left ventricle. The chamber resembles more of a half-moon shape instead of being round like the left ventricle. Furthermore, the muscular mass of the left ventricle normally is more developed than the right. The right ventricle is better able to handle a volume load than the left

Increased venous pressure

Increased hydrostatic pressure and increased filtration

**FIGURE 14.7** ● Increased hydrostatic pressure and increased filtration as seen with congestive heart failure.

and thus is more compliant. Therefore, the finding of cor pulmonale is a serious concern because of the advanced level of disease needed to produce it.

The symptoms of cor pulmonale are related first to the respiratory disease component of the problem, and second to the right-sided heart failure from increased EDV and pressure in the right heart.

### Physiologic Basis of Treatment for Congestive Heart Failure

The goal of the primary care provider in managing the care of patients in CHF is to keep the patient in a compensated state and to prevent decompensation. This is achieved by reducing volume load in the heart in patients who have symptoms of volume overload. Thiazide and loop diuretics help achieve this goal, as do sodium and fluid restrictions. However, treating with diuretics has not proven useful when there are no symptoms of volume overload. The second approach is to maintain myocardial contractility. The major pharmacologic agent to achieve this goal is digitalis. The third goal of treatment is to reduce afterload, which thus reduces the stress on the failing heart. This is accomplished by using drugs of the angiotensin converting enzyme (ACE) inhibitor classification, which produce vasodilation, thus reducing peripheral resistance. CHF patients with cardiac arrhythmias usually require antiarrhythmic agents. A common consensus is that heart failure patients are undertreated. As their symptoms progress, drug dosages can be increased, but this is not always done. Many patients do not receive ACE inhibitors, which have been shown to be helpful in keeping patients from becoming decompensated.

---

● **Pharmacology Update**

Recently, the drug carvedilol has been approved for the treatment of congestive heart failure (CHF) (*http://www.americanheart. org/Heart_and_Stroke_A_Z_Guide/congestc. html*). It is the first beta blocker approved. The drug had both beta blocking, alpha blocking, antioxidant, and vasodilating effects. Recall that excessive adrenergic stimulation damages the heart in CHF. By blocking the sympathetic nervous system, the drug improves left ventricular contractility. The addition of this drug to the pharmacologic protocol has significantly improved survival in CHF patients (Fisher & Moy, 1999).

---

The practitioner needs to evaluate other sources of sodium intake, such as in antibiotics. The non-steroidal anti-inflammatory agents, which many elderly people take for arthritis, can cause renal problems, which then exacerbate the risk for CHF. Teaching these patients how to manage their illness, activity levels, diet, and medications is an important aspect of their management.

## ARRHYTHMIAS

The care of cardiac patients with arrhythmias usually is not part of primary care practice, except in the case of two common arrhythmias: premature ventricular contractions (PVCs) and atrial fibrillation in the elderly.

### Premature Ventricular Contractions

Premature ventricular contractions are abnormal ventricular contractions that arise from an ectopic focus in the ventricle and cause an excitation that produces an early excitation-contraction coupling, resulting in an extra beat (Fig. 14-8). When the ventricle becomes depolarized by a PVC, it is unable to respond to the normal wave of depolarization that arises in the sinoatrial (SA) node. Thus, there is an asynchrony of the heart rate, and the ventricle has an increased EDV after the PVC because of the extra time that has passed, which increases filling from the atria. Therefore, the next normal depolarization wave from the S-A node that finds the ventricle electrochemically responsive produces an increased SV. People perceive a "flutter" sensation in their chests, or a kind of "breathlessness" or "skipping of a beat" when a PVC has occurred. Some patients also experience syncope or chest pain. Most commonly, a PVC is a single event, and the heart rhythm returns immediately to normal. Occasionally, there may be strings of PVCs, and the patient is very aware of the abnormal rhythm. The occurrence of multiple PVCs usually warrants a further evaluation of the patient, since they are more common in patients with CAD. The sensations associated with PVCs can frighten people, causing them to seek help from their primary care provider.

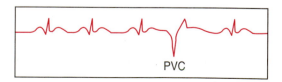

**FIGURE 14.8**  ● Electrocardiogram appearance of extra beat caused by premature venous contraction.

PVCs usually result from fatigue, stress, or ingestion of stimulant drugs such as caffeine or nicotine and occur in most people several times a day without awareness. They also occur in digitalis toxicity, hypocalcemia, and hypokalemia. They produce a drop in cardiac output, which can be significant, particularly in the patient with coexisting cardiac disease. When they occur in an isolated way and can be traced to factors such as caffeine or fatigue, the treatment is simple and obvious. In some settings, patients are treated with antiarrhythmic drugs, although the benefit to a person with no cardiac disease is not well established.

## Atrial Fibrillation

Atrial fibrillation is the most common arrhythmia managed in primary care, with over 1.8 million cases diagnosed in the US. It is seen more commonly in older men, with a prevalence rate as high as 33% in men older than 75 years of age. Many persons with this condition are asymptomatic, and it is diagnosed in only about 5% of these men. This arrhythmia is related to a variety of cardiac disorders such as CAD, valvular heart disease, and hypertension. Any condition that stretches or scars the atria, thus impairing the normal conduction pathway, can produce atrial fibrillation.

The conduction of the impulse from the SA node does not involve a specialized pathway. The impulse spreads over the atrial muscle before it reaches, and is delayed by, the atrioventricular (AV) node. When atrial muscle is damaged, the impulse does not spread in a uniform way, and

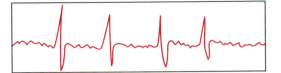

**FIGURE 14.9** ● Electrocardiogram appearance of atrial fibrillation.

chaotic, irregular, and ineffective contractions are the result. The AV node becomes bombarded by numerous stimuli, most of which are too weak to depolarize it and carry the message forward to the ventricles. Those that do depolarize the AV node produce a subsequent ventricular depolarization and contraction. The ventricular rhythm that results can be rapid, normal, or slow, and atrial fibrillation is classified according to the type of ventricular rhythm that it generates. The electrocardiographic appearance of atrial fibrillation is illustrated in Figure 14-9. Atrial contractions, which normally deliver about 25% of the blood from the atria to the ventricles, are weak and ineffective.

The origin of the arrhythmia appears to be in a premature atrial contraction, which triggers the arrhythmia, particularly if the atria is sufficiently enlarged (Simpson, 1997). The arrhythmia can originate from a single, rapidly firing ectopic source or, more commonly, from multiple reentry wavelets (Tse & Lau, 1998). The arrhythmia then produces either a sustained atrial fibrillation or a conversion to normal sinus rhythm. The longer the arrhythmia has been present, the less likely that individuals will convert on their own to normal sinus rhythm.

---

### *CLINICAL VIGNETTE 14.1*

George Stamler is a 75-year-old retiree living in Florida with his 73-year-old wife. He has been previously healthy with just some minor arthritis. He has had bradycardia for about 10 years, with a resting heart rate of 50. An electrocardiogram (ECG) 1 year ago showed sinus bradycardia. He keeps very active, playing golf and participating in a great deal of community service work. His only medical problems have been several skin cancers, which have been surgically removed. He has had several surgeries, including appendectomy, cholecystectomy, and herniorrhaphy. He comes to the primary care provider for his yearly physical examination. His review of systems does not differ significantly from the previous

year's, except that he reports occasional shortness of breath while playing golf. His heart rate today is 90 and irregular. An ECG shows atrial fibrillation with rapid ventricular rate.

Mr. Stamler has developed a common arrhythmia, perhaps perpetuated by his previous bradycardia. He has symptoms of reduced cardiac output with exercise and a too rapid ventricular beat. The atrial fibrillation in this case may be cardioverted. However, only a third of the patients who are cardioverted remain in normal sinus rhythm. If cardioversion is not performed, he will need Coumadin therapy to reduce the coagulability of his blood and thus reduce his increased risk of stroke.

The symptoms of atrial fibrillation are related to whether there is impairment in cardiac output and if coexisting cardiac disease is present. Exercise intolerance, light-headedness, weakness, and chest pains are commonly cited symptoms in patients who are symptomatic. However, many patients are totally asymptomatic, and the discovery of the arrhythmia is an incidental finding. A major concern in atrial fibrillation is the increased risk for stroke. Nearly 20% of ischemic strokes occur in patients with atrial fibrillation. The risk is higher if the patient also has hypertension, left ventricular systolic dysfunction, valvular heart disease, or a history of a prior stroke.

The physiologic basis for treatment is to convert the patient to normal sinus rhythm with cardioversion and drug therapy, which is successful in most patients. However, less than a third remain in normal sinus rhythm for over a year. The other approach is to treat with anticoagulants, thus reducing the risk of thrombi forming in the dilated, fibrillating atria. This is achieved either with aspirin therapy or, more commonly, with warfarin.

## REFERENCES

Anker, S.D. & Rauchhaus, M. (1999). Insights into the pathogenesis of chronic heart failure: Immune activation and cachexia. *Current Opinions in Cardiology, 14* (3), 211–216.

Asai, K., Yang, G.P., Geng, Y.J., Takagi, G., Bishop, S., Ishikawa, Y., Shannon, R.P., Wagner, T.E., Vatner, D.E., Homcy, C.J., & Vatner, S.F. (1999). Beta-adrenergic receptor blockade arrests myocyte damage and preserves cardiac function in the transgenic G(salpha) mouse. *Journal of Clinical Investigation, 104* (5), 551–558.

Cain, B.S., Meldrum, D.R., Dinarello, C.A,. Meng, X., Joo, K.S., Banerjee, A., & Harken, A.H. (1999). Tumor necrosis factor-alpha and interleukin-1 beta synergistically depress human myocardial function. *Critical Care Medicine, 27* (7), 1309–1318.

Caligiuri, G., Liuzzo, G., Biasucci, L.M., & Maseri, A. (1998). Immune system activation follows inflammation in unstable angina: Pathogenetic implications. *Journal of the American College of Cardiology, 32*, 1295–1304.

Colucci, W. & Braunwald, E. (1997). Pathophysiology of Heart Failure. In E. Braunwald (Ed.), *Heart disease: A textbook of cardiovascular medicine* (5th ed.). Philadelphia: W.B. Saunders.

Davidson, M., Kuo, C.C., Middaugh, J.P., Campbell, L.A., Wang, S.P., Newman, W.P., III, Finley, J.C., & Grayston, J.T. (1998). Confirmed previous infection with *Chlamydia pneumoniae* (TWAR) and its presence in early coronary atherosclerosis. *Circulation, 98* (7), 628–633.

Fisher, L.D. & Moye, L.A. (1999). Carvedilol and the Food and Drug Administration approval process: An introduction. *Controlled Clinical Trials, 20* (1), 1–15.

Fowler, M.B., Lasser, J.A., Hopkins, G.L., Minobe, W., & Bristow, M.R. (1986). Assessment of the beta adrenergic receptor pathway in the intact failing human heart. *Circulation, 74*, 1290–1299.

Gersh, B.J., Braunwald, E., & Rutherford, J. (1997). Chronic coronary artery disease. In E. Braunwald (Ed.), *Heart disease: A textbook of cardiovascular medicine* (5th ed.). Philadelphia: W.B. Saunders.

Green, R. (1998). Homocysteine and occlusive vascular disease: Culprit or bystander? *Preventive Cardiology, Summer, 31*–33.

Hajjar, D.P. & Nicholson, A.C. (1995). Atherosclerosis. *American Scientist, 83* (5), 460–467.

Helminen, A., Rankinen, T., Halonen, P., Vaisanen, S., & Rauramaa, R. (1999). Positive and negative life changes and LDL cholesterol. *Journal of Biosocial Science, 31* (2), 269–277.

Kapadia, S.R. (1999). Cytokines and heart failure. *Cardiology Review, 7* (4), 196–206.

Koga, T. & Sasaki, J. (1999). Atherosclerosis. *Nippon Rinsho, 57* (7), 1614–1619.

Kristensen, S.D., Andersen, H.R., & Falk, E. (1999). What an interventional cardiologist should know about the pathophysiology of acute myocardial infarction. *Seminars in Intervention in Cardiology, 4* (1), 11–16.

McCann, B.S., Magee, M.S., Broyles, F.C., Vaughan, M., Albers, J.J., & Knopp, R.H. (1995). Acute psychological stress and epinephrine infusion in normolipidemic and hyperlipidemic men: Effects on plasma lipid and apoprotein concentrations. *Psychosomatic Medicine, 57* (2), 165–176.

McKee, C.D. (1999) Erectile dysfunction. *Drug Store News, 21* (3), 13–41.

Melnick, J.L., Adam, E., & DeBakey, M. (1998) The link between CMV and atherosclerosis. *Infectious Medicine, 15* (7), 479–486.

National Cholesterol Education Program Expert panel (1994). *Second report of the expert panel on detection, evaluation, and treatment of high blood cholesterol in adults.* Washington, D.C.: U.S.: Dept. of Health and Human Services, NIH, NHLBI, 1993, NIH Publication No. 93-3095.

Newby, A.C. & Zaltsman, A.B. (1999). Fibrous cap formation or destruction: The critical importance of vascular smooth muscle cell proliferation, migration and matrix formation. *Cardiovascular Research, 41* (2), 345–360.

Nygard, O., Nordrehaug, J., Refsum, H., Ueland, P., Farstad, M., & Vollset, S. (1997). Plasma homocysteine levels and mortality in patients with coronary artery disease. *New England Journal of Medicine, 337*, 230–236.

Peter, R., Alfredsson, L., Hammar, N., Siegrist, J., Theorell, T., & Westerholm, P. (1998). High effort, low reward, and cardiovascular risk factors in employed Swedish men and women: Baseline results from the WOLF Study. *Epidemiology and Community Health, 52* (9), 540–547.

Redberg, R. (1998). Coronary artery disease in women: Understanding the diagnostic and management pitfalls. *Medscape Women's Health, 3* (5). Available at: http://www.medscape.com.

Simpson, R.J. (1997). Atrial fibrillation. In L. Dornbrand, A. Hoole, & C.J. Pickard, (Eds.), Manual of clinical problems in adult ambulatory care. In *MAXX: Maximum access to diagnosis and therapy: The electronic library of medicine* [CD-ROM]. Philadelphia: Lippincott-Raven Publishers.

Sonnenblick, E.H. & Anversa, P. (1999). Models and remodeling: Mechanisms and clinical implications. *Cardiologia, 44* (7), 609–619.

Tse, H.F. & Lau, C.P. (1998). Electrophysiological properties of the fibrillating atrium: Implications for therapy. *Clinical and Experimental Pharmacology and Physiology, 25* (5), 293–302.

Verhoef, P. & Stampfer, M.J. (1997). Homocysteine: A risk factor for coronary artery disease. *Heart Disease Update, 2*, 1–8.

# Hypertension

Maureen Groer

Hypertension (HTN) is one of the most common illnesses that primary care providers diagnose and manage, being present in close to 50 million Americans. The cost of direct medical expenses for HTN was over $17 billion in 1995, with lost wages and decreases in productivity costing another $6.67 billion (McCarthy, 1997). The presence of this disease often is an incidental finding, either during a routine physical examination or a screening. It also may be discovered by taking a thorough patient history, as it is not uncommon for previously diagnosed hypertensive patients to stop taking medication, either because they believe that they have been "cured," or they were unable to tolerate or afford the prescribed medication. Only 53% of hypertensive patients receive any therapy at all (McCarthy, 1997). Rarely does the hypertensive visit the health care practitioner with minor symptoms such as nosebleeds or headaches, although the common wisdom is that these symptoms are attributed to the disease. The first symptoms of HTN often are an acute cardiac event or a potentially life-threatening stroke, indicating that long-term pathophysiologic damage to target organs has occurred. Because patients usually do not experience symptoms during the early stages of the disease, HTN often is termed the "silent killer." It is a challenge for primary care providers to manage the person with HTN because compliance with lifestyle changes or medications often is difficult for patients who have no overt symptoms of illness.

It is important that the diagnosis of HTN be made according to established standards, using appropriate equipment and proper techniques and diagnostic protocols. Although this may seem elementary, it is instructive to observe the variety of improper approaches and techniques used by various health care personnel to take blood pressure (BP) measurements. The classifications of hypertension for adults according to BP readings are provided in Table 15-1. These BP values are used for patients who are not taking antihypertensive medications and are not acutely ill. If either a systolic or diastolic value is in a different category, the higher category should be used for classifying the patient.

A diagnosis of HTN is made based on the average of two or more readings taken at two or more office visits after the initial finding of high BP. In addition to the categories found in Table 15-1, notice that a BP greater than 130/85 mm Hg in diabetics is considered hypertensive for this group. Another consideration in categorizing the hypertensive patient is the presence of target organ damage from the disease process or the presence of risk factors. Based on these, patients are stratified into risk groups A, B, and C. Depending on how a patient is stratified, the options for treatment differ. For example, a patient in risk group A may have high-normal or stage 1, 2, or 3 HTN but no risk factors such as smoking, dyslipidemia, or diabetes and no measurable target organ damage (such as left ventricular hypertrophy [LVH], nephropathy, or retinopathy). Patients stratified into risk group A may be treated initially, and for long as 1 year, with a program of lifestyle changes and careful monitoring rather than medication. On the other hand, the patient classified into risk group C may have only high-normal BP but target organ damage, which warrants immediate medication treatment along with lifestyle modifications (Sixth Report of the Joint National Committee on Prevention, Detection, Evaluation and Treatment of High Blood Pressure [JNC], 1997).

## TABLE 15.1

### Classification of Hypertension by Systolic and Diastolic Pressures

| Category | Systolic (mm Hg) | Diastolic (mm Hg) |
| --- | --- | --- |
| Optimal | < 120 | < 80 |
| Normal | < 130 | < 85 |
| High normal | 130–139 or | 85–89 |
| Stage 1 HTN | 140–150 or | 90–99 |
| Stage 2 HTN | 160–179 or | 100–109 |
| Stage 3 HTN | > 180 or | > 110 |

HTN, hypertension.

## TYPES OF HYPERTENSION

Hypertension is classified as either primary (essential) or secondary. Essential HTN is the more prevalent and the most likely to be managed in the primary care practice. Secondary HTN, however, must be ruled out when a patient has high BP, although it accounts for less than 10% of HTN. Secondary HTN can be attributed to a pathophysiologic process in an organ or organ system such as the kidneys, the adrenal gland, or the nervous system. For example, a patient with a tumor of the adrenal medulla, a pheochromocytoma, produces bursts of catecholamines that elevate BP to often-remarkable levels. Removal or destruction of the tumor removes the cause of the secondary HTN. On the other hand, essential HTN is considered to be of multifactorial and multigenetic origin and is not a single disease. No single cause has been identified for essential HTN.

## Pathogenesis of Essential Hypertension

Over the years, a variety of potential factors have been identified that contribute to the development of essential HTN. These include genetic influences, sensitivity to dietary sodium, renal abnormalities, abnormalities in the renin-angiotensin system (RAS), increased sympathetic nervous system (SNS) outflow or hyperreactivity, and stress.

### Genetic Influences

The familial nature of essential HTN has been recognized for many years, but it has not been easy to decipher the precise inheritance patterns. Paternal influences are more important than maternal, and the contribution of genetics to risk is in the order of 30% to 60% (Harrap, 1996). Most authorities believe that multiple genes code for the trait of BP and environmental influences interplay with genetic mechanism to cause essential HTN. Animal models of essential HTN have proved useful in understanding how genes interact to cause the disease, but the relevance of rat studies to human illness is always somewhat questionable. In humans, only one genetic locus has been identified in the etiology of essential HTN. The angiotensinogen gene has been postulated to be involved in the etiology of essential HTN through linkage in affected sibling pairs and by the finding of increased risk of HTN associated with polymorphism at the angiotensinogen genetic locus. Preeclampsia also has been found to be associated with the same gene (Lathrop & Soubrier, 1994). Linkage and association studies raise the possibility of a gene on chromosome 1 being involved. It is not known if this gene is part of the angiotensinogen gene or just located near it (Kurtz & Spence, 1993). Another gene suspected in HTN is the angiotensin converting enzyme (ACE) gene. Polymorphisms of this gene have been discovered to be related to an increased risk for acute coronary events, sudden cardiac death, vascular restenosis after angioplasty, and idiopathic and hypertrophic cardiomyopathy. ACE gene polymorphism may affect expression of ACE levels and could be a genetic marker for cardiovascular disease.

Whereas many other genetic loci might be involved in the development of HTN, they have not yet been identified. Genetic differences are being explored at the molecular levels, such as polymorphism of the genes coding for the adrenergic receptor (O'Byrne & Caulfield, 1998)

The genetic risk for HTN is illustrated by the prevalence of the disease in African Americans compared with white Americans. Not only is incidence higher for both males and females and for every age group, the morbidity and mortality related to HTN is significantly greater for African Americans. These patients also are more physiologically resistant to treatment and have more advanced disease when first diagnosed. Undoubtedly, environmental factors such as salt intake, social status, stress, and obesity contribute to development of HTN in African Americans. HTN was virtually unknown in Africa before 1965 (Mufunda & Sparks, 1993) and has been increasing in prevalence. This is most likely related to changing environmental factors, since the rural African communities maintain their normal normotensive levels of BP, whereas urban communities have a higher incidence of HTN. Epidemiologic evidence indicates that the morbidity related to HTN in African Americans could be reduced to that experienced to whites if diagnosis took place earlier and treatment was more uniformly available (Sixth Report of the JNC, 1997).

There are two major genetic theories about how HTN developed as a trait in African Americans. Grim and Wilson (1992) suggest that the conditions of both African life and slavery in America favored the selection of a hereditary trait involving a sodium transport system, which has led to salt sensitivity as the basis for HTN. They suggest that native Africans naturally were low consumers of salt, and during the early years of slavery were not only deprived of salt, but experienced losses of sodium through harsh environmental conditions that led to excess sweating, vomiting, and diarrhea. These conditions favored the genetic retention of traits that enhanced functioning of the RAS to conserve salt. Since then, the diet of Africans in America has become higher in sodium and other electrolytes, leading to a "sensitivity" to salt.

The other theory (Falkner, 1993) purports that the major genetic difference in African Americans is related to insulin-stimulated glucose metabolism, which causes hyperinsulinemia. This leads to a genetic predisposition to HTN, since excessive insulin causes several physiologic responses that could account for its development. Insulin could oppose sodium transport in both renal and smooth muscle cells. Insulin promotes vascular growth and could cause increased peripheral resistance. Vascular hypertrophy from hyperinsulinemia also may lead to enhanced sympathetic reactivity, a phenomenon known to occur in African-American children in response to stressors. However, the genetic loci for these traits have not been identified, and the biochemical and molecular processes remain to be elucidated. Therefore, these theories give only a partial explanation for the genetic influences regulating BP in African Americans.

Even intrauterine factors may be involved in the later development of HTN, since growth deprivation of the fetus during pregnancy has been found to be associated with adult HTN (Law & Shiell, 1996; Kaplan, 1998). Growth retardation may result in a decreased number of available nephrons or filtration surface in later life to handle salt and water loads. Another theory suggests that intrauterine stress may produce high levels of glucocorticoids, which act on the fetus to increase risk for HTN and other diseases associated with intrauterine growth retardation (ischemic heart disease, insulin resistance, and hyperlipidemia) (Nyirenda & Seckl, 1998).

A person's BP tends to track in a particular percentile throughout life. Children at risk for development of HTN later in life can be identified early by the percentile in which their BPs track, although factors such as weight and body mass index (BMI) may be an important influence on BP in children and adolescents. The presence of a prehypertensive state in children sometimes can be identified through hemodynamic factors, tracking percentile, stress responsiveness, and family history (hypertensive parents).

Children of hypertensive parents show several different physiologic differences that can be identified early in life. These children respond to a stressor differently, retaining more sodium than their normal peers. As young adults, these individuals have abnormal left ventricular filling even before a BP increase occurs.

## The Sodium Hypothesis

Excessive sodium intake may play an important role in the development of essential HTN. Sodium promotes volume retention, thus increasing preload and cardiac output (CO). Sodium also may increase vascular tone and reactivity, increase intracellular $Ca^{++}$, promote hyperinsulinemia, and increase plasma catecholamines. High sodium diets often are low in potassium, and the sodium effect on BP may be related to the $Na^+$–$K^+$ ratio in the diet. Evidence suggests that populations with naturally low dietary salt intake have low levels of BP throughout the life span. For most human populations, the dietary sodium intake has increased and the potassium content decreased remarkably in the last 200 years. Human renal physiology evolved concomitant with dietary sodium concentrations that were far less than what is now commonly consumed. The current situation is alarming, since the flavoring and preserving of food with salt is greater than ever before.

It is well known that reducing salt intake for many hypertensive patients results in a lowering of

BP. The concepts of salt sensitivity and salt resistance have arisen with the idea that genetically endowed responses to dietary sodium differ in humans and are associated with HTN risk. An animal model of salt sensitivity, the Dahl rat, has been developed in the laboratory and provides a wealth of information about the genetics and physiology of sodium sensitivity. The inbred sodium-sensitive Dahl rat develops HTN when given a high-sodium diet, but otherwise does not. Thus, the genetic influence is a substrate that allows HTN to develop when certain environmental factors are present.

Sodium sensitivity can be demonstrated in humans by a 10% or more increase in 24-hour BP when going from a low- to high-sodium diet (Gerdts et al., 1998). Approximately 20% of the human population shows this sodium sensitivity response. The physiologic mechanism may be one in which excretion of the sodium load cannot be accomplished through the kidney without an elevation in BP (altered pressure natriuresis). Another physiologic pathway might be a reduction in the sodium sensing mechanisms of the juxtaglomerular apparatus (JGA), so that excessive renin is released. A major question is whether essential HTN arises from a primary kidney abnormality or whether kidney changes occur in response to pathophysiologic mechanisms caused by high BP. When hypertensive patients with renal failure are transplanted with kidneys from nonhypertensive individuals, long-term remission of their HTN occurs, and when recipients receive renal grafts from hypertensive individuals, they are more likely to develop high BP (Kaplan, 1998). These clinical results support an origin for essential HTN in the kidney itself.

The presence of sodium sensitivity is associated with insulin resistance, increased glomerular pressure, microalbuminuria, and lack of a circadian drop in nighttime BP. Cardiovascular events occur more frequently in hypertensive patients who are sodium sensitive (Morimoto et al., 1997).

Membrane-bound cation transport processes have been investigated in HTN. A higher intracellular sodium ion concentration has been shown in persons with genetic heritage from the African gene pool (Cooper & Borke, 1993). A convenient model system to study cation transport is the erythrocyte, a cell that can be easily collected and manipulated in the laboratory. The membrane of erythrocytes (and other cells) from hypertensive animals appears to be altered, and the sodium-hydrogen ion exchange antiporter may be involved in causing the higher intracellular $Na^+$ thought to play a role in essential HTN. Increased activity of this pump raises both intracellular $Na^+$ and pH.

The net effect might be to increase the tone and thickness of vascular smooth muscle cells. This is illustrated in Figure 15-1.

A decreased $Na^+$–$Ca^{++}$ exchange across cell membranes also may occur, leading to increased intracellular $Ca^{++}$. This would increase vascular smooth muscle tone in the walls of arterioles.

## Renin

Figure 15-2 illustrates the RAS. Renin normally is released by the JGA of the kidney in response to decreased blood perfusion and ischemia, decreased afferent arteriolar pressure, or decreased sodium concentration in the cells of the macula densa. Renin is released as a hormone into the circulation and has paracrine effects in the kidney. It has one major extrarenal effect: enzymatic conversion of angiotensinogen to angiotensin I. Angiotensin I then is converted to angiotensin II by ACE, which is a tissue-bound enzyme and the target for one of the major classes of antihypertensive drugs, ACE inhibitors. Angiotensin II has major pressor effects and growth-promoting effects on vascular myocytes, which could lead to vessel wall remodeling. It also stimulates the adrenal cortex to release the hormone aldosterone. Aldosterone then acts on the distal convoluted tubule and collecting duct to increase sodium reabsorption, which promotes osmotic reabsorption of water. This

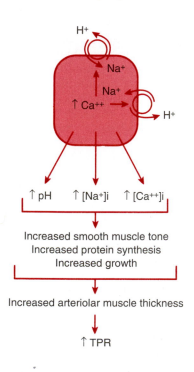

**FIGURE 15.1** ● Increased activity of the $Na^+$-$H^+$ ion exchange antiporter.

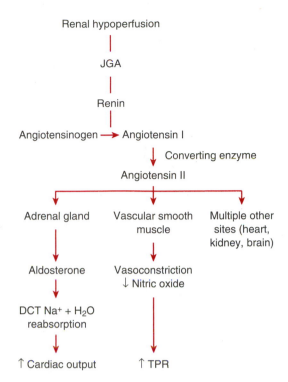

Renal hypoperfusion

|

JGA

|

Renin

|

Angiotensinogen → Angiotensin I

↓ Converting enzyme

Angiotensin II

Adrenal gland    Vascular smooth muscle    Multiple other sites (heart, kidney, brain)

Aldosterone    Vasoconstriction ↓ Nitric oxide

DCT Na⁺ + H₂O reabsorption

↑ Cardiac output    ↑ TPR

**FIGURE 15.2** ● The effects of renal hypoperfusion on the renin–angiotensin–aldosterone system.

increases vascular volume and pressure, and increases sodium concentration in the extracellular fluid.

Because HTN is associated with increased BP being sensed by the JGA, the release of renin in HTN logically should be suppressed, yet most hypertensive patients have normal or elevated renin levels. The cause for this is unexplained but may be related to the presence of ischemic nephrons, increased SNS activity, or abnormal RAS regulation.

Essential HTN is associated with high, normal, or low renin levels. High levels are seen in 10% to 20% of hypertensive patients and are more likely to be exhibited by younger white patients. Such patients have inappropriately high levels of renin in the presence of normal or low dietary sodium and, paradoxically, in the presence of high BP. High plasma renin levels are seen in HTN related to excessive SNS activity, and these patients thus are treated more often with beta blockers or ACE inhibitors (see *Pharmacology Update* section later).

Low renin is seen in about 30% of hypertensive patients, with the remainder having normal plasma renin activity. Older whites, smokers, and African Americans are more likely to have low plasma

renin activity. Low-renin HTN is more likely to be associated with volume-dependent pathophysiologic processes or to be seen in individuals who are likely to be sodium sensitive. Primary care providers should know that low-renin hypertensive patients seem less likely to have cerebrovascular and cardiovascular complications from their high BP. Low-renin HTN often is best treated through diuretics, calcium channel blockers, alpha₁ blockers, and alpha₂ antagonists (see *Pharmacology Update* section later).

### Stress

Chronic stress is believed to play a role in the pathogenesis of essential HTN. The mechanism responsible may be through excessive central SNS drive, increased or inappropriate stress reactivity, or abnormalities in the neurotransmission processes of the SNS. To understand how stress increases long-term arterial BP, recall the anatomic "wiring" of the autonomic nervous system (Fig. 15-3).

Blood pressure is regulated through the SNS and parasympathetic nervous system (PNS), which send efferent output from the brain and spinal cord in nerves that innervate cardiovascular muscle tissue. The vasomotor center in the brain balances sympathetic (SNS) and parasympathetic (PNS) output in response to information received from the baroreceptors. Baroreceptors are pressure-sensitive afferent nerve endings that are located in the carotid artery and aortic arch. Atrial stretch receptors and other volume receptors supply additional information. The baroreceptors are responsible for constantly adjusting arterial pressure in response to postural changes, blood volume, and BP. Fibers from the baroreceptors extend to the vasomotor center in the medulla oblongata, which then sends out efferent fibers through parasympathetic and sympathetic pathways to the heart and blood vessels. There are multiple synapses along these pathways that require neurotransmitters. The parasympathetic pathways release acetylcholine at their neuromuscular terminals, which slows heart rate and causes vasodilation, whereas sympathetic nerves release norepinephrine at their neuromuscular terminals, causing heart rate acceleration, increased cardiac contractility, and increased vascular tone, leading to vasoconstriction of the arterioles and increased peripheral resistance.

Blood pressure fluctuates in all persons around a set point and is physiologically labile in response to internal and external stimuli. The normal arousal response to a perceived threat or challenge is termed the acute stress response and is characterized by an increase in SNS activity. The so-

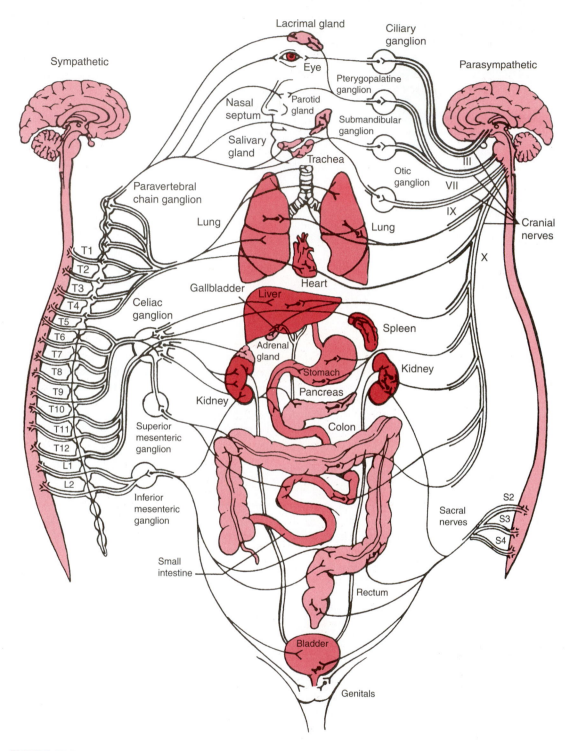

**FIGURE 15.3** ● The autonomic nervous system.

called fight or flight response increases heart and respiratory rates; vasoconstricts arterioles and thus elevates BP; increases blood flow to skeletal muscles, the heart, and the brain; and produces release of epinephrine from the adrenal medulla. This response clearly is an adaptive survival mechanism but could be maladaptive in HTN. HTN could result from excessive vasomotor tone from excessive SNS activity. This is caused theoretically by poorly regulated central brain SNS discharges, dysregulation of the set point around which the baroreceptors respond, or through long-term facilitation of neurotransmitter release of norepinephrine by epinephrine. Some individuals may respond to events in their daily lives by inappropriate, frequent SNS arousal, a phenomenon called hyperreactivity, or the "hot reactor" syndrome. This reactivity may occur even during cognitions and emotional experiences, when there is no need for an arousal response to occur, at least from an evolutionary perspective. Frequent bombarding of the baroreceptors from excessive reactivity to stress may "reset" the baroreceptors to a higher set point.

Primary care providers often observe BP reactivity in patients who experience "white coat hypertension." This is a patient who is normotensive most of the time, but when being measured in the medical office, these individuals have BP in the range of HTN categories. Women and younger people are more likely to show this effect. Monitoring these patients with continuous ambulatory BP monitoring at home and at work while they experience the usual challenges and stressors of daily life has proven to be a useful tool. Many of these patients are reactive to their environment and produce BP elevations throughout the day. Recent research indicates that individuals with white coat hypertension have increased left ventricular mass, indicating increased workload (Owens et al., 1998). However, compared with mild hypertensive patients, those with white coat hypertension have a more benign course (Khattar et al., 1998).

The fact that BP lability and reactivity characterizes some individuals has led to the suggestion that a particular personality type is prone to HTN. Whereas this is true for coronary artery disease, it has not been well documented for hypertensive patients.

The personality variable suggested to play a role in the hypertensive individual is anger suppression and conflict avoidance (Shapiro, 1996). Most of the studies on relationships between behavior, personality, and risk in cardiovascular disease have been carried out only in men. An interesting study of never-treated 40-year-old

women with essential HTN compared with healthy, age-matched normotensive women reports that these women are more likely to be alexithymic and to have difficulties coping with aggression (Nordby et al., 1995). In the study, a psychiatrist was blinded as to which women were normotensive and then conducted interviews, after which he correctly identified whether the individual was normotensive or hypertensive on the basis of personality. In this study, 32 of 46 subjects were correctly identified by the psychiatrist.

There is a body of research on the relationship between chronic stress and HTN. One of the most fascinating studies is one which compared a group of 144 cloistered nuns in Italy with 138 laywomen living in the same geographic area with comparable health habits over a 20-year period (Timio, 1997). BP rose over time in the lay women but remained stable in the nuns. The nuns had higher blood lipids at the end of the 20-year period, but their mean BP was 120/80 mm Hg, whereas the women living in the communities around the nunnery had a mean BP of 162/90. The researchers suggest that the cause of this remarkable difference may be related to the nuns' lack of worry over their survival needs being met, a greater amount of social support, and decreased exposure to environmental factors such as pollution.

In contrast, only a few studies can be found of highly stressed populations developing HTN, such as those showing increased BP in air traffic controllers and in the population of survivors of the Leningrad barricade in World War II. Populations that live in a state of chronic environmental or social stress also have a tendency for higher BPs. These include urban dwellers and African Americans. Many other potential risk factors are found in such populations and confound causality.

### Obesity and Hyperinsulinemia

Obese individuals have an increased risk for HTN, hyperlipidemia, and insulin resistance, leading to hyperinsulinemia. Whether there is a common metabolic defect underlying a syndrome or whether obesity and hyperinsulinemia are steps along the pathway to HTN is unknown. Central obesity (the "apple" shape or upper body distribution of adiposity) is seen more commonly in hypertensive individuals as well as in patients with type 2 diabetes. Research on the newly discovered hormone leptin, which may play a role in obesity, suggests that leptin also may be important in the development of HTN, particularly in women (Suter et al., 1998).

A useful measurement that is easily performed by the primary care provider is the waist circumference. Higher quartiles of waist circumference are markedly correlated with incidence of HTN and type 2 diabetes. For patients with type 2 diabetes, a 23-fold elevation in risk is seen for those in the highest compared with the lowest quartile of waist circumference. Waist circumference appears to be a better predictor of cardiovascular disease than the more traditionally used BMI and waist-to-hip ratio (Okosun et al., 1998).

The mechanisms through which obesity increases HTN risk are most likely related to the enlarged tissue mass that must be perfused and the increased cardiac output of the obese. However, more than 50% of patients with essential HTN have some insulin resistance (Muller-Wieland et al., 1998). Although this might be caused by obesity, nonobese hypertensive individuals also show insulin resistance. Insulin activates the SNS, thus promoting vasoconstriction, raising peripheral resistance, and increasing BP. However, insulin also has a direct vasodilatory effect that opposes the SNS effects. Thus, together, these act in opposition, and BP normally is maintained in the nonobese, nonhypertensive individual. However, in the hypertensive individual, there may be significant insulin resistance, leading to a state of hyperinsulinemia. High basal levels of insulin seem to increase the SNS activity and to downregulate the vasodilatory action, so the net effect is a pressor response to insulin (Kaplan, 1998).

Insulin has other effects that could contribute to the pathogenesis of HTN. These include increased sodium and water reabsorption, a direct growth-promoting effect on smooth muscle cells, and activation of the SNS. Insulin resistance and salt sensitivity may be part of the same syndrome, since several studies show greater insulin resistance in salt-sensitive hypertensive patients (Galletti et al., 1997). In the hypertensive individual, insulin produces a threefold increase in sympathetic activation compared with nonhypertensive individuals. Additionally, activation of the SNS antagonizes insulin-mediated glucose uptake into skeletal muscle cells. There is, therefore, crosstalk between insulin and the SNS, which is altered in the hypertensive individual (Lembo et al., 1996). The relationship between obesity, hyperinsulinemia, and HTN is important and may be the basis for the significant effects of weight loss on reducing BP in the patient with HTN. Weight loss is associated with decreased intracellular calcium, perhaps decreasing the degree of vasoconstriction produced. For each 1% loss of body weight, there is a 1% improvement in insulin sensitivity in the obese, nondiabetic patient.

The effects of obesity and HTN on cardiac damage seem to be greater for women than men. Postmenopausal women who have LVH have poorer prognoses than men of comparable ages and hypertensive levels. Women who are both obese and hypertensive are more likely to have greater wall thickness than nonobese hypertensive women (Kuch et al., 1998).

## PATHOPHYSIOLOGIC CHANGES IN HYPERTENSION

To understand the pathophysiologic disturbances produced by the hypertensive state, it is necessary to clearly understand BP and the variables influencing it. Blood pressure is hydrostatic pressure exerted against the walls of the arteries of the circulatory system and is produced by the force of ejection of a volume of blood from the left ventricle into a network of fairly rigid, noncompliant arterial vessels. These vessels transmit the pressure without much decrement into the widely branching, small-caliber arterioles that disperse the blood into tissue capillaries. The arterioles offer the greatest resistance to the column of blood pushed into them from the heart. The smooth muscle of the arterioles can be constricted or dilated, changing the degree of resistance.

Systolic BP generally reflects cardiac output (CO), whereas diastolic BP reflects peripheral resistance. Mean BP, then, is determined by two influences, CO and total peripheral resistance (TPR), and is given by the following formula:

$$BP = CO \times TPR$$

This equation enables calculation of the mean BP, which is not the average of the systolic and diastolic, but rather the mean arterial pressure measured at any point in time during the cardiac cycle. Since the heart spends a longer time in diastole in a relaxed state as it fills with blood than it does in systole, when the blood is actively ejected from the heart, the mean arterial pressure is about 90 mm Hg. Systolic BP is the pressure in the arteries produced by cardiac systole, whereas diastolic BP is the pressure when the heart is filling.

Cardiac output is defined as the stroke volume in milliliters multiplied by the heart rate in beats per minute. The heart ejects approximately 65% to 70% of the blood in the ventricles at the end of diastole, about 80 mL of blood with each stroke. For a person with a heart rate of 70, the CO then would be 5600 mL/minute. Cardiac contractility is important in determining the stroke volume, as are factors such as preload and afterload. Preload is the volume in the left ventricle at the end of diastole, which stretches the walls of the ventricle. End diastolic volume and stroke volumes are positively related according to Starling's law of the heart. Contractility is an inherent property of cardiac muscle, which is related to the length of muscle sarcomeres; the availability of calcium, oxygen, and metabolic fuels; and the degree of SNS activation. Afterload is the amount of pressure generated in the left ventricle during systole to open the semilunar valve, which is required before the stroke volume can be ejected into the aorta. When there is increased resistance to ventricular empty-ing, such as in situations associated with increased blood viscosity or increased resistance in the ves-sels themselves, afterload is increased and CO may be decreased. Thus, CO can be increased by increased preload, increased contractility, and decreased afterload. Increasing CO produces an increase in systolic BP.

Total peripheral resistance is the total amount of resistance to blood flow offered by the circula-tory system and is measured in peripheral resis-tance units. Most of the peripheral resistance is offered by the arterioles because they branch from the small arteries and subdivide many times into vessels that supply the capillary network, produc-ing a wide surface area of small tubes through which the blood from the major vessels must flow. Recall that flow through a blood vessels is deter-mined by several factors, the most important one being the radius of a vessel. According to Poiseuille's law, pressure varies inversely with radius to the fourth power. Additionally, the smooth muscle of the arterioles is regulated by autoregulatory factors produced by tissues, which relax or contract the muscle. The SNS innervates both arteriolar and venular smooth muscle, releas-ing the neurotransmitter norepinephrine, which acts on adrenergic receptors on this smooth muscle to contract the muscle and thus vasoconstrict. Increasing the amount of peripheral resistance through vasoconstriction would increase the level of diastolic BP.

In physiologic situations, BP is maintained when either CO or TPR changes. For example, when a person exercises, CO increases tremen-dously, which produces an elevation in systolic BP. However, because there is vasodilatation at the arteriolar end of the circulatory system, particu-larly in the muscles and skin, the TPR offered to blood flow drops. Since BP is the product of CO and TPR, with a rise in CO accompanied by a drop in TPR, BP does not rise markedly during exercise.

With HTN, this relationship between CO and TPR must be considered. Blood pressure theoreti-cally could be increased by increases in either of these variables. However, in most hypertensive patients, CO is lower than normal and peripheral resistance is elevated. HTN could be initiated by a rise in CO as a first stage in the process, which might occur with increased preload. For example, salt-sensitive individuals may retain sodium and water, causing excess fluid volume. Stress might produce excessive SNS activity, which would increase myocardial contractility. However, with time, these factors become translated into the most consistent finding in established HTN, elevated peripheral resistance. The physiologic mechanism by which this translation occurs may be through normal autoregulation of the blood supply in tissue beds. If CO increases, blood flow through tissue beds also increases accordingly. But when tissues do not require the nutrients and oxygen being sup-plied at such high levels, a compensatory vasocon-striction occurs through autoregulatory processes. If pathophysiologic changes occur, such as thick-ening in the arteriolar musculature, this rise in TPR remains constant and increases with time, elevat-ing BP through an elevation in TPR. This process is illustrated in Figure 15-4.

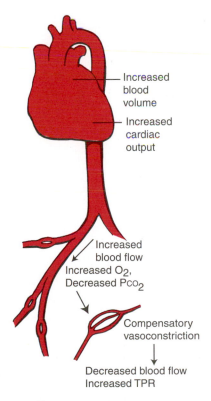

Increased blood volume

Increased cardiac output

Increased blood flow
Increased $O_2$,
Decreased $P_{CO_2}$

Compensatory vasoconstriction

Decreased blood flow
Increased TPR

**FIGURE 15.4** ● Increased cardiac output produces compensatory vasocon-striction, decreased blood flow, and increased total peripheral resistance.

Increased peripheral resistance then seems to be an underlying phenomenon in essential HTN. What variables contribute to this? As discussed previously, vessel radius change influences pressure and flow remarkably. Hypertensive individuals are known to have hypertrophic growth and restructuring of the smooth muscle of the arteriolar walls so that the lumen caliber becomes significantly reduced. There are also changes produced in arteries as well as arterioles that may be related to the direct effects of the high-pressure head in these vessels. Exactly how this vascular wall hypertrophy and remodeling occurs is not known, although several growth factors are suspected to be involved. Another factor, nitric oxide, also is a possible culprit. Nitric oxide synthesis may be defective in hypertensive individuals. Recall that nitric oxide is generated by vascular endothelium and produces vasodilatation in small arteries. Hypertensive vessels may not synthesize adequate amounts of nitric oxide and thus do not adequately vasodilate (Cardillo & Panza, 1998).

These changes in the vessels develop slowly, insidiously, and relentlessly in the person with essential HTN. Years must pass for actual smooth muscle cellular hypertrophy to occur, leading to the thickening of the vessel walls. Aging independently contributes to the progression of these vascular changes. Biochemical and morphologic changes that are part of the aging process cause less endothelial-dependent relaxation in the aorta and small arteries, progressive arteriosclerosis, and accelerated atherosclerosis.

If HTN is treated and a person remains normotensive, amelioration of this slow vascular hypertrophic growth will occur. It is the restriction in blood flow through these damaged vessels that leads to the deleterious target organ effects that cause the morbidity in HTN, and so a slowing down of this process slows down all of these pathophysiologic changes.

## COMPLICATIONS AND END ORGAN DAMAGE IN ESSENTIAL HYPERTENSION

### Arteriosclerosis and Atherosclerosis

Vascular factors in the pathogenesis of HTN, including nitric oxide, have been discussed previously. The presence of blood at higher than normal pressure within the circulatory system can itself produce significant vascular alterations and damage, which compound the disease process. Acceleration of atherosclerotic plaque formation is one of these alterations.

Atherosclerosis begins with the development of a fatty streak in an artery, which ultimately develops into an atheromatous plaque that occludes the vessel and is a site for thromboses (Fig. 15-5). Atherosclerotic plaques occur in large arteries and at bifurcations of arteries. Hypertension is an independent risk factor for atherosclerotic disease, which may be initiated by a proinflammatory state within the arterial wall that results from the generation of reactive oxygen radicals. Mechanical deformation of the arterial wall by the increased pressure stimulates the generation of these damaging oxygen free radical and stimulates the production of proinflammatory proteins (Taylor, 1998). Oxidative stress and inflammation result in endothelial damage, necrosis, and atherosclerotic changes over time.

Elevated glucose levels in both individuals with diabetes and those with hypertension may contribute to the acceleration of atherosclerosis, perhaps through toxic effects on the vascular endothelium. Other risk factors for atherosclerosis in hyperinsulinemic hypertensive individuals are abnormalities in platelet function, clotting factors, the fibrinolytic system, and dyslipidemia (Sowers et al., 1993). The development of atherosclerosis can lead to multiple morbid complications (stroke, coronary artery disease and myocardial infarction, and intermittent claudication).

Arteriosclerosis is another type of vascular damage that occurs in small arteries and arterioles in HTN. Endothelial injury and hyperplasia, as well as hypertrophy, leading to fibrosis of small arteries and arterioles, characterize these lesions. Figure 15-6 shows the types of atherosclerotic and arteriosclerotic lesions that develop in essential HTN.

### Left Ventricular Hypertrophy

The myocardium responds to chronic HTN in ways that lead to both diastolic and systolic abnormalities. Diastolic filling abnormalities occur because the hypertensive heart becomes stiff and unable to use normal Starling mechanisms to increase ejection when diastolic filling increases. This is especially observable when the person with HTN exercises. Left atrial enlargement may be observed in these cases and may be associated with LVH.

Left ventricular hypertrophy occurs in up to half of untreated hypertensive individuals and is an important risk factor for cardiovascular mortality. Whereas left ventricular mass increases as a normal part of aging, in the normotensive elderly, it results from connective tissue degeneration. In

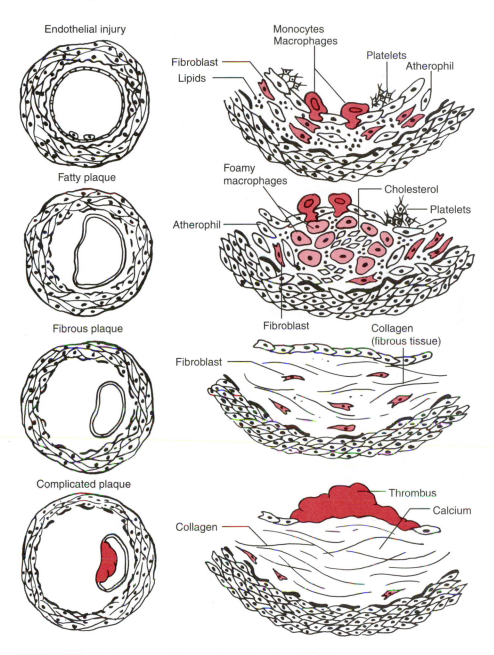

Endothelial injury

Fibroblast
Lipids
Monocytes
Macrophages
Platelets
Atherophil

Fatty plaque

Foamy
macrophages
Atherophil
Cholesterol
Platelets

Fibrous plaque

Fibroblast
Fibroblast
Collagen
(fibrous tissue)

Complicated plaque

Collagen
Thrombus
Calcium

**FIGURE 15.5** ● Formation and progression of the atherosclerotic lesion.

hypertensive patients, LVH is caused by an increase in muscle mass and fibrotic tissue. There is excess deposition of collagen, cellular infiltration, and cardiac myocyte hypertrophy—a process known as *remodeling*. As a person with HTN ages, it is expected that normal aging and HTN are additive in producing significant and pathologic LVH.

The risk of LVH is greatest in obese, postmenopausal women (Kuch et al., 1998). Regardless of treatment, if LVH is in the 95th percentile,

there is two times the risk of morbid cardiovascular events such as congestive heart failure (CHF), myocardial ischemia, and arrhythmias. Reversing the LVH can reduce this risk, and the antihypertensive drugs that are most effective in this regard are the ACE inhibitors and the calcium channel blockers (Schlaich & Schmieder, 1998).

Echocardiography is used to diagnose LVH and to ascertain the geometry of the wall thickness. The wall thickness and ventricular hypertrophy

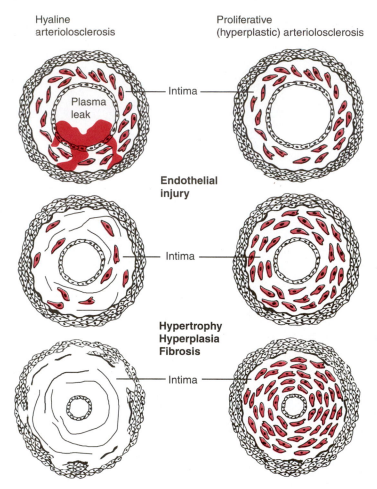

Hyaline
arteriolosclerosis

Proliferative
(hyperplastic) arteriolosclerosis

Intima

Plasma
leak

Intima

**Endothelial
injury**

Intima

**Hypertrophy
Hyperplasia
Fibrosis**

Intima

**FIGURE 15.6** ● Two types of arteriosclerosis: sclerosis and thickening of walls of arterioles. Hyaline arteriosclerosis is associated with benign nephrosclerosis and proliferative arteriosclerosis may be associated with malignant hypertension, nephrosclerosis and scleroderma. (From Schwartz & Ross:. Cellular proliferation in atherosclerosis and hypertension. *Prog Cardiovasc Dis, 26,*:355, 1984.)

take several forms (either eccentric or concentric). When LVH is present, there is elevated wall stress, which reduces systolic performance of the ventricle. Hypertrophy develops as a response to the high TPR and occurs first at the myocellular level, where the stretch in the ventricle produces a stimulation of the synthesis of growth-promoting proteins.

Plasma renin activity appears to be correlated with LVH and may be an important first step for the clinician to ascertain in the hypertensive patient (Koga et al., 1998). Other factors that contribute to the development of LVH include alcohol intake, sodium sensitivity, obesity, blood viscosity, and race (African Americans have increased septum and wall thickness, so they have increased LVH at a lower pressure than do whites).

A major effect of LVH is a diminution in coronary perfusion, since the hypertrophied myocardium eventually is not vascularized adequately, and with reduced capillary density and increased vascular tone, the myocardium cannot be adequately perfused when demand increases, such as during exercise. This leads to coronary artery disease and ischemia, a major factor in causing morbid cardiac complications in the hypertensive patient. HTN is the major risk factor in around 1 million acute myocardial infarctions every year (McCarthy, 1997).

## Congestive Heart Failure

As LVH progresses, diastolic function is disturbed, causing prolonged isovolumic relaxation. This results from the inactivation of actin and myosin that is related to decreased available adenosine triphosphate, which inhibits calcium pumps in the sarcoplasmic reticulum.

LVH can progress to frank CHF in the hypertensive and is particularly prominent in the elderly patient. The progression to CHF is not inevitable if the patient is treated and remains normotensive, but it is not completely preventable either. New research provides a view of HTN as a metabolic syndrome, with HTN being only one aspect of the deleterious processes that can disrupt organ function. Whereas controlling HTN clearly is of enormous benefit, it is not fully protective of end organ damage.

Most patients who develop CHF are hypertensive. The CHF usually develops as the cardiac dilation and inadequate systolic function impairs the heart's ability to eject an adequate fraction of the end diastolic volume. Other cardiovascular complications that are prevalent in HTN include abdominal aortic aneurysms, aortic dissections, peripheral vascular disease, and cerebrovascular disease.

### Stroke

One of the most devastating effects of HTN is the occurrence of a cerebrovascular accident, or stroke. Stroke is the third leading cause of death in the United States, with a mortality rate as high as 50% in patients with HTN. HTN is the principal cause of strokes in people younger than 65 years of age. Transient ischemic attacks (TIAs) also occur at a higher incidence in HTN. Both TIAs and strokes result from cerebrovascular disease, characterized by atherosclerosis and arteriosclerosis of the cerebral arteries, and also from systemic vascular and cardiac disease, which can produce emboli to the cerebral vasculature.

A TIA is produced by temporary ischemia in cerebral tissue caused by a temporary loss of perfusion. Typically, there is a rapid onset and duration of from 2 to 15 minutes, with clearing of symptoms occurring in about the same time frame. Usually, there is no permanent neurologic deficit after a TIA, in contrast to a stroke. The symptoms of a TIA include unilateral weakness or paralysis; difficulty speaking, writing, or calculating; and visual disturbances. The occurrence of a TIA is a serious warning of significant cerebrovascular disease. It portends the eventual development of a stroke in the individual, and up to 40% of patients experiencing a TIA will have a stroke within 5 years.

Strokes occur more frequently with advancing age, and in the elderly hypertensive patient, there may be concurrent cardiac and vascular disease, which affects the physiologic reserves of the individual to recover. The risk of stroke doubles for every decade after age 55 and has a 25% higher prevalence in men. Most strokes in the hypertensive patient are caused by cerebral thrombosis or embolism, with the second most common etiology being intracerebral hemorrhage. The thrombosis begins in an area of the vessels already compromised by atherosclerotic plaque, a common site being the internal carotid artery. The thrombus forms as blood coagulates over the plaque, and a fragment of this clot can travel deeper into the cerebral vessels, causing occlusion and ischemia. A hemorrhage, although less common, may have a more rapid onset and has a higher mortality rate.

### Retinal Disease

The retina of the eye is an important target organ in HTN, and retinopathy is a frequent finding in the hypertensive patient, with as many as 50% of patients showing some incidence of retinal arterial disease. These changes include papilledema, retinal vascular abnormalities, bleeding, infarction (cotton-wool spots), or soft exudates. See Figure 15-7 for examples of these alterations.

The presence of retinopathy also is useful in determining prognosis in sustained HTN. Because the retinal vessels are visible with the aid of the ophthalmoscope, the characteristic retinal markers of hypertensive vascular disease are readily identi-

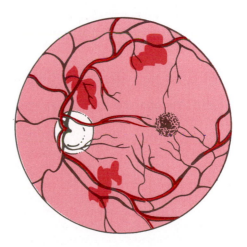

**FIGURE 15.7** ● Hypertensive retinopathy characterized by retinal arterial disease.

fiable. Retinopathy in HTN can be assessed using the Keith-Wagener-Barker scale of stages 0 to 4 (Table 15-2). The retinal vessels can be evaluated for size, narrowing, microaneurysms, appearance of arteriovenous crossings, and tortuosity. The eye grounds can be evaluated for hemorrhages, exudates, and cotton-wool spots. The Keith-Wagener-Barker classification system is commonly used to grade the arteriolar sclerosis, spasms, and bleeding, as well as the presence of exudates and papilledema. This classification is presented in Table 15-2.

The damage in the retinal vessels is thought to be related to the arteriosclerotic process that leads to turbulence in the vessels. Turbulence then produces endothelial damage and sets up a vicious cycle of continuing vascular disease. Cotton-wool spots are early, prognostic retinal lesions resulting from occlusion of the terminal retinal arterioles. The result is acute focal inner retinal ischemia of arteriolar sclerosis and associated changes such as increased arteriolar tortuosity and narrowing.

## Renal Disease

The incidence of end-stage renal disease is increasing, even while cardiovascular mortality is decreasing, presumably because of better treatment of HTN. End-stage renal disease is largely attributable to diabetes and HTN in the United States. Early renal disease often is totally asymptomatic, and if good routine primary care is not provided, a diagnostic marker such as microalbuminemia will not be discovered in the hypertensive patient. Renal disease occurs frequently in HTN, but there is a long-standing dispute among scientists as to whether the renal changes are secondary to HTN or are seen in HTN because the disease itself arises from primary renal abnormalities. The presence of renal complications of HTN is more frequent in African Americans and persons with diabetes. Long-standing HTN itself damages the kidney through several mechanisms, a common one being renal artery stenosis from fibromuscular intimal arteriosclerosis or, in the older patient, atherosclerosis. Renal artery stenosis produces and worsens HTN by many mechanisms, including activation of the RAS. Pharmacologic agents that block the RAS—ACE inhibitors and angiotensin receptor antagonists—seem to be the most effective in treating hypertensive patients with renovascular disease.

The type of early renovascular pathology in HTN is hyaline degenerative nephrosclerosis, which is characterized by sclerotic wall changes in the afferent arteriole produced by the high BPs in these vessels. Nephrosclerosis means "hardening" of the kidney resulting from connective tissue replacement and scarring of the parenchyma. The term usually refers to a disease process that begins in the afferent arteriole but ultimately produces pathologic changes in the glomeruli and the renal interstititium. This process reduces kidney size. Afferent arteriolar nephrosclerosis leads to ischemic damage to the glomerular capillary endothelium, as does high BP itself, which can directly damage the glomeruli. Consequently, mesangial proliferation and collagen synthesis occur, leading to the characteristic "sclerosis" and causing renal insufficiency and renal failure.

Elderly patients may be more at risk for nephrosclerotic damage from HTN because sclerosis of glomeruli occurs as part of natural aging. Compounded with hypertensive nephrosclerosis, the risk of developing renal insufficiency and failure increases with age.

An early sign of renal damage in HTN is the presence of small amounts of albumin in the urine

---

## TABLE 15.2

### The Keith-Wagener-Barker Classification System for Hypertensive Retinopathy

| Degree | Arteriovenous Ratio | Arteriole Focal Spasm | Hemorrhages | Exudates | Papilledema |
|--------|---------------------|-----------------------|-------------|----------|-------------|
| Normal | 3:4 | 1:1 | None | None | None |
| Grade 1 | 1:2 | 1:1 | None | None | None |
| Grade 2 | 1:3 | 2:3 | None | None | None |
| Grade 3 | 1:4 | 1:3 | Present | Present | None |
| Grade 4 | Fine, fibrous cords | Obliteration of distal blood flow | Present | Present | Present |

(microalbuminuria), which may be a later predictor of renal insufficiency and renal failure. Microalbuminuria has been shown to be related to renal vasoconstriction, impaired renal functional reserve abilities, and blunted renal vasodilator responses to ACE inhibitors (Mattei et al., 1997). Other early signs of renal insufficiency include a decrease in the glomerular filtration rate, which is measured with serum creatinine levels and creatinine clearance.

Renal disease, once begun, often progresses inexorably and leads to renal failure. HTN is a major cause of renal failure, and the patient ultimately requires dialysis or transplantation to survive. The cost of renal transplantation is about $12 billion per year (Kobrin & Aradhye, 1997). The nurse practitioner can play an important role in reducing this burden and cost by careful management of the hypertensive patient to prevent the progression and complications of renal failure.

## MALIGNANT HYPERTENSION

Although rarer than in the past, accelerated malignant HTN does occur and is a dangerous, ominous pathophysiologic process. Seen more frequently in African Americans, malignant HTN is the development of high BP values (diastolic greater than 140 mm Hg) over a short period of time, sometimes just a few months, with rapid deterioration of target organs. Characteristic kidney lesions occur, leading to rapid development of renal failure. Acute retinal vascular changes may be observed. LVH and CHF may be present. Although most patients who develop this often-lethal process are diagnosed with HTN, a few will appear in the office in a fulminate hypertensive crisis without having been previously diagnosed. Treatment of preexisting HTN is the most effective way of preventing the occurrence of malignant HTN.

## DEVELOPMENTAL CONSIDERATIONS

### Hypertension in Children and Adolescents

Measurement of BP in infants, children, and adolescents has become a routine part of health care only in the last two decades. It was believed that HTN, particularly essential HTN, was a problem only of adulthood. It is now known that children of hypertensive parents are physiologically different in the ways that they handle a sodium load, respond to stressful stimuli, and in other physiologic parameters. It is also known that the nongenetic roots of essential HTN can be found in health habits and lifestyles that are developed early in life. Finally, on occasion, children and adolescents are found with HTN not caused by any identifiable secondary process, which therefore must be considered essential HTN.

Children's blood pressures must be measured using appropriately sized cuffs. This can be one of the major sources of error in BP measurement in nonpediatrician practices. The use of the fifth Korotkoff sound for the diastolic value is recommended. The BP then is evaluated for the child's age, height, and sex on percentile charts, and, typically, BP tracks in the same percentile throughout childhood and adolescence. Systolic or diastolic BPs between the 90th and 95th percentile are considered high-normal values, and these children may be at higher risk of developing HTN and often are larger, heavier children. Children above the 95th percentile are considered to be hypertensive (National High Blood Pressure Education Program Working Group on Hypertension Control in Children and Adolescents, 1996). After measuring a child within 3 months and continuing to find an elevated BP, the practitioner then must rule out secondary causes such as renal disease, coarctation of the aorta, or diabetes. The true incidence of essential HTN in childhood is unknown, but its frequency is increasing. There are no specific symptoms in children. Key factors in the etiology are family history of HTN and obesity.

### Hypertension in Pregnancy

About 10% of women during their first pregnancy, late in the third trimester, develop preeclampsia, a syndrome characterized by HTN, albuminuria, weight gain, and edema. Hypertensive women who become pregnant continue to have HTN, and some hypertensive women have a superimposed preeclampsia during pregnancy.

The cause of preeclampsia still is unknown, but it appears to be of placental origin and involves endothelial disruption that activates platelets. The HTN may result from increased vascular reactivity. The pathophysiologic processes underlying the symptoms have been well described, with the prominent factor being vasoconstriction. Associated with vasconstriction are vasospasm, ischemia, and fibrin formation, which may further occlude blood vessels. The kidneys, liver, and brain are most susceptible to the effects of preeclampsia, with the onset of eclampsia being diagnosed by the occurrence of a convulsion in the preeclamptic patient. The disease disappears with the termination of the pregnancy, presumably because of removal of the influence of the ischemic placenta.

## Hypertension in the Elderly

Cardiovascular disease is the number one cause of death in the elderly. The elderly may experience the progressive and unremitting damage of HTN for many years, depending on control and compliance, and end-organ damage often is compounded by age-related degeneration. The elderly also have a higher incidence of isolated systolic HTN, especially in those older than 65 years of age. A myth still exists that some degree of HTN is "normal" and even beneficial in the very old. This belief probably arose from the fact that there is excess mortality in elderly people with low BP levels. Low BP, however, may mean something different in an elderly person compared with a younger individual. It may be a sign of malnutrition or chronic disease. In elderly patients with cardiovascular disease, there is a U-shaped curve of cardiovascular mortality with systolic BP. Those with BPs below 120 mm Hg who have preexisting cardiovascular disease may have such poor ejection fractions that they are more at risk for morbid events (Kannel & D'Agostino, 1997). An important clinical question for the primary care provider is related to how low should BP be in the elderly? Postural hypotension may occur as the result of drug therapy and is a concern in terms of perfusion of stenosed coronary arteries or as an etiologic factor in falls in the elderly.

Several research studies support that treatment of both isolated systolic HTN and combined systolic and diastolic HTN in the elderly produce efficacious results, less morbidity, and a longer life. Treatment even in the very elderly (at least until 84 years of age) may prolong life by reducing cardiovascular mortality. Primary care providers should not ignore HTN in the elderly and should treat it in the same manner as with younger patients.

## PHYSIOLOGIC BASIS OF TREATMENT FOR HYPERTENSION

### Lifestyle Modifications

The guidelines for treating HTN put forth by the Sixth Report of the JNC (1997) were used to describe the current approaches to the treatment of HTN. Using these guidelines (see Table 15-1), the primary care provider may prescribe a regimen of lifestyle changes before instituting pharmacologic treatment, particularly in the mild hypertensive patient. The goal of these lifestyle changes is to produce a BP less than 140/90 mm Hg. Even if this BP is not attained, it may reduce the amount of medication needed to control the HTN. Unfortunately, the adherence to a program of modifications in lifestyle usually is difficult and requires diligence and commitment, not only on the part of the practitioner, but also for the patient and the family. Quality of life and general well-being usually improves in patients who make these changes, even if the BP goal is not achieved. The effects of the lifestyle modifications can be additive and could reduce BP levels by 15 to 20 mm Hg or more (Kaplan, 1998). The physiologic rationale for each of these lifestyle modifications is discussed next.

### Weight Loss

Weight loss in the obese hypertensive patient (BMI above 27.8 in men and 27.3 in women) can produce a significant reduction in BP, on the order of a drop of 1 mm Hg for each 1.8 kg of weight loss. Weight loss is known to improve insulin resistance, decrease intracellular calcium, and decrease the cardiovascular and metabolic needs by decreasing body mass. Weight loss also improves dyslipidemia. Therefore, any amount of weight loss is beneficial in HTN. One important phenomenon observed in obese patients is sleep apnea, which affects 2% to 4% of middle-aged adults and can cause resistant diurnal HTN. Some of the signs that a patient may have sleep apnea are obesity, a large neck size (size 17 or higher in men; size 16 or higher in women), daytime sleepiness, and loud snoring. Patients with sleep apnea may have diurnal HTN associated with repetitive stimulation of the SNS. Every time the patient experiences a bout of apnea during the night, it leads to significant respiratory distress, which then causes a SNS arousal, leading to a resistant diurnal HTN.

### Salt Restriction

The patient with HTN is generally advised to reduce dietary sodium to 100 mmol/day (2.4 g of sodium, which is equivalent to 6 g of table salt) (Sixth Report of the JNC, 1997). The normal American diet contains as much as 15 g/day of NaCl. It is not advisable for patients to severely limit sodium (Kaplan, 1998). Sodium reduction must be accomplished by carefully reading labels, since much of the sodium in the diet comes from processed foods. By removing the salt shaker and not adding salt to food during preparation, a low-sodium diet can be achieved. The effects of sodium reduction are most apparent in the elderly and include reduced potassium excretion, which is associated with diuretic use, reduced calcium loss in the urine, and a potential improvement in LVH. Along with sodium reduction, an increase in potassium in the diet is recommended. A high-potassium diet may reduce the dosage needed for HTN control. High-sodium diets tend to be low in potassium. Recommendations of foods high in potassium include green, leafy vegetables, citrus fruits, and bananas. Some epidemiologic evidence exists for a relationship between low dietary calcium and high BP. However, calcium supplementation is not recommended for the reduction of BP, but the perimenopausal woman should add extra calcium to the diet.

An additional, prudent dietary modification that should be suggested for the hypertensive patient is reduction in saturated fats and cholesterol in the diet. This may reduce the risk of atherosclerosis in the patient.

## Smoking Cessation

Smoking is a major risk factor in HTN and cardiovascular disease etiology and progression, and smoking cessation is an important lifestyle adjustment. Every cigarette smoked contains enough nicotine to produce an immediate BP elevation that lasts for 15 to 30 minutes (Kaplan, 1998). The hypertensive patient who smokes is resistant to drug therapy. In short, the use of cigarettes, smokeless tobacco, and cigars must be eliminated in the hypertensive patient. Use of nicotine patches does not appear to produce the same elevation in BP as cigarettes and can be used as an aid to smoking cessation (Sixth Report of the JNC, 1997).

## Alcohol Reduction

Excessive use of alcohol (more than 1 to 2 ounces per day) is another chemical risk factor for HTN. For most individuals, this means two to four alcoholic drinks per day. This amount is greater than that observed to be beneficial to cardiovascular health through an alcohol-induced lowering of blood lipids. Hypertensive patients who drink more than two drinks per day should, therefore, be advised to reduce their consumption, and if sensitive to the pressor effects of alcohol, to drink no more than one alcoholic beverage per day (Kaplan, 1998).

## Stress Management

The pathophysiologic effects of stress have been previously described, and it is logical that removing oneself from stressors might decrease HTN risk. For many people, stress reduction per se is not possible. Rather, they must learn new ways to manage stress and to gain skills in reducing SNS activity. Several techniques to produce SNS relaxation can be advised, such as relaxation exercises, yoga, and biofeedback. There is not, however, a compelling body of evidence showing that stress management techniques produce a significant decrease in BP in HTN. Whereas transitory drops in BP occur with relaxation, a long-term decrease by as much as 20/10 mm Hg with biofeedback has been reported in a small series of patients (Alpert & Rippe, 1996). However, even if long-term BP control is not achievable with relaxation therapies, the well-being and sense of control, as well as potential decreased risk of coronary artery disease through the use of stress management approaches, is significant enough for the practitioner to suggest these techniques for anxious, stressed, hyperreactive, hypertensive patients.

## Exercise

Sedentary individuals have a 1.5 times increased risk of HTN. A program of regular conditioning exercise can, in and of itself, reduce BP in hypertensive patients. Combined with other lifestyle modifications such as weight loss, it can assist the patient in reducing BP to an acceptable level and may reduce the medication needs for patients who eventually will require pharmacotherapy. Mildly hypertensive men who regularly exercise have a significant drop in BP after an exercise session of moderate intensity, and this drop is sustained for up to 13 hours after exercise. Hypertensive patients who are most likely to benefit form a program of regular exercise are sedentary patients who are suspected of having a high level of SNS outflow (Alpert & Rippe, 1996).

The Sixth Report of the JNC (1997) recommends that patients exercise to a level that produces a moderate degree of physical fitness, and suggests 30 to 45 minutes of exercise on most days of the week. Recommended exercise includes brisk walking, but other forms of aerobic activity are acceptable. Before starting the hypertensive patient on an exercise program, a complete health history and physical examination, with particular attention to cardiac health, is required.

## PHARMACOLOGY UPDATE

The physiologic mechanisms by which antihypertensive drugs act are either through the sympathetic nervous system pathways, through renal volume–regulating mechanisms, or through drugs that act on the RAS pathways. The Sixth Report of the JNC (1997) recommends that the first drugs of choice in uncomplicated essential HTN are diuretics and beta blockers. These are the only drugs that have been shown to reduce cardiovascular morbidity and mortality, although many drug trials are in process for the other categories, and definitive answers about long-term efficacy of these drugs are forthcoming. The other drugs available for the treatment of HTN are ACE inhibitors, angiotensin II receptor blockers, alpha blockers, alpha-beta blockers, and calcium antagonists. Table 15-3 describes the physiologic mechanism through which the various categories of drugs work and provides examples of drugs in

## TABLE 15.3

### Physiologic Mechanisms of Various Drugs

| Drug Category | Examples | Mode of Action | When Used |
|---|---|---|---|
| Thiazide diuretics | Chlorothiazide Hydrochlorothiazide | Inhibits $Na^+$ reabsorption at DCT; causes decreased water reabsorption and decreased cardiac output; lowers peripheral resistance (mechanism not known) | Low renin HTN; first-line drug of choice when used in combination with beta blockers for most uncomplicated HTN |
| Loop diuretics | Furosemide Ethacrynic acid | Inhibits $Na^+/K^+/Cl^-$ co-transport in the ascending limb of the loop of Henle; causes decreased water reabsorption and decreased cardiac output | As above; used in patients with renal dysfunction |
| Potassium-sparing agents | Spironolactone | Antagonizes aldosterone; reduces the $K^+$ loss in the urine that is a problem with thiazide and loop diuretics | As above |
| Beta blockers | Atenolol Nadolol Propranol | Acts to block the beta-adrenergic receptors; reduces cardiac output; reduces renin | Used in combination with a diuretic as first-line drug in uncomplicated HTN; particularly effective for high-renin HTN |
| ACE inhibitors | Benezapril Captopril Cilizapril | Reduces level of angiotensin II and thus remove a major vasoconstrictive stimulus; reduces aldosterone levels | First-line drug for diabetics with proteinuria and hypertensive patients with heart failure; used if diuretics and beta blockers not effective; may be less effective in African Americans |
| Angiotensin II receptor blockers | Losartin Valsartin | Removes angiotensin II from its receptor, causing vasodilation and drop in peripheral resistance | Primarily used in patients who do not tolerate ACE inhibitors |
| Alpha blockers | Prazosin Terazosin | Blocks the postsynaptic $alpha_1$ receptors on vascular smooth muscle | Useful in patients with benign prostatic hypertrophy (relaxes tone of prostate); also used in pheochromocytoma |
| Calcium channel blockers (also known as calcium antagonists) | Nifedipine Verapamil | Blocks calcium current in L channels of coronary and peripheral vessels; causes vasodilation | Used in systolic HTN in elderly; used if diuretics and beta blockers not effective |

ACE, angiotensin-converting enzyme; $Cl^-$, chloride; DCT, distal convoluted tubule; HTN, hypertension; $K^+$, potassium; $Na^+$, sodium.

each category, as well as general information about the kinds of patients for whom each category of drug is useful. Practitioners should not use this chart as a guideline for prescribing, since it is not detailed enough. They are advised to carefully review the prescribing guidelines in the Sixth Report of the JNC (1997). This report can be ordered on the World Wide Web at *http://www.intlmedpub.com*. An algorithm for drug prescriptions for hypertensive patients based on the Sixth Report of the JNC is available in Roffman (1998) or in Alpert and Rippe (1996).

---

### ● Case Study 15.1

The following case study exemplifies the pathophysiologic processes in the "silent killer," essential HTN. It illustrates how important it is for the nurse practitioner to review history and clinical data when it is available. It is a good teaching case because the patient is young and appears healthy, and a higher than normal blood pressure might easily be dismissed as a "fluke" finding by a health care provider who does not follow the standard diagnostic protocol.

A 30-year-old African-American man, Mr. Jason Nance, is examined for an insurance physical. He recently changed jobs, and his new employer requires the physical examination. He also states that he has significant financial problems, and he hopes that "you don't find anything wrong because his new job will have a large salary increase associated with it."

#### History

##### Past Medical History

| | |
|---|---|
| Allergies | NKDA |
| Current medications | Frequently takes Tylenol for AM headache; no prescription medications |
| Surgeries | Had fractured leg—surgically pinned at age 12 |
| Injury/Trauma | Had three MVAs between ages 16 and 19; had "concussions," bruises, "nothing serious" |
| Childhood illness | Doesn't know for sure; thinks had immunizations; was never sick as a child |

##### Social History

| | |
|---|---|
| Unmarried | Dates "a lot"; sexually active and uses condoms |
| Tobacco | 2 ppd × 15 years |
| Alcohol | Drinks hard alcohol when he goes out to "party," otherwise has 2 or 3 beers after work at home |
| Social drugs | Admits to drug abuse as teenager. Used marijuana, LSD, cocaine. Was admitted into drug rehab twice. States that he does not use drugs now |
| Caffeine | Has 4 or 5 cups of coffee every morning |
| Exercise | Started jogging recently but gave it up. States he is "too out of shape" |
| Employment | Employed at the computer help desk of a large electronics company. States that his job is extremely stressful, that he works 40 hours a week in his regular employment, and then moonlights 20 to 30 hours a week as a computer service technician. States that he sleeps poorly; awakens frequently |

*(Case study continued on page 304)*

### Family History

| | |
|---|---|
| Mother | 50 years, obese, HTN |
| Father | Deceased of a stroke at age 40 |
| Brother | 25 years old; no health problems |

### 24-Hour Dietary Recall

Breakfast: 3 cups coffee
Lunch: Fast food "Big Burger," fries, shake
Dinner: Chinese buffet at local restaurant, beer
Snack: Donut, candy bar

## Review of Systems

| | |
|---|---|
| General | Weight has been stable since early 20s; no health complaints |
| Skin | No rashes; has dry skin |
| HEENT | Wears glasses and thinks he needs new Rx. Gets blurry vision when he has been working on computer. Gets frequent AM headaches. Denies nosebleeds, dizziness, sore throats |
| Lungs | Has noticed SOB on stair climbing; attributes this to being out of shape. No asthma, bronchitis, pneumonia |
| CV | Has noticed palpitations, especially at work; attributes these to smoking and stress. No chest pain; no prior ECG |
| GI | No N&V; no diarrhea, constipation |
| GU | No dysuria, urgency. No increase in urination Has not had any STDs |
| MS | Denies joint pain, or swelling. States he has underdeveloped leg muscles because he doesn't exercise |
| Neurologic | Denies numbness, tingling, fainting, seizures, weakness |

## Physical Examination

| System | Findings |
|---|---|
| Vital signs | T–98.4°F, P–76, R–16, BP 184/112 Height 6'1", Weight 195 lb |
| General | Alert, friendly, fully oriented. Thin extremities, truncal adiposity, round face; skin warm and dry |
| HEENT | Normocephalic, neck size 17". Cranial nerves intact; TMs intact. Rinne and Weber negative; Hearing normal. Throat negative. No adenopathy; thyroid not palpable; no carotid bruits. Funduscopic exam indicates mild papilledema, multiple cotton-wool spots. A-V nicking in both eyes. Greater in OD |
| Lungs | Clear to auscultation and percussion bilaterally |
| Cardiac | Heart rate irregular. No murmurs. Cardiac borders indicate possible enlarged heart by percussion |
| Abdomen | Soft, nontender, no masses. BS in all 4 quadrants; No CVA tenderness |

*(Case study continued on next page)*

| | |
|---|---|
| GU | Circumcised. No lesions, discharge. Testicles descended bilaterally. No hernias |
| Rectal | Deferred at patient's request |
| Extremities | Pedal pulses absent. Femoral pulses 1+. Radial, brachial pulses 3+. Grip strength good |
| Neurologic | DTRs 3+ in upper and lower extremities. Romberg negative. Sensations intact |

## Laboratory Results

| Test | Result |
|---|---|
| CBC | WNL |
| Chem | BUN 12, creatinine 1.2, total cholesterol 270, triglycerides 200, FBS 115, sodium 144 mEq/L, potassium 3.6 mEq/L |
| Urine | Mod amount sediment, yellow, neg glucose, neg ketones, albumin 1+; pH 5.2 |
| Baseline ECG | Left axis deviation −15 degrees; R wave in limb lead 21 mm |

## Impression

Hypertension, RO secondary causes
RO renal disease
RO coarctation of the aorta
RO Cushing's disease
RO sleep apnea

## Discussion

The decision algorithm for diagnosing HTN is based on three consecutive readings of blood pressure greater than 150/90. This patient has evidence of end-organ damage and stage 3 HTN by initial evaluation. His hypertensive state should be verified by repeated measurements, but the possibility of cardiac, renal, and retinal diseases by physical examination requires immediate work-up of his condition to rule out secondary causes of his HTN.

Renal causes are suspected by the abnormal urinalysis results. Sedimentation and albumin are abnormal and may indicate parenchymal or glomerular disease. Because of his history of traumatic injuries during adolescence, the possibility of parenchymal damage also should be considered, although this is a remote possibility. Microalbuminemia is an early sign of nephrosclerosis. The patient has a normal BUN and creatinine, however. This could, therefore, be functional proteinuria that is transitory, and the nurse practitioner would need repeat urinalysis to confirm. Mr. Nance's creatinine is at the upper limit of normal. It would be important to determine if an earlier creatinine level had been obtained. Mr. Nance has hospital records that could be reviewed. If his creatinine has doubled or tripled in the last few years, even while remaining in the normal range, the nurse practitioner would note this as evidence of potential renal disease.

Coarctation of the aorta needs to be ruled out in this patient for several reasons. He is young, has very high blood pressure, and already has evidence of significant LVH. He also has poorly developed lower limb musculature, absent pedal pulses, and weak femoral pulses. These signs also may indicate PVD. It is important in all young hypertensive patients to take blood pressures in both arms, and in Mr. Nance's case to

*(Case study continued on page 306)*

measure leg blood pressure, which would be reduced by coarctation. A chest x-ray would further aid diagnosis.

Cushing's disease or syndrome needs to be evaluated for this patient because of his round face and truncal obesity, thin limbs, and HTN. Potassium level in this patient is normal, however, and hypokalemia would be present in Cushing's disease. The use of the dexamethasone suppression test to rule out Cushing's disease would be necessary.

Sleep apnea should be suspected as a possible cause of HTN in this patient because of his neck size, his poor sleep performance, and daytime sleepiness. This can be ruled out only by sleep studies.

One important aspect of his history should not be ignored: he admits to drug abuse but denies drug use now. However, HTN in potential drug abusers is common, and drug use should be ruled out by a toxicology screen.

After extensive testing to rule out the above possible secondary causes of HTN, Mr. Nance is diagnosed with essential HTN. There are abundant risk factors for essential HTN in his history and results of physical examination. He is an African-American man with a family history that is suspicious for HTN. He has a poor diet, high in sodium; smokes cigarettes; doesn't exercise; works in a high-stress job; and is experiencing financial and, possibly, personal stress. He abused drugs as an adolescent. He drinks more alcohol than generally is recommended.

The patient's ECG and physical exam suggest LVH. Posterolateral and anterior chest films and echocardiocardiography can determine the extent of LVH. His history of shortness of breath and palpitations may be ominous signs. He also has significant retinal disease, which may account for his blurred vision and headaches. His FBS is above the limits of normal and may indicate a metabolic state of hyperinsulinemia and hyperglycemia. He may be prediabetic.

This patient needs referral to cardiologist and an ophthalmologist for his significant end-organ disease, a program of lifestyle modification, and immediate pharmacotherapy to reduce his blood pressure and reduce the arteriosclerotic damage to his vital organs.

BP, blood pressure; BS, bowel sounds; BUN, blood urea nitrogen; Chem, chemistries; CVA, cerebrovascular accident; DTRs, deep-tendon reflexes; ECG, electrocardiogram; exam, examination; FBS, fasting blood sugar; GI, gastrointestinal; GU, genitourinary; HEENT, head, eyes, ears, nose, and throat; HTN, hypertension; LVH, left ventricular hypertrophy; MVA, motor vehicle accident; NKDA, no known drug allergies; N&V, nausea and vomiting; P, pulse; PVD, peripheral vascular disease; R, respiration; RO, rule out; Rx, prescription; SOB, shortness of breath; STDs, sexually transmitted diseases; T, temperature; WNL, within normal limits.

## REFERENCES

Alpert, J. & Rippe, J. (1996). Manual of cardiovascular diagnosis and therapy (4th ed). In *MAXX: Maximum access to diagnosis and therapy: The electronic library of medicine* (updated August 1997) [CD-ROM]. Philadelphia: Lippincott-Raven Publishers.

Cardillo, C. & Panza, J. (1998). Impaired endothelial regulation of vascular tone in patients with systemic arterial hypertension. *Vascular Medicine, 3* (2), 138–144.

Cooper, R. & Borke, J. (1993). Intracellular ions and hypertension in blacks. In J. Fray & J. Douglas (Eds.), *Pathophysiology of hypertension in blacks*. New York: Oxford University Press.

Falkner, B. (1993). Characteristics of prehypertension in black children. In J. Fray & J. Douglas (Eds.), *Pathophysiology of hypertension in blacks*. New York: Oxford University Press.

Fray, J. & Douglas, J. (Eds.). (1993). *Pathophysiology of hypertension in blacks.* New York: Oxford University Press.

Galletti, F., Strazzullo, P., Ferrara, I., Annuzzi, G., Rivellese, A.A., Gatto, S., & Mancini, M. (1997). NaCl sensitivity of essential hypertensive patients is related to insulin resistance. *Journal of Hypertension, 15* (12 Pt 1), 1485–1491.

Gerdts, E., Lund-Johansen, P., & Omvik, P. (1998). Factors influencing left ventricular mass in salt sensitive and salt resistant essential hypertensive patients. *Blood Pressure, 7* (4), 223–230.

Grim, C. & Wilson, T. (1993). Salt, slavery, and survival: Physiological principles underlying the evolutionary hypothesis of salt-sensitive hypertension in western hemisphere blacks. In J. Fray & J. Douglas (Eds.), *Pathophysiology of hypertension in blacks*. New York: Oxford University Press.

Harrap, S.B. (1996). An appraisal of the genetic approaches to high blood pressure. *Journal of Hypertension, 14* (Suppl. 5), S111–S115.

Kannel, W. & D'Agostino, R. (1997). Blood pressure and cardiovascular morbidity and mortality rates in the elderly. *American Heart Journal, 134* (4), 758–763.

Kaplan, N. (1998). *Clinical hypertension* (7th ed.). Baltimore: Williams & Wilkins.

Khattar, R., Senior, R., & Lahiri, A. (1998). Cardiovascular outcome in white-coat versus sustained mild hypertension: A 10-year follow-up study. *Circulation, 3* (18), 1892–1897.

Kobrin, S. & Aradhye, S. (1997). Preventing progression and complications of renal disease. *Hospital Medicine, 33* (11), 11–40.

Koga, M., Sasaguri, M., Miura, S., Tashiro, E., Kinoshita, A., Ideishi, M., & Arakawa, K. (1998). Plasma renin activity could be a useful predictor of left ventricular hypertrophy in essential hypertensives. *Journal of Human Hypertension, 12* (7), 455–461.

Kuch, B., Muschol, M., Luchner, A., Doring, A., Riegger, G.A., Schunkert, H., & Hense, H.W. (1998). Gender specific differences in left ventricular adaptation to obesity and hypertension. *Journal of Human Hypertension, 12* (10), 685–691.

Kurtz, T.W. & Spence, M.A. (1993). Genetics of essential hypertension. *American Journal of Medicine, 94* (1), 77–84.

Lathrop, G.M. & Soubrier, F. (1994). Genetic basis of hypertension. *Current Opinions in Nephrology and Hypertension, 3* (2), 200–206.

Law, C.M. & Shiell, A.W. (1996). Is blood pressure inversely related to body weight? The strength of evidence from a systemic review of the literature. *Journal of Hypertension, 14*, 935–941.

Lembo, G., Vecchione, C., Iaccarino, G., & Trimarco, B. (1996). The crosstalk between insulin and the sympathetic nervous system: Possible implications in the pathogenesis of essential hypertension. *Blood Pressure, 5* (Suppl. 1), 38–42.

Mattei, P., Arzilli, F., Giovannetti, R., Penno, G., Arrighi, P., Taddei, S., & Salvetti, A. (1997). Microalbuminemia and renal haemodynamics in essential hypertension. *European Journal of Clinical Investigation, 27*, 755–760.

McCarthy, R. (1997). The pharmacologic treatment of hypertension: An update. *Drug Benefit Trends, 9* (9), 71–77.

Morimoto, A., Uzu, T., Fujii, T., Nishimura, M., Kuroda, S., Nakamura, S., Inenaga, T., & Kimura, G. (1997). Sodium, sensitivity and cardiovascular events in patients with essential hypertension. *The Lancet, 350*, 1734–1737.

Mufunda, J. & Sparks, H.V. (1993). Salt sensitivity and hypertension in African blacks. In J. Fray & J. Douglas (Eds.), *Pathophysiology of hypertension in blacks*. New York: Oxford University Press.

Muller-Wieland, D., Kotzka, J., Knebel, B., & Krone, W. (1998). Metabolic syndrome and hypertension: Pathophysiology and molecular basis of insulin resistance. *Basic Research in Cardiology, 93* (Suppl. 2), 131–141.

National High Blood Pressure Education Program Working Group on Hypertension Control in Children and Adoles-

cents. (1987). Update on the task force report on high blood pressure in children and adolescents: A working group report from the National High Blood Pressure Education Program (1996). *Pediatrics, 9*, 649–658.

Nordby, G., Ekeberg, O, Knardahl, S., & Os, I. (1995). A double-blind study of psychosocial factors in 40-year old women with essential hypertension. *Psychotherapy and Psychosomatics, 63*, 142–150.

Nyirenda, M. & Seckl, J. (1998). Intrauterine events and the programming of adulthood disease: The role of fetal glucocorticoid exposure. *International Journal of Molecular Medicine, 2* (5), 607–614.

O'Byrne, S. & Caulfield, M. (1998). Genetics of hypertension: Therapeutic implications. *Drugs, 56* (2), 203–214.

Okosun, I.S., Cooper, R.S., Rotimi, C.N., Osotimehin, B., & Forrester, T. (1998). Association of waist circumference with risk of hypertension and type 2 diabetes in Nigerians, Jamaicans, and African-Americans. *Diabetes Care, 21* (11), 1836–1842.

Oparil, S. & Calhoun, D. (1998). Managing the patient with hard-to-control hypertension. *American Family Physician, 57* (5), 1007–1022.

Owens, P.E., Lyons, S.P., Rodriguez, S.A., & O'Brien, E.T. (1998). Is elevation of clinic blood pressure in patients with white coat hypertension who have normal ambulatory blood pressure associated with target organ changes? *Journal of Human Hypertension, 12* (11), 743–748.

Roffman, D. (1998). Angiotensin II receptor antagonists: Improving selectivity in the management of hypertension. *U.S. Pharmacist, 23* (2), 131–140.

Schlaich, M.P. & Schmieder, R. (1998). Left ventricular hypertrophy and its regression: Pathophysiology and therapeutic approach. Focus on treatment by antihypertensive agents. *American Journal of Hypertension, 11* (11 Pt 1), 1394–1404.

Shapiro, A. (1996). *Hypertension and stress: A unified concept*. Mawah, New Jersey: Lawrence Erlbaum.

The Sixth Report of the Joint National Committee on Prevention, Detection, Evaluation and Treatment of High Blood Pressure. (1997). *Archives of Internal Medicine, 157*, 2413–2446.

Sowers, J.R., Standley, P.R., Ram, J.L., Jacober, S., Simpson, L., & Rose, K. (1993). Hyperinsulinemia, insulin resistance, and hyperglycemia: Contributing factors in the pathogenesis of hypertension and atherosclerosis. *American Journal of Hypertension, 6* (7 Pt 2), 260S–270S.

Suter P.M., Locher, R., Hasler, E., & Vetter, W. (1998). Is there a role for the ob gene product leptin in essential hypertension? *American Journal of Hypertension, 11* (11 Pt 1), 1305–1311.

Taylor, W.R. (1998). Mechanical deformation of the arterial wall in hypertension: A mechanism for vascular pathology. *American Journal of Medical Science, 316* (3), 156–161.

Timio, M. (1997). Blood pressure trend and psychosocial factors: The case of the nuns in a secluded order. *Acta Physiologica Scandinavica Suppl, 640*, 137–139.

# Gastrointestinal and Hepatic Disorders

Maria Cabrera

Maureen Groer

The range of gastrointestinal (GI) and hepatic disorders seen in primary care practice is wide. Common infectious problems include gastroenteritis and hepatitis. Inflammatory disorders include gastroesophageal reflux disorder (GERD), gastritis, peptic ulcer disease (PUD), and irritable bowel syndrome (IBS). Cancers include cancer of the colon. This chapter covers the pathophysiology of major GI and hepatic problems routinely encountered by the primary care provider. Readers are referred to textbooks of medicine for more detailed discussions of less common disorders.

## GASTROENTERITIS

Acute gastroenteritis is one of the most common infectious illnesses treated by the primary care practitioner. These illnesses are particularly common during childhood, are infectious, and can spread rapidly through a community such as a day care center or nursery. Diarrheal illness is the number one infection worldwide, and in developing countries, it is the leading cause of childhood mortality. The incidence of gastroenteritis in the United States is lower, but there are more than 23 million cases per year, accounting for great cost and lost productivity.

The primary organisms responsible for most gastroenteritis in the United States are viruses and bacteria. Viruses account for up to 40% of diarrhea in this country and usually are spread through the fecal-oral route. The etiology of bacterial gastroenteritis often is through food ingestion. Organisms cause gastroenteritis through different pathophysiologic mechanisms, and the body has many host defenses that protect against invasion and infection by dangerous microbes. The three major

viruses causing gastroenteritis are the rotaviruses (groups A, B, and C), enteric adenovirus, and the Norwalk virus. The most common bacterial origin is *Campylobacter jejuni*, which is found in unwashed or poorly cooked chicken and other meats, causing over 2 million cases per year. Table 16-1 indicates the most common microorganisms causing acute gastroenteritis, the route of infection, and the symptoms.

## Pathophysiologic Processes in Gastroenteritis

The host's physiologic responses to microorganisms that cause gastroenteritis depend on factors such as age, prior exposure, immune status, and nutritional status. Virulence and dose of the invading microbe also is an important influence on the pathophysiologic outcome. Many microbes are destroyed in the stomach because of the hydrolytic action of gastric acidity. Microbes that pass through into the small intestine then must compete with the normal flora. The normal flora is the well-established colonization of the gut by organisms that compete with pathogens for nutrients needed for growth; they also secrete short chain fatty acids, which inhibit pathogen growth. Also, much of the secretory IgA in the gut lumen specifically binds to microbial antigens. Bacteria may not need to be ingested or to grow in the intestinal tract to produce pathophysiologic effects. Bacteria produce their damaging effects by secreting enterotoxins, which can be present in contaminated food. So, even if bacteria are destroyed in the stomach, their toxins may not be destroyed, and they then can act on the intestines to cause diarrheal disease. The most common enterotoxin-producing organ-

**TABLE 16.1**

**Microorganisms Causing Acute Gastroenteritis**

| | *Vibrio cholerae, Escherichia coli, Shigella (early), Giardia* | *Shigella, Salmonella, Campylobacter, Entamoeba histolytica* | **Viruses (Rotavirus, Norwalk) or Toxins** (*Staphylococcus aureus, Bacillus cereus*) |
|---|---|---|---|
| Symptoms | Few large-volume stools | Many small-volume stools, tenesmus, fecal urgency | Frequent vomiting and diarrhea, gastroenteritis |
| Site of infection | Small bowel | Large bowel and colon | Small bowel |

(Adapted from Bandres, J. & Dupont, H. [1992]. Approach to the patient with diarrhea. In S. Gorbach, J. Bartlett, & N. Blacklow [Eds.], *Infectious diseases.* Philadelphia: W. B. Saunders.)

ism is the *Staphylococcus*, which causes outbreaks of food poisoning characterized by explosive, watery diarrhea and abdominal cramps. This organism grows well in unrefrigerated food containing mayonnaise and has no odor or taste.

For bacteria to grow and metabolize, they must be able to latch onto the intestinal epithelium, since the normal peristaltic waves and secretions of the gut would flush them through the tract. Some bacteria have pili that bind to specific receptors on intestinal mucosa; they then act locally by secreting their enterotoxins (eg, enterotoxigenic *Escherichia coli*). Other microorganisms attach to and invade intestinal mucosal cells, causing an inflammatory response and cell death (eg, *Shigella*) (Reese & Hruska, 1996). The enterotoxins produced by some pathogenic bacteria act on intracellular processes to increase secretion of fluids and electrolytes into the lumen of the gut. Cholera toxin stimulates adenylate cyclase, which increases cyclic adenosine monophosphate (cAMP). The net effect of increased amounts of intracellular cAMP is large increases in secretion over reabsorption through the intestinal epithelium. The volume of water lost in cholera can be so

great over a short period that it can cause massive hypovolemia and death if fluids and electrolytes are not replaced. *C. jejuni* causes bloody diarrhea because its enterotoxins produce ulcerative lesions, particularly in the colon.

Viruses, on the other hand, always invade cells to produce their pathogenic effects. The most common type of enteric viruses is the RNA rotaviruses, which produce severe diarrheal gastroenteritis in children, usually those younger than 3 years. Rotavirus preferentially infects cells at the tip of the intestinal villi, often killing these cells, thus shrinking the size and disrupting the structural integrity of the villi (Fig. 16-1). Infection with this virus decreases production of digestive enzymes by the intestinal microvilli so that food molecules are not completely digested and thus are osmotically active. A net increase in intestinal secretion occurs, which produces watery diarrhea in infected individuals. Fever, vomiting, and abdominal cramps often accompany this infection (Eastwood, 1997). Enteric adenoviruses also cause diarrheal illness, primarily in children.

The most important etiology of viral gastroenteritis in adults is the Norwalk virus. This also is a

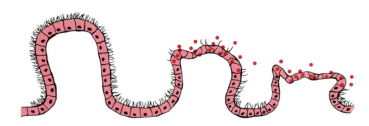

**FIGURE 16.1** ● Villi are disrupted, flattened, and lose cilia due to rotavirus infection.

RNA virus that commonly occurs in epidemic-like patterns, causing infection within contained communities (eg, cruise ships). It is spread in contaminated foods. The virus infects the small intestine, particularly the jejunum, and acts like the rotavirus on villus architecture, decreasing microvilli enzymes as well. Again, this leads to both osmotic diarrhea and a net increased secretion of water and electrolytes into the gut. This type of viral infection spreads among children and adults of all ages.

It is important that the health care provider knows that diarrheal disease is not always caused by infectious gastroenteritis. In elderly patients, laxative abuse is a common etiology, as are other conditions that frequently occur in this population such as diverticular disease, fecal impaction, carcinoma, and diabetic neuropathy (MacLennan et al., 1994). In all patients with symptoms of gastroenteritis, the medical history is the key to diagnosing the etiology and often provides enough clues to determine which organism is causing the symptoms (Reese & Hruska, 1996). Risk factors that should be determined in the history include recent trips, especially international travel (to assess for traveler's diarrhea); use of water from mountain streams when camping; infants and family members in day care centers; elders in chronic care facilities; HIV-positive status; exposure to other sick individuals; exposure to a common source that has caused illness in others (eg, a picnic);

medications (use of antibiotics within the last 6 weeks); exposure to a household pet (especially iguanas and turtles); and recent ingestion of seafood or shellfish (Reese & Hruska, 1996).

## GASTROESOPHAGEAL REFLUX DISEASE

Gastroesophageal reflux disorder is a common illness in the United States. Its major symptom is heartburn—a symptom experienced by many adults. Heartburn is a commonly ignored problem. This lack of concern is encouraged by television advertisements for antacid products advocating self-medication. Because people usually self-medicate for heartburn, the provider may only incidentally discover the presence of the symptom. However, if the heartburn episodes represent GERD, there is often a chronic problem; inflammatory and mucosal changes may lead to stricture, squamous epithelial metaplasia, and Barrett's carcinoma, a malignancy directly related to GERD. Once GERD is established, it is difficult to eradicate completely, and patients frequently have recurrences when they stop treatment.

Gastroesophageal reflux disorder is a condition in which gastric contents reflux through the lower esophageal sphincter (LES) and erode the esophageal squamous epithelium, causing inflammatory and ulcerative lesions. Also, once reflux

---

### CLINICAL VIGNETTE 16.1

Ms. Jennifer Greene is a 22-year-old graduate student who is brought to the clinic by her husband after being up all night with diarrhea and vomiting. Her history is unremarkable except that she attended a church picnic the afternoon before, and within 4 hours after eating potato salad, she vomited profusely. Explosive liquid diarrhea began within 6 hours and was accompanied by intense abdominal cramping. She vomited only once and then began having diarrhea, which she cannot estimate how many times she had. She describes lying on the bathroom floor all night because she was afraid to leave. The stools are green and liquid. She reports less cramping now, 15 hours after the ingestion. Her vital signs are within normal limits, and results of her physical examination are unremarkable except for dry mouth and thirst, increased

bowel sounds, and slight tenderness to abdominal palpation. She has been unable to drink or eat since the day before.

Her history and physical examination suggest food poisoning with preformed enterotoxins because she developed symptoms so rapidly, with vomiting within 4 hours and diarrhea quickly following. It is important to determine if others at the picnic also were ill during the night, since it is unlikely that only a single case of food poisoning occurred. The likely cause of the gastroenteritis is *Staphylococcus aureus,* which produces a heat-stable enterotoxin. She needs to be rehydrated and observed for resolution of her diarrhea, which should occur within a day after the ingestion. Since the enterotoxin is being expelled through the diarrheal stools, she should be encouraged to drink fluids and rest, and should expect to feel better within the day.

has occurred, patients with GERD seem less able to clear refluxed stomach contents from the esophagus (Lieberman, 1997). Whereas most persons, including infants and children, have occasional and even daily reflux, the patient with GERD has more frequent and longer reflux episodes, and thus longer periods of exposure of esophageal mucosa to gastric juice.

The pathophysiologic basis of GERD is related to incompetence of the LES. The LES normally is in a tightly contracted state, except when esophageal peristatic waves travel over it during swallowing, causing relaxation of the sphincter and entry of the food bolus into the stomach. Therefore, it is the major antireflux barrier between the stomach and esophagus. Three potential alterations in the LES cause reflux and GERD. The sphincter itself may be in a less contracted state than normal, and thus more likely to permit acid to reflux back from the stomach as intragastric pressure exceeds esophageal pressure. The sphincter also may relax too frequently and inappropriately. Finally, the sphincter's natural contraction pressure may be overcome by increased intraabdominal pressure brought about by abdominal straining. Once reflux has produced inflammatory damage to the mucosa, depending on the depth of damage to the esophageal luminal wall, the natural resolution of the damage may lead to healing with some degree of fibrosis. Unfortunately, the fibrosis interferes with the ability of the LES to contract normally, and a vicious cycle of incompetence, reflux, inflammation, ulceration, scarring, and further LES incompetence occurs.

The classic symptom of midepigastric, retrosternal burning pain, occurring frequently after a meal and at night, which radiates into the chest (ie, what people refer to as "heartburn") often is accompanied by the taste of acid in the throat. Other signs and symptoms, such as chronic hoarseness and asthma-like symptoms, frequent throat clearing, hiccoughs, dysphagia, and chest pain, may accompany GERD.

Many contributing factors are involved in GERD. Foods often are blamed for episodes of heartburn (chocolate, peppermint, onions, citrus fruits, fats, and caffeine), and alcohol ingestion, exercise, and smoking exacerbate GERD. Several medications also may increase the symptoms (nitrates, oral contraceptives, anticholinergic agents, theophylline) (Lieberman, 1997). In some cases, these factors reduce LES pressure or increase gastric acid secretion. A recent epidemiologic study found that a body mass index greater than 30 kg/m$^2$, having another family member

with heartburn or esophageal or stomach disease, a history of smoking, drinking more than seven alcoholic drinks per week, and many psychosomatic symptoms are associated with symptoms of GERD (Locke et al., 1999). In some patients, GERD seems to be associated with IBS and bronchial hyperresponsiveness. In children with GERD, the symptom may be a chronic cough, which can be misdiagnosed as asthma.

Preventing the long-term sequelae of GERD is a goal of treatment. Esophagitis leading to dysphagia seriously interferes with nutrition and quality of life. Hemorrhagic esophagitis is rare, but it does occur and can lead to perforation. Strictures in the lower esophagus obstruct the passage of food into the stomach and must be surgically treated. Finally, Barrett's esophagus is the presence of a metaplastic conversion of the normal squamous epithelium to columnar cells. These cells are more resistant to acid, and when this process has occurred, the symptoms of GERD may abate. This may presage the development of dysplasia and finally anaplasia, with the highly malignant Barrett's carcinoma being the result.

### Physiologic Basis of Treatment

The physiologic basis of treatment is related to measures that act on LES pressure, gastric acid production, or gravitational influences on reflux. Weight loss, smoking and alcohol cessation, avoidance of foods that aggravate the symptoms, and sleeping in an upright position will all help reduce symptoms. H$_2$ antagonists will resolve symptoms in up to 70%, and proton pump inhibitors in nearly all patients. Agents that increase esophageal motility such as cisapride may also be useful (Williams, 1998). This is a disease that frequently recurs once the above measures are stopped, and the practitioner should consider this in patient management.

### GASTRITIS AND PEPTIC ULCER DISEASE

Chronic superficial gastritis and PUD are the results of chronic inflammatory processes in the stomach and the duodenum. The inflammatory process may lead to the formation of gastric or duodenal ulcers when an imbalance occurs between aggressive and defensive factors of the gastric mucosal layer. A major contributing factor involved in the pathogenesis and management of gastritis and PUD is infection with the *Helicobacter pylori* organism (Fig. 16-2).

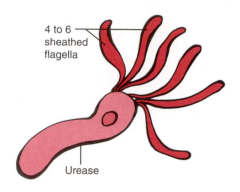

4 to 6
sheathed
flagella

Urease

**FIGURE 16.2** ● *H. pylori* is Gram negative
and spiral shaped.

## Epidemiology

The National Institutes of Health (NIH) published
a report in 1994 stating that 10 of 100 persons in
the United States will experience PUD in their lifetime (NIH, 1994). The NIH also reports that more
than 7000 individuals die of ulcer-related complications each year in the US. It is estimated that half
of the US population is infected with *H. pylori*, the
bacteria responsible for most PUD cases. Most
peptic ulcers are duodenal in the US, but the rate
of gastric ulcers is rising in the 55- to 65-year age
group (Everhart et al., 1998).

The incidence of PUD is highest in the elderly
population, particularly those 75 years of age or
older (Everhart et al., 1998). This probably is the
result of the increased use of nonsteroidal anti-
inflammatory drugs (NSAIDs) in the elderly population to alleviate chronic arthritic pain (Griffin,
1998), although NSAID use has not been associated with an increased risk for infection with *H.
pylori* (Malfertheiner & Labenz, 1998). The type of
gastritis (chemical gastropathy) produced by the
use of NSAIDs consists of petechiae, mucosal erythema, and hemorrhages, with 20% of the patients
presenting with frank ulceration, but the endoscopic appearance of the mucosa does not necessarily correlate with symptoms and is not significantly different from gastritis induced by *H. pylori*
infection (Aabakken, 1999). Gastritis from the use
of NSAIDs is treated by discontinuing the NSAIDs
and sometimes substituting another medication.

The prevalence of *H. pylori* infection has been
associated with low socioeconomic status (Malfertheiner & Labenz, 1998). Children in the US have
a low incidence of *H. pylori* infection compared
with underdeveloped countries. Although *H.
pylori* infection affects all socioeconomic levels, a
higher prevalence of ulcers in the US is related to

low educational levels, yearly household incomes
of less than $20,000, and crowded living condi-
tions. Blacks, Hispanics, and Asians have a higher
incidence of PUD and gastric cancer compared
with whites (Blecker, 1997).

The exact mode of transmission of *H. pylori* is
unknown. *H. pylori* is believed to be transmitted
through the oral-fecal route (Malfertheiner &
Labenz, 1998). A 1994 study reveals that *H. pylori*
also is present in the gut of common household
cats, which suggests that domestic animals may
transmit the disease to humans.

## Risk Factors

The pathogenesis of PUD is believed to involve
multiple risk factors, and many myths abound.
Common risk factors thought to be associated with
the disease are stress, diet, smoking, alcohol, a
positive family history, and use of NSAIDs. The
role of stress in ulcerogenesis still is controversial.
An increase in gastric acid secretion and ulcer formation, producing stress ulcers, is a common finding in patients exposed to high levels of physical
stress from trauma or surgery (Sleisenger & Fordtran, 1997). Psychological stress, on the other
hand, may not be an important risk factor for PUD
(Raeihae et al., 1998).

Another myth is that spicy foods cause ulcers,
but this has been disproved (Rosenstock et al.,
1997). However, food has the potential to neutralize or increase the acid content of the stomach. For
example, milk, often used as an ulcer remedy in
the past, can aggravate ulcers by stimulating stomach acid secretion, thus increasing ulcer pain.
Alcohol use predisposes a person to PUD. Alcohol
causes an increase in gastric acid secretion, which
damages the gastric mucosa and increases the risk
of ulcerogenesis (Raeihae et al., 1998). Caffeine
consumption does not cause PUD, but it is a GI
stimulant. Caffeine increases gastric motility,
which may aggravate a preexisting ulcer.

Smoking is a major risk factor in the development of PUD (Eastwood, 1997). Smoking suppresses the protective mechanism of the gastric
mucosa and potentiates the harmful effects of
aggressive factors such as *H. pylori*. In addition,
smoking increases the time needed to heal ulcers
by enhancing the effects of *H. pylori* infection
(Svanes et al., 1997) and inhibiting the $H_2$ antagonist medications. Recurrent ulcers also are more
likely to occur in smokers.

Using NSAIDs increases the risk of developing
gastritis and PUD, especially gastric ulcers, as well as
the risk of developing the complications of bleeding
and perforation. NSAIDs block the synthesis of

prostaglandins by nonselectively inhibiting the cyclo-oxygenase enzymes (COX-1 and COX-2). Prostaglandins normally participate in the daily repair of the gastric epithelium. Decreased prostaglandins cause decreased protection of the gastric mucosal and therefore an increase in gastritis (Yeomans, 1998).

A family history of PUD is a risk factor for developing PUD. A study conducted in Germany demonstrates that having both a *H. pylori* infection and a positive family history of PUD is associated with an increased risk of developing PUD (Brenner et al., 1998). Therefore, both genetic factors and environment play a role in PUD.

## Pathophysiology

Peptic ulcer disease is a multifactorial disease involving the role of *H. pylori*, gastric juice, and the mucosal defense barriers. Ulcerogenesis usually occurs when there is a deficiency in the protective mechanisms of the gastric mucosa and a rise in the aggressive factors such as *H. pylori* and gastric acid (Sawada & Dickinson, 1997). An increase in unbuffered acid in the duodenum not only is ulcerogenic, but it also causes gastric metaplasia of the duodenal mucosa, which provides a new habitat for *H. pylori*. To better understand the pathogenesis of PUD, a review of gastric acid secretion and the protective mechanisms of the stomach and duodenum follows.

Different regions of the stomach have different physiologic roles in the production of acid, pepsin,

and hormones and in defense of the mucosal barrier. These are diagrammed in Figure 16-3. The upper region of the stomach, the cardia, contains glandular epithelial cells that secrete a layer of alkaline mucus 1 to 5 mm thick. The largest region of the stomach, the corpus, or body, is composed of parietal cells and chief cells. An estimated 1 billion parietal cells are found in the stomach, each able to secrete hydrochloric acid (HCl) and intrinsic factor. The chief cells secrete pepsinogen, which is converted to pepsin, a proteolytic enzyme, in an acidic environment of a pH of 4 or less (Guyton & Hall, 1997). The region of the stomach closest to the duodenum, the antrum, contains G cells, which produce and secrete gastrin. The G cells, which contain many microvilli on their surfaces, release gastrin in response to gastric distention and amino acids in the stomach. Gastrin is a hormone, entering the bloodstream and acting on target cells in an endocrine manner. Gastrin then stimulates HCl and pepsinogen secretion, GI motility, and closure of the LES.

Parietal cells, in the body of the stomach, are located in the secretory glands of the gastric mucosa. The parietal cell membrane contains gastrin, acetylcholine, and $H_2$ receptor sites. These receptor sites play an integral role in the production of gastric acid through the activation of the hydrogen-potassium adenosine triphosphatase ($H^+K^+$ ATPase) pump (Sawanda & Dickinson, 1994). The $H^+K^+$ ATPase pump is located on the parietal cell membrane and releases hydrogen ions into the gas-

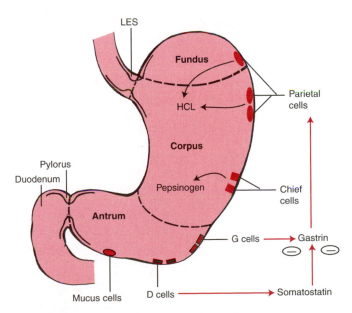

**FIGURE 16.3** ● Anatomy of the stomach and location of cells involved in gastric secretion.

tric lumen, thus producing an acidic environment in the stomach. There are three mechanisms through which the $H^+K^+$ ATPase pump is activated and gastric acid is secreted from the parietal cells (Fig. 16-4). The first involves the release of acetylcholine resulting from cholinergic nerve stimulation from vagus nerve fibers in the stomach. The vagus nerve may be stimulated locally through gastric distention (Sawanda & Dickinson, 1994) or cephalically. Acetylcholine attaches to cholinergic receptor sites on parietal cell membranes, which triggers the release of calcium cations ($Ca^{2+}$). The second mechanism involves the stimulation of G cells by acetylcholine to release gastrin into the circulation. Gastrin binds to its receptor site on the parietal cell membrane and further promotes the release of $Ca^{2+}$ into the parietal cell cytoplasm. The third mechanism involves the stimulation of mast cells by gastrin and acetylcholine to degranulate and release histamine ($H_2$) (Sawanda & Dickinson, 1994). Histamine binds to $H_2$ receptor sites on the parietal cell membrane and stimulates the release of cAMP in the cell. An increase in the concentration of calcium cations and cAMP influences the $H^+K^+$ ATPase pump to release a $H^+$ in exchange for a potassium cation (Guyton & Hall, 1997). Next, the $H^+$ combines with a chloride ion to form HCl; this constitutes the normal gastric acid environment of the stomach.

There are many physiologic gastric acid inhibitory factors. Somatostatin, a hormone secreted by the D cells in the antrum, acts by inhibiting the release of gastrin and histamine. The actions of somatostatin block gastric acid secretion from the parietal cells. However, acetylcholine can block the release of somatostatin. Other hormones, which play a role in inhibiting the release of gastrin, are prostaglandin $E_2$, cholecystokinin (CCK), glucagon, and gastric inhibitory polypeptide. Also, an acidic gastric environment inhibits the release of gastrin from the G cells.

Various defense mechanisms protect the gastric mucosa from damage and ulceration. The gastric mucosa is virtually impermeable to acid because of the phospholipid membrane and close lateral junctions of the epithelial cells that line the stomach. In addition, the epithelial cells secrete alkaline mucus and bicarbonate, which form a protective barrier against pepsin and gastric acid. Mucus and bicarbonate neutralize the acidic pH at the surface of the gastric mucosa. The mucosal epithelial cells regenerate quickly, thus protecting against ulcerogenesis if damage occurs. The gastric mucosa has a rapid blood flow that flushes away any damaging molecules. Prostaglandins also maintain a neutral mucosal environment by stimulating the release of bicarbonate and mucus, preserving blood flow, and repairing mucosal damage. The negative feedback mechanism, which takes place in the duodenum, inhibits the secretion of acid when the acid content of the duodenum is excessive. In addition, the presence of acid in the duodenum stimulates the secretion of the hormone secretin, which increases the output of sodium bicarbonate from the pancreas to neutralize the acid. The pyloric sphincter also functions as a barrier by preventing acid regurgitation into the duodenum.

## Pathogenesis of Peptic Ulcer Disease

The pathogenesis of PUD is associated with various risk factors, and there are three commonly accepted theories of pathogenesis. The first theory suggests that PUD results from an infection with *H. pylori*. The second theory is that a breakdown of the mucosal defense barriers occurs. The last theorizes that an increase in gastric acid secretion causes PUD.

### Helicobacter Pylori

*Helicobacter pylori* is a Gram-negative, spiral-shaped bacteria that has been implicated in the pathogenesis of PUD by causing an antral gastritis. The bacteria releases toxins, cytokines, and enzymes, which produce chronic inflammatory processes. Bacterial products cause neutrophil chemotaxis and activation and epithelial chemokine production. The immune response to the infection is polarized in a TH1 direction (proinflammatory) (Walker & Crabtree, 1998).

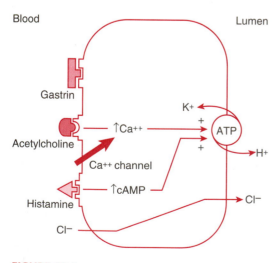

**FIGURE 16.4**  ●  Signals that increase gastric acid secretion.

This bacteria's virulence is determined by the production of a toxin, VacA, and a protein, CagA. Heterogeneity exists among the different strains of *H. pylori*, with the most pathogenic strains expressing certain forms of these two proteins at the highest level. Patients with PUD are more likely to have CagA- and VacA-producing strains than are patients with only gastritis. CagA stimulates a Th1 immune response in the mucosa, which causes further inflammatory effects. VacA becomes more toxic in an acid environment and acts in several ways to enhance pathogenicity, with the major action being inhibition of mucosal repair (Walker & Crabtree, 1998).

Cytokines may be important mediators of PUD. Certainly, *H. pylori* results in cytokine release from the inflammatory cells, which migrate to the sites of infection. In particular, interleukin (IL)-1β, tumor necrosis factor-beta, IL-8, and interferon beta all have been identified as cytokines within the mucosa. Cytokines decrease when the organisms have been eradicated. Cytokines are chemotactic and stimulatory for mononuclear and polymorphonuclear cells by causing the expression of adhesion molecules on the endothelium so that the cells migrate into the mucosa, and then stimulating them to degranulate and release toxic substances and enzymes (Lehmann & Stalder, 1998). IL-8 is secreted as a chemokine from gastric epithelial cells.

*H. pylori* is believed to burrow through the epithelial cells of the gastric mucosa by releasing enzymes. Depending on the host and a variety of factors, the organism may be confined mostly to the antrum of the stomach in some or to the corpus in others. In antral gastritis, the organism causes excess gastrin production, which then stimulates the intact parietal cells in the corpus, causing excess acid production. The D-cell function in the antrum is suppressed, which results in a loss of the somatostatin opposition to gastric acid secretion. If the organism finds a niche in the corpus, the effect is suppression of acid secretion. Antral gastritis is, therefore, more likely to lead to duodenal ulcers. *H. pylori* may sequester itself in niches below the mucosal layers of the stomach, duodenum, or esophagus for a lifetime. However, it attaches only to gastric-type mucosal cells, so significant metaplasia must occur for it to thrive in sites other than the stomach.

*H. pylori* protects itself from the highly acidic gastric environment by producing a protective surface enzyme called urease. Urease is released by microbes that have undergone autolysis, and then the enzyme is adsorbed onto the membrane surfaces of surrounding live microorganisms. Urease hydrolyzes urea to produce ammonia. The high alkalinity of ammonia neutralizes the gastric acidic environment surrounding *H. pylori*, thus permitting continued pathogenic effects on the host. This has been viewed as a kind of communal activity among the members of the bacterial colony (Dunn & Phadnis, 1998).

Cellular and humoral immune responses are activated when the *H. pylori* organism burrows through the epithelium. Once *H. pylori* breaks through the gastric mucosal barrier, the immune response is triggered. This stimulates the release of inflammatory mediators such as cytotoxins, leukocytes, and proteases (Cerda et al., 1995), which causes an acute inflammatory response and tissue injury. Antibodies such as IgG and IgA may be secreted during this time (Damianos & McGarrity, 1997) and can be detected through serologic testing. The effects of gastric acid and pepsin on the breached gastric mucosa, because of *H. pylori*, further potentiates the tissue injury. However, cellular damage of the gastric mucosa is a slow process that often leads to loss of gastric glands, chronic antral gastritis, intestinal metaplasia, and dysplasia (Damianos & McGarrity, 1997). Chronic gastritis eventually may evolve into precancerous atrophic gastritis, and, with time, gastric cancer (Peura, 1997). *H. pylori* is considered a risk factor for developing gastric cancer, especially in certain ethnic groups (Blecker, 1997). An association between gastric lymphomas and *H. pylori* has been reported (Parsonnet et al., 1994). The risks of developing gastric atrophy and gastric carcinoma are eight times greater in PUD patients infected with *H. pylori*. The pathophysiology is related to the development of multifocal atrophic gastritis resulting from inflammatory changes in the stomach itself. The risk is influenced by age when initially infected and the strain of microorganisms and type of CagA marker.

### Duodenal Ulcer

The combined effect of both a high acid output and an infection with *H. pylori* is the suggested pathway through which duodenal ulcers develop. The high acid output is related to an increase in gastrin secretion or an increase in parietal cell mass. Also, abnormally elevated gastrin levels (above 200 pg/mL) have been associated with gastrin-producing adenomas such as Zollinger-Ellison syndrome (Walsh & Dockray, 1994). Other factors, such as rapid gastric emptying or impaired mucosal defense from smoking or inhibition of prostaglandin synthesis, play a role in duodenal ulcer formation. However, the chronic antral gastritis that occurs with a *H. pylori* infection, in addition to this high acid output, leads to duodenitis and, eventually, duodenal ulcers (Peura, 1997).

## Gastric Ulcers

Gastric ulcers also are believed to arise from an impairment in the normal protective mechanism of the gastric mucosa and from the actions of gastric acid. The acid output in gastric ulcer patients has been found to be within or below normal levels (Huang & Hunt, 1996), but slow gastric motility and slow gastric emptying may predispose a person to gastric ulcers (McPhee et al., 1997). Factors that produce gastritis, such as smoking, NSAID use, steroids, or a *H. pylori* infection, are strongly associated with gastric ulcer disease. As discussed previously, *H. pylori* breaches the gastric mucosal barrier and allows the back-diffusion of gastric acidic contents (Huang & Hunt, 1996). This repeated chemical and enzymatic injury leads to gastric ulcer formation.

## Complications

The most serious complications of PUD are bleeding, perforation, and obstruction. These complications, found in approximately 25% of the patients with *H. pylori* in PUD, often have a sudden onset and an increase in the mortality rate if unrecognized or untreated. Complications usually arise from undiagnosed, untreated, or recurrent PUD with or without the use of NSAIDs. Therefore, all patients presenting with complicated ulcer symptoms should be screened for the presence of *H. pylori*, preferably by endoscopy, and appropriate treatment regimen should be initiated as soon as possible.

Bleeding peptic ulcers have the highest mortality rate and require immediate medical attention and treatment. The bleeding occurs from the erosive action of acid and pepsin on the gastric epithelium. The amount of bleeding into the GI tract depends on the blood vessel size and tissue damage. Clinical indications of bleeding are hematemesis, melanotic or dark tarry stool, dizziness, orthostatic hypotension, tachycardia, and decreased hemoglobin and hematocrit counts. Slow and chronic bleeding ulcers usually present with occult blood in the stool as well as low hemoglobin and hematocrit values with symptoms of ane-

mia. Eradication therapy for *H. pylori* decreases the recurrence of bleeding ulcers (Amann & Cerda, 1995). Active GI bleeding with volume depletion requires immediate medical attention and hospitalization for possible blood transfusions, esophagogastroduodenoscopy, or surgery.

A perforation occurs when an ulcer erodes through all of the mucosal and muscle tissue layers of the stomach or the duodenum. The GI contents, such as undigested food, acid, and bacteria, enter the sterile peritoneal cavity. The abdominal cavity and its surrounding tissues respond with an acute inflammatory process known as peritonitis. Ulcer perforations occur less frequently than bleeding ulcers (Laine, 1996). The role of *H. pylori* in ulcer perforation is unknown. Smoking has been identified as an important predisposing factor for developing a perforation (Svanes et al., 1997). The clinical presentation of peritonitis is an acute onset of severe abdominal pain in a patient who appears to be toxic. The physical examination reveals severe rebound tenderness of the abdomen, decreased bowel sounds, signs of hypovolemia, and fever. Also, diagnostic tests such as a chest or an upright abdominal x-ray can detect the presence of free air in the intraperitoneal cavity.

Duodenal or gastroduodenal outlet obstruction is a serious complication of PUD that occurs less frequently than bleeding or a perforation. An obstruction occurs when an ulcer or a tumor forms at the gastroduodenal outlet or in the duodenum. The ulcerogenesis causes an inflammation of the surrounding tissue, muscle spasms, and a narrowing of the duodenum. The clinical presentation of obstruction depends on the degree of narrowing of the gastroduodenal outlet and the delay in gastric emptying (Raeihae et al., 1998). A partial obstruction may present as chronic vomiting after meals, feeling full, or losing weight. A patient with a complete obstruction may present with vomiting after meals and a bloated feeling. The physical examination reveals abdominal distention, noticeable peristaltic movement, hyperactive bowel sounds, an abdominal mass, and possible dehydration. A barium swallow x-ray can detect this complication.

## Clinical Presentation

The classic clinical presentation of PUD usually is a complaint of epigastric pain or discomfort, which is described as chronic, burning, gnawing, sharp, or annoying. The painful ulcer symptoms usually are chronic, lasting a few minutes to even years (Rosenstock et al., 1997). This pain may be caused by the chronic gastritis that often is found with *H. pylori* infection (Fendrick et al., 1997) because of increased levels of gastric acid and gastrin secretion. Pain that is relieved by meals or the use of antacid, or that awakens the patient late at night, usually indicates a duodenal ulcer. The pain results from increased acidity in the duodenum during a fasting state. Gastric ulcers are not alleviated by food or antacids. Patients with gastric ulcers cannot tolerate the normal acid secretions that occur with meals because of the chronic gastritis that usually is present with *H. pylori* infection (Walsh & Dockray, 1994). Epigastric pain from an acute infection with *H. pylori* usually has a short duration and has presenting symptoms similar to those of gastroenteritis (Rosenstock et al., 1997). Other associated symptoms, such as vomiting and

heartburn, are common with *H. pylori* infection, whereas indigestion and feeling bloated contribute to the vague clinical presentation.

Most of the PUD population infected with *H. pylori* are either asymptomatic or have chronic dyspepsia and rarely seek medical attention on initial presentation of symptoms. Unfortunately, these individuals often self-medicate with over-the-counter antacids, Pepto-Bismol, or $H_2$ antagonist drugs. The use of over-the-counter drugs temporarily alleviates the symptoms of ulcers, thus postponing the prompt need for diagnosis and treatment of PUD before the onset of complications arise. Therefore, practitioners must rule out the serious complications of PUD during the history and physical examination or through diagnostic testing.

---

## CLINICAL VIGNETTE 16.2

A 49-year-old Hispanic female presents to the clinic complaining of a burning pain in her epigastric area. She has had this pain intermittently for the last year but was awakened by the pain last night. She took off from work today and came to the clinic because she was afraid that she might be having a heart attack like her neighbor. Her last office visit was 2 years ago.

The evaluation of this patient should begin with arriving at all of the possible differential diagnoses for epigastric pain (Table 16-2). Next, a complete history and a focused examination should be performed, based on the differential diagnoses that need to be ruled out. Finally, the appropriate diagnostic tests, treatment regimen, and referral are made.

The history includes the characteristics of the current illness, allergies, current medication use, past medical history, family history, and recent exposure to communicable diseases. The onset, duration, frequency, quality, quantity, and aggravating and alleviating characteristics of the epigastric pain need to be evaluated. The patient should be questioned regarding any history of cancer, gastrointestinal problems, or cardiovascular problems. Also, her last menstrual period and current use of contraception should be known. Any current use or history of smoking, alcohol, or drugs should be determined if ulcer disease is suspected. Any family history of ulcers, *Helicobacter pylori* infection, cancer, or

cardiovascular problems helps to rule out risk factors for ulcer disease, myocardial ischemia, or malignancy. Current use of over-the-counter or prescription drugs assists the practitioner in differentiating the diagnosis. Finally, a review of systems assists the practitioner to differentiate between all of the possible etiologies. The review of systems for this patient should focus on the cardiovascular, gastrointestinal, psychosocial, nutritional, and elimination patterns.

A focused physical examination should be performed. The general appearance of the patient helps to differentiate an acute presentation of pancreatitis, cholecystitis, myocardial ischemia, or any of the complications of PUD. Orthostatic vital signs should be taken to detect any volume depletion such as that seen with a bleeding ulcer. Weight should be measured, and any decrease in weight should cause suspicion for gastric malignancy. The skin, heart, lungs, abdomen, rectum (for occult blood), and lymph glands should be examined.

In this case, several tests helped to narrow the differential diagnosis. The patient had a 12-lead electrocardiogram to rule out an acute myocardial infarction. The patient had a complete blood count, basic chemistry, amylase, lipase, and a chest x-ray. The diagnosis of PUD was established, but testing for *H. pylori* was not performed.

## TABLE 16.2

### Differential Diagnosis of Epigastric Pain

Myocardial infarction or ischemia
Peptic ulcer disease
Gastroesophageal reflux disease
Gastric cancer
Cholecystitis
Pancreatitis

## Diagnostic Tests

The diagnosis of *H. pylori* can be established through invasive and noninvasive tests. These tests vary in their specificity and sensitivity to accurately detect the *H. pylori* organism. The practitioner should consider the risk to the patient, cost-effectiveness, and ease of administering and interpreting the diagnostic tests in various clinical settings.

The advantages, disadvantages, and approximate range of cost for each test are summarized in Table 16-3. Notice that all of the diagnostic tests, except serologic testing, may have false-negative results if antibiotics, bismuth, or proton pump inhibitor drugs have been used recently by the patient.

The carbon-13 ($^{13}$C) or carbon-14 ($^{14}$C) urea breath test and serology tests are noninvasive. Serologic tests require blood analysis for the presence of elevated IgG and IgA antibody titers to *H. pylori* infection. This blood test is not only accurate and sensitive, but it is widely used for diagnosing *H. pylori* infection in the office. However, the IgG antibody titer may remain elevated for up to 8 months (Fay & Jaffe, 1996) or even years after the eradication of *H. pylori* (Cerda & Yamada, 1995). This means that serologic test results should not be used to document the eradication of *H. pylori* in follow-up visits. The other noninvasive test, the $^{13}$C or $^{14}$C urea breath test, is as sensitive and accurate in diagnosing *H. pylori* as serology tests but is more expensive. This test requires the

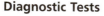

## TABLE 16.3

### Diagnostic Tests

| Test | Advantage | Disadvantage |
|---|---|---|
| Serologic test | Noninvasive<br>Easy to collect in office<br>Inexpensive ($10–$100)<br>Sensitivity 90%–95% for *Helicobacter pylori* | Titers remain elevated > 8 mo<br>Unreliable predictor of *H. pylori* eradication |
| Carbon-13 or carbon-14 urea breath test | Noninvasive<br>Quick and accurate test<br>Sensitivity 90%–95% for *H. pylori* | More expensive ($50–$250) than serologic test because special instruments are required |
| Endoscopy | Accurate diagnosis | Increased discomfort, risk, and cost ($200–$2000) |
| Biopsy urease test | Quick results<br>Inexpensive compared with histology<br>Sensitivity 90%–98% | Requires invasive endoscopy<br>Expensive<br>Risk of procedure to patient |
| Histology | Standard diagnosis for *H. pylori*<br>Sensitivity 70%–95% | Invasive |
| Culture | Used to determine antimicrobial sensitivity in cases of anti-microbial resistance | Invasive<br>Sensitivity 60%–95% for *H. pylori*<br>Delayed results (~7 d) |

patient to ingest a capsule containing both urea and labeled nonradioactive carbon-13 or radioactive carbon-14. If the *H. pylori* organism is present, the urease produced by *H. pylori* hydrolyzes the urea into ammonia and bicarbonate (labeled with $^{13}C$ or $^{14}C$), which is exhaled in the breath as measurable $^{13}CO_2$. The ease of administration and high rate of sensitivity of the urea breath test enhances its use for diagnosing and monitoring *H. pylori* infection (Cerda & Yamada, 1995).

Biopsy, histology, and culture of the gastric mucosa all are invasive diagnostic tests that require endoscopy. Endoscopy may be used to diagnose *H. pylori* infection and to evaluate the severe ulcer symptoms and complications of ulcerogenesis, or to rule out gastric malignancies. Biopsy usually is performed on several gastric mucosal sites, including the antrum, to evaluate the presence of *H. pylori* or gastric cancer. The standard histology test to diagnose *H. pylori* infection mostly has been replaced by the *Campylobacter*-like organism test, a rapid urease test (Fay & Jaffe, 1996). This test is performed by placing the biopsy tissue samples in a urea solution; if *H. pylori* is present, urease hydrolyzes urea and changes the pH and color of the solution, thus confirming the presence of the organism. Culture of the gastric mucosa rarely is obtained because it has a low sensitivity and accuracy, but is reserved mostly for patients in whom the eradication of the *H. pylori* organism has been unsuccessful and antimicrobial sensitivity results are lacking.

Controversy exists regarding which test should be used to diagnose *H. pylori*. The 1994 NIH Consensus Conference suggests that noninvasive diagnostic tests should be used to document the diagnosis of *H. pylori*, but treatment with antimicrobials should be initiated only in patients with ulcers and *H. pylori* infection. This may lead to assumptions that invasive tests are required to treat *H. pylori*. Fendrick, McCort, Chernew, Hirth, Patel, and Bloom (1995) studied alternative management strategies in symptomatic patients with PUD. They conclude that the noninvasive diagnostic tests were less costly and just as effective in diagnosing *H. pylori*, whereas endoscopy was limited to patients with chronic and unresolved symptoms.

Other diagnostic tests for PUD, not specific for *H. pylori*, are complete blood count (CBC), stool hemoccult, and radiology studies. Analysis of the CBC is important in determining a chronic or actively bleeding ulcer. Findings suggestive of acute or chronic GI bleeding are low hematocrit, hemoglobin, and RBC count. A stool hemoccult study, which detects the presence of blood in the stool, is a common test used to confirm GI bleeding. However, it does not differentiate upper from lower GI bleeding. Upper GI series with barium contrast is a reliable radiology test that detects approximately 80% of the ulcers in PUD.

## Physiologic Basis of Treatment

### Nonpharmacologic Management

The nonpharmacologic management of PUD focuses on avoiding any factors that aggravate or slow the healing process of the disease. Patients should be instructed to avoid cigarette smoking because it slows ulcer healing, inhibits the $H_2$ antagonist effects, and increases the chance of ulcer recurrence. Smoking cessation allows the beneficial protective factors of the gastric mucosa to return to normal within a short time (Eastwood, 1997). Alcohol should be avoided because it damages the gastric mucosa. NSAIDs should be avoided because they inhibit the protective effect of prostaglandin on the gastric mucosa. If using NSAIDs cannot be avoided, then a prostaglandin replacement, misoprostol, should be taken along with the NSAID to prevent gastric mucosal damage (Ament & Childers, 1997). The avoidance of specific foods is not believed to be of any value in the treatment of ulcers. The patient should be encouraged to eat nutritionally balanced meals.

### Pharmacotherapy

Treating PUD had been a challenge for many years, until the discovery of *H. pylori* by Warren and Marshall in 1983 (Damianos & McGarrity, 1997). Traditional interventions to treat PUD were aimed at reducing gastric acid using antacids, antisecretory drugs, or, when all else failed, surgery. Currently, many drugs (Table 16-4) and various combinations of treatment regimens are used to treat and eradicate *H. pylori* infection. The regimens differ by success rates, length of therapy, number of pills consumed per day, and cost (Damianos & McGarrity, 1997), thus allowing patient individualization. All treatment regimens consist of one or more antimicrobial agents with one acid antisecretory agent. High *H. pylori* eradication rates—greater than 90%—have been reported with the "triple-therapy" regimen.

The dilemma encountered by practitioners is when to treat PUD, since there is no standard treatment protocol. For this reason, the 1994 NIH Consensus Conference reviewed the diagnostic criteria and treatment regimens and proposed a

## TABLE 16.4

### Drugs for Treating *Helicobacter Pylori* Infection

| Drug Classification | Drug | Mechanism of Action | Common Side Effects | Patient Education |
|---|---|---|---|---|
| Antibiotics | Tetracycline Amoxicillin Metronidazole (Flagyl) Clarithromycin | Eradication of *Helicobacter pylori*: Tetracycline—broad-spectrum bacteriostatic agent Amoxicillin—inhibits bacterial wall synthesis Flagyl—bactericidal Clarithromycin—inhibits bacterial protein synthesis | Tetracycline—diarrhea and photosensitivity Amoxicillin—PCN allergy, diarrhea, candidiasis Flagyl—diarrhea (20% chance), nausea, vomiting, metallic taste in mouth; disulfiram reaction if taken with alcohol Clarithromycin—diarrhea, nausea, headache, bad taste in mouth | Tetracycline Take with bismuth at mealtime Avoid if pregnant Flagyl Do not drink alcohol or take any alcohol compounds while on Flagyl Caution on anaphylaxis reaction |
| $H_2$ antagonists | Cimetidine (Tagamet) Ranitidine (Zantac) Famotidine (Pepcid) Nizatidine (Axid) | Gastric pH by blocking histamine from attaching to $H_2$ receptor site on parietal cells | Diarrhea Constipation Headache Malaise | Take with breakfast or at bedtime Do not take within 1 h of other medicines Stop smoking or do not smoke before bedtime dose of $H_2$ antagonist |
| Proton pump inhibitors | Omeprazole (Prilosec) Lansoprazole (Prevacid) Pantoprazole | Inhibits the release of $H^+$ from $H^+K^+$ ATPase pump | Diarrhea Nausea Headache Abdominal pain (rare) | Take at bedtime on empty stomach |
| Bismuth subsalicylate | Pepto-Bismol | Bismuth—antibacterial property, binds with tetracycline to increase drug delivery to mucosa | Bismuth—black tongue and stools Salicylate—tinnitus | Tongue and stools may turn black Take with tetracycline |
| Antacids | Maalox (OTC) Mylanta (OTC) | Neutralizes gastric acid | Magnesium compounds—diarrhea Aluminum compounds—constipation | Do not take with dietary supplements May decrease absorption of folate, iron, Vit $B_{12}$ (decrease Vit A absorption with magnesium compounds) |
| Barrier agents | Sucralfate (Carafate) | Protective barrier for gastric mucosa without systemic absorption | Constipation (rare) | Do not take with other medicines or Vit supplements Take with full glass of water on empty stomach |
| Prostaglandin | Misoprostol (Cytotec) | Protects gastric mucosa, increases circulation, increases bicarbonate release, decreases gastric acid secretion | Diarrhea Teratogenic in pregnancy | Take with food Do not take with magnesium antacids Avoid if pregnant |

OTC, over-the-counter; PCN, penicillin; Vit, vitamin.

few guidelines in treating and diagnosing *H. pylori*. These guidelines propose that individuals, asymptomatic or symptomatic, should not receive empiric antibiotic therapy unless *H. pylori* infection and ulcer disease have been diagnosed. This indicates that a practitioner should have diagnostic test results confirming the presence of *H. pylori*, but others view this confirmation of ulcers by endoscopy as both costly and unnecessary in the absence of complications.

The goal of treatment is to eradicate the bacterial infection caused by *H. pylori*, alleviate symptoms, decrease the rate of recurrence of the disease, and ultimately cure PUD. Most of these goals can be achieved through the many treatment regimens proposed. Successful eradication of the *H. pylori* organism through a 14-day trial of a bismuth, a metronidazole in combination with tetracycline or amoxicillin, and an antisecretory drug therapy has been generally accepted. Successful eradication—absence of *H. pylori*—may be confirmed 4 weeks after therapy with the rapid urease test.

The practitioner should evaluate many factors when selecting an appropriate treatment approach in a client with diagnosed *H. pylori* infection in PUD. Important factors to consider are the client's likelihood of compliance, prior infection with *H. pylori*, recurrence rate, antibiotic resistance, side effects, and contraindications of drug therapy. In the United States, resistance to metronidazole is approximately 25% (Shubert, 1996), with higher rates of approximately 70% in developing countries (Salcedo & Al-Kawas, 1998).

A 1996 national survey reveals that 50% of primary care physicians (PCPs) empirically treated first-time PUD symptoms with antisecretory agents without testing for *H. pylori* (Aronson, 1998). More impressively, the survey indicates the under-use of antimicrobial agents by PCPs in eradicating *H. pylori* peptic disease in 50% of patients. Since this discovery, the Centers for Disease Control and Prevention have undertaken a public campaign to educate physicians and the general public on *H. pylori* and PUD.

## IRRITABLE BOWEL SYNDROME

Irritable bowel syndrome is a common and frustrating condition frequently seen by health care providers in primary care practices. The symptoms are vague GI pain, bloating and gas, and abnormalities in bowel habits, such as diarrhea or constipation or cycles of both. This illness is common, and patients have marked discomfort, but no uni-

fying pathophysiologic alteration in the GI tract of these patients has been found. IBS has been considered a "functional somatic syndrome" along with a group of other diseases in which consistent pathophysiologic processes have not been discovered. Included in this list, according to Barsky and Borus (1999), are chronic fatigue syndrome, fibromyalgia, Gulf War syndrome, sick building syndrome, repetitive stress injury, multiple chemical sensitivity, and side effects of silicone breast implants. According to these authors, all of these illnesses have significantly higher psychiatric comorbidities than normal controls. Patients with these conditions have unusually high sensitivities to their symptoms and tend to think the worst is going to happen, exaggerate the seriousness of their symptoms, and are pessimistic about their health improving. On the other hand, their pessimism may be well grounded in a lack of responsiveness of health care providers to their symptoms. These patients have tremendous discomfort and often are ignored because so little is available to offer them. Until the pathophysiologic basis for their symptoms is better understood, the treatment often is trial and error and largely supportive. Because the symptoms are difficult to treat, many patients go from one medical provider to another to seek relief.

Patients with IBS have a chief complaint of bloating and chronic abdominal pain, which is felt more frequently in the lower abdomen. The differential diagnosis of this type of pain includes PUD, gallbladder disease, colon cancer, and inflammatory bowel disease (ulcerative colitis or Crohn's disease). Bloating and gas are the predominant symptoms reported by patients (Lembo et al., 1999), and another condition with similar symptoms as commonly misdiagnosed as IBS is lactose intolerance. Therefore, a careful history of food tolerance and the relationship of foods with symptoms is important. The distinguishing characteristics of IBS is that patients report abdominal distension, relief of abdominal pain with bowel movements, looser and more frequent stool accompanying the onset of abdominal pain, passage of mucus, and a feeling of incomplete evacuation of the bowel after a bowel movement (Borum & Brooks, 1997). These patients also have an unusual sensitivity to rectal distension. They do not have melena, foul-smelling stools, fever, anemia, weight loss, and other symptoms that are characteristic of inflammatory bowel disease or cancer.

Because the symptoms of IBS seem to be related to colonic motility, this may be a disease of altered gut motility. Particularly implicated is a decreased vagal cholinergic and an increased sympathetic input to the gut. On the other hand, an alternative explanation is that patients have an increased sensitivity to, or perception of, visceral cues (visceral hyperalgesia). Both of these points of view are supported by some studies and refuted by others (Borum & Brooks, 1998). An integrated biobehavioral model of brain-gut interaction also seems to be a fruitful area for both understanding and treating this illness (Meyer et al., 1999). Based on this approach, targets for future therapy for pain and motility problems of IBS include opiate receptors in the gut and ion channels and receptors within the nervous system. Often, the symptoms of IBS follow a stressful event or an enteric infection. Both of these phenomena could alter local mucosal immunity and affect motility. Patients with IBS also seem more sensitive to the stressors of daily life (Delvaux, 1999).

## Physiology of Treatment

The approach to care of the patient with IBS is to evaluate the need for psychological counseling and stress management, and to provide antidiarrheal, antispasmodic, and anticholinergic drugs to decrease gut motility in patients in whom diarrhea is the predominant symptom. Diet modifications may help, including increasing the fiber in the diet. Foods that produce gas should be avoided, and antiflatulence agents may be used. Caffeine, nicotine, and alcohol should be avoided.

---

## CLINICAL VIGNETTE 16.3

Mrs. Patricia Pearson is a 40-year-old homemaker who comes to the clinic for the first time. She admits to having seen several other providers for her symptoms but states that "no one has helped her condition, and she is getting sicker and sicker." Her past medical history includes two pregnancies and live births, an ulcer, which was successfully treated in her 30s, "bad" premenstrual syndrome, and frequent sinus infections.

Her children are teenagers and are "giving her a lot of trouble." She is currently going through a bitter divorce and admits to having worries about her future and her ability to support herself. She is college educated but has never worked.

Her current condition appears to have developed slowly over the last year. Her complaints are a dragging, constant, bloating and gassy pain, which gets worse and worse until she defecates. However, there are some weeks when she is so constipated that she has only two or three bowel movements over the whole week, and other weeks when she has crampy, diarrhea-like stools all day long. She also reports an uncomfortable, full sensation in her rectum. She appears convinced that she has cancer and has been to three other providers, who have done several tests that ruled out cancer, lactose intolerance, peptic ulcer disease, gallbladder disease, and inflammatory bowel disease. She was told by her last health care provider that her disease was "all in her head" and that she needed psychiatric help.

Mrs. Pearson asks for further testing to determine if she has cancer. She describes her symptoms as "unbearable" and getting worse every day.

Results of her physical examination are unremarkable. She has not lost weight, is not anemic, and has a normal white blood cell count. Her abdomen is soft, bowel sounds are 3+, and she has mild, diffuse tenderness in the lower abdomen. There is no organomegaly and no masses on palpation. Her diagnosis is irritable bowel syndrome.

She is encouraged to keep a food diary to determine if her symptoms are related to certain foods, to stop smoking, and to seek stress management counseling during her highly stressful divorce. Her diet is modified to include at least 30 g of fiber per day, and an antidiarrheal agent is prescribed for the weeks in which the diarrhea symptoms predominate. She will be seen back in the clinic in 3 weeks to determine if these measures are helpful. The practitioner supports her by acknowledging the reality and severity of her symptoms, and tells her that the clinic will review her previous tests, but that her symptoms and findings are not typical of cancer. She is encouraged to log onto *http://www.ibsgroup.org/* for more information about her illness and to join an online support group if she wishes.

# CONSTIPATION

Constipation is a symptom, not a disease, but it is seen so often in primary care practice that the pathophysiologic basis for common types of constipation deserves discussion here. This problem generally does not constitute a major health disruption and may be noticed during a routine physical examination or in the review of systems when the patient has come to the clinic for another complaint.

Constipation usually is defined by the individual rather than by set medical norms. Also, the same definitions are not always used. Constipation is defined in primary care practice as "a bothersome difficulty in initiating or completing defecation" (Johanson, 1997) and usually by passage of less than 35 g of fecal matter per day, which translates to about three bowel movements per week (Sartor, 1997). This usually means that the patient strains while defecating because fecal material has become hard from increased transit time and decreased colonic motility, a cause of constipation called *colonic inertia*. Autonomic neuropathy is believed to be involved in the pathophysiology of slow-transit colonic inertia. The myenteric plexus, which normally controls the endogenous motility of the gut, also may degenerate in some cases. Environmental factors may influence this process, and several have been identified as potentials (Johanson, 1997). Environmental toxins, neurotoxic drugs, environmental chemicals such as insecticides, viruses, and endogenous chemicals such as free radicals and excitatory amino acids all contribute in some way to myenteric degeneration.

The other two common causes of constipation are IBS and pelvic floor dysfunction (PFD). Many other neurologic and endocrine disorders and GI diseases may have constipation as a symptom, but in primary care, chronic constipation usually results from one of the three aforementioned etiologies. PFD is caused by a nonrelaxing pelvic floor, which occurs as the result of pelvic nerve trauma during childbirth or surgery in women. The neurologic damage results in either a state of contraction or lack of relaxation of the puborectal muscle or external sphincter during defecation (De Nuntis et al., 1998). This leads to functional rectal obstruction and constipation, which may explain the disparate female-to-male ratio in the symptom of constipation.

Constipation is a symptom that is mostly self-treated, usually with laxatives. A history of constipation followed by laxative-aided purging sets up a pattern that becomes difficult to break (Sartor, 1997). Any patient who presents with constipation should be carefully evaluated, and a critical part of the assessment is history of the constipation symptom. Women younger than 30 years of age may present with intractable constipation, which is marked by severe colonic inertia. The elderly may develop constipation because of immobility and diet, and then begin a cycle of laxative use, which exacerbates the problem. Multiparous women may have PFD or combinations of PFD and colonic inertia. Irritable bowel syndrome is one of the most common causes of chronic constipation and must be considered.

# HEPATITIS

Viral hepatitis is seen fairly frequently in the primary care office, and it is one of the most common infections worldwide. Good sanitation and hygiene, blood bank protocols, and public health measures contribute to its lower incidence in the United States, but some populations are at high risk for hepatitis. Although at least five distinct viruses cause hepatitis, hepatitis A (HAV), B (HBV), and C (HCV) are the most common in the United States. Hepatitis A is spread through fecal-oral routes, whereas HBV and HCV are spread through blood and sexual contact. All of the hepatitis-causing viruses infect liver cells, producing hepatocellular inflammation and necrosis. These viruses may infect a few individuals without involving the liver, producing a flu-like illness, rashes, fever, and arthralgia. Most persons infected with any of these viruses have a similar clinical presentation, although incubation periods differ, and the diagnosis of the type of hepatitis is made through serologic testing.

## Hepatitis A

Hepatitis A is an RNA virus from the Picornaviridae family. It is environmentally resistant to many virucidal agents such as chlorine bleach, heat, and acid pH; it survives in feces for up to 2 weeks and retains some infectivity at room temperature for up to 4 weeks (Margolis et al., 1997). Hepatitis A has occurred as an epidemic in the United States, with 7- to 10-year cycles. Although it has decreased in importance in the last 2 decades, it still causes about 30% of reported cases of hepatitis (Purcell, 1995). HAV causes an acute infection and rarely produces chronic liver disease, as do HBV and HCV. It is spread through person-to-person contact or can be community acquired, as in day care centers. Endemic areas of HAV in this country include Native American reservations and native Alaskan populations (Purcell, 1997). International travelers should be vaccinated if they travel to endemic areas. The incubation period is 15 to 45 days (median, 28 days). Viral antigen appears in the blood 2 weeks before the onset of jaundice. Specific IgG antibody is found in 20% to 80% of adults, depending on socioeconomic status (it is more likely to be present in lower socioeconomic classes [70% to 80%] than in middle and upper classes [18% to 30%]). This means that many older adults have been exposed to HAV (Reese & Betts, 1996).

The virus infects hepatocytes and can be found in liver macrophages. It is believed that the hepatocellular damage that occurs is not from virus infection per se, but rather from the inflammatory and immune responses to the infected cells. Cytotoxic T cells are implicated in the local hepatocellular damage, and humoral immune responses also are activated with an initial IgM response, followed later by virus-specific IgG (Margolis et al., 1997).

The clinical presentation of HAV includes jaundice, nausea and vomiting, diarrhea, malaise, fever, anorexia, and dark urine. The aminotransferases, aspartate aminotransferase and alanine aminotransferase, often are elevated to levels eight times above normal levels (often more than 1000 U/L) when jaundice appears (Hsu et al., 1995). Normally, the infection runs its course and the virus is cleared, although relapses occasionally occur months after the initial infection.

### Hepatitis B and C

Hepatitis B previously was termed serum hepatitis, and HCV was identified as non-A, non-B hepatitis. The incidence of HBV rose from the 1960s through 1980s and has decreased since the start of the AIDS epidemic. The use of the hepatitis B vaccine has decreased the incidence dramatically in certain populations (Alaskan natives). Populations previously at risk included hemophiliacs and any patient receiving blood or blood products, but these risks also have been dramatically decreased by mandatory testing of blood donors and immunization of patients such as hemophiliacs (Purcell, 1997). Hepatitis B causes an acute infection and may lead to a carrier state, as well as chronic active liver infection. The incubation period is 50 to 180 days.

The incidence of HCV is increasing in the United States. It is an RNA virus belonging to the family Flaviviridae, and there are six major genotypes of the virus. It has high prevalence in groups such as intravenous drug users, dialysis patients,

and persons with high-risk sexual behaviors (Quinn, 1997). Hepatitis C infection has an incubation period of 6 to 7 weeks, but it may range from 2 to 26 weeks (Margolis et al., 1997).

The pathophysiology of this virus, compared with HAV and HBV, is unique in that there is no evidence of protective humoral immunity after infection, and most of those infected develop chronic hepatitis. Liver enzymes are persistently elevated, indicating ongoing hepatocellular necrosis, which ultimately leads to cirrhosis and liver failure. The disease appears to be an important etiologic factor in the development of hepatocellular carcinoma. The clinical presentation of HCV infection is characteristic of mild disease, although some patients become very ill.

Primary care providers were, in the past, more likely to see patients with HAV, but there appears to be a decline in this disease and a rise in HBV and HCV disease.

### CHOLELITHIASIS AND CHOLECYSTITIS

Gallbladder disease and gallstones are prevalent in the United States, with about 20 million people (10% to 15% of the population) having gallstones, most of whom are asymptomatic (Patino & Quintero, 1998). This makes gallstones the most common disease of the digestive system, with health care costs associated with gallstones and cholecystitis greater than $5 billion per year (NIH, 1998). Risk factors for gallstones include high-fat diet, ethnicity (Native Americans have the highest risk, with the Pima Indians having a 70% risk, and African Americans the lowest in the US), gender (higher incidence in female patients), obesity, oral contraceptive use, recent significant weight loss, and pregnancy. Assessment of patients with abdominal pain therefore must include the possible differential diagnosis of cholecystitis, which is inflammation and distension of the gallbladder, resulting in 99% of the cases from obstructive gallstones.

Stones that form in the gallbladder are either black (composed of pure pigment), pure cholesterol (98% cholesterol), or mixed (predominantly cholesterol; 80% are of this type) (Thistle, 1998). Gallstones precipitate from materials in the bile, forming solid masses. The size of stones ranges from tiny sandlike particles to stones the size of a golf ball. For gallstones to form, certain conditions must occur. There usually is gallbladder hypomotility, supersaturation of bile with cholesterol, and a shortened time for aggregation of cholesterol crystals so that gallbladder sludge forms.

Recall that the gallbladder is a reservoir for bile, which is produced in amounts of 600 to 800 mL/day by the liver. Bile consists of water, bile salts, cholesterol, bilirubin, and lecithin. The salts are products of cholesterol metabolism and function as the emulsifier of fat in the duodenum so that micelles can form and be absorbed through the intestinal luminal epithelial membrane. Because bile is needed only during digestion and absorption, it is stored in the gallbladder, where it is concentrated during the fasting state. The gallbladder is stimulated to contract by the duodenal hormone CCK when bile is needed for fat absorption. The bile that is concentrated by both water and electrolyte absorption through the gallbladder mucosa is a thick, mucus-like substance.

Gallbladder motility is regulated by cholinergic input and CCK. If the gallbladder is less motile than usual because of damage from infection or inflammation or decreased somatostatin, which normally stimulates motility, or because of neurologic factors or hypercontractility of the sphincter of Oddi, the gallbladder does not empty adequately, and the remaining bile becomes increasingly concentrated, forming a "sludge." If the bile is high in cholesterol because of a high fat diet or through the actions of estrogen, the bile becomes more saturated and viscous. When the bile becomes thicker, there is a tendency for stasis. Finally, if stasis of bile occurs, the gallbladder continues to absorb water and electrolytes, and the bile pigments, calcium, and cholesterol aggregate, or coalesce, into solid masses.

One of the strongest risk factors for the development of gallstones is recent significant weight loss achieved through a very-low–calorie diet in obese individuals. The risk seems greatest when the diet also is low in fat. The gallbladder is not stimulated to contract under these conditions, which sets the stage for stasis, sludge formation, and stones.

Once gallstones precipitate in the gallbladder, a classic vicious pathophysiologic cycle becomes established. The presence of stones in the gallbladder further impairs normal gallbladder motility and responsiveness to signals, so that continuing stasis and sludge formation are likely. Stones, or gravel-like material, can migrate out of the gallbladder into the cystic duct or common bile duct, where they can then impede bile flow and further aggravate the vicious cycle of stasis and aggregation. Finally, these stones can become large enough to cause obstruction. This not only stops the flow of bile, but also distends the organ, causes inflammation, serves as a nidus for infection, and causes severe pain.

## Clinical Presentation

The presence of gallstones does not necessarily cause symptoms. Only when stones cause obstruction, distension, and inflammation does the patient have symptoms. However, cholelithiasis can be a chronic condition, with intermittent episodes of pain, which often occurs after eating or at night, although attacks can occur without any apparent provocation. Patients report fat intolerance, belching and flatulence, nausea and vomiting, and right upper quadrant pain that often radiates to the back. The pain usually follows a crescendo-decrescendo pattern, but if it persists, the patient is believed to have acute cholecystitis. An acute attack may be marked by systemic symptoms such as malaise and fever. Chronic cholecystitis results in obstruction of bile ducts and progressive damage to the gallbladder. The pancreas also is commonly inflamed in chronic cholecystitis because of obstruction of the pancreatic duct. Jaundice may occur, with light clay-colored stools and dark urine in chronic conditions.

### Physiologic Basis of Treatment

An understanding of the pathophysiology of gallstones provides a basis for prevention, the most important strategy in primary care. Obesity and diet are the two most modifiable risk factors in gallbladder disease.

Once cholelithiasis has occurred, measures can be taken to dissolve stones or to prevent stone formation in high-risk patients, such as a person about to embark on a very-low–calorie diet. Some stones may be chemically dissolved by oral bile acid therapy (ursodeoxycholic acid). However, not all patients benefit from this approach. Those having mild disease with free-floating, cholesterol-type stones no greater than 1.7 cm in diameter and normal serum cholesterol, and who are not pregnant are candidates for oral bile acid therapy (Chopra & Sugarman, 1990). Sound wave lithotripsy still is experimental, as is injecting a chemical into the gallbladder to chemically dissolve stones.

## COLORECTAL CANCER

Primary care providers are in a position to screen for colorectal cancer as part of their ongoing routine patient care. Colorectal cancer is the third leading cause of mortality in the United States. However, after rising for 13 years, the incidence began to drop in 1986, which is related to an increased rate of colonic polypectomy rather than to other epidemiologic factors (Nelson et al.,

1999). The lifetime risk for colon cancer in the United States still is an impressive 5%, with 57,000 deaths per year from this disease (Garay & Engstrom, 1999). Risk factors for colorectal cancer include age, presence of the disease in a first-degree relative, cigarette smoking, the presence of polyps in the colon, ulcerative colitis, alcohol, and high-fat, low-fiber diets. Ninety percent of these cancers occur after 50 years of age, suggesting that the full malignant transformation process requires time and probably is a multistep process.

This type of cancer exemplifies the interaction of genetic risks and environmental insults to susceptible cells in the mucosal lining of the colon or rectum. The stages in the development of colorectal cancer are illustrated in Figure 16-5. The transformation of the colonic mucosa progresses through hyperplasia, adenomatous growth, dysplasia, and anaplasia. Most polyps that become malignant are adenomatous growths that develop into adenocarcinomas, with the degree of malignant potential correlating with size, the degree of dysplasia, and the patient's age. Polyps generally grow slowly, taking 10 to 15 years to undergo full malignant transformation. Oncogenes and tumor suppressor genes appear to be mutated in a sequential order in colorectal cancer.

Certain inherited genes that increase the risk of colorectal cancer have been identified. A dramatic example of genetically inherited risk is the disease familial polyposis coli, an inherited disease in which affected individuals have thousands of polyps throughout the colon, and the risk of malignancy developing in one or more polyps is essentially 100%. The gene that is altered is the APC gene, which regulates apoptosis (programmed cell death) in the colon. If a mutation occurs in this gene, the rate of cell death is disturbed, beginning the tumorigenic process. Another genetic disease

is hereditary nonpolyposis colorectal cancer. In this disease, there is evidence of mutations in certain genes involved in DNA mismatch repair in the colon. When tumors develop in this population, they grow rapidly. APC mutations seem to be the initial step in the multiple steps that occur in all types of colon cancer. Subsequently, mutations in the K-*ras* oncogene and p53 and other suppressor genes occur, probably from exposure to carcinogens in the stool. Typically, colon cancer cells have point mutations in the K-*ras* gene. Also, allele deletion sites have been identified on chromosome 5, 17, and 18 that appear to be involved in malignant transformation of the colonic mucosa (Tabbarah, 1995). Alterations in the p53 gene occur frequently and can be detected in stool samples. The genes involved in colon cancer seem related to regulation of growth of cells and cell cycle.

Aging is associated with increased incidence, and there are several pathophysiologic mechanisms through which advancing age could exert an effect. It is possible that exposure time to carcinogens in food increases with age, or metabolism of carcinogens is altered with age. Cancer of the colon is associated with hyperproliferation, and a natural consequence of aging in the colonic mucosa is increased cell proliferation (Jaszewski et al., 1999).

Symptoms of colorectal cancer often are unremarkable until significant obstruction has occurred. The symptoms that occur also depend on the location of the lesion. There may be vague abdominal pain and anemia in right-sided colon cancer, but rarely is there obstruction. Cancer in the left side often results in constipation, tenesmus, paradoxical diarrhea, and hematochezia, (Chopra & Sugarman, 1990). Weight loss and anemia develop commonly. The most common early sign of colorectal cancer is blood in the

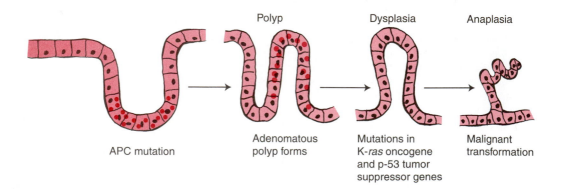

Polyp          Dysplasia          Anaplasia

APC mutation          Adenomatous polyp forms          Mutations in K-*ras* oncogene and p-53 tumor suppressor genes          Malignant transformation

**FIGURE 16.5**  ●  Sequence of changes leading to colorectal cancer.

stool. Another finding is the palpation of a mass on digital rectal probing. Diagnosis generally is made based on a colonoscopy and barium enema.

Colorectal carcinomas are staged according to the Dukes classification (Dukes, 1932). Patients with Dukes stage A have the most favorable prognosis; here, the lesion is in only mucosa and the lymph nodes are negative. Dukes $B_1$ has a 75% to 90% survival, the lesion extends through the muscularis mucosa but not into the serosa, and the nodes are negative. Dukes $B_2$ is when the tumor extends into the serosa with negative nodes. The 5-year survival is 40% to 70%. Dukes $C_1$ through D classifications all have positive nodes. Dukes $C_1$ is when the lesion is only in the bowel wall, whereas Dukes $C_2$ describes a lesion that extends into the serosa. Stage D is when there are distant metastases.

## Pathophysiologic Mechanisms and Prevention

Decreased fiber and increased fat are believed to be important risk factors for colorectal cancer. Fiber is thought to be protective because it dilutes carcinogens in the stool and accelerates stool transit through the colon, thus decreasing mucosal exposure to carcinogens. Wheat fibers may be fermented to short-chain fatty acids such as butyric acid, which may be anticarcinogenic. Broccoli, brussels sprouts, cabbage, and other members of the family Cruciferae also appear to provide anticarcinogenic chemicals in the colon. However, the role of fiber in colon cancer was recently questioned when results were published of a prospective study investigating the relationship between dietary fiber and colon cancer incidence in 88,757 women (Fuchs et al., 1999). These authors found no relationship between these two variables.

The relationship of high-fat diet to colon cancer may result from the effects of bile acids. When bile acids are degraded in the stool, they form products with carcinogenic potential.

A colon cancer–preventive diet is one in which whole grains and fiber are increased, meat and fat consumption is decreased, and foods containing antioxidant vitamins (vitamins A, E, and C) are added. This diet contains several servings a week of cruciferous vegetables and other food sources of anticarcinogens. Extra folate and calcium also is thought to be important because these chemicals may interfere with tumor growth and replication.

The observation that people taking aspirin and other NSAIDs on a regular basis appear to have a decreased incidence of colon cancer has led to several studies that will provide data for the practitioner about recommending a dose of aspirin to decrease risk in the susceptible person (Garay & Engstrom, 1999). The most important interventions by primary care providers to decrease the risk of colorectal cancer are increased screening and early detection.

## REFERENCES

Aabakken, L. (1999). Clinical symptoms, endoscopic findings and histologic features of gastroduodenal non-steroidal anti-inflammatory drugs lesions. *Italian Journal of Gastroenterology and Hepatology, 31,* (Suppl. 1), S19–S22.

Amann, S.T. & Cerda, J.J. (1995). A bleeding ulcer that just won't go away. *Patient Care, December,* 45–46.

Ament, P.W. & Childers, R.S. (1997). Prophylaxis and treatment of NSAID-induced gastropathy. *American Family Physician, 55,* 1323–1332.

Aronson, B. (1998). Update on peptic ulcer drugs. *American Journal of Nursing, 98,* 41–46.

Bandres, J. & Dupont, H. (1992). Approach to the patient with diarrhea. In S. Gorbach, J. Bartlett, & N. Blacklow (Eds.), *Infectious diseases.* Philadelphia: W.B. Saunders.

Barsky, A.J. & Borus, J.F. (1999). Functional somatic symptoms. *Annals of Internal Medicine, 130,* 910–921.

Blecker, U. (1997). *Helicobacter pylori*–associated gastroduodenal disease in childhood. *Southern Medical Journal, 90,* 570–576.

Borum, M. & Brooks, Q. (1997). Irritable bowel syndrome. In J. Johanson (Ed.), *Gastrointestinal diseases: Risk factors and prevention.* Philadelphia: Lippincott-Raven.

Brenner, H., Rothenbacher, D., Bode, G., & Adler, G. (1998). The individual and joint contributions of *Helicobacter pylori* infection and family history to the risk for peptic ulcer disease. *Journal of Infectious Diseases, 177,* 1124–1127.

Brucker, M.C. & Faucher, M.A. (1997). Pharmacologic management of common gastrointestinal health problems in women. *Journal of Nurse Midwifery, 42,* 145–162.

Cerda, J.J., Go, M.F., & Yamada, T. (1995). Peptic ulcer disease: Now you can cure. *Patient Care, December,* 100–117.

Chopra, S. & Sugarman, D. (1990). *Gastroenterology.* Montvale, New Jersey: Medical Economics Co.

Damianos, A.J. & McGarrity, T.J. (1997). Treatment strategies for *Helicobacter pylori* infection. *American Family Physician, 55,* 2765–2774.

De Nuntis, S., Bevilacqua, M., Forlini, G., & Rossi, Z. (1998). Pelvic floor dyssynergia: Videoproctographic analysis and pathologic associations in defecation obstruction syndrome. *Radiological Medicine, 96* (1-2), 73–80.

Delvaux, M.M. (1999). Stress and visceral perception. *Canadian Journal of Gastroenterology, 13* (Suppl. A), 32A–36A.

Dukes, C.E. (1932). The classification of cancer of the colon. *Journal of Pathology, 35,* 323.

Dunn, B. & Phadnis S.H. (1998). Structure, function and localization of *Helicobacter pylori* urease. *Yale Journal of Biology and Medicine, 71* (2), 63–73.

Dunn, B.E., Vakil, N.B., Schneider, B.G., et al. (1997). Localization of *Helicobacter pylori* urease and heat shock protein in human gastric biopsies. *Infections and Immunity, 65,* 1181–1188.

Eastwood, G.L. (1997). Is smoking still important in the pathogenesis of peptic ulcer disease? *Journal of Clinical Gastroenterology, 25* (Suppl. 1), S1–S7.

Evans, A. & Kaslow, R. (Eds.), *Humans* (4th ed.). New York: Plenum Book Co.

Everhart, J.E., Byrd-Holt, D., & Sonnenberg, A. (1998). Incidence and risk factors for self-reported peptic ulcer disease in the United States. *American Journal of Epidemiology, 147,* 529–536.

Fay, M. & Jaffe, P.E. (1996). Diagnostic and treatment guidelines for *Helicobacter pylori. Nurse Practitioner, 21,* 28–35.

Fendrick, A.M., Chernew, M.E., Hirth, R.A., & Bloom, B.S. (1996). Immediate endoscopy or initial *Helicobacter pylori* serological testing for suspected peptic ulcer disease: Estimating cost-effectiveness using decision analysis. *Yale Journal of Biology and Medicine, 69,* 187–195.

Fendrick, A.M., Chernew, M.E., Hirth, R.A., & Bloom, B.S. (1995). Alternative management strategies for patients with suspected peptic ulcer disease. *Annals of Internal Medicine, 123,* 260–268.

Fendrick, A.M., McCort, J.T., Chernew, M.E., Hirth, R.A., Patel, C., & Bloom, B.S. (1997). Immediate eradication of *Helicobacter pylori* in patients with previously documented peptic ulcer disease: Clinical and economic effects. *American Journal of Gastroenterology, 92,* 2017–2024.

Fuchs, C.S., Giovannucci, E.L., Colditz, G.A., Hunter, D.J., Stampfer, M.J., Rosner, B., Speizer, F.E., & Willett, W.C. (1999). Dietary fiber and the risk of colorectal cancer and adenoma in women. *New England Journal of Medicine, 340* (3), 169–176.

Garay, C.A. & Engstrom, P.F. (1999). Chemoprevention of colorectal cancer: Dietary and pharmacologic approaches. *Oncology, 1,* 89–105.

Griffin, M.R. (1998). Epidemiology of nonsteroidal anti-inflammatory drug-associated gastrointestinal injury. *American Journal of Medicine, 104,* 23S–29S.

Guyton, A.C. & Hall, J.E. (1997). *Human physiology and mechanisms of disease* (6th ed). Philadelphia: W.B. Saunders.

Hsu, H., Feinstone, S., & Hoofnagle, J. (1995). Acute viral hepatitis. In G. Mandell, J. Bennett, & R. Dolin (Eds.), *Principles and practices of infectious disease* (4th ed.). New York: Churchill Livingstone.

Huang, J.Q. & Hunt, R.H. (1996). pH, healing rate and symptom relief in acid-related diseases. *Yale Journal of Biology and Medicine, 69,* 59–174.

Jaszewski, R., Ehrinpreis, M.N., & Majumdar, A.P. (1999). Aging and cancer of the stomach and colon. *Frontiers in Bioscience, 4,* D322–D328.

Johanson, J. (1997). Constipation. In J. Johanson (Ed.), *Gastrointestinal diseases: Risk factors and prevention.* Philadelphia: Lippincott-Raven.

Laine, L.A. (1996). *Helicobacter pylori* and complicated ulcer disease. *American Journal of Medicine, 100,* 52S–59S.

Lehmann, F.S. & Stalder, G.A. (1998). Hypotheses on the role of cytokines in peptic ulcer disease. *European Journal of Clinical Investigation, 28,* 511–519.

Lembo, T., Naliboff, B., Munakata, J., Fullerton, S., Saba, L., Tung, S., Schmulson, M., & Mayer, E.A. (1999). Symptoms and visceral perception in patients with pain-predominant irritable bowel syndrome. *American Journal of Gastroenterology, 94* (5), 1320–1326.

Lieberman, D. (1997). Gastroesophageal reflux disease. In J. Johanson (Ed.), *Gastrointestinal diseases: Risk factors and prevention.* Philadelphia: Lippincott-Raven.

Locke, G.R., Talley, N.J., Fett, S.L., Zinsmeister, A.R., & Melton, L.J. (1999). Risk factors associated with symptoms of gastroesophageal reflux. *American Journal of Medicine 106* (6), 6426–6649.

MacLennan, W.J., Watt, B., & Elder, A.T. (1994). *Infections in elderly patients.* London: Edward Arnold.

Malfertheiner, P. & Labenz, J. (1998). Does *Helicobacter pylori* status affect nonsteroidal anti-inflammatory drug-associated gastroduodenal pathology? *American Journal of Medicine, 104,* 35S–42S.

Margolis, H., Alter, M., & Adler, S. (1997). Viral hepatitis. In A. Evans & R. Kaslow (Eds.), *Viral infections of humans.* (4th ed.). New York: Plenum Medical Book Co.

Mayer, E.A., Lembo, T., & Chang, L. (1999). Approaches to the modulation of abdominal pain. *Canadian Journal of Gastroenterology, 13* (Suppl. A), 65A–70A.

McPhee, S.J., Lingappa, V.R., Ganong, W.F., & Lange, J.D. (Eds.) (1998). *Pathophysiology of disease* (2nd ed.). Stamford, CT: Appleton & Lange.

National Digestive Diseases Information Clearinghouse. Gallstones. Available at: *http://www.niddk.nih.gov/health/diget/pubs/gallstns/gallstns.htm.*

Nelson, R.L., Persky, V., & Turyk, M. (1999). Determination of factors responsible for the declining incidence of colorectal cancer. *Diseases of the Colon and Rectum, 42* (6), 741–752.

NIH Consensus Development Panel on *Helicobacter pylori* in Peptic Ulcer Disease. (1994). *Helicobacter pylori* in peptic ulcer disease. *Journal of the American Medical Association, 272,* 65–68.

Parsonnet, J., Hansen, S., Rodriguez, L., et al. (1994). *Helicobacter pylori* infection and gastric lymphoma. *New England Journal of Medicine, 330,* 1267–1271.

Patino, J. & Quintero, G. (1998). Asymptomatic cholelithiasis revisited. *World Journal of Surgery, 22,* 1119–1124.

Peura, D.A. (1997). Ulcerogenesis: Integrating the roles of *Helicobacter pylori* and acid secretion in duodenal ulcer. *American Journal of Gastroenterology, 92,* 8S–16S.

Purcell, R. (1995). Hepatitis viruses: Changing patterns of human disease. In B. Roizman (Ed.), *Infectious diseases in an age of change.* Washington, DC: National Academy Press.

Quinn, P. (1997). Chronic liver disease. In J. Johanson (Ed.), *Gastrointestinal diseases: Risk factors and prevention.* Philadelphia: Lippincott-Raven.

Raeihae, I., Kemppainen, H., Kaprio, J., Koskenvuo, M., & Sourander, L. (1998). Lifestyle, stress, and genes in peptic ulcer disease. *Archives of Internal Medicine, 158,* 698–704.

Reese, R. & Betts, R. (1996). Acute viral hepatitis. In *A practical approach to infectious disease.* Philadelphia: Lippincott-Raven.

Reese, R. & Hruska, J. (1996). Gastrointestinal and intraabdominal infections. In *A practical approach to infectious disease.* Philadelphia: Lippincott-Raven.

Rosenstock, S., Kay, L., Rosenstock, C., Anderson, L.P., Bonnevie, O., & Jorgensen, T. (1997). Relation between *Helicobacter pylori* infection and gastrointestinal symptoms and syndromes. *Gut, 41,* 169–176.

Salcedo, J.A. & Al-Kawas, F. (1998). Treatment of *Helicobacter pylori* infection. *Archives of Internal Medicine, 158,* 842–851.

Sartor, R.B. (1997). Constipation. In L. Dorbrand, A. Hoole, & R. Fletcher (Eds.), *Manual of clinical problems in adult ambulatory care.* Philadelphia: Lippincott-Raven.

Sawada, M. & Dickinson, C.J. (1997). The G cell. *Annual Review of Physiology, 59,* 273–298.

Shubert, M.L. (1996). Pharmacotherapy for acid/peptic disorders. *Yale Journal of Biology and Medicine, 69,* 197–201.

Sleisenger, M.H. & Fordtran, J.S. (1997). *Gastrointestinal disease: Pathophysiology diagnosis treatment* (4th ed.). Philadelphia: W.B. Saunders.

Svanes, C., Soreide, J.A., Skarstein, A., et al. (1997). Smoking and ulcer perforation. *Gut, 41,* 177–180.

Tabbarah, H. (1995). Gastrointestinal cancers. In D. Casciato & B. Lowitz (Eds), *Manual of clinical oncology.* Philadelphia: Lippincott-Raven.

Thistle, J. (1998). Pathophysiology of bile duct stones. *World Journal of Surgery, 22,* 1114–1118.

Walker, M.M. & Crabtree, J.E. (1998). *Helicobacter pylori* infection and the pathogenesis of duodenal ulceration. *Annals of the New York Academy of Science, 859,* 96–111.

Walsh, J.H. & Dockray, G.H. (1994). *Gut peptides: Biochemistry and physiology.* New York: Raven Press Ltd.

Williams, C.N. (1998). Gastroesophageal reflux disease. *Canadian Journal of Gastroenterology, 12* (2), 107–108.

Yeomans, N.D. (1998). New data on healing of nonsteroidal anti-inflammatory drug-associated ulcers and erosions. *American Journal of Medicine, 104,* 56S–61S.

# Common Genitourinary Disorders

Leslie M. Klein

Ramona Scott

Maureen Groer

This chapter discusses some of the most common health problems involving the genitourinary system that are encountered in primary care. Depending on the age and gender of patients in the practice, these problems vary. Urinary tract infections are more common in female patients, whereas benign prostatic hypertrophy (BPH) is obviously a male disease. Sexually transmitted diseases (STDs) are confined to the sexually active population. Because urinary tract infections (UTIs) are the second most common infection in the US and occur in patients of both genders and all ages, the chapter begins with this subject.

## URINARY TRACT INFECTIONS

Urinary tract infections are considered either lower or upper infections, depending on the site. Lower UTIs are infections of the urethra and bladder, and in men, the prostate or epididymis, whereas upper UTIs involve the ureters and kidneys. Another type of classification is route of infection, with uncomplicated UTIs the result of an ascending infection common in sexually active female patients, with *Escherichia coli* the usual infecting organism. An additional characteristic is that these infections respond well to antibiotic therapy. Complicated UTIs often are associated with anatomic or neurologic abnormalities or urologic disease, or recent instrumentation or catheterization of the urinary tract. UTIs also are classified as to whether they are single episodes or are recurrent, which

means an individual has more than three to four infections per year.

Approximately 7 million UTIs occur each year in the United States (Hooton, 1999). In fact, UTIs are the most common bacterial infection occurring in a person's life span, with 43% of females and 12% of males experiencing at least one UTI (Kunin, 1987). There is therefore, particularly in young and middle adulthood, an increased incidence in females. Most UTIs are ascending infections of organisms normally confined to the gastrointestinal tract, so the most common microbe in both complicated and uncomplicated UTI is *E. coli* (60%), with *Enterobacter* and *Enterococcus*, two other colonic organisms, accounting for most of the remaining cases. In complicated UTIs, the range of organisms is wider, with both enteric organisms and *Klebsiella*, *Proteus*, and *Pseudomonas* capable of causing infection.

Because most UTIs that are diagnosed and managed in primary care are uncomplicated lower UTIs, this chapter focuses on the pathophysiology of this condition in detail. Lower UTIs can be either urethritis or cystitis, with one third of women with UTIs having urethritis. The symptoms of urethritis are characteristic of cystitis, but patients have pyuria without bacteriuria. The presentation of urethritis without cystitis should lead the clinician to suspect that the patient may have a STD. In men, chronic prostatitis is a major cause of cystitis and should be suspected in males with recurrent bladder infections.

The common symptoms of cystitis are dysuria, frequency, urgency, malodorous urine, nocturia, suprapubic pain, and fullness. The patient usually is afebrile and does not have systemic involvement in an uncomplicated lower UTI. The persons at highest risk are sexually active females (more than four sexual intercourse episodes per month) (Hooton, 1999), particularly those who use a diaphragm or spermicide, pregnant women, and women who do not urinate after intercourse. Other identified risk factors include ABO blood type and a history of recurrent UTIs. The presence of a short perineum also seems to be an independent risk factor, increasing the likelihood of coliform bacteria traversing the distance between the anus and the urethral meatus.

The risk for UTI is related to both microbial and host defense factors (Ward & Jones, 1996). The microbial factors include virulence, strain, organ specificity, and dose. Whereas many organisms infect the lower urinary tract, the number of microorganisms able to infect the renal parenchyma is limited. Host defenses along the entire urinary tract are important and probably eliminate one third of the potential infections. Thus, the presence of a UTI indicates that the host defenses have been overwhelmed. Urinary flow is a major defense in that ascending organisms are flushed through the tract and removed from the body. Bladder emptying is another consideration, since residual bacteria-containing urine allows for attachment of the bacteria to the bladder mucosa and establishment of bacterial growth. Any condition that impairs bladder emptying or causes retention increases the risk for infection.

Another anatomic defense is appreciated most in the male, in that a longer urethra is an obstacle to ascending infection, which accounts for the male protection from UTIs. The other important aspect of protection relates to the normal flora of the vagina, which is populated with lactobacilli. This flora is believed to compete with other potential pathogens and prevents them from colonizing. Any factor that alters the normally acid pH and normal flora composition of the vagina increases the risk of UTI. These factors include spermicidal creams and diaphragm use, which alters the flora and increases the potential for enteric microbial growth. The atrophic changes associated with low estrogen levels, as occur during the postmenopausal period, also alter the flora and increase risk for UTI in the older woman (Ward & Jones, 1996).

## Pathophysiologic Mechanisms

Lower UTIs tend to be superficial infections of the mucosa, whereas upper UTIs are deeper tissue infections. Lower UTI symptoms are associated with an acute inflammatory response. For the bladder to become colonized by coliform microorganisms, these microbes first must attach to the bladder epithelial cells. *E. coli* have fimbriae that are critical to the adhesion of the microbe to the epithelial cell. The molecule responsible for this is the fimH adhesin on the tips of fimbriae, which attaches to cellular mannose receptors on the superficial facet cells lining the mucosa of the bladder. After attachment, these cells undergo rapid apoptosis and slough off, exposing the underlying mucosal epithelium, leaving it susceptible to infection (Hultaren, 1999). Inflammatory mechanisms in the bladder mucosa initiate the release of cytokines and chemokines, which stimulate migration of macrophages, neutrophils, and lymphocytes, producing two effects: potential clearance of the infection, and the signs and symptoms of cystitis (Svanborg et al., 1999). These events are depicted in Figure 17-1. Cytokine release is a normal defense mechanism in the bladder, with interleukin (IL)-8 and transforming growth factor-beta (TGF-β) being constitutively expressed in bladder epithelium (Hang et al., 1998). When the bladder becomes invaded and infected with *E. coli*, IL-8 production increases and is chemotactic to neutrophils, which migrate from the blood into the bladder epithelium. Cytokines are released both by inflammatory cells and mucosal epithelial cells, causing the classic effects of an inflamma-

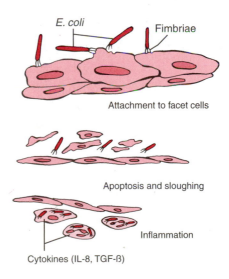

**FIGURE 17.1** ● Attachment of *E. coli* by fimbria to cell receptors initiates apoptosis of cells, which slough off the mucosa, leaving vulnerable cells and producing cytokine-mediated inflammatory and immune processes.

tory response, vasodilation, cellular infiltration, edema, and pain.

Recurrent UTIs are either reinfections with pathogenic enteric organisms or relapses because of partial, incomplete treatment of a preceding infection. Reinfection susceptibility, which usually occurs at least 2 weeks after a previous bladder infection, is an increased ability in susceptible individuals to allow *E. coli* adherence to bladder cells. Relapse usually occurs within 2 weeks of an infection. One possible factor for reinfection relates to antibiotic resistance, which has an increasing incidence. Amoxicillin resistance has increased from 29% to 36% from 1992 to 1996. The same pattern is observed for cephalothin and trimethoprim-sulfamethoxazole (TMP-SMZ) (Gupta et al., 1999). Relapse also is related to a nidus of chronic infection such as renal or prostate infection, or an underlying urologic problem such as a kidney calculi (Ward & Jones, 1996).

Upper UTIs develop because of infection ascending from the bladder through the ureters, although the origin can be hematogenous. Many indigent women with cystitis have concurrent "silent" pyelonephritis (Reller, 1999). Pyelonephritis is renal parenchymal infection that produces fever and chills, dysuria, frequency, pyuria, low back or flank pain, and costovertebral angle tenderness. Again, the causative organism usually is *E. coli*. However, some people with pyelonephritis have no characteristic flank pain or tenderness and often are assumed to have only cystitis. Another consideration is that diabetics with neuropathy may not have pain, even in acute infections. The systemic symptoms of fever and chills are important clues to the presence of bacteria and endotoxins in the blood originating from the infected kidney. A renal abscess can develop in pyelonephritis, causing the same symptoms, but these patients do not respond appropriately to the usual antibiotic therapy and continue to have symptoms after 2 to 3 days of antibiotics. Patients with pyelonephritis, depending on age, health status, and health history, may require hospitalization.

## Developmental Considerations

### Pregnancy

Pregnant women have an increased incidence of both lower and upper UTIs and asymptomatic bacteriuria. There also is an increased incidence in the postpartum period. Pregnancy results in dilation of the ureters and decreased muscle tone of the bladder, and the bladder's position in the pelvis changes to a more abdominal position (Reller,

1999). Significant changes also occur in immune function during pregnancy. The net effect of these hormone-related alterations is an increased risk for both lower and upper UTIs. Pregnant women usually are treated for a longer time (7 to 10 days) than nonpregnant women. If asymptomatic bacteriuria is not treated during pregnancy, nearly half of these women will develop pyelonephritis (Ward & Jones, 1996). Incidence of premature birth increases when women have upper UTIs that remain untreated, so the risk must be decreased by aggressively treating cystitis.

### The Elderly

The urologic problems of elderly persons require special consideration by the primary care provider. Postmenopausal women have an increased risk for UTIs, which is related to estrogen deficit, a risk that can be reduced by topical estrogen application. Estrogen allows lactobacilli to reestablish their dominance and inhibits enteric microorganism growth in the vagina (Raz & Stamm, 1993). Other problems of elderly women increase their propensity for UTIs, such as urinary retention, incontinence, history of UTIs, and previous gynecologic surgery. Elderly men have a higher incidence of UTIs because of prostate disease, which leads to urethral obstruction and urinary retention. The incidence of UTIs is equal when comparing men and women older than 65 years of age, and UTIs commonly are nosocomial (ie, from instrumentation, catheterization) in the elderly. Elderly men and women living in nursing homes and hospitalized elderly patients have an increased risk for UTIs.

The elderly also have an increased risk for asymptomatic bacteriuria (Reller, 1999). This is not treated routinely unless surgery is planned. The bacteriuria disappears and reappears without producing symptoms.

## Diagnosis of Urinary Tract Infection

A patient presenting with symptoms of a UTI requires a careful physical examination, since history alone is not enough to distinguish urethritis from cystitis or prostatitis. A urine sample is required to determine the presence of pyuria (leukocytes and cellular debris) and bacteriuria. The presence of 10 cells/mm$^3$ is considered sufficient to diagnose pyuria. Another common practice is to use the leukocyte esterase dipstick. Bacteriuria may be determined by microscopic examination of spun or unspun urine or a Gram's stain of a drop of unspun urine (Reller, 1999). If the urine is collected properly (midstream clean catch), it should be sterile in healthy persons. A urine culture is not always done in uncomplicated cystitis but is necessary when pyelonephritis is suspected or with complicated or recurrent UTIs.

## Physiologic Basis of Treatment

Guidelines for pharmacologic management of UTIs have been developed by the Infectious Disease Society of America (IDSA) (*http://www.idsociety.org*). One important consideration is the degree of antibiotic resistance in the population being treated by the provider. Resistance to TMP-SMZ is high in Europe and South America, but in the United States, it is low enough to consider this combination to be the standard protocol for acute, uncomplicated cystitis. (Most clinicians have no way of determining the prevalent resistance rates in their locale.) Although it is a popular clinical practice, the IDSA does not recommend single-dose therapy. Three-day therapy with TMP-SMZ usually is recommended. With recurrent cystitis, prophylactic postcoital and continuous TMP-SMZ therapy often is recommended. Women also have the option to self-diagnose and self-treat with antibiotics, which has been shown to be about 85% accurate and 95% effective (Hooton, 1999). For elderly women with cystitis, it is more common to treat with 7 to 14 days of therapy. Males with cystitis also usually require the 7- to 14-day regimen, and if recurrence is present, they need to be urologically evaluated for obstructive uropathy or prostatitis.

Treatment for pyelonephritis is more aggressive: the IDSA (1999) recommends antibiotic therapy for 7 to 14 days. The recommendation for the patient who has mild symptoms is outpatient observation for several hours with antibiotic (often parenteral) therapy, with either TMP-SMZ or a fluoroquinolone. Amoxicillin is added when Gram-positive cocci are seen in the urine. If the patient has a high fever and chills or is vomiting, or if the clinician is concerned about compliance with antibiotic therapy, the patient usually is hospitalized for parenteral therapy.

For the primary care provider, treatment of acute UTI should be accompanied by teaching, since these illnesses often are preventable. Instructions regarding signs and symptoms of UTI should be provided to every at-risk patient. Women should be advised to void before, and particularly after, intercourse. Postcoital antibiotics also are effective in recurrent UTIs. A bad habit of many women is to delay voiding, even in the presence of significant bladder fullness. This increases the contact time of bacteria in the bladder, thus increasing risk for infection. Increasing fluid intake, eating blueberries or cranberries, or drinking cranberry juice also may be helpful, since components in cranberry juice may inhibit the *E. coli* fimbriae adherence to the bladder epithelium. Cranactin tablet may be used instead of juice. The active ingredient in these berries are condensed tannins (proacanthocyanidins). The avoidance of spermicides and diaphragm use in a female patient who is susceptible to recurrent UTIs is another option. Estrogen creams can be effective in the postmenopausal woman who is not on hormone replacement therapy. Finally, basic hygienic practices with regard to cleanliness and wiping from front to back need reinforcement in even the most well-educated person.

## BENIGN PROSTATIC HYPERTROPHY

Benign prostatic hypertrophy is the most common neoplasm seen in aging men and plays a major role

---

### CLINICAL VIGNETTE 17.1

Kathy Holden is a 20-year-old college student who comes to the Student Health Services with complaints of bladder pressure, frequency, dysuria, and "smelly" dark urine of 1 day's duration. She is sexually active, with sexual intercourse "about twice a week" with the same partner. She is on birth control pills, and her partner does not wear a condom. Kathy reports having had bladder infections twice last year. Her vital signs are normal, and her physical examination reveals suprapubic pain, no costovertebral angle tenderness, and no lumbar pain. She does not have vaginal itchiness or discharge, and urethritis is not noted. Her urine sample indicates a positive esterase test, and more than 100,000 bacteria/mL under the oil immersion lens. Gram's stain indicates Gram-negative organisms. There also are red cells in the urine, which is malodorous.

Kathy is taught measures to decrease her risk for subsequent urinary tract infections (UTIs) and is given a 3-day course of Bactrim. Because she does not meet the criteria for recurrent UTIs, she is advised to practice preventive measures and to return to the clinic if her infection does not respond or if symptoms return in the next 2 weeks.

in disrupting the health and well-being of American men. Commonly defined as benign enlargement of the prostate gland, BPH accounts for over 4 million office visits annually and over 370,000 surgical procedures in the United States alone (Kerr, 1997). Although the number of prostatectomies performed for BPH has declined in the last 10 years, transurethral resection of the prostate (TURP) still is the second most common surgery, after cataract surgery, performed on men older than 60 years (Kirby et al., 1998). Clearly, BPH has a tremendous impact on health care costs in America.

## Epidemiology of Benign Prostatic Hypertrophy

Benign prostatic hypertrophy is defined histologically as prostatic cellular proliferation that can be detected clinically by digital rectal examination (DRE) or imaging studies (Kirby et al., 1998). Histologically, BPH affects more than 50% of men in their 50s and more than 80% of men in their 70s. By the ninth decade of life, nearly 100% of men show signs of histologic BPH, with more than 50% of those men developing symptoms of prostatism and requiring medical or surgical management (Kirby et al., 1998). With the US population living longer, the prevalence of BPH is expected to rise.

## Anatomy and Physiology of the Prostate

The prostate gland is a walnut-shaped fibromuscular organ surrounding the prostatic urethra through which urine passes. At birth, the prostate weighs 1 g but enlarges to approximately 20 to 25 g after the onset of puberty and remains at that weight unless BPH develops (McConnell, 1998). Growth of the prostate occurs from puberty until around age 30, at which time prostate growth stops and does not recur histologically until 50 to 60 years of age. The reason for this later-life growth spurt is a topic of debate.

The gland is composed of five distinct anatomic lobes: anterior, posterior, medial, and two lateral lobes. It is further classified into four zones, which are important to ultrasonic examination of the prostate. These include the peripheral, transitional, central, and preprostatic zones (Fig. 17-2). Benign prostatic hypertrophy most commonly occurs in the central and transitional zones, whereas prostate cancer usually is seen in the peripheral zone, the largest zone of the prostate. Cells within the prostate gland are predominantly fibromuscular stromal cells and glandular epithe-

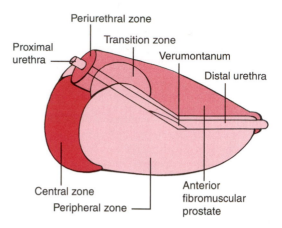

**FIGURE 17.2** ● Three-dimensional diagram showing the anatomical relationships of the zones of the prostate.

lial cells (Fig. 17-3). Cancer occurs within the stromal cells, whereas benign growth occurs in the epithelial cells. The main functions of the prostate gland are to nourish and alkalinize semen and to liquefy seminal coagulum. Proteins secreted by the gland to accomplish this function include prostatic acid phosphatase, prostate-specific antigen (PSA), prostate-specific protein, and beta microseminoprotein. PSA is a glycoprotein found exclusively in the epithelial cells of the prostate and is a widely used screening tool and tumor marker for prostate

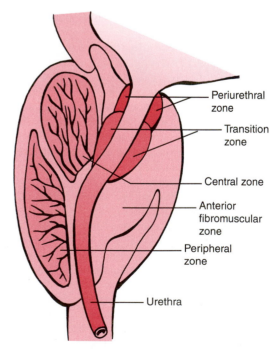

**FIGURE 17.3** ● Sagittal section through the prostate gland.

cancer. In addition, within the prostate, the enzyme 5 alpha-reductase converts testosterone to dihydrotestosterone, a highly potent androgen essential to the development of BPH.

## Etiology and Pathophysiology of Benign Prostatic Hypertrophy

Key factors in the development of BPH are the aging process and the presence of male androgens. BPH does not occur in adolescent or young men, or in men who have been castrated before puberty (McConnell, 1998). BPH occurs equally in men throughout the world without regard to race, with the exception of a low incidence in Japanese men who are thought to have a diet higher in estrogens. It has been shown that Japanese men who migrate to the United States develop BPH at a higher rate than those who remain in Asia, suggesting an environmental or dietary influence (Kirby & Christmas, 1993). There is little evidence to show that smoking, alcohol intake, or other associated disease processes are risk factors for development of BPH. Sexual activity is not believed to be influential in the development of BPH.

BPH has been shown to have a genetic component, probably because of an autosomal dominant gene. Studies show a strong correlation between men with a history of BPH and their first-degree relatives (McConnell, 1998). As many as 50% of men younger than 60 year of age who undergo prostatectomy for BPH have the familial type of the disease, whereas only 9% of those older than 60 may have the genetic form (McConnell, 1998). The gene responsible for familial BPH has not been discovered.

The pathogenesis of BPH is unclear, although the initiating event is thought to be localized proliferation of stromal cells (Steers, 1995). There are numerous theories explaining the basis for the disease, making its development a complex process.

Two theories are the most widely accepted to explain the development of BPH. These include the dihydrotestosterone (DHT) theory and the programmed cell death (apoptosis) theory. The prostate requires adequate levels of testosterone to grow. Circulating testosterone is converted to DHT within the prostate under the influence of 5 alpha-reductase. Then, DHT binds to androgen receptors in a paracrine manner in the epithelial cells of the prostate, resulting in tissue growth. Originally, it was believed that excessive levels of DHT in the prostate caused overgrowth, but this has not been proven. Studies show that DHT levels are the same in hyperplastic glands, as well as normal prostate glands (McPhee et al., 1997).

DHT levels and androgen receptor sites remain high throughout the aging process, therefore, androgen-dependent cell growth continues.

Five alpha-reductase is the enzyme responsible for conversion of testosterone to DHT. Two distinct types of 5 alpha-reductase have been discovered. Type I, found in the skin and liver plays little, if any, role in prostatic function. However, type II 5 alpha-reductase, the predominant prostatic enzyme, is essential for normal growth of the prostate as well as hyperplastic growth. The type II enzyme is secreted primarily by the stromal cells. The role of finasteride (Proscar) and its effect on 5 alpha-reductase inhibition is discussed later.

Apoptosis, or cell death, is a normal physiologic occurrence. Apoptotic cells are phagocytosed by enzymes and other cells, without influence of inflammatory or immune activation. Apoptosis is balanced by growth-promoting events in the normal prostate gland. Numerous growth factors have been found in normal and hyperplastic prostate glands, including TGF, fibroblastic growth factor, and epidermal growth factor. Growth inhibitors also are present in prostate tissue. The balance between these growth factors and growth inhibitors prevents or induces cell proliferation and prevents cell death. Also, the influence of androgens on growth factors may disturb the balance between cell proliferation and cell death.

Another theory explaining the evolution of BPH is the stromal-epithelial interaction theory, or the epithelial reawakening theory. Stromal cells are believed to stimulate epithelial cells to grow, possibly through the influence of androgens and androgen-dependent stromal cells.

Last, the estrogen-testosterone imbalance theory implies that with aging, estrogen and estradiol levels in the plasma increase, whereas circulating testosterone levels decrease, resulting in stromal overgrowth from a higher level of hormone receptors in stromal versus epithelial tissue (Kirby et al., 1998).

Many of the symptoms of BPH are brought on by obstruction or bladder instability, which occurs partly from the aging process. Obstruction by the prostate results in increased pressure within the bladder itself and a reduction in the flow of urine. Obstruction and increased bladder pressures result in changes in the bladder muscle (detrusor muscle) and in bladder function. Initially, the bladder hypertrophies and detrusor pressure increases as a compensatory measure to maintain urine flow. With prolonged obstruction, bladder compliance decreases and emptying is impaired. At this point, urinary retention may occur, either because of bladder decompensation or increased obstruction. Because of bladder decompensation, one third of men who undergo surgical correction of obstruction continue to have significant voiding problems. Visualization of the bladder cystoscopically in a patient with obstructive symptoms clearly shows changes in the bladder surface known as trabeculation. These changes appear as irregular thickening of the bladder lining and the appearance of a "moon surface," indications of muscle hypertrophy secondary to outflow obstruction and detrusor instability.

Other mechanisms that may cause bladder obstruction include decreased contractility of prostate smooth muscle, obstruction resulting from envelopment of the prostatic urethra by enlarged tissue, or median lobe enlargement, which obstructs the bladder neck.

## Pathology of Benign Prostatic Hypertrophy

On gross inspection of a prostate specimen, BPH appears as nodules that may be soft or firm and range from yellow to gray. There also may be evidence of calcification or infarction. Nodules are most commonly seen in the transitional zone but may be present in the periurethral area of the gland. Nodules that protrude into the bladder are referred to as median lobe hyperplasia.

Microscopically, the cells found in BPH nodules are hyperplastic, or increased in cell number.

Most cells examined are epithelial or glandular, with individual cells displaying hypertrophy.

## Symptoms of Benign Prostatic Hypertrophy

Symptoms of BPH are classified as either obstructive or irritative, and they may occur simultaneously. Figure 17-4 illustrates the anatomic position of the prostate in relation to the urologic system. Obstructive symptoms are a result of overgrowth of prostatic tissue, as well as compensatory bladder changes and detrusor instability. These symptoms include impaired urinary stream, hesitancy of urination, a sense of incomplete bladder emptying, and terminal dribbling. Irritative symptoms have a more complex basis. Interference in the muscular sphincter function and instability of the bladder muscle occur as a result of changes in the smooth muscle function of the prostate. Symptoms associated with bladder instability include frequency, urgency, urge incontinence, and nocturia (BPH Guideline Panel, 1994a). Obstructive symptoms occur as a result of impaired distensibility of the prostatic urethra, whereas irritative symptoms occur when there is decreased bladder compliance and instability of the detrusor muscle.

Remember that voiding symptoms of frequency, urgency, and nocturia are likely to send a patient to the provider, but differential diagnosis may include conditions unrelated to BPH. Differential diagnosis should include UTI, urethral stric-

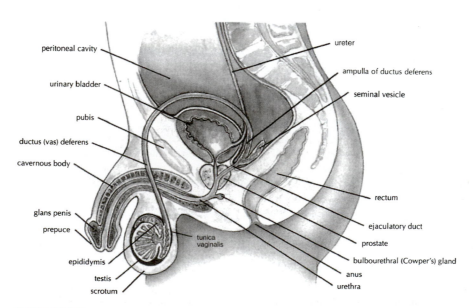

*FIGURE 17.4* ● Location of the prostate gland in relationship to the male urogenital system.

ture, bladder calculi, bladder diverticula, prostatitis, neurogenic bladder, bladder cancer, and prostate cancer. Other possibilities to be considered include diabetes mellitus, cerebral vascular accident, or effects of medications, in particular, anticholinergic medications (Roberts, 1994).

Correlation between prostate size and symptomatology does not always exist.

Mild enlargement of the gland may result in a variety of voiding symptoms, whereas larger gland size may produce only minimal disturbance to a patient's typical voiding pattern. Some men may have few symptoms until they experience an episode of acute urinary retention.

## Complications of Benign Prostatic Hypertrophy

The sequelae of untreated BPH can be serious and potentially irreversible. These complications include urinary retention, bladder decompensation with hypertrophy and trabeculation, bladder diverticula, hydroureter or hydronephrosis, and acute renal failure. Bladder decompensation may be a long-term complication of untreated BPH, even after obstruction is relieved. Additionally, chronic UTI or bladder calculi may result from urinary stasis. The challenge is to determine which patients require treatment and which can be managed with watchful waiting.

Benign prostatic hypertrophy primarily is a quality of life issue. Symptoms may be merely bothersome or may significantly interfere with the patient's lifestyle. The patient and his spouse should be included in determining the need for and the type of treatment.

## Prostate-Specific Antigen Screening

Prostate-specific antigen is a glycoprotein produced by the epithelial cells of the prostate. It is present in both benign and malignant diseases of the prostate. Prostate-specific antigen first was discovered in prostate tissue in 1970 and was able to be measured in the serum in the 1980s (Partin & Coffey, 1998). Serum PSA has become a commonly used tool in screening for prostate cancer and is used as a tumor marker to manage the course of the disease. A Canadian study claims a 69% reduction in prostate cancer mortality in men who are screened yearly (Bankhead, 1998).

Since the initial discovery of serum PSA testing, many improvements have been made in the accuracy rate, and although PSA is not a perfect test, it is a reliable indicator for recognizing who should be evaluated for prostate cancer. PSA lev-

els can be elevated in conditions other than prostate cancer, including BPH, acute and chronic prostatitis, and prostate infarction (Monte & Meyers, 1997). It remains controversial whether significant elevations occur in relation to routine rectal examination or recent ejaculation.

In the past, the universal normal range for PSA has been 0 to 4.0 ng/mL, although this may not be an accurate range for all men, since age and variations in prostate size are not taken into account. It is now known that PSA values increase with age; therefore, a broader range of normal values is being used. Table 17-1 shows reference ranges for age-specific PSA.

Another predictor of prostate cancer is PSA velocity. This tracks changes in PSA levels over a one 1- to 2-year period and is a valuable means of differentiating BPH from prostate cancer in patients with normal PSA values. A rise in the PSA level of more than 0.75 ng/mL/year is suggestive of prostate cancer (Carter et al., 1992). In studies, however, PSA values show variations of 8% to 16%, making a 0.75 increase a refutable value.

An even newer PSA assay, known as percent free PSA, has been found to be the most clinically useful parameter for distinguishing BPH from early, curable prostate cancer. PSA is present in the serum in two clinically important molecular forms: free PSA (unbound) and complexed PSA. Percent free PSA measures unbound PSA and is best used clinically for men with PSA levels in the "reflex range" of 3 to 10 ng/mL. In the reflex range, specificity of the PSA test is enhanced by 25% to 30% without compromising sensitivity (Vashi et al., 1997).

Guidelines for PSA screening, as recommended by the American Urologic Association (AUA), are yearly PSA screening and DRE beginning at age

---

## TABLE 17.1

### Reference Ranges for Age-Specific Prostate-Specific Antigen

| Age | PSA Upper Limit (ng/mL) |
|---|---|
| 40–49 | 2.5 |
| 50–59 | 3.5 |
| 60–69 | 4.5 |
| 70–79 | 6.5 |

PSA, prostate-specific antigen.

50, or at age 40 in African-American men or men with a family history of prostate cancer (BPH Guideline Panel, 1994b).

## Diagnosis

Voiding symptoms may be the initial reason for a patient to seek care from a health care provider, but these symptoms may result from multiple problems other than BPH. The challenge to the primary care provider is to establish that the symptoms result from BPH.

On initial evaluation, a complete history, including urologic history, must be obtained. The history must include other concurrent disease processes such as diabetes, neurologic disorders, cerebrovascular accident (CVA), or lumbar disc problems. In the urologic history, it is essential to include symptoms of UTI, stricture disease, calculus disease, hematuria, or recent instrumentation. A complete list of medications must be obtained, particularly antihistamines and drugs that affect bladder contractility.

Physical examination must include DRE, abdominal examination, genital examination, and focused neurologic examination. Abdominal examination may reveal bladder distention, in which case, a postvoid residual measurement would be necessary, either by catheterization or ultrasonic study. Rectal examination should note rectal tone and any irregularity, nodularity, or induration of the prostate gland. Examination of the penis should be done to rule out meatal stenosis, penile discharge, or penile mass as a cause of the patient's voiding symptoms. Neurologic examination should include anal sphincteric tone, reflexes, sensation, and weakness of the legs associated with lumbar disc disease or neurologic disorders such as multiple sclerosis or Parkinson's disease.

Laboratory studies routinely include urinalysis to rule out microscopic hematuria or other signs of UTI. The presence of hematuria warrants a cytologic study to exclude malignancy. Referral to a urologist for upper tract studies and cystoscopy is indicated in patients with hematuria of unknown cause. Measurement of serum blood urea nitrogen and creatinine should be performed routinely in patients with symptoms of prostatism to rule out renal insufficiency. Renal ultrasound must be performed to evaluate the upper tracts in any patient with BPH and an elevated creatinine level. The PSA value must be obtained, along with rectal examination, for early detection of prostate cancer.

An important tool used in the evaluation of symptoms in a patient with BPH or symptoms of prostatism is the AUA Symptom Index. This seven-item questionnaire rates the severity of the patient's perception of his symptoms and is useful in the management of BPH. The Symptom Index can be repeated periodically to evaluate treatment effectiveness (Table 17-2).

Other optional studies may include uroflow rate, pressure flow studies, ultrasonic post-void residual (PVR), and urethrocystoscopy. These would be the most helpful in patients who may require surgical management.

## Physiologic Basis of Treatment

The severity of the patient's symptoms helps to determine the type of treatment necessary. Patients who are asymptomatic may require no treatment until symptoms arise. Patients with a history of acute urinary retention or other complications may be optimal surgical candidates. For most other patients, either "watchful waiting" or medical management will be the treatment of choice.

Watchful waiting is an appropriate option for many men with BPH, particularly those with an AUA symptom score of less than 7. These patients should be monitored at least yearly to reassess the symptom score and results of DRE and laboratory studies.

Patients with severe symptoms or symptom scores higher than 20 should be referred to a urologist for probable surgical management. Although TURP still is the gold standard of surgical treatment for BPH, many new and less-invasive procedures are available. These include interstitial laser therapy, transurethral incision of the prostate, transurethral laser incision of the prostate, transurethral needle ablation, balloon dilatation, and visual laser ablation of the prostate. Open prostatectomy is indicated for extremely large prostates weighing more than 50 g (Roberts, 1994). Surgical therapy of any type offers the best chance of symptom resolution.

Medical therapy is indicated for patients with mild, moderate, or severe symptoms. Alpha blockers (doxazosin, terazosin, prazosin, and tamsulosin) improve voiding symptoms in 59% to 86% of men by relaxing smooth muscle cells of the prostate and bladder neck (Table 17-3) (BPH Guideline Panel, 1994b). Side effects may include orthostatic hypotension, dizziness, malaise, and nasal stuffiness. Dosage titration is necessary when treatment is begun with all alpha blockers except tamsulosin, because it has no antihypertensive effects. Most men report improvement of symptoms, however, within 1 to 2 weeks. The PSA levels are not affected by using alpha blockers.

Finasteride (Proscar) is a 5 alpha-reductase inhibitor that lowers DHT levels in the prostate by blocking conversion of testosterone to DHT.

**TABLE 17.2** ● ● ●

## Urinary Activities Questionnaire

| | Not at All | Less Than 1 Time in 5 | Less Than Half the Time | About Half the Time | More Than Half the Time | Almost Always |
|---|---|---|---|---|---|---|
| 1. Over the past month or so, how often have you had a sensation of not emptying your bladder completely after you finished urination? | | | | | | |
| 2. Over the past month or so, how often have you had to urinate again less than 2 hours after you finished urinating? | | | | | | |
| 3. Over the past month or so, how often have you found that you stopped and started again several times during urination? | | | | | | |
| 4. Over the past month or so, how often have you found it difficult to postpone urination? | | | | | | |
| 5. Over the past month or so, how often have you had a weak urinary stream? | | | | | | |
| 6. Over the past month or so, how often have you had to push or strain to begin urination? | | | | | | |
| 7. Over the last month, how many times did you most typically get up to urinate from the time you went to bed at night until the time you got up in the the morning? | | | | | | |

(From Barry, M.J., Fowler, F.J. Jr., O'Leary, M.P., et al. 1992. The American Urological Association Symptom Index for benign prostatic hyperplasia. *Journal of Urology, 148*, 1549–1557.)

Its onset of action is slower, with at least 6 months of therapy required before benefits are seen. Finasteride has been shown to reduce prostate size by 20% to 50% within 1 year of treatment (Calciano et al., 1993). Side effects are minimal but include sexual dysfunction and decreased libido. The PSA levels are lowered by as much as 50% in patients taking finasteride. On discontinuance of the drug, symptoms typically return to baseline levels.

Alternative medical therapies have been instituted by some clinicians when treating BPH and prostatism; however, their efficacy is not well documented. The most frequently used of the natural products are saw palmetto, pollen extract, and echinacea. Some studies fail to demonstrate

## TABLE 17.3

### Drugs Used to Treat Benign Prostatic Hyperplasia

#### Dosage of Alpha Blockers

Prazosin 1, 2, or 5 mg BID

Doxazosin 1, 2, 4, or 8 mg QHS

Terazosin 1, 2, or 5 mg QHS

Tamsulosin 0.4 mg after evening meal

*Dosage of 5 Alpha-Reductase Inhibitors*

Finasteride 5 mg QD

BID, twice daily; QD, every day; QHS, every day at bedtime.

an inhibitory action of 5 alpha-reductase, decreased prostate size, or reduction of PSA value. Permixon, a natural agent widely used in Europe but not available in the United States, works similarly to finasteride by blocking 5 alpha-reductase in the prostate (Gray & Allensworth, 1997). Possible mechanisms of action of the natural therapies include an antiestrogen effect, an antiandrogen effect, inhibition of growth factors, and an overall anti-inflammatory effect (Kirby et al., 1998).

## Summary

Benign prostatic hypertrophy is a common medical problem for aging men. Symptoms typically progress over time, and the risk of complications rises. Intervention most likely will be necessary in most men. Symptom severity is highly subjective among men with BPH; therefore, the patient should be included in treatment decisions.

It is the responsibility of the clinician to provide the patient with information about management options and the corresponding associated risks. Patient preference plays an important role in choosing appropriate therapy.

### ● Case Study 17.1

Mr. Ted Gentile, a 62-year-old African-American male, presents to the clinic with complaints of "urinary trouble." He describes a 1-year history of increasing urinary frequency, nocturia × 3 to 4, hesitancy in starting his stream, decreased force of stream, and a sense of urgency. He denies dysuria or hematuria. He is unsure whether he empties his bladder completely. He denies any history of urinary tract infection, genitourinary trauma, recent instrumentation such as catheterization or cystoscopy, and ever having any known STD. Mr. Gentile states that his symptoms are disruptive to his lifestyle, particularly his sleep patterns. He has not seen a health care provider in approximately 3 years and has not had a digital rectal exam in "a few years."

### History

#### Past Medical History

| | |
|---|---|
| Allergies | Allergic to penicillin and sulfa drugs |
| Current medications | Takes occasional aspirin for "arthritis." Was on antihypertensives in the past but stopped them 3 years ago for sexual dysfunction. Occasionally takes Maalox for "upset stomach" |
| Illnesses | Includes hypertension, for which he was on medications, but stopped them on his own 3 years ago because of sexual dysfunction. Also includes history of an ulcer, with no recent exacerbation |
| Surgeries | Includes a cholecystectomy, appendectomy, and ankle surgery for a fractured ankle<br>No history of heart disease, diabetes, or stroke |

*(Case study continued on next page)*

### Family History

| | |
|---|---|
| Father | Died of prostate cancer at age 70, HTN |
| Mother | Died of heart disease at age 67, HTN |
| Brother | Age 60, has diabetes, hypertension, and "prostate trouble" |

### Social History

| | |
|---|---|
| Married | 41 years, has a son and a daughter |
| Employment | Postal worker supervisor; states that his job is "very stressful." He is active in his church. |
| Tobacco | Started smoking at age 17 and smoked 1½ ppd for 30 years, quit approximately 15 years ago |
| Alcohol | Drinks 4–6 beers on the weekend |
| Exercise | Relaxes with walking, occasional swimming, and reading |
| Sexual history | Patient is potent but experienced impotency while on BP medications in the past. He is happily married in a monogamous relationship. He denies any history of STDs |

### Dietary History

States that he eats "too much." He does not follow any particular diet but avoids salt because of his blood pressure

## Review of Systems

| | |
|---|---|
| General | Weight has been stable over the past few years. States his appetite is good. Denies fatigue, malaise, fever or night sweats. He feels that he is in overall good health |
| Skin | No history of skin diseases, rashes, pruritis, or skin lesions |
| HEENT | Denies headache, vertigo, or syncope. No difficulty with vision, although vision is corrected to 20/20. Last eye examination was 2 years ago. No earaches, tinnitus, or drainage from ears |
| | States that he does have "hay fever" symptoms in the spring, for which he takes OTC decongestant/antihistamines. No difficulty swallowing, sore throat, or hoarseness |
| Neck | No history of thyroid disease or goiter. No limitations of movement |
| Respiratory | Quit smoking 15 years ago. Denies SOB, chronic cough, or asthma. No other history of lung disease. Last CXR was 3 years ago |
| CV | No history of heart murmur, chest pain, or palpitations. Hypertension diagnosed 3 years ago but patient discontinued antihypertensives on his own. Last ECG was done 3 years ago at the time of his physical. Has never had a 2-D echocardiogram |
| GI | Long history of dyspepsia and was diagnosed with an ulcer many years ago. Denies dysphagia, pyrosis, or nausea. Bowel movements are regular with no significant diarrhea or constipation. No history of rectal bleeding. Gallbladder was removed over 20 years ago |

*(Case study continued on page 342)*

| GU | States his voiding problems began 1 year ago and have worsened in severity over the last 2 or 3 months. Describes frequency, urgency, nocturia × 3–4, hesitancy, and slow stream. No history of prostatitis, UTI, or STD. No history of kidney stones. Denies penile discharge, testicular pain, or inguinal hernia. He does not perform self-testicular examination on a regular basis |
| MS | Fractured ankle playing sports many years ago, for which he underwent surgery. States he has "arthritis" in his knees, hands, and shoulders, for which he takes aspirin occasionally |
| Neurologic | No history of seizures, stroke, or syncope. No numbness or tingling of extremities. Denies mental status changes |
| Hematologic | Never had a tendency toward bleeding or excessive bruising. Has never received a blood transfusion |

## Physical Examination

| System | Findings |
| --- | --- |
| Vital signs | T-98.2°F P-80 R-20 BP-170/96 Height = 5'11", Weight = 179 lb |
| General | Well-developed, well-nourished black male in no acute distress. Appears younger than stated age |
| HEENT | Normocephalic. Wears glasses. PERRLA. TMs clear bilaterally without erythema or fluid. Nares patent bilaterally. Throat clear |
| Neck | Supple with no palpable nodes |
| Heart | Regular sinus rhythm. PMI @ 5th ICS midaxillary line. No murmur, thrill, or gallop appreciated |
| Lungs | Clear to auscultation, bilaterally. Breath sounds equal |
| Abdomen | Soft, nontender. Bowel sounds present in all quadrants. Old, well-healed surgical scars present. Bladder nontender and nonpalpable |
| Genitalia | Normal, circumcised male. Testes palpable bilaterally, nontender, and without masses. No penile discharge present |
| Rectal | Normal rectal tone. No masses noted. Prostate smooth, nontender, and symmetrically enlarged without palpable nodularity |
| Extremities | No cyanosis, clubbing, or edema. Pedal pulses 2+ bilaterally |
| Neurologic | Cerebellar function intact. Grips equal bilaterally and DTRs 2+ bilaterally in all extremities |
| GU | Patient was asked to complete an AUA symptom index to evaluate his urinary symptoms, with a score of 17 (moderate). A postvoid residual of 175 mL was obtained by urethral catheterization |

## Laboratory Studies

| Test | Result |
| --- | --- |
| 1. Urinalysis | WNL, no hematuria or pyuria present |
| 2. BUN | 20 |

*(Case study continued on next page)*

3. Creatinine          1.7
4. PSA                Results pending

### Differential Diagnosis

1. Benign prostatic hypertrophy
2. Prostate cancer (positive family history), PSA pending
3. Prostatitis
4. UTI
5. Bladder calculus
6. Urethral stricture
7. Hypertension, BP elevated today, history of hypertension in the past

### Impression

1. BPH vs prostate cancer. Will await results of PSA. DRE reveals enlarged prostate but not suspicious of cancer
2. Probable hypertension
3. Osteoarthritis
4. History of PUD

### Plan

1. Will initiate Hytrin therapy to see if voiding symptoms improve and to lower BP. Begin with 1 mg QHS × 3 days, then increase to 2 mg QHS. May require titration to 5 mg
2. Will await PSA result. If elevated, may refer to urologist for possible prostate ultrasound
3. Moniter BP. May require additional therapy if remains elevated
4. Acetaminophen for arthritis pain in view of ulcer history
5. Counseled patient on avoidance of antihistamines because of potential for urinary retention

AUA, American Urologic Association; BP, blood pressure; BUN, blood urea nitrogen; CV, cardiovascular; CXR, chest x-ray; 2-D, two-dimensional; DRE, digital rectal examination; DTRs, deep tendon reflexes; ECG, electrocardiogram; GI, gastrointestinal, GU, genitourinary; HEENT, head, eyes, ears, nose, and throat; HTN, hypertension; ICS, intercostal space; MS, musculoskeletal; OTC, over-the-counter; PERRLA, pupils equal, round, regular to light accommodation; PMI, point of maximal impulse; PSA, prostate-specific antigen; PUD, peptic ulcer disease; QHS, every day at bedtime; SOB, shortness of breath; STD, sexually transmitted disease; TMs, tympanic membranes; UTI, urinary tract infection.

## SEXUALLY TRANSMITTED DISEASES

Among all of the pathogens known to infect humans, those causing STDs present the more challenging cases for the primary care provider. Some of the STDs can be diagnostic puzzles, but all challenge the psychosocial and, occasionally, ethical or moral aspects of primary care. The following sections of this chapter include descriptions and discussions of the major STDs, as well as vaginitis.

## Types and Terminology

Many different pathogens are sexually transmissible, even when the usual route of infection is non-sexual. An example is cytomegalovirus infection. Other diseases, such as herpes simplex type 1, usually occur as a STD, with the exception of a congenitally acquired disease. Table 17-4 lists distinctive sexually transmissible pathogens. Because it is beyond the scope of this chapter to discuss each pathogen, here the practitioner is provided with an understanding of the most common STDs and

## TABLE 17.4

### Most Common Sexually Transmissible Pathogens

| Bacteria | Viruses | Protozoans and Fungi | Ectoparasites |
|---|---|---|---|
| *Neisseria gonorrhoeae* | Human immuno-deficiency virus (HIV) | *Trichomonas vaginalis* | *Pthirus pubis* |
| *Chlamydia trachomatis* | Herpes simplex virus | *Entamoeba histolytica* | *Sarcoptes scabiei* |
| *Mycoplasma hominis* | Human papillomavirus | *Giardia lamblia* | |
| *Mycoplasma urealyticum* | Hepatitis A, B, and C | *Candida albicans* | |
| *Treponema pallidum* | Cytomegalovirus | | |
| *Gardnerella vaginalis* | Molluscum contagiosum | | |
| *Mobiluncus cinaedi* and *Mobiluncus fenneliae* | | | |

vaginitis, the causative pathogens, and diagnosis and treatment.

### Chlamydia Trachomatis

Chlamydiae are widespread, pathogenic organisms well adapted for persistence and survival. These microbes are infectious, easily transmissible, and adept at escaping normal host immune mechanisms (Manire & Wyrick, 1986). The genus *Chlamydia* (from the Greek word for cloak) has four species, *C. psittaci*, *C. pecorum*, *C. pneumoniae*, and *C. trachomatis*, with the latter two able to infect humans. With regard to STD, *C. trachomatis* can cause several different diseases, depending on which biovar of the organism is present and which host cell it infects.

The *Chlamydia* genus is unique among bacteria primarily because of its peculiar growth cycle, which forces it to be an intracellular obligate parasite. *C. trachomatis* has the following features: (1) DNA and RNA, (2) a continuous cell envelope similar to Gram-negative bacteria, (3) prokaryotic ribosomes and synthesis of its own proteins and nucleic acids, (4) a limited number of metabolic systems, and (5) susceptibility to a wide range of antibiotics. The host cell, however, provides the necessary adenosine triphosphate for full functioning (Braude, 1986).

### Growth Cycle of *Chlamydia*

Figure 17-5 illustrates the unique growth cycle of *Chlamydia*. The cycle contains five basic elements involving two major developmental

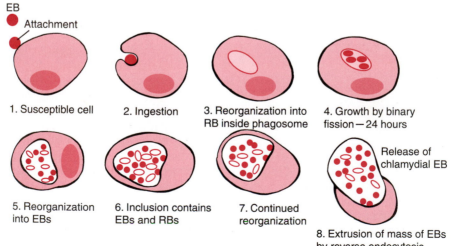

1. Susceptible cell
2. Ingestion
3. Reorganization into RB inside phagosome
4. Growth by binary fission—24 hours
5. Reorganization into EBs
6. Inclusion contains EBs and RBs
7. Continued reorganization
8. Extrusion of mass of EBs by reverse endocytosis

Release of chlamydial EB

EB
Attachment

**FIGURE 17.5**  ●  The growth cycle of *C. trachomatis*.

forms: the elementary body (EB) and the reticulate body (RB). The elementary body is small (350 nm in diameter) with an electron-dense center and is adapted to the extracellular environment. The RBs are larger (1 μm in diameter) with flexible cell walls, and they cannot survive outside of the host. The growth cycle steps are described as follows:

1. The EB attaches to the host cell using a mechanism that has not been fully understood but may involve microvillus projections.
2. The EB then is ingested into the host cell by phagocytosis into an endosomal vacuole.
3. Morphologic change of the EB into the RB begins within 6 to 8 hours after entering the cell—another process not well understood.
4. In the fourth stage of the cycle, maturation and differentiation of the RBs occur. From 8 to 24 hours after entry into the host cell, the RBs replicate by binary fission, after which some reorganize into infectious EBs.
5. Finally, the host cell becomes so damaged and depleted that it ruptures, releasing EBs.

### Epidemiology

Chlamydial infections have been reported worldwide. In the United States, *C. trachomatis* is the most common reportable STD, with 4 to 5 million new cases per year at a cost of $2 to $4 billion (Centers for Disease Control [CDC], 1997). The success of *C. trachomatis* as a pathogen may be linked to the fact that it has 18 major serovars, accounting for several diseases (Schachter, 1999). Although most of these diseases are sexually transmitted, trachoma and congenital infection are exceptions.

### Pathophysiology

The pathogenesis of chlamydial infections has not been fully explained, but the immune response of the host may hold the key to understanding the diseases produced by *Chlamydia*. Depending on which serovars are involved, *C. trachomatis* may involve lymphoid tissues or squamocolumnar-columnar epithelial cells. An inflammatory response is characterized by numerous and varied types of inflammatory cells into the affected tissues. Polymorphonuclear leukocytes (PMNs) are the predominant cells in the acute stage of infection, whereas lymphocytes dominate in subacute and chronic stages of disease. The current theory of chlamydial disease involves specific heat-shock proteins (HSP6O), which produce hypersensitivity responses in the host. The fact that women with tubal-factor infertility secondary to *C. trachomatis* infections have increased levels of antibody to *Chlamydia* HSP6O lends significant credibility to this theory (Toye et al., 1993).

### Clinical Manifestations

*Infections in Men.* *C. trachomatis* is a major cause of nongonococcal urethritis (NGU) and postgonococcal urethritis in 30% to 50% of cases in heterosexual men (Braude et al., 1986). Symptoms include burning and stinging with micturition and a clear-to-milky urethral discharge. Although less common, proctitis and epididymitis attributable to *C. trachomatis* have been reported (Palella & Murphy, 1997).

*Infections in Women.* In women, mucopurulent cervicitis is the most common manifestation of *C. trachomatis* infection. Most women are asymptomatic, however, and the astute practitioner must have a high index of suspicion in the young, sexually active population. Careful inspection of *cervical*, not vaginal mucus, revealing greater than 30 PMNs per high power field is strongly suggestive of chlamydial infection. The most serious sequelae of *C. trachomatis* infection in women is pelvic inflammatory disease (PID), with an incidence of up to 40% causing infertility in up to 20% secondary to salpingitis (Palella & Murphy, 1997). Other infections in women include bartholinitis, urethritis, and endometritis. *C. trachomatis* also may be responsible for some cases of preterm labor.

### Other Chlamydial Infections

Reiter's syndrome occurs mostly in men and is a triad of urethritis, conjunctivitis, and arthritis. It also may have characteristic mucocutaneous lesions. Interestingly, 60% to 70% of those with Reiter's syndrome are positive for the HLA-B27 haplotype (Keat et al., 1978).

Fitz-Hugh-Curtis syndrome is an inflammation of the liver capsule, not the parenchyma proper. Thus, it is referred to as perihepatitis. Signs and symptoms include right upper quadrant pain from swelling. Purulent and fibrous exudate appear, but adhesions are a late manifestation. This syndrome is thought to be a hyperimmune response to *C. trachomatis*. Some organisms travel transperitoneally, but others may travel by lymphatic and hematogenous routes. The syndrome occurs in up to 10% of women with salpingitis and is frequently confused with cholecystitis.

Lymphogranuloma venereum is rare in the United States and is caused by the L1, L2, or L3 serovars of *C. trachomatis*. The most common clinical presentation is inguinal, usually with unilateral lymphadenopathy. Proctocolitis or inflammation of perianal tissues also can occur.

Trachoma is endemic in hot, dry, poverty-ridden countries. Characterized by a chronic inflammation, it can contribute to blindness if left untreated. Infants born to mothers infected by *C. trachomatis* may develop ophthalmia neonatorum or chlamydial pneumonia. Up to a third of infants born to infected mothers develop inclusion conjunctivitis, which can cause blindness, whereas as many as 10% of infants develop pneumonitis. Both diseases have a later onset (up to 3 months) than gonorrhea.

### Diagnosis

Because of its intracellular nature, *C. trachomatis* cannot be grown on artificial media, thus requiring McCoy or HeLa cell tissue cultures, which are expensive and time-consuming (Palella & Murphy, 1997). Currently, DNA probes and enzyme-linked immunosorbent assays (ELISAs) have acceptable sensitivities and are faster and less costly. Accurate diagnosis by urine tests have been disappointing because of low sensitivity (Stamm, 1999). Serologic testing is not used clinically for detection of chlamydial infection.

### Physiologic Basis of Treatment

As with any disease, treatment depends on many variables, including age, the organ system affected, and severity of symptoms. *C. trachomatis* infection manifests itself in many ways. Fortunately, no drug-resistant strains have been discovered. By following the 1998 STD Treatment Guidelines from the CDC, the practitioner may choose from the following list of drugs to treat *C. trachomatis* infection in its various forms: azithromycin, doxycycline, erythromycin, ofloxacin, or amoxicillin.

## Neisseria Gonorrhoeae

### History and Introduction

Gonorrhea has been recognized as a disease in humans for centuries, as evidenced by several ancient writings. The book of Leviticus in the Bible gives rules for controlling the spread of gonorrhea. First named by Galen in 130 AD (gonos-seed; rhoia-flow), it was Albert Neisser who first described and named the organism *Neisseria gonorrhoeae* in 1879 (Braude, 1986). The colloquial term "clap" most likely was coined from the district in Paris where prostitutes were housed, Les Clapier. Despite its long history and multiple treatment regimens, *N. gonorrhoeae* remains an important pathogen, causing much distress in humans, its only known host.

Nine of the 10 species of *Neisseria* are cocci, and all colonize humans, although *N. gonorrhoeae* always is considered a pathogen. It is aerobic, Gram-negative, usually forms in pairs with each coccus being 0.6 to 1.5 μm in diameter, and has the appearance of a coffee bean (Levi, 1997). Often described in the literature as a fastidious organism, *N. gonorrhoeae* requires specific conditions in temperature (36° or 37°C), humidity (50%), and $CO_2$ (3% to 10%) for growth. Using various types of identification methods, researchers have discovered over 70 different types of *N. gonorrhoeae* (Palella & Murphy, 1997). An additional characteristic of the different colonies of *N. gonorrhoeae* that is helpful in identification is opacity or transparency (Sparling, 1999).

### Pathogenesis

Three basic steps are involved in the pathogenesis of *N. gonorrhoeae* infection: (1) attachment of diplococci to epithelial cells, (2) penetration into or between epithelial cells, and (3) destruction of epithelial cells (Gutman, 1995).

Playing an integral role in pathogenesis is the membrane structure of the bacterium. The most important parts of the rugose cell membrane are the pili, filamentous structures with three regions. Pili are known to undergo complex antigenic and phase variations, contributing to the virulence of a particular strain of *N. gonorrhoeae* (Sparling, 1999).

In addition to pili, various proteins and lipo-oligosaccharides (LOS) are involved in aiding the gonococcus to cause disease in the host organism. Por proteins (*Porins*) damage the cell membrane and affect PMN destruction of *N. gonorrhoeae* (Levi, 1997). *Opa* proteins assist adherence of cells in a colony and adhesion of gonococci to epithelial cells. Antibody response is produced by yet another porin protein, P111. Notice that *N. gonorrhoeae* infection produces IgA proteases, which may affect the mucosal immune response ability (Braude, 1986). The effect of LOS is to trigger an intense inflammatory response, which induces most of the damage caused in PID (Levi, 1997). Finally, other proteins are responsible for iron or oxygen repression, further debilitating the host.

### Epidemiology

Most (77%) of reported cases of gonorrhea occur in persons in the 15- to 29-year age range. Race is another important variable, with 81% of reported cases in 1993 being female African Americans (Palella, 1997). Higher rates of gonorrhea infection are reported in the Southeast and in urban areas of the United States, but overall, rates have fallen since the mid-1970s (Levi, 1997). With regard to epidemiology, practitioners need to be aware of gonorrhea's seasonal variations. Higher rates are noted in late summer and lower rates in late winter and early spring, with resistant strains occurring more often in the latter group (Reynolds et al., 1979).

Transmission efficiency depends on several factors including gender, anatomic site, and strains of bacteria. As with most STDs, the rate of gonorrhea transmission is higher from male to female than vice versa. Any sexual contact that involves receiving infected semen, whether vaginal, anal, or oral, is risky for the receiver.

## Clinical manifestations of *Neisseria gonorrhoeae*

***Infections in Men.*** Gonococcal urethritis is the most common infection caused by *N. gonorrhoeae*, with 80% to 90% of men developing symptoms of purulent discharge and burning within 2 weeks of exposure (Levi, 1997). Gonorrhea produces more dysuria than NGU, and its incubation period is shorter. Pharyngitis, however, tends to be asymptomatic and is more common in homosexual men, who also are at increased risk for gonorrheal proctitis. With the advent of modern antibiotic therapy, complications such as epididymitis are rare.

***Infections in Women.*** Because gonococcus attacks only noncornified columnar or cuboidal epithelial cells, the endocervical canal is the site of predilection in women. When colonization is high, the female urethra and the Bartholin and Skene's glands also may be affected. Early symptoms of gonorrheal infection in women are rare and mild and may include increased vaginal discharge, menorrhagia, or dysfunctional uterine bleeding. The clinician must remember that gonorrhea attracts leukocytes, forming pus, so that any clinical sign such as mucopurulent cervicitis should be evaluated, even if the patient has no symptoms.

In 10% to 17% of untreated cases, the organism ascends, causing PID, which occurs most often during or just after menses, when the mucus barrier is diminished (Scott et al., 1999). The tubes become red and swollen, usually bilaterally, as the muscularis and serosa are inflamed. If pus comes out the end of the tubes, the patient can have peritonitis with secondary tubal occlusion and adhesions.

Because of the inherent difficulty with culture media, many clinicians prefer to use DNA probes to detect *N. gonorrhoeae*. Serologic tests are available but are more helpful in the complicated cases, such as disseminated gonococcal infection. No matter which method is used for detection, remember that the detection method is no better than the specimen obtained. When taking urethral specimens, make sure that the patient has not voided recently, since urine dilutes the specimen. The urethra may be gently stripped to produce a specimen if necessary. For cervical specimens, the swab should be inserted 1 to 2 cm into the canal and rotated for 10 seconds. Anal specimens are obtained in a similar manner, but care must be taken to avoid fecal contamination.

## Physiologic Basis of Treatment

When treating infections caused by *N. gonorrhoeae*, notice that up to 40% of persons infected with gonorrhea have concomitant chlamydial infection. Therefore, the CDC recommends *dual* treatment for any patient infected by gonorrhea or chlamydia. The drugs of choice for treatment of uncomplicated cases are cefixime, ceftriaxone, ciprofloxacin, or ofloxacin plus azithromycin or doxycycline. Alternative regimens include spectinomycin, single-dose cephalosporin, or single-dose quinolone. Most of these drugs take into account the strains of penicillin-resistant gonococcus.

## Syphilis

## History and Introduction

The disease caused by *Treponema pallidum* was named syphilis after a fictitious hero invented by Girolamo Fracastoro in 1530 in his poem, "Syphilis sive de Morbo Gallico" (Graham, 1951). An epidemic arose in Europe in the late 15th century, coinciding with Columbus's voyages. Others argue that Biblical and ancient Chinese writings describe the disease now called syphilis. No matter what the true origin, the disease continues, despite the most powerful weapon against it, penicillin.

Discovered by Schaudinn and Hoffmann in 1905, *T. pallidum* is one of 13 species of *Treponema*, although only two others, *Treponema pertenue* (causing yaws) and *Treponema carateum* (causing pinta) are infectious to humans. *T. pallidum* is a spirochete bacteria, 6 to 20 μm in length, with a diameter of 0.01 to 0.18 μm and is Gram negative. Using an electron microscope, scientists have determined *T. pallidum* to have outer and inner membranes and a cell wall, although the outer membrane lacks the usual lipopolysaccharide of most Gram-negative bacteria (Hardy et al., 1983). The three periplasmic flagella at each end of the bacterium are responsible for its motility.

## Pathogenesis

*T. pallidum* generally enters the human host through mucosal surfaces or microabrasions in the skin. The mechanism by which the bacteria attaches to and enters various cells is not clear, but within a few hours, numerous treponemes are present in regional lymph nodes near the site of inoculation (Stamm, 1999). The primary lesion of syphilis occurs at the site of inoculation 2 to 6 weeks (mean, 3 weeks) from initial infection. Known as a chancre, this lesion is painless and well circumscribed, with a hard base 1 to 2 cm in diameter. From this lesion, the treponemes can be collected and observed using dark-field microscopy.

The chancre is an area of intense cellular warfare, with necrosis of the ulcer arrive plasma cells, lymphocytes, and histiocytes, and, eventually, obliterative endarteritis (Stamm, 1999). The host eventually destroys enough treponemes to allow healing of the primary lesion by immune responses, but enough bacteria survive to cause chronic infection and various stages of syphilis. Many theories exist as to why the immune system of the host cannot clear the bacteria, but the most popular explanation is the limited number of surface-exposed transmembrane proteins on *T. pallidum* (Domingue, 1997).

### Epidemiology

In the Western world, syphilis incidence peaked around World War II, then declined until the late 1970s, had a brief rise, and declined again until the mid 1980s. The last increase was attributed to sex-for-drugs behavior, which also led to a rise in congenital syphilis (Palella, 1997). Recently, syphilis cases have been on the decline, with only 16,787 reported U.S. cases in 1995 (Musher, 1999).

### Natural Course of Untreated Syphilis

Three large studies of the clinical manifestations of untreated syphilis have been done in this century. They are the Oslo study from 1890 to 1910 by Boeck, the Tuskegee study from 1932 to 1972 by the US Public Health Service, and the Roahn study from 1917 to 1941, which was based entirely on a review of autopsy materials from the Yale University School of Medicine. The Tuskegee study received national criticism, which resulted in a recent presidential apology to survivors of the study.

Although many 19th century descriptions of the natural course of syphilis exist, these studies aided clinicians in recognizing and understanding the stages of the disease. With the exception of congenital disease, syphilis always is transmitted sexually by a person during the first few years of infection (Sparling, 1999). There are four stages of syphilis, each with its unique characteristics and treatment strategies.

*Primary Stage.* As discussed previously, the primary chancre occurs, on average, 3 weeks from exposure at the site of the inoculum. The practitioner must be suspicious of a nonpainful ulcer that is larger than the typical herpes simplex virus (HSV) lesion. Some lesions in nongenital sites such as the anus may have an atypical appearance

(Sparling, 1999). These heal within a few weeks, but the host is infectious at this time.

*Secondary Stage.* The secondary stage of syphilis is a systemic illness with variable manifestations. Signs and symptoms occur within a few weeks or months (mostly 3 to 6 weeks) of the primary lesion and may include low-grade fever, fatigue, pharyngitis, headache, lymphadenopathy, and characteristic rash. This maculopapular rash mostly appears on the palms of the hands and soles of the feet—an important clue for primary care practitioners who often are presented with mysterious rashes. Condylomata, which are large, raised, gray-white lesions near the site of inoculation, also may be present (Musher, 1999). Other, rarer signs and symptoms of secondary syphilis include "patchy" alopecia, hepatitis, and a nephrotic syndrome (Sparling, 1999).

*Latency Stage.* When a patient has serologic evidence of syphilis but no clinical signs, the disease is staged as latent. This stage has been arbitrarily divided into early latent (of 1 year or less duration) or late latent (over 1 year's duration). Secondary relapses of up to 25% were noted in the Oslo study during the early latent phase (Sparling, 1999). Patients in the late latent stage are not thought to be as contagious.

*Tertiary Stage.* If left untreated, syphilis claims most of its victims, in terms of morbidity and mortality, in the tertiary stage. This stage occurs in approximately one third of untreated patients. One half of these have benign disease, one fourth have cardiovascular disease, and one fourth have neurologic disease (Swartz, 1999).

Late benign syphilis involves various manifestations of nodular and noduloulcerative lesions known as gummas. They have a characteristic gross and microscopic appearance, and although classified as benign, these lesions can cause significant cutaneous and osseous tissue destruction (Swartz, 1999). From the Oslo and Tuskegee studies, it was learned that gummas appeared from 2 to 40 years after the onset of the initial infection.

The aorta is the most commonly affected vessel in cardiovascular syphilis, usually in the ascending region. As many experienced clinicians know, aortic aneurysm often is difficult to diagnose because of its various presentations. Another manifestation of cardiovascular syphilis, aortic valvular disease, requires only a good stethoscope to raise suspicion a significant problem.

Neurosyphilis is classified in four ways: asymptomatic, meningeal, parenchymatous, and gummatous. Although the spectrum of clinical manifestations of neurosyphilis is broad, a common finding may be a small vessel vasculitis

(Sparling, 1999). Briefly, meningitis resulting from *T. pallidum* infection may present clinically with cranial nerve palsy and signs of increased intracranial pressure (Swartz, 1999). The cerebrospinal fluid is aseptic but has a positive rapid plasma reagin (RPR) reaction. Neurosyphilis always should be considered in the young adult with a CVA. Parenchymatous neurosyphilis presents as a combination of psychiatric and neurologic disorders ranging from confusion and personality changes to tremors and the rare Argyll Robertson pupils (small, fixed pupils) (Swartz, 1999). Another manifestation of parenchymatous neurosyphilis is tabes dorsalis, with a variety of signs and symptoms occurring in the fifth and sixth decades of life.

The gummas of neurosyphilis are rare but have been reported in the cerebrum and spinal cord (Swartz, 1999).

### Congenital Syphilis

Most of the statistics involving risks of a fetus having syphilis are quoted from the Oslo study, in which almost half of babies born to infected mothers were symptomatic. One fourth also were seropositive, whereas one fourth were disease free or recovered spontaneously (Palella & Murphy, 1997). Current theory holds that congenital syphilis can occur after maternal infection at any gestation, with the fetus of later gestations being more at risk. Congenital syphilis can be a cause of spontaneous abortion before 20 weeks' gestation because of the failure of the fetus to mount an immune response (Radolf, 1999).

When a newborn is infected with *T. pallidum*, almost every fetal organ may be involved. The most common sites affected are the liver, kidneys, bone, pancreas, spleen, lungs, heart, and brain. "Snuffles," cutaneous lesions, "saber shins," and Hutchinson teeth are a few of the obvious signs of congenital syphilis. If CDC guidelines for screening and treatment in pregnancy are followed, the incidence of congenital syphilis should continue to decrease.

### Diagnostic Methods

Primary syphilis can be positively diagnosed only by observing the *T. pallidum* spirochete using dark-field microscopy. Unfortunately, most clinical sites do not have access to this technique, and as previously noted, many patients do not present with a primary lesion. Therefore, serologic testing is used most often to establish the diagnosis of syphilis.

The two basic types of serologic testing are nontreponemal and treponemal. Evolving from the original work by Wassermann in 1906, nontreponemal tests are the venereal disease research labora-tory (VDRL) and RPR tests. The VDRL test is a slide microflocculation test, as is the RPR card test (Palella & Murphy, 1997). Both the VDRL and RPR tests are reported as the reciprocal of the highest dilution of serum that precipitates with antigen. Pregnancy, as well as diseases such as lupus, can produce a low-dilution false-positive result. Results of the nontreponemal tests always are positive if the patient has had syphilis, even if treated.

The two most common treponemal serologic tests are the fluorescent treponemal antibody absorption test (FTA-ABS) and the microhemagglutination-Treponema pallidum test. The FTA-ABS is a modified test for diagnosing congenital syphilis. Any nontreponemal screening test must be confirmed by one of the treponemal tests before a patient can be properly treated and counseled. Other emerging tests involve polymerase chain reactions (PCR) and ELISA.

### Treatment

Penicillin is the *only* highly successful treatment for syphilis at any stage. The dosages and formulations of penicillin vary by stage of the disease. So effective is penicillin that the CDC recommends desensitization, if necessary, so that adequate treatment may be ensured. Follow-up serologic testing is required to monitor the success of therapy.

## Bacterial Vaginosis

### History and Introduction

Bacterial vaginosis (BV) is the most common cause of vaginal symptoms in women of reproductive age. It is not a classic STD because it is not found as a symptomatic disease in men and is found in women who are not sexually active. However, BV is more common in sexually active women, and sexual transmission in lesbian couples has been documented (Berger et al., 1995).

Historically, BV has been known by several names, including leukorrhea and "the whites." Pioneering work by A.H. Curtis and R. Schroder established the fact that BV is a vaginal, not uterine, disease and most likely results from a shift in normal vaginal flora. Many researchers continued to search for a specific bacteria that cause BV, and in 1955, the name *Gardnerella vaginalis* vaginosis was used to describe BV. *Haemophilus vaginalis* vaginitis was the name chosen by Gardner and Dukes, who originally discovered the *G. vaginalis* bacteria (Gardner & Dukes, 1955). In 1984, the term *bacterial vaginosis* was proposed in Sweden and currently is accepted because it reflects the polymicrobial nature of the condition and the lack of an inflammatory response (French & McGregor, 1997).

### Etiology and Pathogenesis

To understand how BV affects the host, it is important to review the composition of the normal vaginal flora. In 1894, Doderlein first discovered lactobacilli, which are acid-producing Gram-positive rods, the predominant flora of the vagina. These microorganisms protect the vagina from STDs (Hillier, 1999). This protective role is the result of the $H_2O_2$ produced by some strains of lactobacilli, as well as their lactic acid production. Many other bacteria are found as a part of the normal vaginal flora, including anaerobic Gram-negative rods, *G. vaginalis*, and *Mycoplasma urealyticum* (Hillier, 1999).

When lactobacilli prevalence is decreased, the vagina becomes susceptible to the growth of many different types of bacteria, resulting in BV. The most common types of bacteria replacing lactobacillus are *G. vaginalis*, anaerobes, and *Mycoplasma hominis*. The most common anaerobes found in BV are *Prevotella bivia*, *Bacteroides ureolyticus*, and *Fusobacterium nucleatum* (Hillier, 1999). It is the replacement of lactobacilli by a mixed flora of bacteria usually present in small amounts in the vagina that causes BV.

This change in vaginal flora may be initiated by coitus, which introduces a set of organisms (Hillier, 1999). Currently, however, there has not been a host factor identified that increases the likelihood of developing BV. The characteristic "fishy" odor associated with BV is thought to result from the presence of trimethylamine produced by *Mobiluncus* bacteria. Increased levels of IL-1α and prostaglandins are found in the cervical mucus of women with BV (Hillier,1999).

### Clinical Manifestations and Diagnosis

Increased vaginal discharge and malodor are the usual presenting symptoms in women with BV. The odor may be first noted after coitus, when the high pH of semen produces amines when mixed with the abnormal vaginal flora. This symptom may be distressing to women from a hygienic standpoint.

Whereas local vaginosis symptoms are at best annoying and at worst psychologically disturbing, it is the ascension of BV into the upper genital tract that causes the most physical morbidity. Although it is difficult to prove a causative role, the microflora isolated from the upper genital tract in women with PID is consistent with that of BV (Sweet, 1995). Some studies show a link between endometritis and BV. Noting an association of increased postoperative infection and BV, some clinicians use prophylactic treatment before gynecologic surgery. Substantial controversy still exists about the possible role of BV in cervical cancer, and investigations are ongoing.

Of all possible complications of BV, preterm birth has received the most recent attention. The first study to establish a role of BV in preterm labor was by Minkoff and coworkers (1984). The association of BV with chorioamnionitis and amnionitis has been substantiated by other studies, and the current standard of most obstetric practitioners is to screen for BV at the first obstetrical visit and treat as needed.

The diagnosis of BV is straightforward and requires only a good microscope, potassium hydroxide, and a few minutes of the clinician's time. The discharge produced by BV is homogeneous with a gray-to-white color and a pH above 4.5. When the vaginal fluid is mixed with KOH, it emits the classic positive "whiff test." Clue cells are specific for BV (Fig. 17-6). These are epithelial cells that have a stippled or "moth-eaten" cell margin. Other methods of diagnosis, such as Gram's stain and the newer rapid card tests, are available but are less specific and less sensitive than wet preparations.

### Physiologic Basis of Treatment

The treatment of choice for BV is oral metronidazole because of its efficacy against anaerobes. This discovery was made by Pheifer and colleagues in 1978. Various regimens have been studied, but a 7-day oral treatment is superior to shorter regimens and achieves a cure rate of greater than 80%. Because the side effects of oral therapy may be intolerable to some patients, intravaginal metronidazole is available with similar cure rates. Another intravaginal preparation is a 2% clindamycin cream, which also has an acceptable cure rate. The cost of the vaginal preparations is up to three times the cost of generic metronidazole.

The CDC does not recommend treatment of male partners of women with BV. The American College of Obstetricians and Gynecologists recommends treatment of pregnant women with oral metronidazole after the first trimester.

## Trichomoniasis

### Introduction

*Trichomonas vaginalis* is one of three species of trichomonads infecting humans and is the one that is sexually transmitted. Trichomonads are eukaryotic, flagellated protozoans that have over 100 species. Donne first described *T. vaginalis* in 1836, but until the last 30 years, it was regarded as a harmless entity.

### Biology of *Trichomonas Vaginalis*

The growth and multiplication of *T. vaginalis* depend on an optimum pH of 4.9 to 7.5 in a temperature between 35° and 37°C (Kneger & Alderete, 1999). The size and shape of *T. vaginalis*

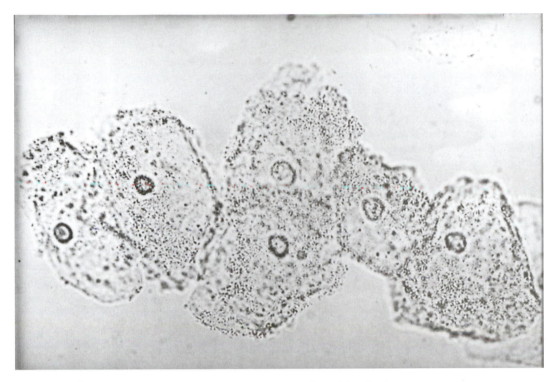

**FIGURE 17.6** ● Microscopic appearance of clue cells, seen in bacterial vaginosis.

varies, but overall it has an ovoid shape with a mean length of 15 μm. Four anterior flagella provide an erratic motility, whereas a fifth flagellum extends underneath the organism. Reproduction occurs by mitotic division and longitudinal fission every 8 to 12 hours. *T. vaginalis* is able to phagocytose bacteria and viruses, and even leukocytes and erythrocytes.

### Epidemiology and Transmission

Several studies indicate that *T. vaginalis* mostly is a STD (Kneger & Alderete, 1999). It can live outside of the body for 45 minutes, but fomite transmission is considered rare. Therefore, high-risk groups for *T. vaginalis* are sex workers and prison inmates. The disease can be transmitted heterosexually as well as homosexually.

Prevalence rates in women in the general population are 5% to 10%. When other STDs are present, the risk increases up to 50%. In men, prevalence rates overall are similar to women, 5% to 15%. As with women, if men have a coexistent STD, such as NGU, the risk of infection with *T. vaginalis* increases (Kneger & Alderete, 1999).

### Pathogenesis and Clinical Manifestations

*T. vaginalis* may have from two to eight serotypes, which may explain why some infections are more tenacious than others. The most obvious host response to *T. vaginalis* is the increased production of neutrophils. The infection also elicits cellular, humoral, and secretory immune responses but does not confer immunity to repeated episodes. In the natural history of the disease, trichomoniasis may be removed by leukocytes and the complement pathway.

In women, *T. vaginalis* produces symptomatic green, frothy discharge with pruritus in about 50% of infections. A rare but specific sign of trichomoniasis is "colpitis macularis" or "strawberry cervix" in which small punctate cervical hemorrhages may be seen. Chronic infection can be present, as well as more severe signs and symptoms such as abdominal pain. *T. vaginalis* has been associated with premature rupture of membranes (Read & Klebanoff, 1997).

In men, *T. vaginalis* is less symptomatic and can clear spontaneously because of the antitrichomonal properties of prostatic fluid (Kneger & Alderete, 1999). When symptomatic, men exhibit urethritis-type symptoms. In rare cases, *T. vaginalis* is associated with penile ulcers and balanitis.

### Diagnosis

Wet preparations demonstrate live, motile trichomonads is 60% to 70% of infections (Rein, 1990). Staining methods and Pap smears are slightly less accurate than wet preparations. Culture techniques remain the "gold standard" for diagnosis of infection with *T. vaginalis*.

### Physiologic Basis of Treatment

Metronidazole is the drug of choice for trichomonal infection. Multiple versus single-dose regimens have been used. Other treatments such as clotrimazole or nonoxynol-9 have been used with some effectiveness. Resistant strains of *T. vaginalis* to standard metronidazole doses have been reported and require persistence on the part of the practitioner and patient to eliminate.

## Human Papilloma Virus

### History and Introduction

As with many STDs, human papilloma virus (HPV) was recognized as early as the first century AD. The first clues to the oncogenic potential of HPV were provided in the 1930s, and now HPV is known to be a contributing factor in cervical cancers (Bosch, 1995).

There are over 100 different HPV types, with 35 types known to infect the human genital tract (zur Hausen, 1996). Human papilloma viruses are small (60-nm diameter), naked, icosahedral particles with double-stranded, circular DNA. Because they cannot be grown in tissue culture, little is known about the virus's life cycle. The HPV does have a role in the etiology of anogenital cancers. The changes in cell function caused by HPV proteins involve unchecked proliferation of cells and decreased ability to eliminate damaged cells.

### Epidemiology and Prevalence

Human papilloma virus is the most common viral STD and is three times more common than HSV (Palella & Murphy, 1997). Using PCR-based methods, the prevalence of HPV among women with normal Pap smear results is estimated at 16.2%. Similar prevalence rates have been found in healthy men (Koutsky & Kiviat, 1999). Human papilloma virus is more common in younger, sexually active persons. As many as 50% of sexually active adults have one or more HPV types, most of which are unrecognized and benign (Koutsky & Kiviat, 1999).

### Pathogenesis

The infection of the host with HPV begins with the entry of the virus into basal cells of differentiating squamous epithelium. After the virus has entered the cells, it produces proliferation of all layers of the epithelium except the basal layer and results in characteristic acanthosis, perikeratosis, and hyperkeratosis (Zhang, 1997). As previously mentioned, unchecked proliferation may explain the oncogenic role of HPV. Incubation periods and maximum infectivity periods are difficult to determine

and may be months or years. The HPV is thought to be more infectious with newer lesions. Infectivity also may be transient.

### Clinical Manifestations

Human papilloma virus can manifest itself in visible warts and nonvisible squamous intraepithelial lesions (SILs) of the cervix. Although SILs can be detected in any genital epithelial sample, most have limited clinical significance. Therefore, the importance of regular Pap smears in the sexually active female patient cannot be overemphasized.

Most individuals with genital warts present with a new "bump" or growth. Often, this is accompanied by an itching or burning sensation. In men, these growths can be on the penis, scrotum, meatus, or perianal area. In women, the most common sites are the introitus, vulva, perineum, and perianal area. Vaginal warts are less common but can occur. Unlikely sites also include lips, tongue, or palate. Warts may have various morphologic appearances from the cauliflower-like condylomata acuminatum to the flat-topped macular warts, which have a higher chance of becoming cancerous (Fig. 17-7).

The oncogenic potential of HPV depends of the viral type. Human papilloma virus types 16, 18, 31, and 45 are responsible for most squamous cell carcinomas of the genital tract, whereas types 6 and 11 are more common but less dangerous. Several recent studies have explored using DNA probes to guide management of abnormal findings from Pap smears (Adam, et al., 1997).

Finally, HPV can be a congenital disease. Recurrent respiratory papillomatosis expressed in neonates and children is known as juvenile-onset RRP and was recognized as early as 1871. The disease usually presents as persistent hoarseness but may occur as an airway emergency. Human papilloma virus types 6 and 11 are the etiologic agents. Unlike HPV 11 of the cervix, RRP involving HPV 11 may progress into malignancy. The estimated risk for papillomatosis for a newborn from an HPV-infected mother is 1:100, and cesarean section does not prevent transmission (Kashima et al., 1999).

### Physiologic Basis of Treatment

Knowing that HPV cannot be eradicated in the host, the clinician must limit the damage caused by the virus. Most patients find warts aesthetically, and in some cases, psychologically disturbing. Patients commonly express feelings of shame and embarrassment, and most want the warts to be removed.

Various destructive compounds are available to the practitioner. Podophyllin resin and trichloroacetic and bichloroacetic acids are

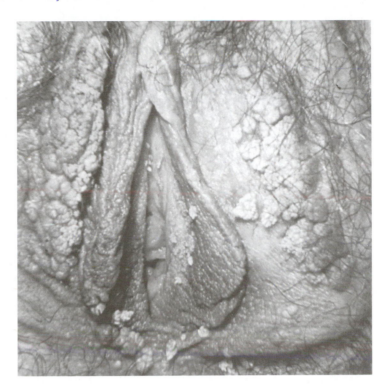

**FIGURE 17.7** ● Appearance of vaginal warts.

provider-applied treatments. Other destructive provider-applied treatments are cryotherapy, electrosurgery, laser vaporization, or excision. The lesions also can be injected with interferon or 5-fluorouracil. All of these regimens are painful, and cure rates range from 32% to 88% (Koutsky & Kiviat, 1999).

Patient-administered methods include podofilox gel or solution and imiquimod cream. Podofilox is a purified form of podophyllin and can be used in pregnancy. Imiquimod cream stimulates interferon and can cause local irritation.

When a SIL is present, management depends on the severity of the lesion. An experienced colposcopist is essential to proper management of SILs of the genital tract. Loop electrode excision procedure and cryotherapy have been used extensively to treat SILs (Copas, 1999).

## Herpes Simplex Virus

### History and Introduction

Clinical manifestations of the herpesviruses have been recognized by clinicians for at least 25 centuries (Corey & Wald, 1999). Beginning with the recognition of "cold sores," various physicians have been aware of the herpesvirus as a STD when the same types of lesions appeared on the genitalia. Perhaps few STDs carry the stigma associated with HSV in modern society after epidemics in the 1970s and 1980s.

Herpesviruses are numerous, with over 100 identified types, although only 8 are known to infect humans (Roizman & Baines, 1991). They are large viruses that have a glycoprotein envelope and contain double-stranded DNA with 125,00 to 250,000 base pairs. There are three subfamilies of herpesviruses. The alpha herpesviruses are rapidly dividing and neurotropic and infect a variety of cells in culture. This subfamily includes HSV-1, HSV-2, and varicella-zoster virus, which are the most commonly recognized. The beta herpesviruses, which include cytomegalovirus, HSV-6, and HSV-7, have a slower replication, and the types of cells affected are restricted. Finally, the gamma herpesviruses are lymphotrophic and affect a narrow range of cells in culture. They include Epstein-Barr virus and HSV-8, which is associated with Kaposi's sarcoma.

### Structure and Replication

When viewed with an electron microscope, the herpesviruses appear six sided because of the icosahedral capsid, which is 100 to 125 nm in diameter. The capsid contains viral proteins and the DNA genome. Surrounding the capsid is a fibrous tegument, which is in turn surrounded by a lipid-containing envelope with glycosylated protein spikes (Sokol & Garry, 1997).

The herpesviruses replicate like all obligate intracellular parasites. The steps include (1) attachment to a cellular receptor, (2) penetration by fusion of the virion envelope with the cellular membrane, (3) uncoating of the virus into the nucleus of the host cell, (4) gene expression, (5) viral DNA synthesis, and, finally, (6) assembly and egress of virions. The herpesviruses kill the host cells. This is not the end of the virus, however. A distinguishing characteristic of the herpesviruses is their ability to develop latency in the host for the life of the host. The mechanisms by which this latency occurs are not fully understood, but the site of latent HSV is in the sensory ganglia of the nerves supplying the site of initial infection (Fraser & Valyi-Nagy, 1993). Other types of herpesviruses reside in the latent state in different sites (Pertel & Spear, 1999).

### Epidemiology and Prevalence
By using improved assays that allow identification of type-specific antibodies for HSV-1 and HSV-2, a clearer picture is emerging of the prevalence of HSV. For the HSV-1 virus, studies show a 50% to 80% prevalence among adults (Guinan, 1988). Two U.S. studies have tested a random and representative sample of the population for the presence of HSV-2 antibodies, and they showed a seroprevalence of 16.4% to 21.7% of adults (Corey & Wald, 1999). In the 19- to 39-year age group, HSV-2 occurs most often, with African-American women experiencing up to an 80% lifetime incidence (Fleming, 1997).

### Pathogenesis
Because HSV becomes quickly inactive at room temperature, the usual transmission is through close contact with an infected person who is shedding virus at a mucosal site. Once the surface is infected, focal necrosis occurs with degeneration of cells and the production of mononucleated giant cells and eosinophilic intranuclear inclusions (Corey & Wald, 1999). Polymorphonuclear cells respond initially, followed by macrophages and lymphocytes.

### Diagnosis
One of the first things a practitioner learns to appreciate about HSV infection is that "herpes hurts." The lesions of HSV usually are painful, and all of the lesions are in the same stage of eruption and healing. A laboratory diagnosis is preferable to support clinical signs.

To collect a sample for HSV isolation, the vesicular lesion must be scraped well with a Dacron swab and properly transported in the correct media. Serologic diagnosis of HSV remains difficult because some assays make it difficult to distinguish between HSV-1 and HSV-2 antibodies. Serologic tests are more useful in determining past infection because the difference in acute and convalescent titers is small in HSV infection.

### Physiologic Basis of Treatment
Knowing that a cure does not exist for HSV, the goals of therapy revolve around limiting the severity of the outbreak, preventing serious sequelae, and preventing recurrence. Acyclovir was the first antiviral developed for HSV infection. An ester of acyclovir, valacylovir, recently has been marketed and has more bioavailability than plain acyclovir. Famciclovir, a prodrug of penciclovir, also is a newer drug that is effective against HSV. All of the antivirals can be given episodically or daily for suppression. Knowing that the incidence of asymptomatic shedding may be underestimated, practitioners should counsel their patients regarding the use of antivirals for suppression of HSV outbreaks. Along with local infection, the HSV enters sensory and autonomic nerve root ganglia, where latency is established. The mechanism behind reactivation is unknown but may involve decreased immune surveillance.

### Clinical Manifestations
Herpes simplex virus has a variety of expression. Various terms have been used to identify an initial infection versus a recurrent one. The clinical syndrome associated with an initial, or primary, infection, usually is more severe than a recurrent episode. Whether the lesion is oral or genital, a primary infection has an incubation period of 2 to 7 days and produces a cluster of small vesicles that ulcerate after 3 to 5 days (Fig. 17-8). Systemic complaints of flu-like symptoms and adenopathy occur in up to 70% of primary cases (Sokol & Garry, 1997). The length of time to healing is about 3 weeks. Recurrent infections are less common with HSV-1 and less severe overall. Thought to be rare, an individual may have a mild initial infection and a more severe clinical episode later. This type of outbreak is termed first-episode, nonprimary HSV.

Unfortunately, painful local lesions are not the only expression of HSV. Cervical infection can occur, sometimes with no other symptom than urinary retention. Cervical infection may lead to congenital HSV, but over 70% of infants with neonatal HSV are born to women without signs or symptoms of disease (Whitley, 1980). The risk of neonatal infection with primary HSV infection of the mother is 50%, and the risk of death or serious morbidity in these infants also is 50% (Sweet, 1995). Among mothers with recurrent HSV infection or prior history of HSV-1 infection, the risk of congenital infection is substantially decreased.

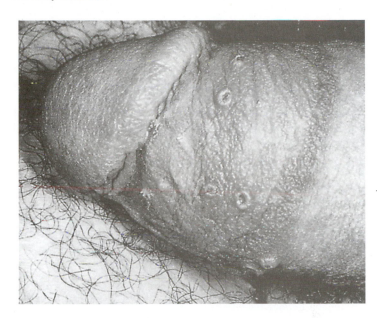

**FIGURE 17.8** ● Herpetic penile ulcers.

Some rare complications of HSV in adults include aseptic meningitis, autonomic nervous system dysfunction, transverse myelitis, and disseminated infection. When the patient is immunocompromised, HSV infection can lead to serious complications and even death.

## Candidiasis

### Introduction and Epidemiology

Three of four women are estimated to have at least one episode of vulvovaginal candidiasis (VVC) in their lifetime (Hurley & DeLouvois, 1979). Cures for "yeast" infections are advertised on television, in magazines, and by word of mouth. Although morbidity is rare, VVC is irritating, and patients seek rapid cures from practitioners and over-the-counter medications. Debate exists as to whether *Candida* are a part of the normal vaginal flora, since some studies indicate a 20% positive culture rate in asymptomatic women (Goldacre et al., 1979).

### Microbiology

Most yeast strains that infect the vagina are of the *Candida albicans* species. Of the non-albicans species, *Candida glabrata* and *Candida tropicalis* are the next most common causes of VVC. Some authors claim an increase in non-albicans VVC, whereas others have not confirmed this trend (Horowitz et al., 1992; Sobel et al., 1995).

No strain tropism for VVC has been found among the more than 200 strains of *C. albicans* (Odds, 1987). Using newer DNA probe technology, however, scientists may discover reasons why some women are plagued by recurrent infections, whereas others have only one or two lifetime episodes. *Candida* organisms exhibit dimorphism. Blastospores are responsible for transmission and spread, whereas mycelia (germinated form) are responsible for symptomatic disease (Sobel, 1999).

### Pathogenesis

Adherence to vaginal epithelial cells is the first step in colonization of *Candida* in the vagina. The albicans strains seem to do this better than non-albicans strains. Germination of *Candida*, which allow higher colonization, is facilitated by increased estrogen and glycogen levels (Sobel, 1990). The questions of how *Candida* causes the patient to become symptomatic and why some patients have recurrent disease have not yet been answered fully.

The body responds to *Candida* with an inflammatory response, but PMNs usually are not numerous in the vaginal fluid in cases of VVC. The overall composition of vaginal flora may inhibit colonization of *Candida*. Responses by IgM, IgG, and SIgA are noted after acute episodes of VVC, but their protective role is unknown (Mathur et al., 1977). Cell-mediated immunity may have a role in the severity or recurrence of VVC (Fidel, 1993).

### Predisposing Factors

Pregnancy has been well documented to be a predisposing factor for VVC, with highest colonization in the third trimester. Low-dose oral contraceptives do not increase the risk for VVC, nor do barrier methods (Foxman, 1990). Women with diabetes mellitus have higher rates of *Candida* colonization than nondiabetics. Some protocols for management of recurrent VVC call for glucose testing, but this testing is not advocated in normal, healthy women because of an extremely low yield (Sobel, 1999). Traditionally, use of antibiotics has been viewed as a predisposing factor for VVC, but newer studies challenge this observation (Cotch et al., 1998). Therefore, automatically providing a prescription for an antifungal agent with every antibiotic prescription is unwarranted.

### Infection Sources

When women with recurrent VVC were studied, 100% had rectal culture results positive for *Candida*. Thus, the question is, does *C. albicans* have an intestinal reservoir, or is the rectal colonization a reflection of contamination? The question has not been fully answered.

Also, 20% of male partners of women with recurrent VVC have penile colonization of *Candida*. This is more likely in uncircumcised men. Although *Candida* may be sexually transmitted, this may not have any influence over the pathogenesis of infection (Sobel, 1999).

### Clinical Manifestations

Vulvar pruritus is the most common symptom of candidiasis. Vaginal discharge may be minimal but, if present, may be cottage cheese–like in character. Labial and vulvar edema, erythema,

and soreness often are present, and the patient may present with a "bladder infection" because of external dysuria. On speculum examination, a curdy, nonhomogeneous discharge may be present in the vaginal rugae, which may appear inflamed.

In men with symptomatic disease, a transient, postcoital rash and pruritus are the most common symptoms. Balanoposthitis has been reported.

### Diagnosis and Treatment

Using a simple wet preparation with saline and KOH should successfully diagnose most symptomatic infections. The practitioner should remember the nonhomogeneous nature of mycelia distribution and carefully review one or, possibly, two slides. The microscopic appearance of yeast forms are seen in Figure 17-9. In the patient with recurrent disease with negative findings on microscopic study, a fungal culture for *Candida* may prove valuable.

Azoles, either oral or topical, are the first-line drugs of choice for candidiasis, all proving to be 80% to 90% effective. Some oral agents have the risk of hepatotoxicity, but patients appreciate the convenience. Oral and topical azoles may be used on a sustained or pulsed basis for recurrent cases. No agent is 100% fungicidal when treating VVC.

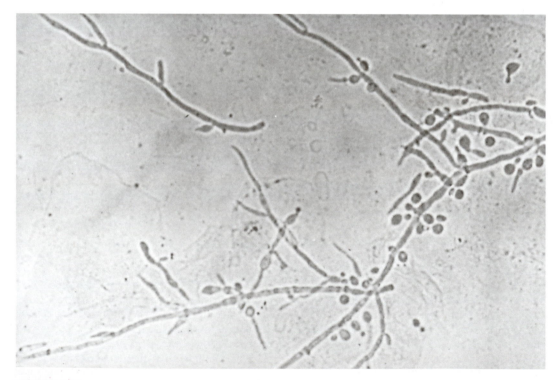

***FIGURE 17.9***  ●  Yeast forms seen under the microscope.

In resistant strains, unconventional treatments such as boric acid or Gentian violet may be necessary.

## Molluscum Contagiosum

### History and Introduction

Molluscum contagiosum (MC) is a common, benign, papular lesion of the skin that is sexually transmitted in adults. It was first described by Bateman in 1817, who named the condition after a common term for pedunculated lesion, "molluscum." He thought the transmission or "contagiosum" to be from fluid expressed from the lesions (Douglas, 1999). A century later, MC was found to be a virus belonging to the poxvirus family, with cellular inclusions and elementary bodies. The virus is brick shaped and small, with a biconcave viral core and linear, double-stranded DNA (Porter et al., 1992). As with HPV, MC cannot be grown in cell culture, so the knowledge of its life cycle is limited.

### Pathophysiology

Molluscum contagiosum virus (MCV) has two subtypes, MCV-1 and MCV-2. Both enter the cell by phagocytosis and undergo changes resulting in free virus cores (Douglas, 1999). Infection with MCV occurs only in the epidermis. Transmission occurs through skin-to-skin contact or fomites, as is often the case with children, in whom the disease is common. The changes in the skin caused by MCV are well described. The classic lesions usually are 3 to 5 mm and are dome shaped, with an umbilicated center. These lesions contain focal areas of hyperplastic epidermis surrounding lobules, filled with debris and degenerating molluscum bodies (Douglas, 1999).

### Epidemiology and Clinical Manifestations

For sexually transmitted MCV, young sexually active teens and adults exhibit the highest prevalence. The disease in these individuals usually is limited to the thighs, groin, buttocks, and lower abdominal wall. The umbilicated lesions occasionally grow up to 10 to 15 mm and are termed "giant molluscum."

The incubation period for MCV averages 2 to 3 months, and the average duration of individual lesions is 2 months, but the MCV may persist for 2 years (Douglas, 1999). Average hosts may have 10 to 20 lesions, whereas immunocompromised patients may have hundreds. In 10% of patients, a complication known as "molluscum dermatitis" may appear, causing a large eczematoid reaction that clears as the lesion clears.

### Diagnosis and Treatment

Usually, the diagnosis of MCV is made by observation alone. If in doubt, the practitioner can examine the white, caseous material from the lesion's core using Gram stain. The cells demonstrate pathognomonic, enlarged epithelial cells with intracytoplasmic molluscum bodies (Kwitten, 1980).

Because of the benign and self-limiting course of MCV, the therapy of choice is "tincture of time." If the lesions are bothersome or the patient insists on removal, this can be accomplished with excisional curettage, electrodesiccation, or chemical agents. A randomized, controlled trial found podophyllotoxin cream to be superior to placebo (Syed et al., 1994).

## Ectoparasites: Scabies and Lice

### Introduction

Of the many different types of parasites affecting humans, *Sarcoptes scabiei* and *Pthirus pubis* are the two most common sexually transmitted forms. Both have a worldwide distribution affecting millions per year. With rare exceptions, neither causes serious morbidity or mortality, but both cause severe pruritus. Each has slightly different pathophysiologic features, which are discussed separately in the following sections.

### Scabies

***Introduction.*** Scabies has been afflicting humans for centuries, but it was Von Hebra in 1868 who first proved the relationship between the mite and the disease (Platts-Mills, 1999). The name scabies is derived from the Latin, scabera, "to scratch," which accurately describes the most common symptom. Scabies mites are members of the class that includes spider, ticks, and chiggers.

***The Organism.*** The adult female mite is 400 μm long, and the male is half her length. Both are eyeless with hairs on the dorsum of the head that allow for sensory input. There are four pairs of legs on the adult forms. The mites can move rapidly on the skin at a maximum rate of 2 to 5 cm/minute (Platts-Mills & Rein, 1999). The female mite is the one that burrows into the skin through the stratum granulosum by biting parts called chelicerae (Billstein & Mattaliano, 1990). Soon after entering the skin, the female is fertilized by the male and begins laying eggs about 40 hours after fertilization. She continues laying 2 to 4 eggs per day while burrowing 0.5 to 5 mm per day. Along with an average of 20 to 40 eggs in her life span, the female also deposits fecal pellets into the burrows, which may produce most of the immune response in the host (Platts-Mills & Rein, 1999). These pellets are termed scybala. The time from fertilization to adulthood is 14 days, during which five stages occur. Scabies larvae and mites feed on a living dermis, not blood.

*Epidemiology.* Scabies have been known to occur in epidemics in intervals of 10 to 30 years and were pandemic in the world wars (Burkhart, 1983). Depending on the location, the prevalence may be as low as 2% or as high as 70% (Borchardt, 1997). The transmission requires prolonged contact and is more likely when partners spend the night together. Nonsexual transmission within a household can occur.

*Pathogenesis.* The relationship of IgE in response to scabies infestation has been studied (Hoering & Schroeter, 1980). The cellular infiltration in the dermis affected by scabies shows indications of hypersensitivity reactions. These reactions are similar to those noted with dust mites.

*Clinical Manifestations.* The most common sites of burrows are the webs of the fingers, followed by the sides of the hands and volar wrists. Genital sites include the penis, scrotum, and buttocks. The breasts and nipples may be involved in women. Atypical presentations such as nodular scabies or Norwegian (crusted) scabies can occur. The pruritus associated with the burrows is intense and may become generalized.

*Diagnosis.* Common fountain pen ink rubbed over the affected skin may help to identify burrows after the ink is wiped off with alcohol. A hand lens also is helpful. The skin may be scraped with a number 15 blade, and the scrapings placed on a slide with immersion oil to look for mites, eggs, or fecal pellets.

*Physiologic Basis of Treatment.* The drug of choice is 5% permethrin cream. It is applied and removed in 12 hours. Alternatives include lindane 1% (which has had reported toxicity), 25% solution of benzyl benzoate, and 10% crotamiton cream. Treating the the environment and contacts is essential for eradication of the infestation. Sexual contacts and family members need to be treated as soon as the index case is confirmed. Bedding and clothing should be washed in hot water.

## Pediculosis Pubis

*Introduction.* As with scabies, lice have been infesting humans for centuries. *Pediculus humanus* var. *capitis* has been found in archaeologic digs worldwide. Of the three forms that infest humans, *Pediculus humanus* var. *capitis* (head lice), *Pediculus humanus* var. *corporis* (body lice), and *Pthirus pubis* (pubic lice), only the latter is commonly transmitted sexually. *P. humanus* var. *corporis* is the only variety to cause disease in humans. The organism transmits typhus fever, trench fever, murine typhus, and epidemic relapsing fever (Borchardt, 1997). In this chapter, only *P. pubis* is discussed.

*The Organism.* Pubic lice are 3 to 4 mm with a body that appears similar to that of a crab, hence the colloquial term for pediculosis pubis, "crabs." The French colloquial term is "pallons d'amour," translated butterflies of love. The most notable difference in head lice and pubic lice is the grasping ability of the claws. Each louse's claw is uniquely designed for the diameter of its respective body area. Pubic lice are seldom found in scalp hair and vice versa for head lice. The oval shape of the African-American hair shaft also makes lice less common in this population.

Lice require blood for growth. They feed by using a stylet in their mouthparts to penetrate the skin, and their saliva prevents clotting at the site. Pubic lice are the most vulnerable of all lice and rarely live over 24 hours off the host (Billstein, 1999).

The life cycle of lice have five stages, all of which occur on the host. By simple metamorphosis, the egg (or nit) passes through three nymphal stages into the reproductively mature adult. The eggs of pubic lice are small, 0.8 by 0.3 mm. They hatch within 5 to 10 days, and the nymph matures over the next 8 to 9 days. The mature adult mates within 10 hours and continues for the life of the organism. The female lays about four eggs per day by gluing the eggs to the hairs. The maximum distance covered by the pubic louse is 10 cm/day, slower than the body louse.

*Epidemiology.* Since sexual transmission is the most common route of spread, sexually active adults are most at risk for infestation with *P. pubis*. Pediculosis pubis frequently is present with other STDs, with some STD clinics reporting 37% prevalence (Judson, 1980). Nonsexual transmission has been documented from bedding and toilet seats but is rare.

*Diagnosis.* The clinician is admonished to be alert for "moles that move." The lice are seen easily with a magnifying lens as reddish brown specks. If doubt exists, examination under a low-power microscope should reveal nits or adult forms.

*Physiology of Treatment.* The CDC recommends using 1% permethrin cream applied to affected areas and washed off after 10 minutes to treat pediculosis pubis. A 1% lindane shampoo is another treatment but is not recommended for pregnant or lactating women or children. Both should used 7 to 10 days after initial treatment. Bedding and clothing should be washed in hot water. Nonwashable items may be sprayed with pyrethrin piperonyl butoxide–containing disinfectants.

# REFERENCES

Adam, E., et al. (1998). Is human papillomavirus testing an effective triage method for detection of high-grade (grade 2 or 3) cervical intraepithelial neoplasia? *American Journal of Obstetrics, 168* (6), 1235–1244.

Bankhead, C. (1998). PSA screening linked to 69% reduction in death. *Urology Times, 26,* 1.

Berger, B.J., et al. (1995). BV in lesbians: A sexually transmitted disease. *Clinics in Infectious Disease, 21,* 1402.

Bergman, J.J., et al. (1984). Clinical comparison of microscopic and culture techniques in the diagnosis of *Candida vaginitis. Journal of Family Practice, 18,* 549.

Billstein, S.A. (1999). Pubic lice. In K.K. Holmes, et al. (Eds.), *Sexually transmitted diseases* (3rd ed.). New York: McGraw-Hill.

Billstein, S.A. & Mattaliano, V.J. (1990). The nuisance of sexually transmitted diseases: *Molluscum contagiousum,* scabies, and crab lice. *The Medical Clinics of North America, 74* (6), 1487–1505.

Borchardt, K.A. (1997). Lice. In K.A. Borchardt & M.A. Noble (Eds.), *Sexually transmitted diseases: Epidemiology, pathology, diagnosis, and treatment.* Boca Raton, FL: CRC Press.

Borchardt, KA. (1997). Scabies. In K.A. Borchardt & M.A. Noble (Eds.), *Sexually transmitted diseases: Epidemiology, pathology, diagnosis, and treatment.* Boca Raton, FL: CRC Press.

Bosch, F.X., et al. (1995). Prevalence of human papilloma virus in cervical cancer: A worldwide perspective. *Journal of the National Cancer Institute, 87,* 796.

BPH Guideline Panel. (1994a). AHCPR quick reference guide for clinicians: Benign prostatic hyperplasia. Diagnosis and treatment. *Journal of the American Academy of Nurse Practitioners, 4,* 167–174.

BPH Guideline Panel. (1994b). Practical briefings: Clinical news you can put into practice now. *Patient Care, 6,* 18–27.

Braude, A.I., Davis, C.E., & Fierer, J. (Eds.) (1986). *Infectious diseases and medical microbiology* (2nd ed.). Philadelphia: W.B. Saunders.

Burkhart, C.G. (1983). Scabies: An epidemiological reassessment. *Annals of Internal Medicine, 9,* 498.

Calciano, R.F., Resnick, M.I., Schmidt, J.D., & Soloway, M.S. (1993). Finasteride and other options for BPH. *Patient Care, 7,* 14–34.

Carter, B.H., Pearson, J.D., Metter, J., Brandt, L.J., Chan, D.W., Andres, R., Fozard, J.L., & Walsh, P. (1992). Longitudinal evaluation of prostatic specific antigen levels in men with and without prostate cancer. *Journal of American Medical Association, 267,* 2215–2220.

Centers for Disease Control. (1997). *Chlamydia trachomatis* genital infection United States, 1995. *MMWR, 46,* 193–198.

Copas, P.R. (1999). Treatment of female genital intraepithelial neoplasia with cryotherapy. *Operative Techniques in Gynecologic Surgery, 4,* 99–102.

Corey, L. & Wald, A. (1999). Genital herpes. In K.K. Holmes, et al. (Eds.), *Sexually transmitted diseases* (3rd ed.). New York: McGraw-Hill.

Cotch, M.F., et al. (1998). Epidemiology and outcomes associated with moderate to heavy *Candida* colonization during pregnancy. *American Journal of Obstetrics, 178* (2), 374.

Cunningham, F.G., MacDonald, P.C., & Gant, N.F. (1989). *Williams obstetrics* (18th ed.). Norwalk, CT: Appleton & Lange.

Domingue, G.J. (1997). Syphilis. In K.A. Borchardt & M.A. Noble (Eds.), *Sexually transmitted diseases: Epidemiol-*

*ogy, pathology, diagnosis, and treatment.* Boca Raton, FL: CRC Press.

Douglas, J.M. (1999). Molluscum contagiosum. In K.K. Holmes, et al. (Eds.), *Sexually transmitted diseases* (3rd ed.). New York: McGraw-Hill.

Fidel, P.L. (1993). Systemic cell mediated immune reactivity in women with recurrent vulvovaginal candidiasis. *Journal of Infectious Disease, 168,* 1458.

Fleming, D.T. (1997). HSV-2 in the United States 1976–1994. *New England Journal of Medicine, 337,* 1105–1111.

Foxman, B. (1990). The epidemiology of vulvovaginal candidiasis: Risk factors. *American Journal of Public Health, 8,* 329.

Fraser, N.W. & Valyi-Nagy, T. (1993). Viral, neuronal, and immune factors which may influence herpes simplex virus latency and reactivation. *Microbial Pathology, 15,* 83–91.

French, J.I. & McGregor, J.A. (1997). Bacterial vaginosis: History, epidemiology, microbiology, sequelae, diagnosis, and treatment. In K.A. Borchardt & M.A. Noble (Eds.), *Sexually transmitted diseases: Epidemiology, pathology, diagnosis, and treatment.* Boca Raton, FL: CRC Press.

Gardner, H.L. & Dukes, C.D. (1955). *Haemophilus vaginalis* vaginitis: A newly defined specific infection previously classified "nonspecific vaginitis." *American Journal of Obstetrics and Gynecology, 69,* 962.

Goldacre, M.J., et al. (1979). Vaginal microflora in normal young women. *British Medical Journal, 1,* 450.

Graham, H. (1951). *Eternal Eve.* Garden City, New York: Doubleday & Co.

Gray, M. & Allensworth, D. (1997). Medical management of benign prostatic hyperplasia. *Urologic Nursing, 17,* 137–141.

Guinan, M., et al. (1988). Genital herpes simplex virus infection. *Epidemiology Reviews, 7,* 127–146.

Gupta, K., Scholes, D., & Stamm, W. (1999). Increasing prevalence of antimicrobial resistance among uropathogens causing acute uncomplicated cystitis in women. *Journal of the American Medical Association, 281* (8), 736–738.

Gutman, L.T. (1995). Gonococcal Infection. In J.S. Remington & J.O. Klein (Eds.), *Infectious diseases of the fetus and newborn infant.* Philadelphia: W.B. Saunders.

Hang, L., Wullt, B., Shen, Z., Karpman, D., & Svanborg, C. (1998). Cytokine repertoire of epithelial cells lining the human urinary tract. *Journal of Urology, 159* (6), 2185–2192.

Hardy, P.H., Jr., & Levin, J. (1983). Lack of endotoxin in *Borrelia hispanica* and *Treponema pallidum. Proceedings of the Society for Experimental Biology and Medicine, 174,* 47.

Hillier, S.L. (1999). Bacterial vaginosis. In K.K. Holmes, et al. (Eds.), *Sexually transmitted diseases* (3rd ed.). New York: McGraw-Hill.

Hillier, S.L. (1999). Normal vaginal flora. In K.K. Holmes, et al. (Eds.), *Sexually transmitted diseases* (3rd ed.). New York: McGraw-Hill.

Hooton, T. (1999). Uncomplicating urinary tract infections. Available at: http://www.medscape.com.

Horowitz, B.J., et al. (1992). Evolving pathogens in vulvovaginal candidiasis: Implications for patient care. *Journal of Clinical Pharmacology, 32,* 248.

Hultgren, S. (1999). Bad bugs and beleaguered bladders. *Program and Abstracts from the 39th ICAAC, September 1999, San Francisco, CA. Symposium 136B,* 1356.

Hurley, R. & DeLouvois, J. (1979). Candida vaginitis. *Postgraduate Medical Journal, 55,* 645.

Isenberg, S.J., et al. (1995). A controlled trial of povidone-iodine as a prophylaxis against ophthalmia neonatorum. *New England Journal of Medicine, 332,* 562.

Judson, F.N. (1980). Comparative prevalence rates of sexually transmitted diseases in heterosexual and homosexual men. *American Journal of Epidemiology, 112,* 836–843.

Kashima, H., et al. (1999). Recurrent respiratory papillomatosis. In K.K. Holmes, et al. (Eds.), *Sexually transmitted diseases* (3rd ed.). New York: McGraw-Hill.

Keat, A.C., et al. (1978). Role of *Chlamydia trachomatis* and HLA-B27 in sexually acquired reactive arthritis. *British Medical Journal, 1,* 605.

Kerr, R. (1997). Benign prostatic hyperplasia. *Urology Times, 25,* (Suppl.), 3–10.

Kirby, R. & Christmas, T. (1993). *Benign prostatic hyperplasia.* London: Mosby-Yearbook Europe.

Kirby, R., McConnell, J., Fitzpatrick, J., Roehrborn, C. & Boyle, P. (Eds.) (1998). *Textbook of benign prostatic hyperplasia.* Oxford: Isis Medical Media.

Kneger, J.N. & Alderete, J.F. (1999). Trichomonas vaginalis and trichomoniasis. In K.K. Holmes, et al. (Eds.), *Sexually transmitted diseases* (3rd ed.). New York: McGraw-Hill.

Korn, A.P., et al. (1995). Plasma cell endometritis in women with symptomatic bacterial vaginosis. *Obstetrics and Gynecology, 85,* 387–390.

Koutsky, L.A. & Kiviat, N.B. (1999). Genital human papillomavirus. In K.K. Holmes, et al. (Eds.), *Sexually transmitted diseases* (3rd ed.). New York: McGraw-Hill.

Kunin, C. (1987). *Detection, prevention and management of urinary tract infections.* Philadelphia: Lea & Febiger.

Kwitten, J. (1980). Molluscum contagiosum: Some new histologic observations. *Mt. Sinai Journal of Medicine, 47,* 583–588.

Levi, M.H. (1997). Current concepts in the laboratory diagnosis of gonorrhea. In K.A. Borchardt & M.A. Noble (Eds.), *Sexually transmitted diseases: Epidemiology, pathology, diagnosis, and treatment.* Boca Raton, FL: CRC Press.

Manire, G.P. & Wyrick, P.B. (1986). The chlamydiae. In A.I. Braude, C.E. Davis, & J. Fierer (Eds.), *Infectious diseases and medical microbiology* (2nd ed.). Philadelphia: W.B. Saunders.

Mathur, S., et al. (1977). Humoral immunity in vaginal candidiasis. *Infections and Immunology, 15,* 287.

McConnell, J. (1998). Diagnosis of benign prostatic hyperplasia. In P. Walsh, A. Retik, D. Vaughn, & A. Wein (Eds.), *Campbell's urology.* Philadelphia: W.B. Saunders, 1429–1445.

McPhee, S.J., Lingappa, V.R., Ganong, W.F., & Lange, J.D. (1997). *Pathophysiology of disease: An introduction to clinical medicine.* Stamford: Appleton & Lange.

Minkoff, H., et al. (1984). Risk factors for prematurity and premature rupture of membranes: A prospective study of the vaginal flora in pregnancy. *American Journal of Obstetrics and Gynecology, 150,* 965.

Monte, J.E. & Meyers, S.E. (1997). Defining the ideal tumor marker for prostatic cancer. *Urologic Clinics of North America, 24,* 247–252.

Musher, D.M. (1999). Early syphilis. In K.K. Holmes, et al. (Eds.), *Sexually transmitted diseases* (3rd ed.). New York: McGraw-Hill.

Odds, F.C., Webster, C.E., Riley, V.C., Fisk, P.G. (1987). Epidemiology of vaginal *Candida* infection. Significance of numbers of vaginal yeasts and their biotypes. *European Journal of Obstetrics Gynecology and Reproductive Biology, 25*(1), 53–66.

Palella, F.J. & Murphy, R.L. (1997). Sexually transmitted diseases. In S.T. Shulman, et al. (Eds.), *The biologic and clinical basis of infectious diseases* (5th ed.). Philadelphia: W.B. Saunders.

Palella, F.J. & Murphy, (1997). Sexually transmitted diseases. In S.T. Shulman, et al. (Eds.), *The biologic and clinical basis of infectious disease* (5th ed.). Philadelphia: W.B. Saunders.

Partin, A. & Coffey, D. (1998). Molecular biology, endocrinology and physiology of the prostate and seminal vesicles. In P. Walsh, A. Retik, D. Vaughn, & A. Wein (Eds.), *Campbell's urology.* Philadelphia: W.B. Saunders, 1381–1428.

Pertel, P.E. & Spear, P.G. (1999). Biology of herpeviruses. In K.K. Holmes, et al. (Eds.), *Sexually transmitted diseases* (3rd ed.). New York: McGraw Hill.

Pheifer, I.A., et al. (1978). Nonspecific vaginitis: Role of *Haemophilus vaginalis* and treatment with metronidazole. *New England Journal of Medicine, 298,* 429.

Platts-Mills, T.A. & Rein, M.F. (1999). Scabies. In K.K. Holmes, et al. (Eds.), *Sexually transmitted diseases* (3rd ed.). New York: McGraw-Hill.

Porter, C.D., et al. (1992). *Molluscum contagiosum virus.* In L. Archard (Ed.), *Molecular and cell biology of sexually transmitted diseases.* London: Chapman & Hall.

Radolf, J.D., et al. (1999). Congenital syphilis. In K.K. Holmes et al. (Eds.), *Sexually transmitted diseases* (3rd ed.). New York: McGraw-Hill.

Raz, R. & Stamm, W. (1993). A controlled trial of intravaginal estriol in postmenopausal women with recurrent urinary tract infections. *New England Journal of Medicine, 329* (11), 753–756.

Read, J.S. & Klebanoff, M.A. (1993). Sexual intercourse during pregnancy and preterm delivery: Effects of vaginal microorganisms. The vaginal infections and prematurity study group. *American Journal of Obstetrics, 168,* 514.

Rein, M.F. (2000). Trichomonas vaginalis. In G.L. Mandell, J.E. Bennett, & R. Dolin (Eds.), *Mandell, Douglas, and Bennett's principles and practices of infectious diseases.* (5th ed.). Philadelphia: Churchill Livingston.

Reller, L.B. (1999). The patient with urinary tract infection. In R. Schreier (Ed.), *MAXX: Manual of nephrology.* Philadelphia: Lippincott Williams & Wilkins.

Reynolds, G.H., et al. (1979). The national gonorrhea therapy monitoring study: II. Trends and seasonality of antibiotic resistance of *Neisseria gonorrhea. Sexually Transmitted Diseases, 6* (Suppl.), 103.

Roberts, R. (1994). Benign prostatic hyperplasia: Assessing severity, helping patients choose among management options. *Consultant, 7,* 1077–1085.

Roizmann, B. & Baines, J. (1991). The diversity and unity of herpesviridae. *Comparative Immunology and Microbiology of Infectious Diseases, 14,* 63–70.

Schachter, J. (1999). Biology of *Chlamydia trachomatis.* In K.K. Holmes, et al. (Eds.), *Sexually transmitted diseases* (3rd ed.). New York: McGraw-Hill.

Scott, J.R., DiSaia, P., Hammond, C.B., & Spellacy, W.N. (Eds.) (1999). *Danforth's obstetrics and gynecology* (8th ed.). Philadelphia: Lippincott Williams & Wilkins.

Sobel, J.D. (1990). Vaginal infections in adult women. *The Medical Clinics of North America, 74* (6), 1573.

Sobel, J.D. (1999). Vulvovaginal candidiasis. In K.K. Holmes et al. (Eds.), *Sexually transmitted diseases* (3rd ed.). New York: McGraw-Hill.

Sobel, J.D., et al. (1995). Single dose fluconazole compared with conventional topical therapy of *Candida* vaginitis. *American Journal of Obstetrics, 172,* 1263.

Sokol, D.M. & Garry, R.F. (1997). Herpesvirus. In K. Borcharjt & M.A. Noble (Eds.), *Sexually transmitted dis-*

*eases: Epidemiology, pathology, diagnosis, and treatment.* Boca Raton, FL: CRC Press.

Sparling, P.F. (1999). Natural history of syphilis. In K.K. Holmes, et al. (Eds.), *Sexually transmitted diseases* (3rd ed.). New York: McGraw-Hill.

Sparling, P.F. (1999). Biology of *Neisseria gonorrhea.* In K.K. Holmes, et al. (Eds.), *Sexually transmitted diseases* (3rd ed.). New York: McGraw-Hill.

Stamm, L.V. (1999). Biology of *Treponema pallidum.* In K.K. Holmes, et al. (Eds.), *Sexually transmitted diseases* (3rd ed.). New York: McGraw-Hill.

Steers, W.D. (1995). Benign prostatic hyperplasia. *Disease of the Month, 41,* 437–500.

Svanborg, C., Godaly, G., & Hedlund, M. (1999). Cytokine response during mucosal infections: Role in disease pathogenesis and host defence. *Current Opinions in Microbiology, 2* (1), 99–105.

Swartz, M.N., et al. (1999). Late syphilis. In K.K. Holmes, et al. (Eds.), *Sexually transmitted diseases* (3rd ed.). New York: McGraw-Hill.

Sweet, R.L. (1995). Role of bacterial vaginosis in pelvic inflammatory disease. *Clinics in Infectious Disease, 20,* (Suppl. 2), 5271–5272.

Sweet, R.L. & Gibbs, R.S. (1990). *Infectious diseases of the female genital tract.* Baltimore: Williams & Wilkins.

Syed, T.A., et al. (1994). Topical 0.3% and 0.5% podophyllotoxin cream for self-treatment of molluscum contagiosum in males: A placebo-controlled, double-blind study. *Dermatology, 189,* 65.

Toye, B., et al. (1993). Association between antibody to the Chlamydial heat-shock protein and tubal infertility. *Journal of Infectious Diseases, 168,* 1236.

Vashi, A.R., Wojno, K.J., Henricks, W., England, B.A., Vessella, R.L., Lange, P.H., et al. (1997). Determination of the reflux range and appropriate cut points for percent free prostatic specific antigen in 413 men referred for prostatic evaluation using the AxSym system. *Urology, 49,* 19–27.

Ward, T. & Jones, S. (1996). Genitourinary infections. In R. Reese & R. Betts (Eds.), *MAXX: Infectious disease: A practical approach.* (4th ed.). Philadelphia: Lippincott-Raven.

Whitley, R.J., et al. (1980). The natural history of HSV infection of mother and newborn. *Pediatrics, 66,* 489.

Zhang, M.Z., et al. (1997). *Condyloma acuminatum.* In *Sexually transmitted diseases: Epidemiology, pathology, diagnosis, and Treatment.* Boca Raton, FL: CRC Press.

Zur Hausen, H. (1996). Roots and perspectives of contemporary papillomavirus research. *Journal of Cancer Research and Clinical Oncology, 122,* 3.

# Common Menstrual and Menopausal Disorders

## Leslie M. Klein

## Carolyn J. Moore

The first part of this chapter describes the pathophysiology of common problems related to the menstrual cycle, and the second half focuses on the pathophysiologic effects of menopause. Many women prefer to ask their primary care providers for routine gynecologic and reproductive health care. In the course of that care, the practitioner may discover problems that do not require referral to specialists but can be managed in the primary care practice. Included in this category are menstrual cycle–related distress and pain disorders such as dysmenorrhea and premenstrual syndrome (PMS). Unfortunately, women with these disturbing and occasionally debilitating disorders sometimes are not taken seriously, and their conditions are not adequately treated. A holistic orientation to women's health provides a useful framework for helping patients with these types of problems.

Menopause is increasingly being recognized as a time in life in which many pathophysiologic problems develop from estrogen deficit. Here, the mechanism are reviewed through which estrogen deficit causes osteoporosis, cardiovascular diseases, and other problems. Because many women are unable to or choose not to take hormone replacement therapy (HRT), the practitioner must understand the underlying biologic basis for these various postmenopausal illnesses.

*The authors thank Karen K. Nickell, MSN student, for her review of literature on endometriosis, and Dava Shoffner, RN, PhD, for critiquing the section on menopause.*

## MENSTRUAL CYCLE DISORDERS

### Dysmenorrhea

The origin of the word "dysmenorrhea" is from the Greek, meaning "difficult monthly flow." Today, the term dysmenorrhea is used to denote the pain that frequently accompanies menstruation. Various studies estimate the prevalence of dysmenorrhea to be from 30% to 93%, depending on the definition used and the population studied. The incidence of severe and disabling dysmenorrhea usually is cited at around 10% to 15% (Smith, 1993). Dysmenorrhea is the largest single reason for lost work hours among menstruating women. It was estimated in 1985 that dysmenorrhea was responsible for 600 million hours of lost work time annually (Dawood, 1985).

Dysmenorrhea is categorized as either primary or secondary. Primary or functional dysmenorrhea usually begins 6 to 12 months after menarche and is associated with ovulatory menstrual cycles. Secondary dysmenorrhea is associated with the presence of pelvic pathology, most commonly endometriosis. Secondary dysmenorrhea, depending on the type of pelvic dysfunction involved, may begin with the first menstrual cycle but usually occurs later in life. Thus, the onset of menstrual pain several years or more after menarche usually indicates secondary dysmenorrhea (Dawood, 1990).

### Secondary Dysmenorrhea

Sudden and severe dysmenorrhea beginning at menarche is rare, and congenital defects in müllerian tube structure should be suspected. The dysmenorrhea in these cases is caused by an outflow obstruction requiring surgical correction. However, dysmenorrhea secondary to endometriosis also has been known to occur at or shortly after menarche (Dawood, 1985).

Other causes of secondary dysmenorrhea include pelvic inflammatory disease (PID), ovarian cysts, uterine polyps, uterine adenomyomas, pelvic adhesions, and ovarian cancers (Dawood, 1990). Intrauterine devices placed for birth control were a significant cause of dysmenorrhea when this type of contraception was commonly used. Careful physical examination and appropriate laboratory testing reveal most of these underlying problems. A laparoscopic examination is usually necessary to confirm the diagnosis of endometriosis.

## Endometriosis

Endometriosis is characterized by the presence of extrauterine endometrial tissue implants on the ovaries, fallopian tubes, ureters, peritoneum, and outer surfaces of the uterus (Damewood et al., 1997). It is a disorder that affects 10% of reproductive-aged women and is an important cause of infertility. Ectopic tissues are implanted in adjacent structures after endometrial seeding most probably through retrograde menstruation. These tissue implants respond to the cyclic influences of the female hormones just like the uterine endometrium, and the menstrual release of blood and prostaglandins from this tissue causes the associated pain. However, retrograde menstruation is a common phenomenon, and individuals who develop endometriosis react differently to the extrauterine glands and stroma, possibly through an autoimmune type of reactivity. Reduced numbers of cytotoxic and natural killer (NK) cells, increased T-suppressor cells, and increased peritoneal macrophages are involved. Macrophages secrete transforming growth factor-beta, which promotes angiogenesis and inhibits NK cell function (Corwin, 1997). The net effect is inflammation, pain, scarring, and distortion of tissue implants, which may contribute to infertility. The degree of pain is not related to the extent of endometriosis. Dyspareunia is a frequent co-complaint in women who have dysmenorrhea secondary to endometriosis, as are infertility and chronic pelvic pain (Schroeder & Sanfilippo, 1999).

### Primary Dysmenorrhea

The onset of primary dysmenorrhea usually coincides with the initiation of ovulatory cycles 6 to 12 months after menarche. Symptoms sometimes lessen, at least temporarily, after the birth of a

---

## CLINICAL VIGNETTE 18.1

Ms. Johnson is a 33-year-old married female, G2 P1, who presents to the clinic complaining of menstrual pain.

History of present illness: She states that over the last 18 months she has had increasing pain with menstruation that has caused her to miss work and limit her activities. The pain is cramping and continues throughout her menstrual flow, although it is worst on the first 3 days. Ibuprofen helps some. Upon questioning, she states that she has also recently begun to experience pain with intercourse.

Past medical history: No significant illnesses; no previous surgeries. Takes no routine medications except a daily multivitamin. Menarche age 12, cycle length regular at 29 to 30 days, menstrual flow is usually light to moderate. Did experience mild to moderate dysmenorrhea as adolescent and young adult but this was easily treated with over-the-counter medications and decreased significantly after the birth of her child. Her 7-year-old daughter was born vaginally at full term after an uncomplicated pregnancy and labor. Last Pap smear was 3 years ago.

Family history: Her mother and older sister have both had hysterectomies, but Ms. Johnson does not know why.

Physical examination: Within normal limits except for a fixed retroverted uterus.

Laboratory results: Complete blood count and differential are normal. Cervical cultures for gonorrhea and chlamydia are negative. CA-125 is mildly elevated. Pap smear is normal.

Assessment: History and exam are compatible with endometriosis. In the absence of dyspareunia, a 3-month trial of prescriptive strength nonsteroidal anti-inflammatory drugs is appropriate.

Plan: Referral to a gynecologist for diagnostic laparoscopy and treatment.

child (Dawood, 1985). Nearly every menstruating woman experiences menstrual discomfort on occasion. In some women, this dysmenorrhea is severe and disabling, leaving them unable to function for 24 to 72 hours a month. In most women with primary dysmenorrhea, the pain begins with the onset of menstrual flow and recedes after 24 to 48 hours.

Risk factors for dysmenorrhea have been studied, but results are inconclusive. Several studies have attempted to correlate the severity of dysmenorrhea with lifestyle factors such as diet, amount of exercise, smoking, and alcohol use. A longitudinal study of 195 college women failed to find a significant correlation between dysmenorrhea and smoking, alcohol use, or exercise (Harlow & Park, 1996). Harel, Biro, Kottenhahn, and Rosenthal (1996) found that using fish oil supplements decreased the severity of dysmenorrhea and postulated that a diet heavy in red meat increased menstrual pain, whereas other studies (Johnson et al., 1995; Cintio et al., 1997) found no correlation between diet and dysmenorrhea. Exercise has been shown to decrease the severity of dysmenorrhea symptoms in some studies (Hightower, 1997), but exercisers do not seem to have a decreased incidence of dysmenorrhea (Johnson et al., 1995; Jarrett et al., 1995).

### Pain

Psychosocial variables such as stress, general perceptions of health (Jarrett et al., 1995), menstrual attitudes, emotional reactions at menarche (Shaver et al., 1987), knowledge base about menstruation, and maternal menstrual discomfort (Campbell & McGrath, 1997) have not been shown to have any correlation with the severity of menstrual pain or with the tendency to self-medicate for menstrual pain. In these studies, the only variables that were consistently correlated with medication use were severity and duration of menstrual symptoms. The major factors affecting the severity of dysmenorrhea are physiological.

The chain of physiologic events that leads to menstrual pain begins with the buildup of endometrial tissue during the proliferative and secretory phases of the menstrual cycle. Progesterone, released by the corpus luteum, has a major influence on endometrial composition; hence, the correlation of dysmenorrhea with ovulatory cycles. As the secretory phase ends and menstrual flow begins, phospholipids are released from the cell walls of the sloughing endometrium. These phospholipids are converted by phospholipase $A_2$ to arachidonic acid. Cyclooxygenase then acts on arachidonic acid to produce cyclic endoperoxides and 5-hydroperoxyeicosatetraenoic acid (5-

HPETE). Cyclic endoperoxides are, in turn, acted on by several enzymes to generate prostaglandins and thromboxanes, whereas 5-HPETE is converted to leukotrienes, most notably leukotrienes B and C. The major prostaglandins produced in the human uterus are $PGE_2$, a vasodilator, and $PGF_{2\alpha}$. Hypercontractility and vasoconstriction are caused by $PGF_{2\alpha}$, whereas the leukotrienes are potent vasoconstrictors. Both substances sensitize nerve endings (Smith, 1993). Menstrual pain is a result of the sensitized nerve endings and uterine ischemia caused by hypercontractility of uterine smooth muscle and vasoconstriction (Fig. 18-1).

Women with dysmenorrhea have increased levels of $PGF_{2\alpha}$ in menstrual fluid compared with normal controls (Pickles et al., 1965; Powell et al.,

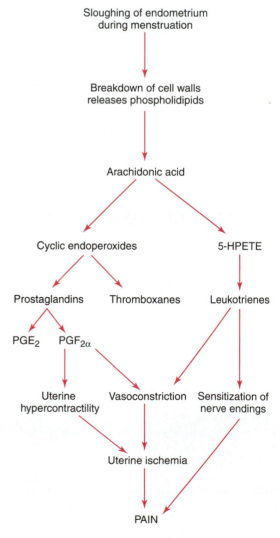

**FIGURE 18.1** ● Physiologic pathways of menstrual pain.

1985). Phospholipid metabolism may be increased in the uterine wall in dysmenorrhea, which leads to an accumulation of arachidonic acid metabolites. These, in turn, cause pain.

The reason for the difference in prostaglandin levels is not known. A study of menstrual pain and limitation conducted on Australian twins by Treloar, Martin, and Heath (1998) concludes that up to 77% of menstrually induced activity limitations can be explained by genetic factors.

Primary care providers should realize that most women view menstrual pain as a natural and expected event. Even women with severe and disabling dysmenorrhea view themselves as healthy (Jarrett et al., 1995) and may not report dysmenorrhea. Also, most women tend to self-treat menstrual symptoms rather than to seek help from a health care provider. Therefore, the clinician must question women of reproductive age regarding the degree of dysmenorrhea, efficacy of self-care measures, and degree of limitation caused by dysmenorrhea. Adolescents and women who report frequently or even occasionally missing work or school or in whom self-care measures are not effective then may be identified and treated.

### Physiologic Basis of Treatment

Standard treatments for primary dysmenorrhea include combination oral contraceptives (COCs) and antiprostaglandins. Of the antiprostaglandins, the most useful and best tolerated are the non-steroidal anti-inflammatory drugs (NSAIDs). If one NSAID does not prove effective in a 3-month trial, another from a different class can be used. The COCs are ideal in women who also need birth control and have no contraindications. If both COCs and NSAIDs have been tried without relief, the client should be reevaluated for secondary causes. Referral of these cases may prove necessary.

Other treatments that have been advocated for use in dysmenorrhea include transcutaneous electrical nerve stimulation (TENS), low-dose nitroglycerin patches, acupuncture, acupressure, fish oil supplements, and the Chinese herb dong quai. Dong quai contains a carcinogen and an agent that can cause photodermitis and is not recommended (Therapeutic Research Center, 1998). Acupuncture is widely used for menstrual disorders in the Far East, but a controlled study failed to show effectiveness (Helms, 1987). Acupressure likewise has failed in a controlled trial (Mahoney, 1993). Fish oil supplements (Harel et al., 1996) and nitroglycerin patches (Pittrof et al., 1996) have shown some promise but still are investigational. Several studies have proven TENS to be effective for menstrual pain (Milsom et al., 1994; Kaplan et al., 1994); it is an alternative for women who have contraindications to COCs or prefer not to use medications. Regular aerobic exercise may be helpful and should be advocated in any case for its multiple beneficial effects.

### Premenstrual Syndrome

Premenstrual syndrome was first identified in 1931 by Frank, who termed the condition premenstrual tension. It captured popular attention in 1980 when it was successfully used as a defense in a murder trial. Since then, it has been the subject of intermittent research and popular speculation. Many different definitions, theories, and treatments have been proposed, most of which have since proven to be inaccurate or ineffective. Only in the last 10 years has PMS become a well-defined and treatable condition.

Over 150 different symptoms have been ascribed to PMS over the last 60 years. Painstaking research, which was conducted by Mortola and his associates at the University of California at San Diego, has defined a specific set of symptoms that characterize the PMS experience. Affective symptoms of irritability, depression, and fatigue occur in most women with PMS, along with physical symptoms such as bloating, breast tenderness, and headache. Other common affective and behavioral symptoms include labile mood, crying spells, social withdrawal, difficulty concentrating, and oversensitivity. Other physical symptoms that frequently occur in women with PMS include acne, food cravings, appetite changes, and gastrointestinal (GI) upset (Mortola, 1997a).

More important than the nature of the symptoms is their timing. Symptoms must be present during the luteal phase of the menstrual cycle and be greatly decreased or absent in the follicular phase to support a diagnosis of PMS. Because retrospective reporting has not been accurate in quantifying premenstrual changes, prospective reporting of daily symptoms throughout at least two complete, unmedicated menstrual cycles is required. A simple and reliable recording tool is the Calendar of Premenstrual Experiences (COPE), which is available from the Department of Reproductive Medicine at the University of California, San Diego (Mortola et al., 1990). Other tools also are available, and a less formal symptom diary also can be used.

Many women experience some symptoms of PMS. Only 20% to 25% of women do not notice any premenstrual changes. Of the remainder, 20% to 40% of women experience occasional diffi-

## CLINICAL VIGNETTE 18.2

Ms. Crawford is a 19-year-old college freshman who reports to the university clinic complaining of menstrual cramping that is severe enough to cause her to miss class for a day or two almost every month.

History of present illness: Ms. Crawford reports that she has experienced severe cramping at almost every period for the last 4 years. The pain is intense and cramplike and lasts 36 to 48 hours. Ibuprofen and heat help a little. She has dealt with this in the past by taking 200–400 mg of ibuprofen two or three times a day and "Going to bed with a heating pad until I feel better." She is requesting assistance at this time because "missing a day or two of classes every month is affecting my grades."

Past medical history: Usual childhood illnesses. No serious illnesses. Had "tubes in ears" at age 3, no other surgeries. No current medications. Does not smoke. Reports an occasional beer or two on weekends. Gravida 0. Menarche at age 13, regular cycles averaging 26 to 28 days, moderate flow lasting 5 to 7 days. Not currently in a relationship, reports one sexual partner in high school. Has never had a Pap smear.

Family history: Noncontributory.

Physical Examination: Normal findings.

Laboratory results: Hemoglobin 10 mg/dL, hematocrit 32, remainder of complete blood count and differential within normal limits. Cervical cultures for gonorrhea and chlamydia are negative. Pap smear is normal. CA-125 is normal.

Assessment: Severe primary dysmenorrhea and mild anemia.

Plan: Ms. Crawford has no contraindications or objections to combination-type oral contraceptives (COCs). She is begun on a low-dose 28-day formulation. She is warned that COCs do not prevent STDs. She is advised to continue to take ibuprofen as needed, to take a daily multivitamin with iron, and to increase her aerobic exercise. A follow-up visit is scheduled in 3 months.

Follow-up: Ms. Crawford reports the pain has eased up a lot and that she did not miss any classes last month. Her flow is also lighter and shorter, and her hemoglobin is now 12 mg/dL. She states she has taken ibuprofen once or twice a day during the last two periods but is still having breakthrough pain. COCs are continued and her nonsteroidal anti-inflammatory drug is changed to a prescription dose of naproxen. She is instructed to start taking the naproxen at the onset of menstruation and continue it around the clock for 48 hours rather than to wait until pain becomes severe. This regimen proves to be effective and Ms. Crawford experiences a pain-free period for the first time in 4 years.

---

culty with PMS symptoms, 10% to 20% have moderate premenstrual symptoms that may cause lifestyle disruptions, 10% to 20% have severe PMS with lifestyle dysfunction, and 2% to 5% meet the criteria specified in the DSM-IV for premenstrual dysphoric disorder (PMDD) (Mortola, 1992b).

PMS and PMDD probably represent two points on a continuum rather than distinct conditions. The criteria for PMDD specify that 5 of 11 mostly affective and behavioral symptoms must have occurred during the last week of the menstrual cycle in most of the woman's cycles for the preceding year and that another affective disorder is not present. Depression, anxiety, irritability, or labile mood must be included in the symptom set. Physical symptoms are grouped together and counted as one of the required five symptoms (Freeman et al., 1996).

## Epidemiology and Pathophysiology

Researchers have not been able to determine any definitive risk factors for PMS. It usually begins in the mid-20s and can continue through the fourth decade of life (Woods et al., 1997). Menopause, whether natural or induced, always ends PMS. Some women experience a reduction in symptom severity while taking oral contraceptives (OCs), but most do not. In some cases, PMS has been induced by using OCs or other hormonal therapies. Oral contraceptives may provide a more advantageous hormonal environment for the few women who do obtain relief with their use (Mortola, 1994).

Stress is correlated with PMS but is not a causative factor (Beck et al., 1990). Women with PMS do not manifest high levels of stress when tested during their follicular phase. It seems that

PMS causes stress rather than the reverse. Wide-scale screening using the Minnesota Multiphasic Personality Inventory likewise shows that personality factors are not a causative factor in PMS (Mortola, 1997a). Women with a negative affect frequently report PMS symptoms but do not differ from normal controls in rates of PMS when daily prospective ratings are used for diagnosis (Akker et al., 1995). One feminist viewpoint, that PMS is a sociopolitical construct invented to repress women, is unlikely in view of the more definitive research available. Biologic factors seem to play the biggest role in PMS etiology.

The pathophysiologic processes involved in PMS appear to be a result of complex interactions between ovarian hormones, neurotransmitters, endogenous opioids, and the autonomic nervous system. The pathway involved is not clear, and research is continuing. The fact that the neurobehavioral symptoms are a result of defects in the mechanisms regulating the neurotransmitter serotonin (5-hydroxytryptamine) is strongly implied by laboratory and animal studies. It was thought until recently that the luteal surge of progesterone might be responsible for initiating PMS symptoms, since progesterone had been found to affect both the serotonin and γ-aminobutyric acid neurotransmitter systems. A study using the progesterone antagonist RU 486 did not support this hypothesis (Chan et al., 1994). It seems likely at this point that the relative serotonin deficiency found in women with PMS is initiated by cyclic variations in one or more of the ovarian hormones, probably in combination with idiosyncratic variations in central nervous system sensitivity to these hormones (Mortola, 1997). The fact that multiple controlled research trials (Diegoli et al., 1998; Mortola, 1997; Ozren et al., 1997; Steiner et al., 1995; Sunblad et al., 1997; Wood et al., 1992) have established the effectiveness of selective serotonin reuptake inhibitors (SSRIs) in relieving the affective and behavioral symptoms of PMS in most women further supports this hypothesis.

## Differential Diagnosis

Many other disorders mimic the symptoms of PMS, so the differential diagnosis is critical. Medical conditions that must be ruled out include anemia, diabetes mellitus, hypothyroidism, chronic fatigue syndrome, and collagen vascular diseases. Hormonal imbalances, such as those found in perimenopause, hyperprolactinemia, hypoandrogynism, hypothyroidism, or hypoglycemia, should also be investigated. Laboratory tests that may be helpful in ruling out these disorders include a complete blood count, urinalysis, blood chemistries, thyroid-stimulating hormone levels, and other hormonal assays.

Conditions that frequently have a premenstrual exacerbation also may be confused with PMS. For example, women who experience migraine headaches may find that they occur more frequently in the premenstrual period. Irritable bowel syndrome, asthma, and psychiatric disorders also may have premenstrual exacerbations (Freeman et al., 1996). Premenstrual exacerbation of a psychiatric disorder is the diagnosis most frequently mistaken for PMS. Completing a psychiatric screening of the client during her postmenstrual or follicular phase is important in avoiding this error. The definitions of PMS and PMDD include the stipulation that a psychiatric disorder other than PMDD is not present.

Neophyte practitioners may question taking the time to establish an accurate diagnosis when distinguishing between PMS and premenstrual exacerbation of a depressive disorder, since an SSRI is likely to make the client feel better in either case. Some clients prefer to carry a diagnosis of PMS, since it presents less of a social stigma than does depression. The importance of establishing a diagnosis is more understandable when treatment options are clarified. Whereas SSRIs are helpful for many persons, they are not uniformly effective in all cases of depression or PMS. In clients with depression, another class of antidepressants may be more effective. For those with PMS, antidepressants from other classes are not effective.

Therefore, the use of a daily symptom rating tool such as the COPE is essential before initiating treatment. The COPE has been established as reliable in serial studies, with a false-negative rate of 2.8% and a false-positive rate of less than 1% when used as recommended throughout two consecutive, unmedicated menstrual cycles (Mortola et al., 1990). In a client with PMS, COPE scores during the client's luteal phases will be at least twice as high as scores during the follicular phases. Luteal scores should total at least 42, whereas follicular scores should be less than 40. An affective disorder should be suspected if follicular phase COPE scores are greater than 40. Clients who have a luteal score that is 30% to 50% higher than their follicular score and yet whose luteal score still is under 40 may be considered to have subclinical PMS.

When using other tools or a symptom diary to establish the accuracy of a presumptive diagnosis of PMS, careful consideration of the symptoms as well as their timing and severity is essential. Affective or behavioral symptoms should be absent or minimal in the follicular or postmenstrual phase

## CLINICAL VIGNETTE 18.3

Melissa Storm is a 29-year-old married female who presents to the nurse practitioner requesting treatment for premenstrual syndrome (PMS).

History of present illness: Ms. Storm reports that she becomes so depressed in the week before her period that it is difficult for her to function. She states that she has had this problem for about 18 months, since weaning her 2 1/2-year-old daughter. She had also experienced some postpartum depression after her daughter's birth that "never really went away." She says that she is tired all the time and doesn't sleep well but is able to function fairly well except for the week just before her period starts. She is presently 25 days into her menstrual cycle.

Past medical history: Ms. Storm had the usual childhood illnesses. She had an appendectomy at age 14; no other surgeries. She denies any health problems and takes no medications. Her immunizations are up to date. She is a G1 P1 and had an uncomplicated pregnancy and delivery. She has regular periods 27 to 29 days apart. She did not menstruate for the 11 months that she breastfed her daughter.

Family history: Ms. Storm is adopted.

Psychosocial: Ms. Storm does not work outside the home. Her husband is an advertising executive. She reports that her husband is understanding and supportive but that "he is getting tired of this too." Her adoptive parents live nearby and have been helping with childcare and errands when Ms.

Storm is having trouble coping. She denies any drug or alcohol abuse problems. She denies any suicidal ideation.

Physical examination: Ms. Storm is 12% below her ideal weight. She is pale and listless, speaks hesitantly, and does not make eye contact. Her clothing is drab, her hair is limp, and she is not wearing any makeup or jewelry. Findings are otherwise unremarkable.

Laboratory results: Complete blood count, urinalysis, TSH, T4, and blood chemistries are all normal.

Plan: The importance of an accurate diagnosis is explained to Ms. Storm and she agrees to keep the "Calendar of Premenstrual Experiences" (COPE) for the next two menstrual cycles. She is instructed to call sooner if her difficulties increase and to schedule her return appointment during her postmenstrual week.

Diagnosis: When Ms. Storm arrives for her follow-up appointment, she is somewhat more animated, making occasional eye contact with the practitioner. She is wearing pastel clothing and lipstick. The COPE score totals over the previous two cycles are 42 during the follicular phase and 56 during the luteal phase. A Beck's depression index administered on this date reveals a mild depression. Ms. Storm's diagnosis is premenstrual exacerbation of depressive disorder.

Treatment: Ms. Storm is prescribed fluoxetine 20 mg daily and is referred to a licensed clinical social worker for counseling. Regular aerobic exercise is recommended. Appropriate follow-up is arranged.

---

and present to a significant degree in the luteal phase of at least two consecutive, unmedicated menstrual cycles to justify a PMS diagnosis (Mortola, 1992a).

After a diagnosis is established, the practitioner next should consider the severity of the symptoms and the effects on the client's functioning. A client with mild or subclinical PMS may benefit from a combination of education, support, and lifestyle changes. Clients who have moderate to severe PMS with lifestyle disruptions may need immediate pharmacologic treatment, whereas clients who meet the criteria for PMDD may need therapy that is beyond the scope of the nurse practitioner. Lifestyle disruptions in PMS are evidenced by (1) marital or relationship discord confirmed by the

client's partner, (2) difficulties in parenting as evidenced by behavioral disturbances in the children, (3) legal difficulties, (4) confirmed poor work or school performance, or (5) suicidal ideation (Mortola, 1997a). Criteria for PMDD may be found in the DSM-IV.

### Physiologic Basis for Treating Premenstrual Syndrome

During the assessment process, any woman who meets DSM-IV criteria for major depressive disorder, bipolar disorder, or PPD should be referred for psychiatric evaluation and consultation. Anyone exhibiting depression should be carefully questioned regarding suicidal ideation. If the client admits active suicidal thoughts or plans, she

## CLINICAL VIGNETTE 18.4

Joyce Jones is a 35-year-old single female who presents to her primary care provider requesting "something for my nerves before I go crazy or kill someone!"

History of present illness: Ms. Jones reports that she becomes oversensitive, easily angered, and irritable every month before and during her period. She says that she has had complaints from her coworkers about her moodiness and that her partner knows "to just leave me alone when I get like this." She also drives aggressively during this time and is barely able to control episodes of road rage. It is worse some months and better some months. She also complains of bloating and intense cravings for chocolate and sweets during this time.

Past medical history: Ms. Jones had chickenpox and recurrent ear infections as a young child. She also had an episode of meningitis at age 12, for which she was hospitalized. She had "tubes in ears" twice before age 4 and a tonsillectomy at age 5; no other surgeries. Her immunizations are up to date. She has never been pregnant, had menarche at age 11, and menstruates regularly on a 28 to 30 day cycle. She has mild persistent asthma for which she uses a cromolyn inhaler QID and an albuterol inhaler PRN; no other medications.

Family history: Ms. Jones' mother is 51 and healthy; her father is 55 and has hypertension. Her maternal grandmother died of a stroke at age 68; her maternal grandfather is 85 and has Alzheimer's. She doesn't know anything about her paternal grandparents. She has a younger sister who is healthy.

Psychosocial: Ms. Jones is a lesbian and has been in a committed relationship for 9 years. She manages a clothing store; her partner is a nurse. She denies any drug or alcohol abuse but states that she drinks socially. She does not smoke. She does not exercise regularly but does walk her dog for a short distance daily.

Physical examination: Ms. Jones is about 20% over her ideal weight. A few wheezes are noted on auscultation of lung sounds. All other findings are within normal limits.

Laboratory results: Complete blood count, urinalysis, TSH, T4 are all normal. Random glucose is slightly elevated at 125; other chemistries are normal.

Plan: Ms. Jones will keep the Calendar of Premenstrual Experiences (COPE) for the next two menstrual cycles, during which she is to avoid or minimize her alcohol use. She is scheduled to return in 2 weeks, during her follicular phase, to complete a Minnesota Multiphasic Personality Inventory (MMPI) and undergo a 3-hour glucose tolerance test. She is also asked to bring confirmation from her partner or her assistant manager that her premenstrual moods are disrupting these roles.

Diagnosis: The 2-hour glucose is 141. MMPI results are nominal. COPE scores are 55 in the luteal phase and 24 in the follicular phase. The COPE scores also reveal that although Ms. Jones reported that her symptoms continued throughout her period, they actually dropped precipitously once she began to menstruate. Both Ms. Jones' partner and coworker confirm disruptive premenstrual mood changes. Ms. Jones has moderate premenstrual syndrome (PMS) with lifestyle disruption. She is also at risk of developing diabetes.

Treatment: Ms. Jones is counseled regarding appropriate lifestyle changes. Regular aerobic exercise will reduce her risk of diabetes and can improve her PMS symptoms. Dietary changes and weight loss are also recommended. She is started on fluoxetine 20-mg daily and instructed to report any adverse side effects and to return for follow up in 2 months.

should not simply be referred, but ideally should be accompanied to the appropriate treatment facility. Alternatively, the client can be asked to contract not to make any attempt at suicide while psychiatric care is being arranged.

Women who do not meet DSM-IV criteria for major affective disorders may be appropriately treated by the nurse practitioner. Before choosing a treatment regimen, the level of distress caused by the client's PMS must be ascertained. Clients in whom PMS symptoms do not cause significant disruptions in activities or relationships may be able to manage their PMS nonpharmacologically. Simply being reassured that PMS is a real condition with a biologic cause can be therapeutic. The client can be empowered to deal with her symptoms proactively through a combination of education and lifestyle changes.

Lifestyle changes that have proven beneficial to women with PMS include regular aerobic exercise; an adequate amount of sleep; decreasing the intake of salt, caffeine, and alcohol; and consuming a balanced diet of 60% complex carbohydrates, 20% protein, and 20% fat (Youngkin & Davis, 1998). Other suggestions that may prove beneficial include asking friends and family for support, participating in support groups or counseling, and stress management programs. Simply encouraging the client to rearrange her activities to allow extra rest during her premenstrual week and to defer more challenging or stressful activities to the postmenstrual period can prove salutary.

Such alternative practices as reflexology (Jackson, 1995), transcendental meditation, and Yoga (Ansley, 1998) have reported success in the treatment of PMS. Light therapy also is a possible treatment, since up to 25% of women with PMS report seasonal variation in severity of symptoms (Pray, 1998). Because the placebo response can be high in PMS, clients may be encouraged to try any treatment of interest that does not have harmful potential. Megadoses of B vitamins and evening primrose oil do not fall into the harmless category, however (Mortola, 1994).

If these changes do not provide the client with adequate symptom relief, or if significant lifestyle disruption already is present, medications are indicated. The SSRIs are indicated as first-line PMS medications. Although SSRIs are not always effective for the physical symptoms of PMS, it is the affective symptoms that cause the most distress (Barnhart et al., 1995). The choice of SSRIs should be made with the individual client's needs in mind. Smaller doses than those used in depressive disorders generally are effective, for example, 10 to 20 mg of fluoxetine per day versus the 20- to 60-mg per day dose commonly used to treat depression. Studies indicate that when depression is not present as a comorbid condition, fluoxetine and, possibly, other SSRIs may be as effective when dosing is confined to the luteal phase. This dosing plan can decrease cost and incidence of side effects for clients in whom these factors are a concern (Mortola, 1997b).

If anxiety is a primary symptom and SSRIs are not effective, anxiolytics should be considered. Benzodiazepines should be prescribed with caution, since addiction and abuse are possible. Alprazolam can be prescribed during the luteal phase only, and the client should be weaned at a rate of 25% per day after menses begin. This dosing schedule is effective at relieving symptoms while avoiding dependence and withdrawal (McComb, 1999). If addiction is a concern, buspirone may be prescribed. Buspirone must be taken throughout the menstrual cycle for 2 to 6 weeks before full effectiveness is reached (Freeman et al., 1996). The client should be cautioned in this respect.

If neither the SSRIs nor anxiolytics, in conjunction with lifestyle changes, provide the PMS client with sufficient symptom relief, she may be a candidate for medical oophorectomy. In this mode of therapy, gonadotropin-releasing hormone (GnRH) agonists are prescribed. These medications cause a downregulation of pituitary sensitivity to luteinizing hormone (LH) and follicle-stimulating hormone (FSH) and lead to a cessation of hormone production by the ovary (Mortola, 1997b). The client should be cautioned as to the potential risks of such treatment, including menopausal symptoms and the increase in long-term risks of heart disease, osteoporosis, and possibly Alzheimer's disease. If she elects to pursue this option, she should be referred to a gynecologist with experience in this mode of therapy.

Other medications occasionally are used when physical symptoms are severe. Spironolactone, a potassium-sparing diuretic, can be prescribed during the luteal phase for bloating. Subjective feelings of bloating have not been found to correlate well with actual weight gain, however, and the client should be advised to try increasing exercise and water intake to provoke a natural diuresis before a trial of diuretics is indicated (Mortola, 1994).

Because premenstrual symptoms affect most women at some point, the primary care provider can expect to hear complaints of these symptoms on a regular basis. No one PMS therapy is suitable to all women, but most women who have PMS can find relief through one or more of these therapies. The primary care provider is in a prime position to help women who are affected by PMS to improve their health and functional ability.

## MENOPAUSE-ASSOCIATED DISORDERS

Menopause is an assured event in the life of a woman as she ages. The transition from reproductive to nonreproductive years can be a time of anticipation and relief for some women, whereas for others it brings connotations of aging and loss of womanhood. Primary care providers encounter many women who are entering this phase of their lives, so they must be prepared to manage the health care challenges of menopause and to provide care that prevents its complications.

Since the life expectancy of women is increasing, more women will experience menopause.

More than 1 million women in the United States experience menopause each year, and with the average life expectancy being nearly 80 years of age for American women, many women will spend one third of their lives in menopause (Levine, 1998).

For some women, menopause brings with it a sense of satisfaction, content, and a new meaning to relationships. For others, it is seen as a time of loss. Some women view menopause as an end to their childbearing years and an end to their sexuality. To others, menopause signifies the onset of the aging process. For most women, however, menopause is seen as a natural stage in the life process, a common bond shared between mothers, daughters, sisters, and friends. Menopause should not be viewed by health care providers as a negative experience, but as a new phase in a woman's life that promises new rewards and challenges. It allows providers the perfect opportunity to deliver woman-centered care to the aging woman while promoting a lifetime of positive health maintenance practices.

## Stages of Menopause

As a woman ages, the frequency of ovulation begins to decline, and levels of estrogen and progesterone steadily decrease. This results in changes in the menstrual cycle. After a while, menstruation ceases completely, and estrogen levels fall dramatically. This process is known as menopause.

Perimenopause is the period immediately before and after the cessation of menses. This period lasts roughly 4 years; however, anovulatory cycles may occur as much as 10 years before menopause (Speroff et al., 1994). During anovulation, hormonal levels may become erratic, leading to irregular and heavy menstrual cycles. Other symptoms that may occur during the perimenopausal period include hot flashes, vaginal dryness, insomnia, mood swings, and memory loss. During this phase, bone loss begins to occur as a result of lower estrogen levels, which may later lead to osteoporosis. Health care choices made during this time may have a significant impact on a woman's health in later years.

Menopause is defined as the cessation of menses for 12 consecutive months. It can be further defined as natural, artificial, or hormonal menopause. Natural menopause is an inevitable event occurring as a result of decreased ovarian function in the presence of adequate gonadotropin stimulation. On average, natural menopause occurs between the ages of 48 and 55 years, with 95% of women having reached menopause by age 55 (Beckmann, et al., 1997). The mean age for natural menopause is 51 years (Voda, 1997). Artificial menopause occurs as a result of surgical removal of the uterus or both ovaries. It may also occur in women who have undergone chemotherapy or radiation therapy. Hormonal menopause occurs in women who have previously used sex hormones such as estrogens or progestins. Women who have used hormone therapy during the perimenopausal phase experience menopause 1 to 2 years later than nonhormone users (Harper, 1990).

Approximately 1% of women will experience menopause before 40 years of age; this is known as premature menopause or premature ovarian failure. Etiologies of premature ovarian failure include chemotherapy, radiation, autoimmune disorders, infection, metabolic disorders, chromosomal abnormalities, ovarian ischemia, and trauma.

Several other factors are associated with early onset of menopause. Cigarette smokers have been shown to reach menopause 1 to 2 years earlier than nonsmoking women (Youngkin & Davis, 1998). Living at high altitudes also is correlated with earlier onset of menopause (Speroff et al., 1994). Thinner women seem to experience menopause at an earlier age, presumably because of the correlation between body fat and estrogen production. Some women who have undergone abdominal hysterectomy without oophorectomy may experience symptoms of premature menopause. For many women who have had hysterectomies, menopause may occur 3 to 5 years earlier than the mean age for natural menopause (Beckman et al., 1997). This is believed to result from compromised ovarian blood flow at the time of surgery or from the lack of hormonal stimulation that the uterus normally infers on the ovaries (Speroff et al., 1994).

Several factors are associated with delayed menopause including uterine leiomyomas, diabetes mellitus, breast cancer, and endometrial and cervical cancer (Mezrow & Rebar, 1990). Women who have used estrogen during the perimenopausal period may experience menopause 1 to 2 years later than women who have not (Harper, 1990).

Although it is commonly believed that mothers and daughters experience menopause at the same approximate age, little evidence supports this. Age of menarche does not correspond to age at onset of menopause.

## Physiologic Events

Approximately 8 million oocytes develop in the female fetus during the gestational period, yet by birth the number has decreased to about 1 million. The number of oocytes present in the female declines rapidly from birth, so that by puberty only about 400,000 are present. This process is known as atresia. By age 35, a woman may have only 100,000 eggs left, and by the onset of menopause, this number has declined to less than 10,000 (Dawood, 1993). About 400 eggs are ovulated during the reproductive years (Beckman et al., 1997).

Menstruation is the result of a complex interactive process between the hypothalamus, the anterior pituitary gland, the ovaries, and associated target organs. The hypothalamus secretes GnRH, in turn stimulating the anterior pituitary gland to secrete the gonadotropic hormones known as FSH and LH. The action of FSH and LH occurs in the ovaries. Theca cells surrounding the oocyte are stimulated by LH to produce androgens, estrogens, and progesterone. Ovulation occurs under the influence of FSH and LH.

Three types of estrogens are produced in the body: estrone ($E_1$), estradiol ($E_2$), and estriol ($E_3$). Of these, estradiol is the most potent and most abundant estrogen produced in the premenopausal years, whereas estrone becomes the most common in the postmenopausal years. Estrone and estradiol are the estrogens that have been implicated in the development of breast and ovarian cancer, whereas estriol is noncarcinogenic. Estriol is a less potent form of estrogen, which is converted in the liver from estrone. A small amount of estriol is secreted by the ovary. Estradiol is produced by the granulosa cells of the ovarian follicles and is dependent on FSH. Throughout the aging process, estradiol levels, progesterone levels, and follicular activity decline, thus interrupting the negative feedback system in the anterior pituitary that controls ovulation and menstruation. The pituitary gland in turn releases FSH and LH to stimulate the ovaries to increase hormonal production.

Estrogen is secreted cyclically from the ovaries throughout the menstrual cycle and is responsible for the normal sexual maturation of the female. Estrogen levels peak just before ovulation and during the middle of the luteal phase, promoting endometrial proliferation in preparation for pregnancy. Estrogen plays a role in the process of ovulation, implantation of the fertilized ovum, maintenance of pregnancy, and lactation. In addition, estrogens stimulate maturation of the vagina, uterus, fallopian tubes, and breasts during embryonic development and during puberty. Skeletal growth, fat distribution, axillary and pubic hair growth, and skin pigmentation occur as a result of estrogen production.

Additionally, estrogen exerts many effects outside of the reproductive system. Bone resorption, or the loss of bone, occurs at a slower rate under the influence of estrogen, thus the onset of menopause contributes to the development of osteoporosis in postmenopausal women by increasing the rate of bone loss. Estrogens have a positive effect on the cardiovascular system by increasing high-density lipoprotein (HDL) levels and lowering low-density lipoprotein (LDL) and total cholesterol levels. Other cardioprotective effects of estrogen include vasodilation of the vessels, increased left ventricular filling, and increased stroke volume. Adversely, estrogens increase triglyceride levels and promote coagulation of the blood by increasing plasminogen levels and factors II, VII, IX, and X. With the onset of menopause, the risk of cardiac disease greatly increases, making cardiovascular disease the leading cause of morbidity and mortality in the aging female (Youngkin & Davis, 1998). Estrogen is thought to protect against Alzheimer's disease and dementia as well. The mechanism of action is believed to be a direct effect in the brain, possibly increased cerebral blood flow and increased production of neurotransmitters.

Ovarian changes precede the onset of menopause. After age 35, fewer follicles are present, and production of estrogen and progesterone by the ovaries begins to decline. The remaining oocytes become resistant to the effects of FSH. Normally during the monthly menstrual cycle, FSH levels increase to stimulate the developing follicle to produce more estrogen. Higher estrogen levels, in turn, decrease FSH stimulation, a negative feedback in the hypothalamus-pituitary axis. With the perimenopausal phase, when estrogen levels are declining, plasma levels of FSH begin to rise. At the onset of menopause, FSH levels become much higher. Changes in the menstrual cycle occur gradually in response to fluctuating hormone levels until ovarian failure eventually occurs. At this point, menstruation ceases and menopause has begun.

After menopause, the theca cells in the ovarian stroma continue to produce hormones in the absence of follicles and estrogen under the influence of LH. The adrenal glands continue to produce androgens at the premenopausal rate. The androgens, androstenedione and testosterone, are the major hormones present in postmenopausal women. The ovarian thecal cells in postmenopausal women produce about twice as much testosterone as those of premenopausal women (Beckman et al., 1997). An exception to this is in premenopausal women who undergo oophorectomy, at which time there is a 50% decrease in plasma testosterone levels (Goldzieher, 1997). Approximately 95% of androstenedione is produced by the adrenal glands, whereas 5% is produced from the ovaries in postmenopausal women (Brenner & Mishell, 1991). Androstenedione is converted in the fatty tissues to estrone, the most common form of estrogen produced in menopausal women. Estrone levels are higher in women with higher body fat distribution, resulting from a higher conversion rate of androstenedione to estrone. Therefore, obese women experience fewer symptoms of hypoestrogenemia than do thinner women, and the incidence of osteoporosis is lower. At the same time, obese women are more likely to develop endometrial hyperplasia or adenocarcinoma as a result of higher levels of androstenedione (Brenner & Mishel, 1991).

After menopause, the ovaries become scarred, atrophied, and fibrotic and no longer produce estrogen. Estrogen remains measurable in the blood, however, given the conversion of androgens to estrogens. Whereas the plasma levels of androgens decline after menopause, there is an overall increase in androgenicity because of lowered estrogen levels.

## Clinical Presentation

Declining estrogen levels may produce several bothersome symptoms, which may impact a woman's quality of life. Symptoms of estrogen deficiency may occur during the perimenopausal phase; however, the severity of symptoms increases with complete ovarian failure. Although menopause is inevitable, producing a variety of untoward effects, only about 40% of women find its symptoms intolerable enough to seek help from their provider (Noble, 1996).

The first indication that a woman is entering the perimenopausal phase may be a change in menstrual cycles such as irregularity, menorrhagia, or oligomenorrhea. During this time, FSH levels begin to rise, indicating a decline in ovarian function. Hot flashes may begin to occur. Vasomotor symptoms occur in up to 95% of menopausal women (Wehrle, 1996). Several hypotheses explain the causes of hot flashes, including a surge in LH levels, changes in the hypothalamus brought on by the GnRHs, the relationship between estrogen levels and the metabolism of catecholamines, and, possibly, a surge in prostaglandins (Harper, 1990). Hot flashes may last up to several minutes per episode and may occur up to 20 times per day. They may be associated with an intense feeling of warmth in the face, neck, and chest, flushing of the

skin, sweating, palpitations, shaking, and anxiety. Typically, hot flashes are worse at night and may occur in response to food or alcohol intake. In general, hot flashes resolve spontaneously within 5 years of the onset of menopause if estrogen replacement therapy is not prescribed (Beckman et al., 1997).

Sleep disturbances, including insomnia and frequent awakenings, are a common occurrence in menopausal women and may result from nocturnal hot flashes. It also may take longer to fall asleep. Sleep deprivation may lead to irritability, fatigue, mood disturbance, and difficulty with relationships.

The most bothersome effects of menopause occur in the urogenital tract. The tissues of the genital tract are estrogen dependent. With the loss of estrogen, major changes occur in the genitalia and urinary tract. Loss of pubic hair occurs, and the external genitalia become smaller and thinner, but the most obvious changes occur in the vagina itself. The vagina becomes shorter, thinner, and less elastic. The vaginal epithelium becomes thin, pale, and friable. Atrophy of the vaginal mucosa may induce symptoms of urinary frequency, urgency, dysuria, and incontinence. Many women may become more susceptible to urinary tract infections because of changes in the urethral epithelium. In addition, the pH of the vagina changes, becoming less acidic and more conducive to yeast vaginitis. Blood flow to the vagina is decreased, resulting in diminished vaginal secretions, which makes sexual intercourse painful and difficult. Postcoital bleeding may occur as a result of irritation and loss of lubrication. The uterus, cervix, and ovaries become smaller, comparable to prepubertal size, whereas pelvic musculature weakens and frequently leads to uterine, bladder, or rectal prolapse.

The effects of menopause and estrogen deprivation on female sexuality vary from woman to woman. Several factors may combine to cause a decrease in sexual function including vaginal atrophy, diminished vaginal lubrication, and decreased libido. Response to sexual stimulation and orgasm also may be altered. These changes may occur as a result of lowered estrogen levels, as well as altered androgen levels.

Many women associate menopause with psychological symptoms including irritability, mood swings, depression, crying spells, memory lapses, and difficulty concentrating. Controversy exists as to whether these symptoms are a result of decreasing estrogen levels or other events that a woman may be experiencing. Sleep deprivation also may contribute to feelings of moodiness, irritability, and a general sense of fatigue. Studies fail to consistently support the view that menopause negatively affects mental well-being (Speroff et al., 1994). Estrogen replacement has been shown to be effective in improving these symptoms, however. In addition, emotional support and counseling may be beneficial. Nurse practitioners must not use stereotyping to perpetuate the myth that menopause brings on psychological disorders, but instead must realize that other factors in a woman's life may be responsible for psychosocial issues.

Changes in the skin also occur with the onset of menopause. Estrogen plays an important role in maintaining healthy skin and hair. With declining levels, many women notice thinning of the skin and hair, loss of skin elasticity, increased wrinkling, and dryness of the skin and scalp. Hyperpigmentation, or "age spots," may occur as a result of melanocyte proliferation. Sweat gland activity decreases, making the skin more sensitive to changes in temperature. Hirsutism, or increased facial hair, may occur as a result of altered androgen levels in combination with declining estrogen levels.

The breasts are target tissues for estrogen, and as a result of estrogen deprivation, the breasts undergo changes with the onset of menopause. The glandular tissue of the breasts gradually is replaced with adipose tissue, and elasticity is diminished, making the breasts appear smaller and flattened.

Some women may report dry mouth, bad taste, and decreased saliva after entering menopause. Atrophy of the gums and buccal mucosa may occur with estrogen deprivation, making dental caries and gum disease a more frequent occurrence

in the aging. Common symptoms of menopause are listed in Table 18-1.

## Long-Term Effects

### Osteoporosis

One of the most debilitating consequences of menopause is osteoporosis, the loss of bone density. Osteoporosis is characterized by decreased bone mass and increased susceptibility to bone fractures. The 1993 Consensus definition of osteoporosis is "a systemic skeletal disease characterized by low bone mass and microarchitectural deterioration of bone tissue, with a consequent increase in bone fragility and susceptibility to fracture" (Consensus Development Conference, 1993). The pathophysiology of osteoporosis involves both inadequate peak bone mass and bone loss. Peak bone mass develops during the age range of 15 to 25 years and is maintained during the premenopausal years in healthy women (Kessenich & Rosen, 1996). Factors that influence the development of peak bone mass include nutrition, calcium intake, endocrine secretions, exercise, and ethnic and genetic factors. Bone loss increases during periods of estrogen deprivation and at menopause. In women with long periods of amenorrhea, peak bone mass may never been attained, leaving these individuals at an even greater risk for osteoporosis during postmenopausal years. The estradiol deficiency causes this phenomenon. Women who are amenorrheic because of low body weight or who are lactating for prolonged periods have long periods during which they are estrogen deficient.

Bone is constantly remodeled in healthy people in response to stresses and strains, but bone loss is equal to bone formation so that peak bone mass is

---

## TABLE 18.1    ● ● ●

### Common Symptoms of Menopause

| *Skin* | *Genitourinary* | *Breasts* |
|---|---|---|
| Thinning of skin and hair | Dyspareunia | Reduced size and support |
| Dryness of skin | Vaginal itching | Softening |
| Decreased sweating | Decreased lubrication | *Metabolic* |
| Loss of elasticity | Yeast infections | Hot flashes |
| Wrinkling | Frequency/Urgency | *Psychiatric* |
| Hyperpigmentation | Urinary incontinence | Irritability |
| Graying of hair | Uterine/Bladder prolapse | Insomnia |
| Hirsutism | | Mood swings |
| Dry mouth | | Decreased concentration |

maintained. Under the influence of a variety of factors, including parathyroid hormone and estrogen, bone resorption results from osteoclast activity, and bone formation results from stimulation of osteoblast activity. Bone remodeling is dynamic, with temporary bone remodeling units being initiated and remodeled every 10 seconds (Parfitt, 1981). In a given remodeling unit, osteoclasts excavate a cavity, which then is filled with new bone produced by osteoblasts. The remodeling process is initiated by the osteoblast, which releases cytokines that stimulate osteoclast activity. In menopause, the type of osteoporosis that develops is termed type I, in which osteoclast activity seems to become uncoupled from the osteoblast regulation and occurs in excess. The cavities formed by osteoclasts within bone remodeling units remain empty of new bone, thus weakening the skeletal matrix. Furthermore, excess calcium from excess bone resorption enters the extracellular fluid, and calcium is lost from the body through the kidney. Type II osteoporosis is part of normal aging, and the causative mechanism is senescence of osteoblast function (Kessenich & Rosen, 1996). Factors other than age alone that influence this type of osteoporosis include immobility and decreased calcium and vitamin D intake or absorption.

Osteoporosis can develop rapidly during the menopausal years, with the greatest acceleration of bone loss occurring in early menopause, when estrogen is abruptly withdrawn from influencing skeletal resorption and growth. Interleukin (IL)-1 increases at menopause and may be blocked by estrogen. When estrogen is withdrawn, IL-1, IL-6, and tumor necrosis factor-alpha all are increased in skeletal tissue, and these cytokines are osteoclastogenic. Multiple cytokines may be involved in osteoporosis, and estrogen replacement therapy is thought to reduce their activity.

Bone mass density reaches a peak at around age 30, then normally begins to decline at a rate of 0.5% per year compared with 1% to 2% per year in postmenopausal women (Beckman et al., 1997). Most of the total bone loss in women occurs in the first 3 to 5 years after menopause (Wehrle, 1996). The most significant bone loss occurs in the hip and vertebral spaces, making fractures of the hip and spine a common and costly complication in postmenopausal women. The numbers of hip fractures are expected to increase sixfold by the year 2050 to over 6 million per year (Cooper et al., 1992).

Risk factors for developing osteoporosis (Table 18-2) include Caucasian race, slender build, long-term steroid use, positive family history, nulliparity, early menopause, and low bone mass at the onset of menopause. Additionally, avoidable risk

| TABLE 18.2  |
|---|
| **Risk Factors for Development of Osteoporosis** |
| Slender build |
| Caucasian or Asian descent |
| Positive family history |
| Low calcium intake |
| Excessive caffeine intake |
| Sedentary lifestyle |
| Early menopause/oophorectomy |
| Nulliparity |
| Alcohol abuse |
| Smoking |
| Prolonged steroid use |
| Drug-induced amenorrhea (GnRH inhibitors) |
| High sodium intake |
| High protein intake |

GnRH, gonadotropin-releasing hormone.

factors include smoking, alcoholism, excess caffeine intake, insufficient calcium intake, and lack of exercise. Protective factors against development of osteoporosis include African-American race, obesity, multiparity, and use of oral contraceptives.

Initially, osteoporosis is an asymptomatic disease. Loss of height may the first sign of osteoporosis, which results from bone loss in the anterior vertebral bodies. This may be characterized by the classic kyphosis, or Dowager's hump, frequently noted in elderly women. Back pain may be the initial complaint of the patient; however, radiologic studies may fail to reveal significant or obvious changes until late in the disease process. Compression fractures of the spine or fractures of the hip and wrist may be the presenting symptom and may occur spontaneously or after even a minor trauma.

## Cardiovascular Disease

An additional concern facing postmenopausal women is that of cardiovascular disease. Aging women have a higher risk of developing coronary artery disease, cerebrovascular accident, hypertension, and peripheral vascular disease because of estrogen deprivation. Heart disease is the number one cause of morbidity and mortality in women older than age 50 and accounts for more than 500,000 deaths each year. These influences are discussed in Chapter 14. Death from myocardial infarction (MI) occurs more frequently in postmenopausal women than in men of comparable age, whereas premenopausal women rarely experience MIs. Most MIs are a result of atherosclerosis in the large vessels, which is attributable to changes in lipid metabolism.

Total cholesterol, LDL, and triglyceride levels rise significantly after menopause, whereas HDL levels and HDL-LDL ratios decrease, combining forces to contribute to plaque formation in the vessels. Hyperlipidemia is a known risk factor for development of cardiovascular disease; therefore, these changes in the lipid profile represent less cardioprotective capability in postmenopausal women compared with those women who have yet to reach menopause.

Estrogen also has an effect on clotting factors, in particular, factor VII, and may play a role in clot formation. As a result of thromboses, ischemic events may occur more commonly in women on HRT.

### Clinical Diagnosis

A diagnosis of menopause can be made based largely on the patient's menstrual history and symptoms. Thorough history taking is an important tool in planning the care of women who are entering menopause. Physical examination can be useful in assessing hypoestrogenic states; however, laboratory studies are helpful in making a definitive diagnosis.

The FSH levels may begin to rise in the perimenopausal period when menstrual cycles are becoming more erratic. LH and estradiol levels remain normal during this phase. Shortly after the onset of menopause, FSH levels rise dramatically and LH levels become mildly elevated in comparison. These levels remain elevated for a period of 1–3 years following menopause, at which time they begin to show a gradual, slight decline. Generally speaking, FSH levels of > 30 are indicative of menopause (Speroff, Glass & Kase, 1994).

Serum estradiol levels, normal during the perimenopausal phase, begin to fall after the onset of menopause. Measurable amounts of estrogen remain in the blood as a result of androstenedione conversion to estrone. As a result of lowered estrogen levels, the androgen-estrogen ratios change dramatically, producing symptoms of hirsutism.

In addition to elevated gonadotropin levels, vaginal cytology smears may be used as a measure of estrogen status. In the presence of hypoestrogenic states, parabasal cells are seen in vaginal secretions.

### Physiologic Basis of Treatment

When a diagnosis of menopause is suspected, the important decision of using HRT must be consid-

ered. It is well documented that estrogen therapy provides relief of menopausal symptoms and protection against osteoporosis, cardiovascular disease, and Alzheimer's disease. Risks and benefits must be weighed with each individual patient, since estrogen therapy is not without its risks.

The objectives in using HRT in menopausal women are relief of aggravating symptoms and protection from long-term complications such as osteoporosis and cardiovascular disease. Before considering HRT, a woman's complete health history, including family history, lifestyle habits, smoking habits, alcohol use, risk factors, vital signs, and physical examination, must be obtained. Additionally, Pap smear, mammogram, and lipid profile are essential before initiating HRT. The primary care provider must communicate openly with a patient who is considering HRT, explaining all risks involved and working collaboratively with her in determining if she is an appropriate candidate for HRT. Risk factors for development of heart disease, osteoporosis, breast cancer, endometrial cancer, deep vein thrombosis, and pulmonary embolism must be addressed. Contraindications to the use of estrogen replacement therapy are listed in Table 18-3.

### Short-Term Effects

Without question, estrogen replacement therapy relieves the major symptoms of menopause. Hot flashes subside quickly. Vaginal and urethral atrophy is reversed, vaginal dryness is improved, and

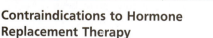

## TABLE 18.3

### Contraindications to Hormone Replacement Therapy

*Absolute*
Hormone-related cancer
Hormone-induced thromboembolism
History of pulmonary embolism
Undiagnosed vaginal bleeding
Pregnancy
Active liver disease

*Relative*
Chronic liver disease
Extremely elevated triglycerides
History of breast cancer
History of endometrial cancer
Endometriosis

urinary symptoms are relieved. Sexual desire may be improved with estrogen replacement in some women.

The psychological effects of menopause including mood swings, depression, and irritability also improve with estrogen replacement, and sleep returns to a more normal pattern. Many women report a general sense of well-being when HRT is used.

Additional benefits of estrogen therapy include improvement in the skin changes associated with menopause. Buccal mucosal atrophy is reversed, helping to prevent periodontal disease.

Short-term effects of estrogen replacement therapy may provide relief of symptoms and make the transition into menopause a more comfortable one; however, it is the long-term protection against major disease that should promote serious consideration of its use.

### Long-Term Effects

Use of estrogen is the most effective means of preventing osteoporosis and cardiovascular disease in postmenopausal women (Speroff et al., 1994). Studies show that estrogen also provides protection against development of dementia and Alzheimer's disease. In a study of more than 13,000 women by the Leisure World Cohort, long-term estrogen users had a 50% reduction in their risk for developing Alzheimer's compared with nonusers (Pagininni, 1996). Several older and smaller studies consistently demonstrate a significant reduction in the risk of Alzheimer's disease in women who have taken HRT.

Osteoporosis and its related fractures are a major cause of mortality and morbidity in postmenopausal women. Estrogen therapy slows the rate of bone resorption, thus preventing bone loss and possibly increasing bone density. Studies show that women who are not treated with estrogen after menopause may lose as much as 5 inches of height, whereas women who do receive estrogen therapy report no changes in height. When estrogen therapy is instituted, the rapid rate of bone loss seen in postmenopausal women quickly returns to premenopausal rates and remains at these levels as long as therapy is maintained. With discontinuation of therapy, protection against osteoporosis is lost.

Postmenopausal women are at much higher risk of developing cardiovascular disease in the absence of estrogen replacement therapy. Studies show that women who take estrogen after the onset of menopause have a 50% less chance of developing heart disease than those who do not (*Clinical Reviews*, 1997).

Mortality and morbidity is higher in postmenopausal women with heart disease than in men of comparable age. Before menopause, mortality from heart disease is higher in men than in women; however, after menopause, this difference is reversed. More than half of all deaths in women older than 50 years are attributable to heart disease (Wehrle, 1996).

Also, the incidence of death from acute MI is greater in postmenopausal women than in men. In addition, the incidence of cerebrovascular accident and hypertension increases in women after menopause. Hormone replacement therapy has been shown in many studies to reduce cardiovascular mortality by 50% (Youngkin & Davis, 1998). No studies have shown that estrogen may be indicated in preventing hypertension or CVA (Youngkin & Davis, 1998). It is thought, in general, that estrogen users live 1 year longer than nonusers (Pagininni, 1996).

Changes in the lipid profile that occur after menopause are responsible for the drastic increase in the incidence of heart disease in women. Estrogen replacement therapy increases HDL levels and lowers LDL and total cholesterol levels, helping to stave off cardiovascular disease. Estrogen can increase triglyceride levels, although this appears to be a modest increase and is not believed to significantly contribute to the development of atherosclerosis. In addition, estrogen has a direct effect on arterial and venous walls and on blood flow through the vessels, which also may be beneficial in preventing coronary artery disease.

The use of estrogen also may be beneficial in postmenopausal diabetics. However, its use has not been widely promoted: diabetics are prescribed estrogen therapy less than half as often as nondiabetics (Lehmberg & Cohen, 1998). Glucose intolerance and insulin resistance have been reported in women who use oral contraceptives, but women who use HRT have shown overall improvement in glycemic control (Lehmberg & Cohen, 1998). Postmenopausal diabetics are at greater risk of developing heart disease and lipid disorders. Estrogen therapy may significantly improve lipid profiles in diabetics, just as in nondiabetics, thus providing extra protection against heart disease.

In summary, estrogen is the first-line treatment choice in reducing vasomotor symptoms and urogenital symptoms in postmenopausal women. It also is helpful in reversing skin changes and improving mood disturbances. It is, however, most helpful in exerting a protective effect against osteoporosis and cardiovascular disease. Whereas many benefits can be obtained with the use of estrogen, there also are serious risks involved with its use, which must be weighed against the benefits achieved.

## Estrogen Risks

The use of estrogen has been heavily debated among medical professionals. This controversy began in the early days of HRT, when estrogen was associated with the development of endometrial cancer in women who used it without progesterone or progestin opposition. Under the influence of estrogen, the endometrial lining proliferates, leading to hyperplasia, and may progress to adenocarcinoma. However, by opposing the estrogen with progesterone or progestin therapy, the endometrium continues to shed and proliferation is inhibited. Progesterones are effective in preventing endometrial hyperplasia whether taken continuously or cyclically. The addition of progesterones is not necessary if the woman has undergone previous hysterectomy. Estrogen is contraindicated in any woman with a history of endometrial cancer or undiagnosed vaginal bleeding. Any postmenopausal women with vaginal bleeding should be referred for evaluation. In addition, any woman older than 55 years of age who has yet to reach menopause and still is experiencing menstruation may be at increased risk of developing endometrial malignancy and should be referred to a gynecologist for evaluation (Brenner & Mishell, 1991).

Another important area of controversy in the use of estrogen is breast cancer. Breast cancer is the most common cancer among American women, affecting one of every nine women (Speroff et al., 1994). Risk factors for development of breast cancer include early menarche, nulliparity, late childbearing, and late menopause, implying that breast cancer is associated with estrogen production.

Studies examining the relationship between HRT and development of breast cancer produce inconsistent findings. Some large studies suggest that women who have used estrogen for more than 10 years may have a slightly increased risk for breast cancer; however, most researchers believe that the benefits of estrogen therapy clearly outweigh this risk. Remember that death from heart disease exceeds death related to breast cancer in women. Clinical breast examination and mammography should be included in the initial workup for any woman considering estrogen therapy and should be an essential part of annual health maintenance. Any woman with an undiagnosed breast mass should refrain from using estrogen.

Since clotting factors are altered by estrogen, thromboembolism is more prevalent among oral estrogen users. Estrogen is contraindicated in women with active thromboembolism or thrombophlebitis. Women with a remote history of thrombotic disorders can safely use transdermal estrogen, since this delivery route has no effect on clotting factors (Beckman et al., 1997).

Other risks associated with estrogen use include increased incidence of gallbladder disease and gallstones. The mechanism of action occurs by inhibition of bile acid synthesis and increased cholesterol saturation in biliary secretions (Dawood, 1993). Triglyceride levels may rise significantly, increasing the risk of pancreatitis during treatment. The use of transdermal estrogen may decrease the risk of gallbladder and pancreatic disease, since the liver is bypassed.

## Side Effects

In addition to these potential risks, estrogen use may produce a variety of untoward side effects, therefore any woman considering its use must be informed of possible adverse reactions. Common side effects include nausea and vomiting, breast tenderness and enlargement, vaginal bleeding, fluid retention, and weight gain. Asthma, epilepsy, and migraines may be exacerbated with the use of estrogen. Benign uterine fibroids also may increase in size with the use of HRT (Oestrich, 1995).

## Use of Androgens in Menopause

Several areas of the brain are important to sexual functioning, libido, and sexual response. These include the pituitary, the hypothalamus, the cerebral cortex, and the limbic system. Sexual libido, or the lack of, may be attributable to androgen production and the effects of androgens on the brain.

Testosterone in women is produced by the ovaries, the adrenal glands, and peripheral conversion of androstenedione. The use of exogenous testosterone may lead to suppression of endogenous testosterone production because of the negative feedback mechanism associated with the hypothalamus-pituitary axis (Levine, 1998). Long-term safety of its use has not been well documented.

However, women who have not responded to estrogen therapy alone may benefit from the addition of testosterone to the therapeutic regimen. This may be given along with the estrogen therapy or by itself. The addition of androgen therapy to the treatment regimen has been shown to be effective in improving sexual pleasure (Wehrle, 1996).

## Alternatives to Hormone Replacement Therapy

The use of estrogen may be contraindicated in some women for many reasons, or a woman may have personal reasons for choosing not to use HRT. For these women, patient education and supportive care are important.

Alternative therapies are available that may lessen the effects of hypoestrogenemia and protect against the long-term consequences of menopause. These should be presented and thoroughly discussed with any woman who is experiencing menopause symptoms.

In treating hot flashes, it may be helpful to incorporate exercise, relaxation methods, and use of lightweight clothing. Avoidance of cigarettes, alcohol, caffeine, and hot spicy foods may also aid in alleviating bothersome symptoms. Herbal remedies of ginseng, lime blossom, evening primrose oil, and vitamin E have been reported to be successful in treating hot flashes. The prescription medications propranolol (Inderal), clonidine, and naproxen (Naprosyn) also have been used, although the indications for their use do not include hot flashes (Wasaha & Angelopoulos, 1996).

Pelvic floor strengthening may be achieved through Kegel exercises and may help to reduce urinary symptoms. Topical estrogen cream may be applied to the urinary meatus to relieve symptoms of dysuria and urgency; however, it should not be used as a vaginal lubricant for intercourse, since absorption by the partner may occur. Dyspareunia and vaginal dryness may be relieved with water-soluble vaginal lubricants.

Anxiety-related symptoms may be improved by a regular exercise program, stress-reduction methods, a healthy diet, and rest. Use of phytoestrogens, or naturally occurring estrogen-like substances, may provide some relief of symptoms. These are found in plants such as alfalfa, basil, parsley, beans, licorice, and soybean products.

To reduce the risk for osteoporosis, patients should be instructed to eat a calcium-rich diet. This can be achieved through dietary measures or supplements. Several factors interfere with the absorption of calcium including caffeine, aluminum-containing antacids, and a diet high in protein (Youngkin & Davis, 1998). The recommended daily allowance (RDA) for calcium in women younger than 65 years who are taking HRT is 1000 mg/day, and for women who are not taking HRT or who are older than 65, the RDA is 1500 mg. Calcium is best absorbed when taken with meals. Addition of vitamin D supplements also enhances absorption of calcium.

Weight-bearing exercise and resistance training are essential for further protection against osteoporosis and heart disease. Exercise builds new bone and prevents demineralization of bone. Moderate exercise (30 to 60 minutes per day, 4 to 5 days per week), including walking, jogging, tennis, biking, swimming, and weight training, produces beneficial long-term effects and should be promoted to all women.

Smoking contributes to the development of osteoporosis by reducing bone density and also is a strong risk factor for cardiovascular disease. Smoking cessation should be strongly encouraged.

An alternative to estrogen, known as a selective estrogen receptor modulator, is available to protect against osteoporosis in women who cannot or do not want to take HRT. Raloxifene HCl (Evista) works in the same way as estrogen to prevent bone loss and rebuild bone mass; however, it does not provide relief of menopausal symptoms. Side effects include hot flashes, leg cramps, and blood clots.

Other preparations that are effective in preventing osteoporosis, yet provide no other benefits for postmenopausal women, include alendronate (Fosamax) and calcitonin-salmon (Miacalcin) nasal spray.

### Treatment Regimens

The goals of estrogen therapy are to alleviate symptoms of ovarian failure and to protect against the long-term complications associated with it. Several treatment options are available when a patient elects to use estrogen replacement therapy. To minimize the risks and side effects associated with estrogen use, the smallest dose that provides relief of symptoms is recommended.

Estrogen can be delivered either orally or transdermally and also is available in vaginal preparations, which may be used to relieve vaginal symptoms (Harper, 1990). Oral estrogens are available as natural, conjugated, or synthetic estrogens. Natural estrogens, which include micronized estradiol, are converted to estrone in the liver. Because of the first-pass effect, oral estrogens are less potent than transdermal estrogens, which do not pass through the GI tract.

Several treatment options are available when using estrogen therapy. In women who have undergone hysterectomy, estrogen can be used alone. In women who have an intact uterus, opposition with progesterone is essential to induce endometrial shedding. Progesterones may be used intermittently, that is, 10 to 14 days of the month in addition to daily estrogen, or continuously in a daily dose combined with estrogen. Combination preparations are available in oral or transdermal form that contain both conjugated estrogen and medroxyprogesterone and are taken daily throughout the month.

Estrogen therapy also may be used in conjunction with androgen therapy, especially in women who complain of loss of libido. However, remember that other factors in the relationship may be contributing to sexual dysfunction, and sexual counseling may be indicated. Side effects of androgen therapy include hirsutism, acne, and enlarged clitoris. In women with an intact uterus, androgen therapy must be combined with progesterone therapy. Several combination regimens are available containing either esterified estrogen or conjugated estrogen, along with methyltestosterone.

Transdermal estradiol patches that bypass the liver are another form of estrogen delivery. In women with an intact uterus, opposition with medroxyprogesterone must be added. Transdermal estrogen provides rapid relief of hypoestrogenic symptoms without fluctuations in estrogen levels. This type of delivery system is ideal for women with a history of clotting or liver disorders and can be used safely in women who cannot take oral estrogens (Youngkin & Davis, 1998). Transdermal estrogen is equal to oral estrogen in protecting against osteoporosis; however, protection against cardiovascular disease has not been determined.

Transvaginal estrogen preparations are available in the form of a vaginal cream or as an estrogen-releasing vaginal ring. These forms of estrogen therapy are indicated primarily for relief of urogenital symptoms; however, they are systemically absorbed and must be used with the same contraindications that apply to oral estrogens. The same side effects that are seen with oral estrogens also are seen with vaginal estrogen preparations. Estrogen vaginal creams may be used in conjunction with oral estrogen when vaginal symptoms are not relieved by oral estrogen. Dosages may be decreased over time when adequate tissue revascularization has taken place (Kent, 1994). The estrogen ring consists of a small, flexible silicone ring that continuously releases estradiol directly into the vaginal wall. The ring is effective for 90 days, at which time it must be replaced, and does not interfere with intercourse. These preparations provide excellent relief of vaginal and urinary symptoms, but little protection against osteoporosis or cardiovascular disease.

## Summary

Primary care providers must educate aging female patients about the normal and abnormal symptoms of menopause. Patients who are informed about their health care choices can better understand the importance of preventive care and can take the proper steps to protect themselves from long-term, debilitating diseases.

Menopause should not be a time of dread for women, but instead an opportunity to become involved in their own health care, a chance to grow in relationships, and a time to experience fulfillment and satisfaction.

### ● Case Study 18.1

A 52-year-old white female presents to the clinic for an annual physical. She has not been seen by a provider in 2 1/2 years, and her chief complaints today are insomnia, irritability, and crying spells. She states that these symptoms began about 1 year ago. She assures you that she is not feeling depressed.

#### History

##### Past Medical History

| | |
|---|---|
| Allergies | PCN |
| Current medications | Multivitamin, occasional OTC sleeping aids |
| Surgeries | Cholecystectomy, appendectomy, T&A |
| Childhood illness | Usual childhood illnesses. Last tetanus shot was 4 years ago. Annual flu vaccine |

##### Social History

| | |
|---|---|
| | Married × 31 years with 3 children |
| Tobacco | Nonsmoker |
| Alcohol | Drinks alcohol socially |
| Caffeine | Heavy caffeine use, 5–6 coffee/cola/day |
| Exercise | Walks 3 miles 3–4×/week |

*(Case study continued on next page)*

*Family History*

| | |
|---|---|
| Mother | HTN, MI, osteoporosis |
| Father | MI, DM |
| Sister | Breast cancer at age 48; breast cancer in PGM and aunts |

*24-Hour Recall*

Breakfast: Bagel, juice, 2 cups coffee
Lunch: Turkey sandwich, yogurt, cola
Snack: Banana, 2 oatmeal cookies, cola
Supper: Chicken/pasta, salad, ice cream

## Review of Systems

| | |
|---|---|
| General | Weight gain of 5 lb since last visit. "Night sweats" × 1 year |
| Skin | No rashes. "Age spots" on hands |
| HEENT | Occasional headache |
| CV | Occasional palpitations. No chest pain |
| Breasts | Performs BSE. Last mammogram 2 years ago |
| Respiratory | No cough, SOB, DOE |
| GI | Occasional indigestion, relieved by antacids. No change in bowel habits |
| GU | LMP 18 months ago. C/O urinary urgency and dysuria × several months. Decreased vaginal lubrication and pain with intercourse |
| MS | Arthritis in hands. No edema |
| Neurologic | Difficulty with concentrating at times. No numbness or weakness |
| Psychological | Denies depression, sadness, withdrawal, or anxiety. Insomnia × 1 year. Experiences mood swings and irritability frequently. Frequent crying spells "for no reason" |

## Physical Examination

| System | Findings |
|---|---|
| Vital signs | T-97.5°F P-72 R-20 BP-128/76 Height-5'7", Weight-135 lb |
| General | Thin WF in NAD. Alert & oriented |
| Skin | No rashes or suspicious lesions noted. Hyperpigmented areas on both hands |
| HEENT | PERRLA. EOMs intact. TMs normal. Pharynx without redness. No cervical adenopathy. Thyroid without enlargement or nodularity |
| CV | RSR without murmur |
| Breasts | Soft, no nodules. No nipple discharge |
| Lungs | CTA |
| Abdomen | Soft, flat, + bowel sounds. No organomegaly |
| Back | No CVA tenderness |
| Pelvic | External genitalia normal. Vagina is pale pink with loss of rugation. Cervix friable. Uterus is small, freely movable. Ovaries noted. Pap done. No tenderness |
| Rectal | No masses noted. Hemoccult negative |

*(Case study continued on page 382)*

| | |
|---|---|
| Extremities | No edema. Pedal pulses 2+ bilaterally. Numerous small varicosities present LE |
| Neurologic | Intact. DTRs 2+ and equal bilaterally |

### Laboratory Studies

| Test | Result |
|---|---|
| Chem 22 | WNL except cholesterol 24 |
| CBC | Hgb/Hct 13.1/41 |
| U/A | pH 7, dipstick negative |
| ECG | NSR with one PVC present |
| FSH | 68 mIU/mL |

## Impression

Healthy postmenopausal female
Excessive caffeine intake
Hypercholesterolemia

## Discussion

This patient is experiencing numerous symptoms consistent with menopause. Her last menstrual period was 18 months ago. Other symptoms include "night sweats," irritability, insomnia, urinary symptoms, and dyspareunia.

Her physical examination reveals atrophic vaginal changes, evidenced by pale pink vaginal mucosa and cervical friability. Her laboratory studies show elevated FSH and cholesterol levels.

The patient's risk factors for serious disease include a strong family history of heart disease and a first-degree relative with breast cancer. Risk factors for developing osteoporosis include a positive family history, Caucasian race, thin build, excessive caffeine intake, and poor calcium intake.

Further workup should include a mammogram, a DEXA bone density measurement, and a fasting lipid profile. After the results of these tests are obtained, the patient should return to discuss the use of HRT for treatment of her symptoms and as a preventive measure against heart disease and osteoporosis, given her multiple risk factors. However, this must be used with caution, considering a family history of breast cancer.

She is encouraged to reduce her caffeine intake and to increase her calcium intake. She is advised to begin taking a calcium supplement (1500 mg/day) and a "baby aspirin" each day. She is encouraged to continue her current exercise regimen and to add resistance training to her program.

*BP, blood pressure; BSE, breast self-examination; CBC, complete blood count; C/O, complains of; CTA, clear to auscultation; CV, cardiovascular; CVA, costovertebral angle; DEXA, dual energy x-ray absorptiometry; DM, diabetes mellitus; DOE, dyspnea on exertion; DTRs, deep tendon reflexes; ECG, electrocardiogram; EOMs, extraocular movement; FSH, follicle-stimulating hormone; GI, gastrointestinal; GU, genitourinary; Hgb, hemoglobin; Hct, hematocrit; HEENT, head, eyes, ears, nose, and throat; HRT, hormone replacement therapy; HTN, hypertension; LE, lower extremity; LMP, last menstrual period; MI, myocardial infarction; MS, musculoskeletal; NAD, no apparent distress; NSR, normal sinus rhythm; OTC, over-the-counter; P, pulse; PCN, penicillin; PERRLA, pupils equal, round, reactive to light accommodation; PGM, paternal grandmother; PVC, preventricular contraction; R, respiration; RSR, regular sinus rhythm; SOB, shortness of breath; T, temperature; T&A, tonsillectomy and adenoidectomy; TMs, tympanic membranes; U/A, urinalysis; WF, white female; WNL, within normal limits.*

# REFERENCES

Ansley, D. (1998). Premenstrual syndrome. Available at: http://onhealth.com/ch1/resource/conditions/fulltext/item, 463.asp. Accessed July 18, 1999.

Barnhart, K., Freeman, E., & Sondheimer, S. (1995). A clinician's guide to the premenstrual syndrome. *Medical Clinics of North America, 79* (6), 1457–1472.

Beck, L., Gevirtz, R., & Mortola, J. (1990). The predictive role of psychosocial stress on symptom severity in premenstrual syndrome. *Psychosomatic Medicine, 52* (5), 536–543.

Beckmann, C., Ling, F., Barzansky, B., Bates, G., Herbert, W., Laube, D., & Smith, R. (1997). *Obstetrics and gynecology* (2nd ed.). Baltimore: Williams & Wilkins.

Brenner, P. & Mishell, D. (1991). Menopause. In D. Mishell, V. Davajan, & R. Lobo (Eds.), *Infertility, contraception, and reproductive endocrinology*. Boston: Blackwell Scientific Publication.

Campbell, M. & McGrath, P. (1997). Use of medication by adolescents for the management of menstrual discomfort. *Archives of Pediatric and Adolescent Medicine, 151* (9), 905–913.

Chan, A., Mortola, J., Wood, S., & Yen, S. (1994). Persistence of premenstrual syndrome during low-dose administration of the progesterone antagonist RU 486. *Obstetrics and Gynecology, 84* (6), 1001–1005.

Cintio, E., Parazzini, F., Tozzi, L., Luchini, L., Mezzopane, R., Marchini, M., & Fedele, L. (1997). Dietary habits, reproductive and menstrual factors and risk of dysmenorrhea. *European Journal of Epidemiology, 13*, 925–930.

*Clinical Reviews.* (1997). Hormone replacement therapy: Weighing the hazards and rewards. *Clinical Reviews, 7,* (9), 53–72.

Consensus Development Conference. (1993). *American Journal of Medicine, 94*, 646–650.

Cooper, C., Campion, G., & Melton, L.J. (1992). Hip fractures in the elderly: A world-wide projection. *Osteoporosis International, 2*, 285–289.

Corwin, E.J. (1997). Endometriosis pathophysiology, diagnosis and treatment. *The Nurse Practitioner, 22* (10), 35–57.

Damewood, M., Kresch, A., & Metzger, D. (1997). Current approaches to endometriosis. *Patient Care, 31* (1), 3–44.

Dawood, M. (1985). Dysmenorrhea. *The Journal of Reproductive Medicine, 30* (3), 154–167.

Dawood, M. (1990). Dysmenorrhea. *Clinical Obstetrics and Gynecology, 33* (1), 168–178.

Dawood, M. (1993). Menopause. In L. Copeland, J. Jarrell, & J. McGregor (Eds.), *Textbook of gynecology*. Philadelphia: W.B. Saunders.

Diegoli, M., da Fonseca, A., Diegoli, C., & Pinotti, J. (1998). A double-blind trial of four medications to treat severe premenstrual syndrome. *International Journal of Gynecology and Obstetrics, 62*, 63–67.

Freeman, E., Kielich, A., & Sondheimer, S. (1996). PMS: New treatments that really work. *Contemporary OB/GYN, 41* (2), 25–41.

Goldzieher, J. (1997). Postmenopausal androgen therapy. *The Female Patient, 22*, 42–44.

Harel, Z., Biro, F., Kottenhahn, R., & Rosenthal, S. (1996). Supplementation with omega-3 polyunsaturated fatty acids in the management of dysmenorrhea in adolescents. *American Journal of Obstetrics and Gynecology, 174* (4), 1335–1338.

Harlow, S. & Park, M. (1996). A longitudinal study of risk factors for the occurrence, duration, and severity of menstrual cramps in a cohort of college women. *British Journal of Obstetrics and Gynaecology, 103* (11), 1134–1142.

Harper, D. (1990). Perimenopause and aging. In R. Lichtman & S. Papera (Eds.), *Gynecology well woman care*. Norwalk, CT: Appleton & Lange.

Helms, H. (1987). Acupuncture for the management of primary dysmenorrhea. *Obstetrics and Gynecology, 69* (1), 51–55.

Hightower, M. (1997). Effects of exercise participation on menstrual pain and symptoms. *Women & Health, 26* (4), 15–27.

Jackson, A. (1995). Alternative update: Premenstrual syndrome. *Nursing Times, 91* (3), 64.

Jarrett, M., Heitkemper, M., & Shaver, J. (1995). Symptoms and self-care strategies in women with and without dysmenorrhea. *Health Care for Women International, 16*, 167–177.

Johnson, W., Carr-Nangle, R., & Bergeron, K. (1995). Macronutrient intake, eating habits, and exercise as moderators of menstrual distress in healthy women. *Psychosomatic Medicine, 57* (4), 324–330.

Kaplan, B., Peled, Y., Pardo, J., Rabinerson, D., Hirsh, M., Ovadia, J., & Neri, A. (1994). Transcutaneous electrical nerve stimulation (TENS) as a treatment for dysmenorrhea. *Clinical Experiences in Obstetrics and Gynecology, 21* (2), 87–90.

Kent, H. (1994). Clinical management of atrophic vaginitis. *Menopause Management, 6* (3), 12–15.

Kessenich, C. & Rosen, C. (1996). The pathophysiology of osteoporosis. In C.J. Rosen (Ed.), *Osteoporosis: Diagnostic and therapeutic principles*. Totowa, New Jersey: Humana Press.

Lehmberg, P. & Cohen, S. (1998). The benefits of HRT for women with diabetes. *The Clinical Advisor for Nurse Practitioners, May,* 30–41.

Levine, S. (1998). The sexual consequences of perimenopause and menopause: Is a decline in sexuality inevitable despite hormone therapy? *Women's Health in Primary Care, 6,* (1), 509–513.

Mahoney, D. Acupressure and its use for dysmenorrhea: Unpublished doctoral dissertation. Texas Women's University, Denton, TX, 1993.

McCombs, J. (1999). Dysmenorrhea and premenstrual syndrome: Drug Store News [Continuing Education]. Available at: http://www.drugstorenews.com/ce/96_5_lesson.htm. Accessed July 18, 1999.

Mezrow, G. & Rebar, R. (1990). The Menopause. In W. Droegemueller & J.J. Sciarra (Eds.), *Gynecology and obstetrics* (vol. 1). Philadelphia: J.B. Lippincott.

Milsom, I., Hedner, N., & Mannheimer, C. (1994). A comparative study of the effect of high-intensity transcutaneous nerve stimulation and oral naproxen on intrauterine pressure and menstrual pain in patient's with primary dysmenorrhea. *American Journal of Obstetrics and Gynecology, 170*, 123–129.

Mortola, J. (1992a). Assessment and management of premenstrual syndrome. *Current Opinion in Obstetrics and Gynecology, 4*, 877–885.

Mortola, J. (1992b). Premenstrual syndrome. *The Western Journal of Medicine, 156* (6), 651.

Mortola, J. (1994). A risk-benefit appraisal of drugs used in the management of premenstrual syndrome. *Drug Safety, 10* (2), 160–169.

Mortola, J. (1997a). Premenstrual syndrome. In C. Bardin (Ed.), *Current therapy in Endocrinology and metabolism* (pp. 251–256). St. Louis: Mosby.

Mortola, J. (1997b). From GnRH to SSRIs and beyond: Weighing the options for drug therapy in premenstrual syndrome. *Medscape women's health, 2*. Available at: http://www.medscape.com/Medscape/WomensHealth/

journal/1997/v02.../wh3074.mortola.htm. Accessed August 21, 1999.

Mortola, J., Girton, L., Beck, L., & Yen, S. (1990). Diagnosis of premenstrual syndrome by a simple, prospective, and reliable instrument: The calendar of premenstrual experiences. *Obstetrics and Gynecology, 76* (2), 302–307.

Noble, J. (1996). *Textbook of primary care medicine* (2nd ed.). St. Louis: Mosby.

Oestrich, S. (1995). A closer look at hormone replacement therapy. *Advance for Nurse Practitioners, January,* 10–14.

Ozeren, S., Corakci, A., Yucesoy, I., Mercan, R., & Erhan, G. (1997). Fluoxetine in the treatment of premenstrual syndrome. *European Journal of Obstetrics and Gynecology, 73,* 167–170.

Pagininni, A. (1996). What a woman needs to know: Long term risks and benefits of estrogen replacement therapy. *Advance for Nurse Practitioners, 52* (March), 22–25.

Parfitt, A.M. (1981). Bone remodeling in the pathogenesis of osteoporosis. *Resident Staff Physician, December,* 60–72.

Pickles, V., Hall, W., Best, F., & Smith, G. (1965). Prostaglandins in endometrium and menstrual fluid from normal and dysmenorrheic subjects. *Journal of Obstetrics and Gyneacology of the British Commonwealth, 72,* 185–192.

Pittrof, R., Lees, C., Thompson, C., Pickles, A., Martin, J., & Campbell, S. (1996). Crossover study of glycerol trinitrate patches for controlling pain in women with severe dysmenorrhea. *British Medical Journal, 312,* 884.

Powell, A., Chan, W., Alvin, P., & Litt, I. (1985). Menstrual PGF-2alpha, PGE-2 and TXA-2 in normal and dysmenorrheic women and their temporal relationship to dysmenorrhea. *Prostaglandins, 29* (2), 273–290.

Pray, S. (1998). PMS: A disorder that is diagnosable. *U.S. Pharmacist, 23* (9). Available at: http://www.medscape.com/jobson/USPharmacist/1998/v23.n09/usp2.../usp2309.01.pray-03.htm. Accessed July 14, 1999.

Schroeder, B. & Sanfilippo, J. (1999). Dysmenorrhea and pelvic pain in adolescents. *Pediatric Clinics of North America, 46* (3), 555–571.

Shaver, J., Woods, N., Wolf-Wilets, V., & Heitkemper, M. (1987). Menstrual experiences: Comparisons of dysmenorrheic and nondysmenorrheic women. *Western Journal of Nursing Research, 9* (4), 423–444.

Smith, R. (1993). Cyclic pelvic pain and dysmenorrhea. *Obstetrics and Gynecology Clinics of North America, 20* (4), 753–764.

Speroff, L., Glass, R., & Kase, N. (1994). *Clinical gynecologic endocrinology and infertility* (5th ed.). Baltimore: Williams & Wilkins.

Steiner, M., Steinberg, S., Stewart, D., Carter, D., Berger, C., Reid, R., Grover, D., & Streiner, D. (1995). Fluoxetine in the treatment of premenstrual dysphoria. *New England Journal of Medicine, 332,* 1529–1534.

Sundblad, C., Wikander, I., Andersch, B., & Eriksson, E. (1997). A naturalistic study of paroxetine in premenstrual syndrome: Efficacy and side-effects during ten cycles of treatment. *European Neuropsychopharmacology, 7,* 201–207.

Therapeutics Research Center. (1998). Fifty common herbs and their potential interactions with regular drugs. *Pharmacist's Letter.* Document no. 130901.

Treloar, S., Martin, N., & Heath, A. (1998). Longitudinal genetic analysis of menstrual flow, pain, and limitation in a sample of Australian twins. *Behavioral Genetics, 28* (2), 107–116.

van den Akker, O., Sharifian, N., Packer, A., & Eves, F. (1995). Contribution of generalized negative affect to elevated menstrual cycle symptom reporting. *Health Care for Women International, 16,* 263–272.

Voda, A. (1997). *Menopause, me and you: The sound of women pausing.* New York: Harrington Park Press.

Wasaha, S. & Angelopoulos, F. (1996). What every woman should know about menopause. *American Journal of Nursing, January,* 24–32.

Wehrle, K. (1996). Perfect timing for a healthy life: What to expect during perimenopause. *Advance for Nurse Practitioners, November,* 18–26.

Youngkin, E. & Davis, M. (1998). *Women's health: A primary care clinical guide* (2nd ed.). Stamford, CT: Appleton & Lange.

# Common Disorders of the Musculoskeletal System

Maureen Groer

Timothy Jones

This chapter describes several common musculoskeletal disorders seen in primary care patients. The range of such musculoskeletal disorders is wide. Injuries commonly bring people to their health care provider. Chronic degenerative conditions that lead to pain and deficits in mobility also are frequently observed. These disorders usually are not difficult to diagnose. This discussion begins with fibromyalgia syndrome (FMS) and chronic fatigue syndrome (CFS), which are, on the other hand, among the more baffling disorders involving the musculoskeletal system.

## FIBROMYALGIA

Fibromyalgia is a *syndrome* characterized by widespread muscle aches, pain, stiffness, fatigue, and sleep disturbances. It is a form of nonarticular rheumatism that has been described since the 17th century (Yunus, 1994). Clinical examination reveals tender points, tenderness in skin folds, skin hyperemia, reticular skin discoloration, and, rarely, swelling in the fingers (Yunus, 1994; Wolfe et al., 1990; Campbell et al., 1983). The American College of Rheumatology defines FMS as a history of widespread pain and pain in one of 18 tender point sites on digital examination. The tender points are indicated in Figure 19-1. Patients also often have sleep disturbances, fatigue, and depression. All other neurologic and laboratory tests usually give negative results (Yunus, 1994; Wolfe et al., 1990). Fibromyalgia may be present in association with other diseases (eg, systemic lupus erythematosus and hepatitis C

viral infection) (Bennet, 1997a; Buskila et al., 1997). A difficult differential diagnosis may be myofascial pain, which is a syndrome of trigger points that elicit referred pain on palpation (Auleciems, 1995). In myofascial pain syndrome (MPS), the pain usually is axial and localized, and without the other associated symptoms of FMS such as fatigue (Auleciems, 1995). Also, considerable overlap exists between FMS and CFS. Many patients with CFS also have muscle pain and even trigger point tenderness. Depression also is common to both illnesses. Both CFS and FMS exist on a continuum of symptoms and have similar underlying pathophysiologic processes. Both may follow a viral illness and have immune dysfunction and cytokine-mediated effects associated with them. Both may represent disorders in which patients are unusually sensitive to somatic symptoms (see Irritable Bowel Syndrome in Chapter 16).

Fibromyalgia and myofascial pain sydrome are two distinct syndromes with one element in common: chronic pain with no structural, anatomic, or known organic cause. Muscle pain affects about 4% to 11% of the population, and 3.4% of women and 0.5% of men in the United States meet the full criteria for the diagnosis of FMS (although many more probably are undiagnosed or misdiagnosed) (Wolfe et al., 1995). Whereas symptoms may progressively improve with time, studies show that symptoms do not completely disappear in most patients (Kennedy & Felson, 1996). Table 19-1 compares FMS and MPS, and Table 19-2 indicates the differential diagnoses to be considered

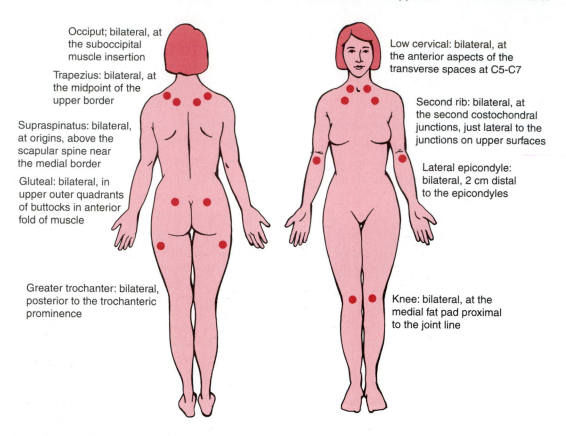

Occiput; bilateral, at the suboccipital muscle insertion

Trapezius: bilateral, at the midpoint of the upper border

Supraspinatus: bilateral, at origins, above the scapular spine near the medial border

Gluteal: bilateral, in upper outer quadrants of buttocks in anterior fold of muscle

Greater trochanter: bilateral, posterior to the trochanteric prominence

Low cervical: bilateral, at the anterior aspects of the transverse spaces at C5-C7

Second rib: bilateral, at the second costochondral junctions, just lateral to the junctions on upper surfaces

Lateral epicondyle: bilateral, 2 cm distal to the epicondyles

Knee: bilateral, at the medial fat pad proximal to the joint line

**FIGURE 19.1** ● Location of tender points in fibromyalgia. Palpation of these points produces localized, exquisite pain.

for both MPS and FMS (Rakel, 1997). Chronic fatigue syndrome is further discussed later in this chapter.

## Pathogenesis

The pathogenesis of FMS is unknown, although several theories have been proposed. Muscle pain usually is deep and aching, poorly localized, and may be referred to other tissues (eg, fascia, tendons, other muscles) (Bennet, 1997b). Muscle pain derives from mechanical, chemical, and ischemic stimulation of nociceptors (ie, free nerve endings) (Bennet, 1997b). Pain travels along nerve pathways stimulated by neurotransmitters such as substance P along C fibers (Yunus, 1994). Inhibitory neurotransmitters of pain include serotonin, norepinephrine, γ-aminobutyric acid (GABA), and enkephalins (Yunus, 1994).

Alterations in the energy supply to muscle tissue cause muscle pain from overuse or ischemia of normal muscle tissue (Mense, 1990; Olsen & Park, 1998). These are thought to contribute to a

decreased pain threshold, increased response to painful stimuli, and continued pain after a painful stimulus (Bennet, 1997b).

The complex interrelationships of symptom generation in FMS are illustrated in Figure 19-2.

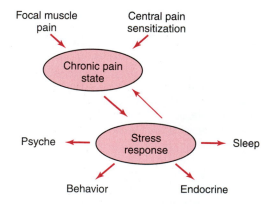

**FIGURE 19.2** ● Many factors interact in the pathophysiology of fibromyalgia to create a cycle of pain-fatigue-pain.

## TABLE 19.1

**Comparison of Features of Fibromyalgia and Myofascial Pain Syndrome**

| Features | FMS | MPS |
|---|---|---|
| Musculoskeletal pain | Widespread | Regional |
| Tender points | Multiple, widespread | Few, regional |
| Referred pain | + | ++ |
| Fatigue | ++++ | ++ |
| Poor sleep | ++++ | ++ |
| Paresthesias | +++ | ++ |
| Headaches | +++ | ++ |
| Irritable bowel | ++ | + |

FMS, fibromyalgia; MPS, myofascial pain syndrome.
(Modified from Yunus, M. [1994]. Fibromyalgia syndrome and myofascial pain syndrome: Clinical features, laboratory tests, diagnosis, and pathophysiologic mechanisms. In E. Rachlin [Ed.], *Myofascial pain and fibromyalgia* [p. 22]. St. Louis: Mosby-Year Book.)

### Histologic Changes

Many studies examine muscle tissue from patients with FMS. In general, there are no unusual findings other than atrophy in muscle tissue. Some research suggests that the areas of tenderness have decreased high-energy phosphates (Bennet, 1997b) or decreased capillary flow. Release of chemical pain–promoting substances such as bradykinin, substance P, $K^+$ ions, and prostaglandins (Bennet, 1997b) then results. These substances are thought to increase nociception. Microtrauma to muscle tissues from exertion, caused by high levels of calcium in the sarcolemma, also is thought to contribute to fibromyalgic pain (Bennet, 1997b). Electromyographic studies show a decrease in the relaxation phase of muscles after exertion, possibly causing a reduced blood flow to those muscles (Bennet, 1997b). This may partly explain the existence of pain after exercise in patients with FMS. These findings suggest a more focal cause of pain rather than a global pain origin (Bennet, 1997b).

Atrophy of muscle fibers (type II) and ragged red fibers are seen in FMS (Yunus, 1994). Collagen cross-linkage also may be reduced, possi-

## TABLE 19.2

**Differential Diagnoses for Fibromyalgia and Myofascial Pain Syndrome**

| Fibromyalgia | Myofascial Pain Syndrome |
|---|---|
| Depression | Costochondritis |
| Hypothyroidism | Trochanteric bursitis |
| Polymyalgia rheumatica | Anserine bursitis |
| Polymyositis | Posterior cervical MFTP |
| Other autoimmune diseases | Upper trap MFTP |
| | Lateral epicondylitis |
| | Middle trapezius MFTP |
| | Supraspinatus MFTP |
| | Gluteus minimus and multifidus MFTP |
| | Impingement syndrome |

MFTP, myofascial trigger point.

bly leading to a restructuring in the extracellular matrix and collagen deposition around nerve fibers. This is proposed to reduce the pain threshold of these fibers (Sprott et al., 1997). The oxygenation of muscle tissues is decreased (Yunus, 1994), possibly from a fall in oxygen saturation during sleep (Lario et al., 1996). These findings in muscle tissues are not conclusive and are nonspecific. Other changes in tissue include an increased number of connective tissue mast cells and increased IgG deposits in the dermal-epidermal junction specific to collagen bundles (Enestrom et al., 1997). The presence of the mast cells may be responsible for potent pain mediators such as histamine and substance P (Enestrom et al., 1997). Future studies may find more specific pathology in muscle tissues or surrounding tissues.

Some preliminary research findings of brain function by single photon emission computed tomography and positron emission tomography scanning show decreased function of the caudate in FMS (Mountz et al., 1998). A decreased activation of the thalamus to acute pain and hyperalgesia from higher levels of activation in the cingulate cortex also has been reported (Mountz et al., 1998).

## Sleep

Most patients with FMS have a sleep disturbance, which may contribute greatly to the distress and intensity of disease. With a sleep disturbance, the sleep-pain-tension cycle mounts, creating a cycle that may be difficult to control. The primary defect may be a sleep disorder, which results ultimately in biochemical and cytokine-mediated changes that produce the musculoskeletal effects.

Sleep disturbances affect circadian rhythms and the hypothalamic-pituitary axis. Sleep deprivation studies are known to produce musculoskeletal pain in subjects (Yunus, 1994). Most common is an alpha wave intrusion during stage 4 delta sleep (Bennet, 1997b). Because this does not occur in all patients with FMS, it is not known if this is an associated problem or a contributing factor in FMS pain. This can be explained by the numerous causes of sleep disturbance in FMS (eg, restless leg syndrome, pain) (Bennet, 1997b). Other sleep disturbances include sleep apnea, a 50% decrease in rapid eye movement (REM) sleep, an absence of stage 3 or 4 sleep, and altered chronobiology (Bennet, 1997b; Yunus, 1994). The frequency of sleep disturbances in FMS is great enough to mandate empirical treatment.

## Neuroendocrinology

The hypothalamic-pituitary-adrenal (HPA) axis also has been found to function abnormally in patients with FMS (Bennet, 1997b; Yunus, 1994; Crofford, 1998). Because neurotransmitters and hormones are distributed throughout the body, this hypothesis could explain the widespread distribution of musculoskeletal pain and symptoms. Neuroendocrine abnormalities may be one of the most important or predominant features of this multifactorial disease. Abnormalities include decreased urinary free cortisol levels with a blunting of the evening cortisol trough (Bennet, 1997b; Crofford, 1998). Insulin-like growth factor-I (IGF-I, or somatomedin C) levels also are low in some patients (Bennet, 1997b; Crofford, 1998). The disturbance in stage 4 sleep, as described earlier, may be the cause of the low levels of IGF-I (Bennet, 1997b; Crofford, 1998). Other neurohormones found to be out of balance include plasma histidine (histamine precursor), methionine (precursor of *S*-adenosylmethionine), and tryptophan (serotonin precursor).

An imbalance of neurotransmitters, such as serotonin and norepinephrine, may play a pathophysiologic role (Russell, 1998). This is indicated by the widespread pain that has a focal origin but spreads to other tissues (Bennet, 1997b; Mense, 1990). Substance P, a neurotransmitter involved in the transmission of pain, may be involved in the pathophysiologic mechanisms (Yunus, 1994; Russell, 1998). Elevated levels of substance P have been found in the cerebrospinal fluid (Yunus, 1994; Russell, 1998). Decreased serum levels of tryptophan and tryptophan transport molecules also have been reported. Cerebrospinal 5-hydroxyindoleacetic acid (serotonin metabolite) is decreased in studies of patients with FMS (Yunus, 1994). Researchers have shown that hyperalgesia occurs when there is a failure of serotonergic pathways, leading to hyperactivity of *N*-methyl-D-aspartate receptors and activating production of nitric oxide (Nicolodi et al., 1998). Other metabolites of norepinephrine and dopamine are decreased in patients with FMS compared with controls (Yunus, 1994; Russell, 1998), but levels of the sleep hormone melatonin appear normal (Press et al., 1998). The source of the increased levels of neurotransmitters may be upregulation of genetic transcription after cellular and molecular changes (Bennet, 1997b). Some studies have found a possible link with an autoimmune process of anti–5-hydroxytryptamine antibodies (Klein & Berg, 1995). Stage 4 (REM) sleep is altered by abnormalities in serotonin and somatomedin C. Pain and pain amplification is influenced by the neurotransmitters serotonin, norepinephrine, histidine, methionine, and tryptophan. It is not known whether the neuroendocrine abnormalities are a result of genetics, trauma, infection, or other causes (Yunus, 1994).

Patients with FMS appear to have an unusual sensitivity to cold-induced vasospasm. When compared with normal subjects or people with low back pain, FMS patients have a greater vasospastic response to the application of cold and a more intense sensation of pain (Lapossy et al., 1994).

## Peripheral Attributions

Localized muscle trauma develops into widespread musculoskeletal pain in FMS (Yunus, 1994). Indirect trauma to muscle tissue from activities such as spinal stress and poor posture may contribute to this (Yunus, 1994). Deconditioning of muscles, microtrauma, and sympathetic hyperactivity have been shown to be secondary to the processes involved in the disease process (Yunus, 1994).

## Stress

Stress and psychological dysfunction are common in FMS. About half of patients have a lifetime history of depression (Bennet, 1997b). Stress, anxiety, panic, poor coping, perceived low quality of life, and operant condition are some of the psychological issues found. Sexual, physical, and emotional abuse or neglect may play a role in the development and maintenance of the disease (Walker et al., 1997). As with other findings in FMS, it is not known if these are primary or secondary problems (Bennet, 1997b).

The pathophysiologic mechanisms and interactions in FMS are depicted in Figure 19-3. In this model, the disorder arises from a heterogeneous neurohormonal dysfunction that leads to a vicious fatigue-pain-fatigue cycle.

## Physiologic Basis of Treatment

### Exercise and Cognitive-Behavioral Treatment

Cognitive-behavior modalities, performed by a multidisciplinary team, can provide a reduction in the stress-pain cycle by reducing feelings of helplessness, restructuring negative patterns of thought, and providing coping strategies for pain (Alarcon & Bradley, 1998).

Exercise can be beneficial in FMS, since up to 80% of patients with FMS are physically deconditioned and develop a cycle of physical inactivity with pain (Feiffenberger & Amundson, 1996).

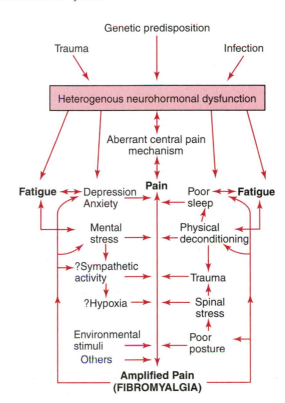

**FIGURE 19.3** ● Probable pathophysiologic mechanisms in fibromyalgia syndrome (FMS) showing various interacting factors. The most important mechanism in FMS most likely involves neurohormonal dysfunctions. (Yunnus, M.B. [1994] Fibromyalgia syndrome and myofascial pain syndrome, Table 1–3. In Rachlin, E. [Ed.]. Myofascial pain and fibromyalgia. St. Louis, C.V. Mosby Co. p. 15.)

Exercise improves FMS primarily by an improvement in the self-perception of wellness (Alarcon & Bradley, 1998). Pain may be worse at first after the initiation of an exercise program but improves with further reconditioning (Feiffenberger & Amundson, 1996). Cardiovascular fitness training is effective in raising pain thresholds (Alarcon & Bradley, 1998), and flexibility exercise programs may produce improvements in pain and conditioning (Alarcon & Bradley, 1998; Goldenberg, 1997). Whatever the exercise program, it should be low-impact, aerobic health training lasting for 30 minutes, performed 3 to 4 times a week (Bennet, 1997b). This should be reached in a period of 6 to 12 months (Bennet, 1997b).

### Antidepressants and Neurochemical Regulators

Most of the hypotheses for FMS revolve around imbalances in neurotransmitters, particularly serotonin. With this in mind, medical therapeutics should be directed toward boosting these levels to inhibit pain perception. The selective serotonin reuptake inhibitors (SSRIs) have been shown to be effective in small studies (Goldenberg et al., 1996). The tricyclic compounds, such as amitriptyline and imipramine, have shown good effects on pain control, stiffness, and improvement in sleep in FMS (Alarcon & Bradley, 1998; Goldenberg et al., 1996; Feiffenberger & Amundson, 1996). However, their effects may diminish with time and have no effect on sleep physiology or point tenderness (Alarcon & Bradley, 1998; Feiffenberger & Amundson, 1996). The administration of SSRIs and tricyclics together may provide overall improvement in pain and sleep (Alarcon & Bradley, 1998; Goldenberg et al., 1996). Some studies have shown that ondansetron (a 5-HT$_3$ receptor antagonist) and tropesitron are effective in decreasing the intensity and distribution of pain only when serum serotonin levels were not altered (Alarcon & Bradley, 1998). Ondansetron improves not only pain, but also tender points, headaches, and general functioning (Goldenberg, 1997).

## Analgesics

Tramadol is a non-opioid, non-NSAID analgesic safe for long-term use (Bennet, 1997b). With tramadol, studies report up to an 80% decrease in pain. There have been reports of abuse or misuse of this medication, but statistically speaking, the number is insignificant. Tramadol works in two fashions: (1) inhibition of the reuptake of norepinephrine and serotonin at the synapse, the two transmitters involved in pain inhibition, and (2) stimulation of mu-2 opioid receptors (United States Pharmacopeial Convention Drug Information [USP DI], 1998). Stimulation of the mu-2 opioid receptor inhibits pain by an unknown mechanism. Scheduled use of this medication probably is most effective in FMS because of its chronic nature and the mechanism of action of tramadol.

## Benzodiazepines

Benzodiazepines can be beneficial in select patients with FMS. These medications can relieve the muscle spasms, anxiety, and insomnia associated with FMS. Additionally, they increase the activity of GABA, a neurotransmitter involved in the inhibition of pain (Bennet, 1997b; Yunus, 1994; USP DI, 1998). Diazepam is a choice benzodiazepine in FMS because of its long half-life (reduced problems associated with withdrawal of medication) and high efficacy in relief from muscle spasm (USP DI, 1998).

## Muscle Relaxants

Cyclobenzaprine is a related tricyclic compound that works by inhibiting the reuptake of norepinephrine and serotonin (Feiffenberger & Amundson, 1996). Single daily doses at bedtime have been shown to control the symptoms of FMS, including point tenderness, sleep disturbances, and pain (Alarcon & Bradley, 1998; Feiffenberger & Amundson, 1996). Cyclobenzaprine may be more effective in combination with ibuprofen (Alarcon & Bradley, 1998).

## Growth Hormone

Growth hormone has been shown to improve quality of life, IGF-I levels, and muscle pain scores in a 9-month treatment study (Alarcon & Bradley, 1998).

## Alternative Treatments

Ice and heat are viable options in providing quick relief (20 to 30 minutes); however, their effects are short lived. Massage, acupuncture, and passive stretching of muscles also provide similar relief (Bennet, 1997b). A combination of these therapies probably is the best option.

Trigger point injections with lidocaine, methylprednisolone, or both may provide relief in specific painful areas (Bennet, 1997b).

---

### ● Case Study 19.1 ·

Christine Nordstrom, a 29-year-old divorced laborer and part-time student, presents for follow-up of complaints of neck and shoulder pain for 2 years. Christine describes her pain as dull and nonradiating and states that it gets worse as the day goes on. She has neck stiffness and a perceived decrease in lateral range of motion. She denies any recent trauma; however, when she was 15, she was involved in a motor vehicle accident that caused a whiplash injury and had her arm in a sling for a few weeks. She gets little relief

*(Case study continued on next page)*

from Tylenol or ibuprofen and has had the most relief with heating pads. She has been taking the Relafen, which was prescribed on her last visit, without any relief. She also has soreness in her knees and frequent tension-type headaches.

## History

### Past Medical History

| | |
|---|---|
| Allergies | No drug allergies |
| Current medications | Birth control pills |
| Surgeries | Tonsillectomy as a child, wisdom teeth extraction as a child |
| Childhood illness | Chicken pox as a child. No chronic illnesses or other health problems |

### Social History

| | |
|---|---|
| Marital | Divorced, no children |
| Tobacco | Smokes 12 cigarettes/day for last 10 years |
| Employment | Full-time night shifts at a local shipping company loading boxes. She is trying to go back to college part-time for a degree in computer programming. |

### Family History

| | |
|---|---|
| Mother | Osteoarthritis and hypertension |
| Father | Died of lung cancer at age 63 |
| Siblings | No illnesses |

## Review of Systems

| | |
|---|---|
| General | No weight changes. Complains of being tired all the time |
| Skin | Negative |
| Neurologic | Negative. Denies any paresthesias, vertigo, or syncope |
| HEENT | Occasional allergic rhinitis |
| CV | Negative |
| Respiratory | Negative |
| GI | Has intermittent gastrocolic diarrhea and cramps about once a week. No pyrosis or melena |
| MS | No weakness of muscles. Her knees swell and become sore with running in sports. Denies any fasciculation or atrophy. She exercises sporadically, just an occasional game of tennis or softball. States her back frequently hurts, especially after work. She usually just sleeps it off. Denies any swelling in any other joints |
| Endocrine | Negative |
| Hematologic | Negative |
| Psychosocial | States she often feels sad or depressed. Is under a lot of stress with work and harassment by her ex-husband. She also has to make mortgage and college tuition payments. She denies any panic, psychosis, crying, or suicidal ideation |

*(Case study continued on page 392)*

## *Physical Examination*

| System | Findings |
| --- | --- |
| Vital signs | T-98.4°F HR-79 RR-18 <br> BP-123/84 <br> Height 5'8", Weight 176 lb |
| General | No distress, posture slumped, good hygiene and dress |
| Skin | Warm, dry, intact, no rashes |
| Neurologic | DTRs-bicep 2/2, tricep 2/2, radial, 2/2, knee 2/2, ankle 2/2 and brisk. CN II-XII grossly intact. Negative Romberg |
| HEENT | Fundi negative, EOMI, conjunctivae pink, no sinus tenderness, tympanic membranes negative, no lymph nodes, throat clear, thyroid nonpalpable. Neck with full ROM, and hyperextensibility. Tender to palpation at 8 points along occiput, down through the trapezius, without referral of pain |
| Thorax | Lungs clear, HRRR. No spinal tenderness, no anterior chest tenderness to palpation. 4 tender points to palpation at low back, no fullness |
| Abdomen | Negative |
| Extremities | Peripheral pulses palpable, no edema. Negative talen and phalens tests, some mild pain with Apley scratch test, negative painful shoulder arc, no reduction of power. Tenderness to palpation at 2 lateral knee points bilaterally. Straight leg raises negative, can heel and toe walk |

## *Laboratory Studies*

| Test | Result |
| --- | --- |
| 1. Arthritis panel | Negative |
| 2. CBC | Normal |
| 3. TSH | Normal |

## *Impression*

Fibromyalgia syndrome

## *Plan*

1. Physical therapy referral for exercise program and stretching exercises
2. Ibuprofen 600 mg TID
3. Xanax 0.5 m TID
4. Ultram 50 mg 1–2 tablets every 6 hours as needed
5. Use ice rubdowns as needed
6. Return to clinic in 2 weeks
7. Other treatment options:
   - Guaifenesin 600 mg BID (to reduce phosphate deposits)
   - High-protein, low-carbohydrate diet

BP, blood pressure; CBC, complete blood count; CN, cranial nerve; CV, cardiovascular; DTRs, deep tendon reflexes; EOMI, extraoccular muscles intact; GI, gastrointestinal; HEENT, head, eye, ear, nose, and throat; HR, heart rate; HRRR, heart rate and rhythm regular; MS, musculoskeletal; P, pulse; RR, respiration rate; T, temperature; ROM, range of motion.

# CHRONIC FATIGUE SYNDROME

Chronic fatigue is a common symptom in primary care practices, accounting for 10 to 15 million visits to medical offices each year (Komaroff, 1994). It is also likely that many people with significant and even debilitating fatigue do not visit their health care provider for help, feeling that their fatigue is the result of work, stress, and lifestyle. Most of the patients who ultimately are diagnosed with CFS have been experiencing chronic symptoms for years. When a patient presents with a chief complaint of fatigue, the first diagnosis to be ruled out is depression. Organic illness such as hypothyroidism, hypotension, or cancer, which cause fatigue, also must be considered. When psychiatric and organic etiologies have been excluded, the diagnosis of CFS may be possible.

## Diagnostic Criteria

Diagnostic criteria for CFS vary from country to country. The United States criteria were developed by the Centers for Disease Control (CDC) in 1988 and were criticized as being narrow. New criteria were released in 1993 and categorize CFS as a subset of chronic fatigue, which is a subset of persistent fatigue. The new criteria for diagnosis are the following:

1. Clinically evaluated, unexplained persistent or relapsing chronic fatigue that is of new or definite onset (ie, not lifelong), is not the result of ongoing exertion, is not substantially alleviated by rest, and results in substantial reduction in previous levels of occupational, educational, social, or personal activities.
2. The concurrent occurrence of four or more of the following symptoms: substantial impairment in short-term memory or concentration; sore throat; tender lymph nodes, muscle pain; multijoint pain without swelling or redness; headaches of a new type, pattern, or severity; unrefreshing sleep; and postexertional malaise lasting more than 24 hours. These symptoms must have persisted or recurred during 6 or more consecutive months of illness and must not have predated the fatigue (*http://www.cdc. gov/ncidod/diseases/cfs/defined2.htm*).

## Symptoms

Fatigue has many manifestations and definitions. Fatigue can be described as a *feeling* or as a *decrement in performance* (Wessely et al., 1998). Some authorities consider CFS fatigue to result from neuromuscular disease. However, the myalgia and pervasive fatigue of CFS is unlike other muscular types of fatigue. The fatigue described by patients with CFS is a *feeling* that is greater than that experienced by the ordinary person after a lack of sleep or excessive exercise. It is profound, debilitating fatigue, not "sleepiness," and it becomes worse with physical or mental efforts throughout the day. Nevertheless, there is evidence of a sleep disorder in affected persons. In CFS, patients complain of waking unrefreshed from a night's sleep. Many CFS patients take more than 1 hour to fall asleep, and most wake in the night for more than 1 hour.

Whereas the fatigue felt by patients is their overriding concern, other symptoms are present and bothersome and bring people to their primary care providers with great frequency. Sore throat, muscle aches, fevers, and depression may require frequent visits. Designated the "yuppie flu" because it occurs frequently in professional and upper socioeconomic status groups, some providers are reluctant to make the diagnosis because of skepticism about the reality of the disorder. Recent epidemiologic evidence indicates that this "yuppie" association is artifactual, and CFS can be found across all social classes when the CDC Diagnostic Criteria are used properly (Wessely et al., 1998).

## Pathogenesis

### Infection

Many patients with CFS report the onset of symptoms after a viral illness or blood transfusion, which has led to theories pointing to chronic viral illness, such as chronic Epstein-Barr viral (EBV) infection. Occasionally, CFS appears in an epidemic-like pattern. In addition, certain infectious illnesses have sequelae characterized by fatigue, such as brucellosis and influenza. Attention has been focused on chronic EBV infection (chronic mononucleosis) as a cause of CFS. Chronic fatigue syndrome was described as a chronic EBV infection in 1982, but several later studies did not confirm a relationship between symptoms and the presence of elevated EBV antibody titers. Many patients diagnosed as having chronic EBV infection also were found to have significant psychiatric comorbidity (Fekety, 1998).

Other microorganisms speculated to be involved in CFS include yeasts, other herpesviruses, retroviruses, and *Borrelia burgdorferi* (the agent that causes Lyme disease).

No uniform evidence of a specific microbial agent has been causally associated with CFS.

What could account for both the viral associations and immunologic alterations commonly observed in CFS patients is the stress and fatigue experienced as the result of experiencing a chronic, debilitating, profoundly distressful illness.

### Immune Changes

A variety of immunologic aberrations is seen in CFS. A new nomenclature has appeared, terming the illness *chronic fatigue and immune deficiency syndrome*. Not all patients show the same immunologic pattern, however. Whereas lymphadenopathy is a frequent finding, only about one third of patients have a lymphocytosis. T cells are found to be abnormal in some CFS patients, but the nature of the abnormality has been difficult to elucidate. One finding is that the number of T cells bearing the CD45RA and CD45RO markers is significantly reduced in CFS. This might be evidence of chronic antigenic exposure of lymphocytes, since similar patterns are seen in autoimmune diseases such as lupus erythematosus and multiple sclerosis (Strober, 1994). In addition, CFS lymphocytes usually show reduced proliferative responses in vitro to antigenic stimulation and are less able to secrete cytokines such as interferon gamma (IFN-$\gamma$) and interleukin (IL)-2 when stimulated (Strober, 1998).

Another immune cell that has been studied in CFS is the natural killer (NK) cell. The NK cells are actively cytolytic cells that do not require restriction of the major histocompatibility complex and presumably would be involved in attacking virally infected cells if this occurred in CFS. Several studies demonstrate changes in NK cell number and NK cell functional activity. The literature generally suggests a decreased number of some types of NK cells in CFS and a decreased cytolytic ability of these cells (Strober, 1998).

A problem with the research data is that no consistent relationship between the immunologic alterations and fatigue symptoms has been established.

### Cytokines

Cytokines have long been suspected of being partly responsible for the symptoms of CFS. These symptoms in many ways mimic the sickness behavior elicited by proinflammatory cytokines. The level of IFN-$\gamma$ appears to be normal in CSF, but levels of other proinflammatory cytokines have been elevated in several studies. Transforming growth factor beta may be elevated in patients, and it becomes even more elevated after exercise (Chao et al., 1990). Nevertheless, there are no consistent and reproducible abnormalities in cytokines that explain a distinct immunologic aberration in the disease.

### Neuroendocrine Changes

Neuroendocrine alterations suggest increased central serotonergic function and reduced adrenal axis function in CFS. The primary defect may be a reduced drive of the HPA axis and a resultant hypoadrenalism. A reduced adrenal gland size was found in CFS patients compared with normal controls in one study (Scott et al., 1999). A relatively new treatment approach is the use of low-dose hydrocortisone, which seems to significantly reduce fatigue in many patients (Cleare et al., 1999).

## Physiologic Basis of Treatment

Because a single etiology has not been found for CFS, the treatment approaches are empirical and range from bizarre nutritional practices to more proven interventions. Patients with this illness often are frustrated and go from one provider to another seeking treatments. Patients often use alternative medicines, as evidenced by the many sites on the World Wide Web for herbal remedies and nutrient additives available for CFS.

Antidepressants such as the SSRIs may be helpful in patients who have comorbid depression and in patients with sleep disorders and pain. Increasing brain serotonin may address a neurochemical abnormality in CFS. However, use of antidepressants is not considered a first-line choice of medication for most CFS patients (Wessely et al., 1998).

Whereas a variety of immunotherapies have been attempted in CFS, no one approach has been shown to be beneficial. Immunoglobulins, leukocyte extracts, and IFN-$\gamma$ are some of the immunotherapies that have been attempted and discarded.

Many patients are helped by psychological counseling or behavioral therapy. These patients also seek information and are often knowledgeable about their disease and current treatments and research. One site that patients may find useful for the most up-to-date information is *http://www-hsl.mcmaster.ca/tomflem/cfs.html*.

The major treatment advocated by many clinicians for patients with CFS is rest and reduction in exercise. Nevertheless, exercise probably should be one of the major recommended approaches for patients with FMS. In a few well-designed exercise interventions, CFS patients subjectively improved. Rest may be harmful in the long run, leading to increasing sedentariness, deconditioning, and weight gain.

The primary care provider is thus faced with little in the pharmacopoeia that can be helpful, other than antidepressants, and should consider referral for cognitive-behavioral therapy and tolerable exercise programs.

## NECK AND BACK PAIN

Neck and low back pain are prevalent problems and are the second most common type of pain for which people seek care. Neck pain affects about 10% of the general population and is commonly caused by degenerative disc disease or arthritis. Low back pain usually results from sprains, disc disease, or osteoarthritis changes. However, many other etiologies are possible, and both neck and back pain do not always have a musculoskeletal origin. Kidney disease, for example, can cause back pain, and referred pain from visceral disease may cause neck pain (Gore, 1998). This chapter focuses on the musculoskeletal types of back and neck pain.

### Low Back Pain

Four of five adults experience an episode of low back pain during their lifetime. It is the major cause of work place disability and lost productivity, most commonly occurring between 30 and 50 years of age. Societal costs of low back pain are enormous, on the order of $80 billion per year.

### Anatomy

Vertebral anatomy involves complex structures and relationships that become disturbed in conditions causing low back pain. Figure 19-4 illustrates a lumbar vertebral segment. The intervertebral disc has an external ligamentous structure and an internal soft pulp, called the nucleus pulposus. The function of the disc is to connect adjacent vertebrae and act as a shock-absorbent material. The facet joints also are important. Their function is to connect the chain-like vertebral column into a single anatomic structure that allows persons to bend and move. Facet joints are subject to degenerative osteoarthritis. The nerve roots leave the spinal cord through foramen. Notice that the nerve roots could be compressed if there was a change in the size or shape of the disc, or if arthritic changes such as spurs and osteophytes impinged on the nerves as they exit the spinal cord.

### Disc Degeneration

The intervertebral discs are composed of the strong, external, round ligament, the annulus, and the soft, gelatinous, internal nucleus pulposus (see Fig. 19-4). The nucleus is cartilaginous, containing collagen, proteoglycans, and other proteins. It

---

### CLINICAL VIGNETTE 19.1

Marilyn Brown is a 28-year-old librarian who presents to the primary care clinic with a self-diagnosis of chronic fatigue syndrome (CFS). She has read popular literature and has surfed the World Wide Web for information. She describes her symptoms as exhaustion—so severe that she can hardly get through the day. She is asking to go on long-term disability from her position because she feels she can no longer work. At work, she gets confused and forgetful and makes many errors. She had been active socially, at work, and in recreation until a sudden onset of fatigue began about 3 months ago. Her symptoms have become progressively worse. She has not seen a health care provider about these symptoms until today. Ms. Brown describes waking in the morning completely unrefreshed. She also reports early morning awakening. She drags through the day, and any activity, either mental or physical, wears her out. She also describes frequent sore throats, headaches, and generalized myalgia. On examination, she is found to meet the DSM-IV criteria for depression, and results of her physical examination are normal except for 2+ cervical adenopathy. She meets the Centers for Disease Control criteria for CFS, although the only observable *physical* finding is adenopathy. Results of all laboratory studies are normal.

This patient presents a challenge in that the provider should be cautious about potential malingering in a highly intelligent and well-informed patient. On the other hand, she presents a classic pattern of CFS, and it is reasonable for her to wish to be classified as disabled, since CFS patients often are unable to work.

Pharmacologic treatment for her depression is imperative. She also may be a candidate for low-dose hydrocortisone and an exercise intervention.

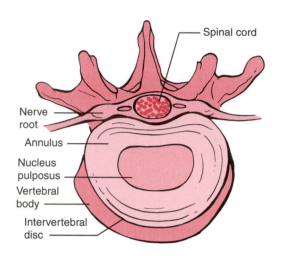

**FIGURE 19.4** ● Anatomical relationships in the lumbar area between the vertebral bones and intervertebral disc. The disc is composed of the outer annulus and inner nucleus pulposis.

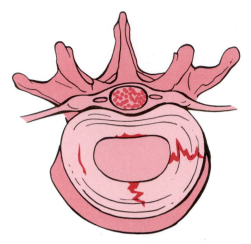

**FIGURE 19.5** ● Annular tears.

is well hydrated in younger people (up to 90%) but loses water, along with proteoglycans, with aging. It normally has the approximate consistency of crabmeat and acts, in a cushion-like manner, as a shock absorber when loads are applied to the spine. Normally, the nucleus imbibes water as the disc compresses, but as degeneration occurs, it is less able to do this, becoming stiffer and more compressible. With degeneration, the distinction between the annulus and the nucleus is lost, and both structures become fibrous, dry, and stiff. Degeneration of these structures leads to disc disease and various pain syndromes. The cause of degeneration is unknown, but it is not just a natural aging process. The disc becomes frayed, dehydrated, and subject to tears in the annulus (radial, rim, and concentric tears all are possible). Annular tears are depicted in Figure 19-5. Once these tears appear, an inflammatory granulomatous process ensues, which ultimately leads to fibrosis. Fibrotic changes cause the disc to become thin and narrow. Tears allow the soft nucleus material to herniate, causing pressure on nerve roots (Fig. 19-6). The types of disc extensions that then occur include annular bulging, or herniations, which are asymmetric protrusions of the nucleus pulposus, or complete extrusion of the pulposus through a tear. Bits of nuclear material can form blebs off of the extruded material and become sequestered outside of the disc. These changes then produce compression on nerve roots, with resultant pain and radicular symptoms. An additional problem is arthritic degenerative changes, such as osteophytes that develop at the disc-bone junction

(Fig. 19-7). These further inflame and compress nerve roots.

Theories about the pathogenesis of disc degeneration suggest that there may be a primary biochemical disorder in disc chondrocytes. Enzymes from chondrocytes that degrade the cartilaginous matrix may be secreted in excess, leading to morphologic and functional alterations in the disc. Most implicated are the matrix metalloproteinases, excessive prostaglandin E, nitric oxide, and IL-6 (Kang et al., 1996). As in osteoarthritis, the process of degradation exceeds the synthesis of matrix, leading to weakening, tearing, and thinning of the disc (Corrigan & Maitland, 1998). The scarring that occurs as annular tears are repaired produces a decrease in strength of the annulus.

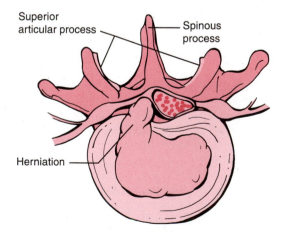

**FIGURE 19.6** ● Herniation of nucleus pulposis causing pressure on neurologic structures.

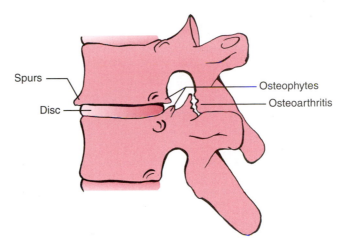

Spurs

Disc

Osteophytes

Osteoarthritis

**FIGURE 19.7** ● Osteoarthritis of the spine with osteophytes compressing a nerve root.

Factors that predispose to disc degeneration include gender and age. The process occurs earlier in men than in women and begins in the 20s, peaking in the 40s. Thus, the degeneration is not caused by senescence. Trauma is not a common reason for a disc rupture, except in a disc that already is compromised by these degenerative processes. Years of heavy lifting, prolonged standing or sitting, and significant obesity increase the likelihood of disc disease, whereas exercise and activity generally promote healthy disc nutrition (Corrigan & Maitland, 1998). Research suggests a strong genetic influence on disc degeneration. In a study of monozygotic and dizygotic twins, the influence of heredity, when all of the other just-mentioned risk factors were controlled, was high: 74% at the lumbar spine and 73% at the cervical spine (Sambrook et al., 1999).

### Symptoms

Symptoms of disc degeneration depend on the location and severity. However, many clinicians note that there often is little relationship between radiographic findings and severity of symptoms. In the early stages, there are no symptoms because the disc itself is avascular and lacks nerve supply. Only when nerve compression occurs do symptoms appear. Pain is felt as a deep, local aching in the back, but it may be referred to the buttock. Bending often causes the pain to be severe, since this motion produces compression of the disc and causes it to bulge distally toward nervous tissue. Symptoms can develop acutely if a herniated disc occurs, an injury in which an acute annular tear results in protrusion of the nucleus pulposus, producing a space-occupying lesion that compresses nerve roots and may cause local inflammation. The injury may occur during vigorous exercise or after an event as innocuous as a sneeze. Back pain

occurs immediately, often with muscle spasm. This is followed by the development of unilateral leg pain. Sciatica commonly results from pressure on the nerve roots that ultimately come together in the large sciatic nerve. Sciatic pain often is described as sharp, nagging, pain with sensory changes occurring in a pattern related to the corresponding dermatome (Corrigan & Maitland, 1998). Numbness, pain, and weakness are the result. Table 19-3 depicts the effects of nerve root compression in the spine at different levels. Localization of symptoms helps to determine the site of disc damage and nerve root compression.

### Physiologic Basis of Treatment

Low back pain tends to resolve within 3 to 6 weeks, *with or without treatment*. Interventions to reduce the pain include 2 to 3 days of bed rest, application of ice to reduce inflammation, and taking NSAIDs and muscle relaxants in patients with severe muscle spasms. Early ambulation is encouraged because patients can quickly become deconditioned, which may lead to a positive, vicious cycle of further pain and disability. Obesity and cigarette smoking are factors that increase the incidence of disc disease and should be addressed with the patient. Strengthening of the abdominal muscles helps to protect the back, and persons should be taught proper ways of bending and lifting to protect the back from further injury. Physical therapy can help patients in both acute and chronic stages of degenerative disc disease. Surgery is used only in severe, stubborn cases, and includes laminectomies, discectomies, and spinal fusion.

A cause for immediate concern in a patient presenting with acute low back pain is evidence of spinal cord compression, which can lead to the *cauda equina* syndrome. In this situation, a large herniation of the nucleus pulposus fills the spinal

## TABLE 19.3

### Lumbar Disc Herniation

| Disc | Root | Pain and Paresthesias | Sensory Loss | Motor Loss | Reflex Loss |
|------|------|----------------------|--------------|------------|-------------|
| L3-L4 | L4 | Anterior thigh, inner shin | Anteromedial thigh, down along shin to inner side of foot | Quadriceps | Knee jerk |
| L4-L5 | L5 | Radiating down outer side of back of thigh and outer side of calf, across dorsum of foot to great toe | Outer side of calf and great toe | Extensor hallucis longus | None |
| L5-S1 | S1 | Radiating down back of thigh and outer side and back of calf, to foot and lesser toes | Outer side of calf, outer border of foot and lesser toes | Gastrocnemius, and occasionally muscles of eversion of foot | Ankle jerk |

(From Hinton, R. [1995]. Backache. In M. Samuels [Ed.], *Manual of neurological therapeutics*. In *MAXX: Maximum access to diagnosis and therapy: The electronic library of medicine* [CD-ROM]. Philadelphia: Lippincott-Raven Publishers.)

canal and compresses the cord itself, rather than nerve roots, causing pressure and inflammation and leading to severe weakness in the legs and feet, as well as incontinence. This is a surgical emergency requiring immediate referral and intervention.

### Spinal Stenosis

In spinal stenosis, the entire spinal canal may become narrower. It is most commonly seen in persons older than 60 years of age and can cause severe disability. It occurs most frequently in the lumbar vertebrae, where chronic disc degeneration and arthritis lead to hypertrophy of the facet joints. The L3-4 and L4-5 joints are the most commonly involved (Jenny & Katcherside, 1994). A World Wide Web site of practical usefulness for the health care provider is *http://www.cdc.gov/niosh/homepage.html*, which provides latest research and treatment guidelines on back injuries, as well as *http://www.ahcpr.gov*, which publishes management plans and guidelines.

### Back Sprain

Back sprain, or *facet syndrome*, occurs after a sudden motion, a fall, or lifting of a heavy object, leaving the individual in acute pain, often bent to one side, and restricted in movement. Paraspinal muscles and ligaments are more subject to sprain

as an individual ages. Sprained muscles tend to go into spasm and become stiff, and people then protect them from painful stretching through posture and movement. Rest is helpful for the early few days after an acute muscle sprain, and these types of injuries generally resolve with conservative treatment.

### Neck Pain

Neck pain is common in the general population, and, like low back pain, common etiologies include degenerative disc disease and arthritic changes in both the disc-bone articulation and the zygapophyseal joints. There are seven cervical vertebrae, and C-5, C-6, and C-7 are most frequently the origin of symptoms. Crepitus, pain, limitation of motion, and radicular neurologic symptoms may occur. When the cervical nerve roots are compressed, pain, motor, reflex, and sensory deficits occur along the distribution of the nerve (radiculopathy). Table 19-4 depicts the signs and symptoms associated with lateral herniation of a cervical disc.

## INFLAMMATORY MUSCULOSKELETAL CONDITIONS

Although practitioners occasionally see patients who have experienced skeletal trauma leading to fracture, mostly these patients are seen in the

---

### CLINICAL VIGNETTE 19.2

Mark Grover is a 29-year-old married stockbroker who is brought to the office by his wife after experiencing a back injury while playing basketball. He explains that his back pain occurred after a pivot move and was so severe that he fell to the floor in pain. He appears to be bent to one side and walks gingerly. On palpation, he is tender at L4. He has a history of back strains, is about 30 lb overweight, and admits to smoking a pack per day.

He has a normal neurologic examination, and a negative straight leg-raising test. X-rays are not indicated, and magnetic resonance imaging would be useful only if his pain does not resolve. He is advised to rest for the next day or two, apply ice packs for 20 minutes to the affected area every 4 hours, take ibuprofen for pain, and return if he is not better within a week. His diagnosis is acute low back sprain.

---

emergency room and require orthopedic specialty care. The discussion in this chapter is limited to chronic inflammatory musculoskeletal injuries and conditions because it is this type of patient who seeks primary care. Two models of this sort of injury are provided: plantar fasciitis and carpal tunnel syndrome.

### Plantar Fasciitis

A common complaint in active individuals, obese persons, and older, sedentary individuals is heel pain. The plantar fascia (aponeurosis) is the site of most common heel pain, and it becomes chronically inflamed. This thick, broad band of dense connective tissue originates at the os calcaneus tuberosity and then fans out, dividing into five longitudinal bands that insert into the skin, the metatarsophalangeal joints, and base of the phalanges (Fig. 19-8). It plays an important function in stabilizing the foot and maintaining the arch of the foot during weight-bearing activities. The heel is tender to touch medially, where the fascia inserts into the os calcaneus, and people may have severe limitations of activity because of pain. The described pain is severe, localized heel pain that spreads into the plantar fascia and is worse on awakening. After activity, the pain resolves somewhat, but later in the day, it becomes more noticeable. The pain also increases with exercise.

The pathophysiology is believed to be a chronic degenerative and reparative processes caused by stress overload on the fascia (Cooper, 1997). People with a cavus foot are more likely to stretch this fascia and overload the structure. Runners who repetitively strike their heel on the ground, along with repetitive hyperextension of the toes, produce stress that can lead to microtears in the aponeurosis. This then initiates an inflammatory response, ultimately leading to degenerative changes. Many people with this condition also have a heel spur,

---

## TABLE 19.4 ● ● ●

### Cervical Disc Herniation

| Disc | Root | Pain and Paresthesias | Sensory Loss | Motor Loss | Reflex Loss |
|------|------|----------------------|--------------|------------|-------------|
| C4-C5 | C5 | Neck, shoulder, upper arm | Shoulder | Deltoid, biceps | Biceps |
| C5-C6 | C6 | Neck, shoulder, lateral aspect of arm, radial aspect of forearm to thumb and forefinger | Thumb, forefinger, radial aspect of forearm, lateral aspect of arm | Biceps | Biceps, supinator |
| C6-C7 | C7 | Neck, lateral aspect of arm, ring and index finger | Forefinger, middle finger, radial aspect of forearm | Triceps, extensor carpi ulnaris | Triceps, supinator |
| C7-T1 | C8 | Ulnar aspect of forearm and hand | Ulnar half of ring finger, little finger | Intrinsic muscles of the hand, wrist extensors | None |

(From Hinton, R. [1995]. Backache. In M. Samuels (Ed.), *Manual of neurologic therapeutics.* In *MAXX: Maximum access to diagnosis and therapy: The electronic library of medicine* [CD-ROM]. Philadelphia: Lippincott-Raven Publishers.)

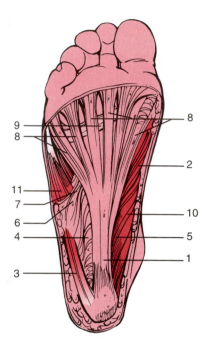

**FIGURE 19.8** ● Plantar aponeurosis.
*(1)* Central component, ie, plantar fascia,
*(2)* Medial component, *(3)* Lateral
component, *(4)* Lateral plantar sulcus,
*(5)* Medial plantar sulcus, *(6)* Lateral crux,
*(7)* Medial crux. *(8)* Superficial longitudinal
tracts, *(9)* Transverse superficial tract,
*(10)* Abductor hallucis muscle, and
*(11)* Abductor digiti quinti muscle.
(Sarrafian, S.K. [1983]. *Anatomy of the
foot and ankle.* Philadelphia: JB Lippincott.)

but it is not known if the spur initiates the injury or results from inflammation and fibrosis. A complicating factor can be the occurrence of plantar nerve entrapment from edema and inflammation.

Plantar fasciitis can be resistant to recovery, with patients experiencing pain from this condition for months to years. Injection of steroids, ice application, strapping, and rest all are used with variable success. Orthotics may be helpful for the runner. Rarely is surgery required, and it is typical for a patient to suddenly notice that the pain has disappeared without any treatment at all. The primary care provider will encounter this chronic inflammatory musculoskeletal condition often in practice.

## Carpal Tunnel Syndrome

Carpal tunnel syndrome is an excellent model of a musculoskeletal injury that may be caused by repetitive trauma. It is the most common entrap-

ment injury seen in primary care practices. It has a higher incidence in middle-aged women and in persons with obesity, hypothyroidism, pregnancy, and certain autoimmune conditions. Computer operators, secretaries, athletes, gardeners, and any individual who repetitively flexes and extends the wrist is at risk. The median nerve becomes entrapped between the flexor tendons and median carpal ligament because of inflammatory tendinitis. This entrapment of the median nerve affects the conduction velocity and leads to pain—particularly at night, which awakens the patient—and paresthesias of the thumb, index, and middle finger. Motor deficits also may occur, leading to atrophy and weakness in the hand muscles. Tapping of the median nerve at the wrist causes a positive Tinel's sign (pain or tingling in the index and middle finger) or a positive Phenal's sign, which is an increased severity of numbness when the hand is flexed. The disorder is seen most commonly in middle-aged women.

Carpal tunnel syndrome often is treated successfully by the primary care provider, thus avoiding surgery. Weight loss, treatment of underlying disorders, avoidance of the repetitive activity that has caused or aggravated the condition, and splinting of the wrist all are useful approaches. Treatment of pain with NSAIDs and a daily dose of vitamin B$_6$ are suggested pharmacologic approaches.

## REFERENCES

Alarcon, G. & Bradley, L. (1998). Advances in the treatment of fibromyalgia: Current status and future directions. *The American Journal of the Medical Sciences, 315* (6), 397–404.

Auleciems, L. (1995). Myofascial pain syndrome: A multidisciplinary approach. *Nurse Practitioner, 20* (4), 18–31.

Bennet, R. (1997a). The concurrence of lupus and fibromyalgia: Implications for diagnosis and management. *Lupus, 6,* 494–499.

Bennet, R. (1997b). The fibromyalgia syndrome. In W. Kelley, E. Harris, S. Ruddy, & C. Sledge (Eds.), *Textbook of rheumatology* (vol. 1, 5th ed.). Philadelphia: W.B. Saunders Company.

Buskila, D., Shnaider, A., Neumann, L., Ziblerman, D., Hilzenrat, N., & Sikuler, E. (1997). Fibromyalgia in hepatitis C virus infection. *Archives of Internal Medicine, 157* (24), 2497–2500.

Campbell, S., Clark, S., Tindall, E., Forehand, M., & Bennett, R. (1983). Clinical characteristics of fibrositis. *Arthritis and Rheumatism, 26* (7), 817–824.

Chao, C., Janoff, E., Hu, S., et al. (1990). Altered cytokine release in peripheral blood mononuclear cell cultures from patients with the chronic fatigue syndrome. *Cytokine, 3,* 292–298.

Cleare, A.J., Heap, E., Malhi, G.S., Wessely, S., O'Keane, V., & Miell, J. (1999). Low-dose hydrocortisone in chronic fatigue syndrome: A randomised crossover trial. *Lancet, 353* (9151), 455–458.

Cooper, P. (1997). Current concepts on the management of heel pain. *Medscape Orthopaedics and Sports Medicine, 1* (10). www.medscape.com.

Corrigan, B. & Maitlan, G.D. (1998). *Vertebral musculoskeletal disorders.* Oxford: Butterworth Heinemann.

Crofford, L. (1998). Neuroendocrine abnormalities in fibromyalgia and related disorders. *The American Journal of the Medical Sciences, 315* (6), 359–366.

Enestrom, S., Bengtsson, A., & Frodin, T. (1997). Dermal IgG deposits and increase of mast cells in patients with fibromyalgia: Relevant findings or epiphenomena? *Scandinavian Journal of Rheumatology, 26,* 308–313.

Feiffenberger, D. & Amundson, L. (1996). Fibromyalgia syndrome: A review. *American Family Physician, 53* (5), 1698–1704.

Fekety, R. (1994). Infection and chronic fatigue syndrome. In S. Straus (Ed.), *Chronic fatigue syndrome.* New York: Marcel Dekker.

Goldenberg, D. (1997). Fibromyalgia, chronic fatigue syndrome, and myofascial pain syndrome. *Current Opinion in Rheumatology, 9,* 135–143.

Goldenberg, D., Mayskiy, M., Mossey, C., Ruthazer, R., & Schmid, C. (1996). A randomized, double-blind crossover trial of fluoxetine and amitriptyline in the treatment of fibromyalgia. *Arthritis and Rheumatism, 39* (11), 1852–1859.

Gore, D. (1998). The epidemiology of neck pain. *Medscape Orthopaedics and Sports Medicine, 2* (5). www.medscape.com

Hinton, R. (1995). Backache. In M. Samuels (Ed.), *Manual of neurological therapeutics.* In *MAXX: Maximum access to diagnosis and therapy: The electronic library of medicine* [CD-ROM]. Philadelphia: Lippincott-Raven Publishers.

Jenny, A.B. & Ketcherside, W.J. (1994). Neurosurgical emergencies In R.J. Stine, C.R. Chudnofsky, & C.K. Aaron (Eds.), *A practical approach to emergency medicine.* In *MAXX: Maximum access to diagnosis and therapy: The electronic library of medicine* [CD-ROM]. Philadelphia: Lippincott-Raven Publishers.

Kang, J.D., Georgescu, H.I., McIntyre-Larkin, L., Stefanovic-Racic, M., Donaldson, W.F., III, & Evans, C.H. (1996). Herniated lumbar intervertebral discs spontaneously produce matrix metalloproteinases, nitric oxide, interleukin-6, and prostaglandin $E_2$. *Spine, 21* (3), 271–277.

Kennedy, M. & Felson, D. (1996). A prospective long-term study of fibromyalgia syndrome. *Arthritis and Rheumatism, 39* (4), 682–685.

Klein, R. & Berg, P. (1995). High incidence of antibodies to 5-hydroxytryptamine, gangliosides and phospholipids in patients with chronic fatigue and fibromyalgia syndrome and their relatives: Evidence for a clinical entity of both disorders. *European Journal of Medical Research, 1,* 21–26.

Komaroff, A.L. (1994). Clinical presentation and evaluation of fatigue and chronic fatigue syndrome. In S. Straus (Ed.), *Chronic fatigue syndrome.* New York: Marcel Dekker.

Lapossy, E., Gasser, P., Hrycaj, P., Dubler, B., Samborski, W., & Muller, W. (1994). Cold-induced vasospasm in patients with fibromyalgia and chronic low back pain in comparison to healthy subjects. *Clinical Rheumatology, 13* (3), 442–445.

Lario, B., Valdivielso, J., Lopez, J., Soteres, C., Banuelos, J., & Cabello, A. (1996). Fibromyalgia syndrome: Overnight falls in arterial oxygen saturation. *American Journal of Medicine, 101,* 54–60.

Mense, S. (1990). Psychology of nociception in muscles. In J. Fricton & E. Awad (Eds.), *Advances in pain research and therapy. Vol. 17: Myofascial pain and fibromyalgia.* New York: Raven Press.

Mountz, J., Bradley, L., & Alarcon, G. (1998). Abnormal functional activity of the central nervous system in fibromyalgia syndrome. *The American Journal of the Medical Sciences, 315* (6), 377–384.

Nicolodi, M., Volpe, A., & Sicuteri, F. (1998). Fibromyalgia and headache: Failure of serotonergic analgesia and N-methyl-D-aspartate–mediated neuronal placidity. Their common clues. *Cephalgia, 18* (Suppl. 21), 41–44.

Olsen, N. & Park, J. (1998). Skeletal muscle abnormalities in patients with fibromyalgia. *The American Journal of the Medical Sciences, 315* (6), 377–384.

Press, J., Phillip, M., Neumann, L., Barak, R., Segev, Y., Abu-Shakra, M., & Buskila, D. (1998). *The Journal of Rheumatology, 25* (3), 551–555.

Rakel, R. (1996). *Saunders' manual of medical practice.* Philadelphia: W.B. Saunders Company.

Russell, I. (1998). Advances in fibromyalgia: Possible role for central neurochemicals. *The American Journal of the Medical Sciences, 315* (6), 377–384.

Sambrook, P.N., MacGregor, A.J., & Spector, T.D. (1999). Genetic influences on cervical and lumbar disc degeneration: A magnetic resonance imaging study in twins. *Arthritis and Rheumatism, 42* (2), 366–372.

Scott, L.V., Teh, J., Reznek, R., Martin, A., Sohaib, A., & Dinan, T.G. (1999). Small adrenal glands in chronic fatigue syndrome: A preliminary computer tomography study. *Psychoneuroendocrinology, 24* (7), 759–768.

Sprott, H., Muller, A., & Heine, H. (1997). Collagen crosslinks in fibromyalgia. *Arthritis and Rheumatism, 40* (8), 1450–1454.

Strober, W. (1994). Immunological function in chronic fatigue syndrome. In S. Strauss (Ed.), *Chronic fatigue syndrome.* New York: Marcel Decker.

United States Pharmacopeial Convention (USP DI). (1998). United States pharmacopeial convention drug information. Vol. 1. In *MAXX: Maximum access to diagnosis and therapy: The electronic library of medicine,* [CD-ROM]. Philadelphia: Lippincott-Raven Publishers.

Walker, E., Keegan, D., Gardner, G., Sullivan, M., Bernstein, D., & Katon, W. (1997). Psychosocial factors in fibromyalgia compared with rheumatoid arthritis: II. Sexual, physical, and emotional abuse and neglect. *Psychosomatic Medicine, 59,* 572–577.

Wessely, S., Hotopf, M., & Sharpe, M. (1998). *Chronic fatigue and its syndromes.* Oxford: Oxford University Press.

Wolfe, F., Ross, K., Anderson, J., Russell, I., & Herbert, L. (1995). The prevalence and characteristics of fibromyalgia in the general population. *Arthritis and Rheumatism, 38*(1), 19–28.

Wolfe, F., Smythe, H., Yunus, M., Bennet, R., Bombardier, C., et al. (1990). The American College of Rheumatology 1990 criteria for the classification of fibromyalgia. *Arthritis and Rheumatism, 33* (2), 160–172.

Yunus, M. (1994). Fibromyalgia syndrome and myofascial pain syndrome: Clinical features, laboratory tests, diagnosis, and pathophysiologic mechanisms. In E. Rachlin (Ed.), *Myofascial pain and fibromyalgia.* St. Louis: Mosby-Year Book.

# Common Hematologic Disorders

Maureen Groer

This chapter describes the most common hematologic disorders seen in the primary care practice. Included are the more common anemias and acute infectious mononucleosis. Because it is routine practice to do a blood screening as part of the physical examination, hematologic abnormalities often are discovered when these results are reviewed by the provider. For example, iron deficiency anemia may manifest as an unanticipated decrease in hemoglobin or hematocrit values. Leukocyte and platelet disorders may show up in the same way, through routine blood screening. At other times, illnesses are symptomatic, and the astute practitioner needs to diagnose the patient based on history and results of the physical examination and blood tests. An example of the latter scenario is acute infectious mononucleosis. This chapter begins with a discussion of the most common hematologic abnormality, iron deficiency anemia.

## IRON DEFICIENCY ANEMIA

There are 20 million individuals with iron deficiency anemia in the United States alone. Depletion of iron reserves, which is a precursor to the development of anemia, may be present in more than a third of apparently healthy menstruating or childbearing women. Iron deficiency anemia is the most common anemia worldwide and in the US. The prevalence, approaching 50% in some groups, is higher is lower socioeconomic status groups, menstruating women, and pregnant and lactating women, and in children younger than 2 years of age. The primary care provider usually will discover anemia during routine examinations because people often are not symptomatic if the anemia has developed slowly. Fatigue, shortness of breath, palpitations, bounding pulse, lack of endurance, widened pulse pressure, systolic ejection murmur, and light-headedness are common signs and symptoms.

This type of anemia develops because an inadequate amount of iron is available for normal erythropoiesis. Hemoglobin synthesis in erythrocytes requires iron, which is delivered to the bone marrow from either dietary sources or body iron reserves. An important aspect of this disease is the recognition that anemia usually results when the body stores of iron are depleted. Dietary sources of iron are meats, eggs, and some vegetables. Little bioavailable iron is present in grains, which, for many populations, are the staples of their diets. Thus, a half a billion people in the world have iron deficiency anemia.

## Iron Transport and Metabolism

Dietary iron is present in several molecular forms, which influences the ability of the gastrointestinal tract to absorb iron. The most absorbable form is heme iron, which is derived from animal sources. Heme then is enzymatically broken down in the duodenal cells into iron, which is attached to the transporter molecule *transferrin*. Trivalent ($Fe^{3+}$) and divalent ($Fe^{2+}$) forms of iron, present in plant foods, require an acid gastric environment to become solubilized for entry into intestinal luminal cells. Transferrin binds iron in the gastrointestinal tract and then circulates in the blood, delivering iron where it is needed (Fig. 20-1). The amount of iron absorbed is regulated by the amount of iron stores, the rate of erythropoiesis,

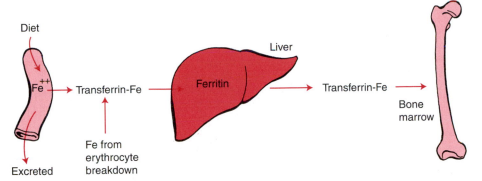

**FIGURE 20.1** ● Iron transport and storage.

the concentration and type of iron in the diet, and dietary factors that enhance or inhibit iron absorption. The latter includes intake of vitamin C, which increases iron absorption, and inhibitors, including calcium, phytates, tannins, and polyphenols (*Morbidity and Mortality Weekly Report* [MMWR], 1998).

Transferrin first binds to erythroid precursor cell receptors and then is phagocytosed. Inside the cells, the high acidity of the phagolysosome causes the iron to dissociate from transferrin. The iron then is transported to mitochondria, where it is enzymatically inserted into the protoporphyrin molecule. Synthesis of globin is determined partly by the concentration of heme synthesized in the cell. Because erythroid precursor cells have transferrin receptors, iron is delivered at the appropriate point in erythropoiesis. Erythropoietin stimulates this process markedly.

Transferrin also brings iron to storage sites if it is not needed for erythropoiesis or other cellular functions. Iron in the storage pool is mostly in the form of ferritin, a water-soluble molecule found in highest concentration in the liver. Men have about 1000 mg of iron stored in the liver, which is available when necessary, whereas women have about 600 mg. When iron either is lost in excess or is taken in inadequate amounts in the diet, the stored iron is transferred by transferrin to the bone marrow. Depletion of iron stores occurs before iron deficiency anemia develops. Another source of iron is through breakdown of erythrocytes by the reticuloendothelial system (RES). About one fifth of the iron in erythrocyte hemoglobin is recirculated to bone marrow for hemoglobin synthesis. This form of iron is the major pool of iron used in erythropoiesis. The phagocytic cells of the RES release the iron from degraded hemoglobin, then transferrin carries it to either the bone marrow or liver stores.

## CAUSES OF IRON DEFICIENCY

### Excessive Loss of Iron Over Intake

The dietary intake of iron in the normal American adult is about 15 to 18 mg/day, and only about 10% of that amount normally is absorbed (Ungaro, 1999). Men are able to store more iron than women, and thus women are more likely to develop iron deficiency anemia. The major storage form is ferritin, although a small amount is stored as hemosiderin. A measure of stored iron is the serum ferritin levels. A serum ferritin level of less than 12 μg/L indicates that no iron is stored, and levels above 15 μg/L still may not be sufficient to meet erythropoietic demand (Cavill, 1999).

### Developmental Considerations

Normal losses of iron (1 mg/day) include losses through stool, skin, and mucosal cells, which are shed from the surfaces of epithelia and have a life span of only 3 to 4 days. Menstruating women lose, on the average, 0.3 to 0.5 mg/day, and during pregnancy, the maternal iron lost to fetal growth is 3 mg/day (Bothwell & Charlton, 1981). Childhood is another time when iron demands often exceed iron stores. About 9% of children aged 1 to 3 years are iron deficient, with 3% having iron deficiency anemia (MMWR, 1998). During childhood, diet is the major factor responsible for iron deficiency. Cow's milk has less bioavailable iron than breast milk, and early introduction of cow's milk may lead to anemia. Cow's milk also causes an enteropathy in very young children's intestines that can lead to impairment of iron absorption and even blood loss. Adolescents are another group at risk for inadequate iron stores and anemia. This results from increased iron needs for growth and menstruation and poor diet with inadequate iron intake. All of these risk groups benefit from iron supplementation of their diets.

## Blood Loss

Chronic blood loss is the largest cause of iron deficiency anemia in adults. The leading cause of gastrointestinal bleeding across the world is parasitic infestation (hookworm, whipworm). Anatomic abnormalities such as Meckel's diverticulum and colonic arteriovenous malformations are other causes. Gastritis, peptic ulcer disease, and inflammatory bowel disease produce erosive, bleeding lesions that can result in iron deficiency. Any adult with occult or frank blood in the stool must also be evaluated for bowel malignancy.

## Chronic Illness

Anemia occurs more frequently in people who have a variety of chronic diseases. The anemia of chronic illness is related to general debilitation, poor nutrition, and competition for nutrients in the bone marrow. Shortened erythrocyte life span, decreased bioavailability of iron, and decreased bone marrow function are etiologic factors in this type of anemia. The anemias of chronic illness tend to be normocytic and reticulocytopenic. Anemia is a common finding in patients with cancer, chronic infections such as tuberculosis, and chronic inflammatory conditions such as rheumatoid arthritis. Unexplained anemia in a patient with no evidence of blood loss is a sign of potential underlying chronic disease or infection.

## Symptoms

Symptoms of iron deficiency anemia generally do not appear until the hemoglobin value falls below 10 mg/dL. If anemia develops rapidly because of blood loss, the symptoms are different than in the chronically anemic patient. Elderly patients often manifest the illness differently, with an increased incidence of angina pectoris, for example. Younger patients often are asymptomatic with mild anemia. However, all patients exhibit symptoms on exertion when the hemoglobin level is less that 7 mg/dL. Symptoms include shortness of breath, light-headedness, fatigue, weakness, palpitations, dizziness, tinnitus, irritability, and difficulty sleeping. Patients may notice a bounding pulse, and the pulse pressure may be widened from peripheral vasodilation. A systolic ejection murmur also is common. All of these symptoms are related to tissues hypoxemia. The patient may appear pale, and a common technique to quickly assess the possibility of anemia is to note if the conjunctiva or creases of the hands appear paler than normal.

In severe and chronic anemia, epithelia are disrupted and patients have stomatitis and glossitis. The tongue may appear swollen, smooth, and shiny. Fingernails may be so soft that they develop concave spooning (*koilonychia*). These symptoms are rare in the United States but are commonly seen in third world countries.

An unusual but common symptom in iron deficiency anemia is pica. Pica is a craving for non-food substances such as laundry starch, clay, dirt, and ice. Pica is a cultural expectation in certain parts of the southern United States, particularly during pregnancy. No reason for pica is known, although one explanation is that the individual is seeking sources of iron to alleviate the anemia. However, many of the substances that people ingest bind dietary iron and actually decrease its absorption. Another type of pica that has relevance is the ingestion of chips of lead paint from peeling walls. In this type of pica, seen in infants and small children, lead-based paint enters the system and competes with iron for absorption through the gastrointestinal tract. Iron is inadequately absorbed, and lead then deposits in hematopoietic tissues and directly impairs erythropoiesis by inhibiting enzyme systems involved in heme production. Children with elevated lead levels are seen in every socioeconomic group, and a common early finding is iron deficiency anemia.

Chronic iron deficiency anemia is believed to adversely influence the growth and development of children. Depriving young experimental animals of iron causes irreversible changes in behavior and brain neurotransmitters (Walter, 1994). In human infants, a variety of cognitive, psychomotor, behavioral, and balance abnormalities occur with iron deficiency. Some studies indicate that reversal of the anemia ameliorates the neurologic and developmental effects, whereas other studies dispute this finding. When a child develops iron deficiency anemia, there is an increased likelihood that other nutritional and environmental deficiencies are present, so it may not be possible to determine the true etiology of the developmental delays (MMWR, 1998). There is evidence that irreversible changes in cognitive performance, persisting through the school-aged years, may occur in infants who had severe iron deficiency anemia (Walter, 1994).

Iron deficiency anemia during pregnancy has adverse effects on the developing fetus. Iron depletion occurs in most pregnant women who are not taking dietary supplementation, and guidelines for prevention of anemia universally recommend that pregnant mothers take supplemental iron. Severe anemia is associated with an increased incidence of preterm birth, low birth weight, and perinatal complications in iron-deficient mothers.

## Hematologic Effects of Iron Deficiency

As iron stores become depleted, erythropoiesis becomes increasingly disturbed. An increase occurs in the concentration of erythrocyte protoporphyrin, a precursor to hemoglobin. The red blood cells initially are normocytic, but as the deficiency continues, they become microcytic and hypochromic. This causes a decrease in the blood of both the hemoglobin concentration (less than 13 g/dL for men; less than 12 g/dL for menstruating women; less than 11 g/dL for pregnant women) and the hematocrit. The range of erythrocyte size, measured by the red cell distribution width (RDW), is wide and is important in making the diagnosis. The reticulocyte count is another indicator, with reticulocytopenia usually being present. The reticulocyte count is a measure of bone marrow function, with an increase indicating a stimulation of erythropoiesis resulting from acute blood loss, for example. A decreased count, as is found in iron deficiency anemia, indicates depressed erythropoiesis.

The erythrocytes formed in the iron deficient bone marrow are small and pale and have a variety of shapes (poikilocytic). The cells have decreased membrane fluidity, which makes them more likely to hemolyze. Thus, the anemia is compounded by an ongoing hemolysis.

## Clinical Tests for Iron Deficiency Anemia

Whereas hemoglobin and hematocrit are excellent and easy screening tests, the best laboratory indicator of iron deficiency anemia is low serum ferritin level, with a level of 10 ng/dL or lower indicating anemia. For every microgram per liter of serum ferritin, approximately 10 mg of iron is stored in the liver and other sites. Serum ferritin is therefore an index of body stores of iron. Another parameter is the total iron binding capacity, which is increased but has a decreased saturation. This is because the level of transferrin, the molecule that transports iron, is increased, but the quantity of iron it holds is markedly decreased. Serum iron levels also are decreased. A newer indicator, which seems to be an accurate diagnostic test for iron deficiency anemia, is a high concentration of the serum transferrin receptor. The mean cell volume (MCV) also is a useful indicator, since it is a parameter of cell size and generally is decreased in iron deficiency anemia. However, a decreased MCV also is observed in other types of anemia. As mentioned previously, the RDW indicates variability in cell size, which is a common finding in iron deficiency.

Several considerations are important when the primary care provider is making the diagnosis of iron deficiency anemia. One is race, since blacks have, on average, slightly lower hemoglobin and hematocrit levels. Asians, whites, and Native Americans have similar values (MMWR, 1998). Another consideration is altitude and cigarette smoking, since both of these factors shift physiologic adaptations to chronically decreased oxygen concentrations. Therefore, the baseline values are higher in these individuals, and adjustments need to be made before diagnoses can be accurate.

## Physiologic Basis of Treatment

The physiologic basis for treatment is to restore the body reserves of iron and to make an adequate amount of iron available for normal erythropoiesis. The cause of the anemia must be determined and addressed. In most cases, the treatment of choice is oral iron supplementation in the form of ferrous sulfate, 300 mg, three times per day with meals. Although most patients tolerate this approach, the gastrointestinal irritation caused by oral iron supplements may be disturbing enough to require the use of enteric tablets or parenteral iron administration. Patients should be advised to take iron supplements with meals if the gastrointestinal symptoms are severe but to be cautious about foods that could bind iron (eg, bran, tea). In addition, using antacids should be discouraged because reducing the gastric acidity decreases total iron absorption. Taking additional vitamin C with the iron tablets assists in iron absorption. The response to iron therapy should be an observable reticulocytosis by the 10th day of treatment. The hemoglobin concentration should rise to normal levels within 6 to 8 weeks, but iron stores remain depleted. Therefore, an additional 4 to 6 months of iron therapy usually is necessary (Ungaro, 1999).

The primary care provider should consider primary prevention as a strategy to reduce the incidence of iron deficiency anemia in at-risk patients. For children younger than 2 years of age, the parents should be advised about the dietary sources of iron for their child. For pregnant women, iron supplementation is routine. Another important approach is screening at-risk populations (low-income children, adolescent girls, nonpregnant menstruating females) for hemoglobin and hematocrit levels.

## MEGALOBLASTIC ANEMIA

Another common anemia seen in the primary care practice is megaloblastic anemia, which mostly results from atrophic gastritis in the elderly. Vitamin $B_{12}$ or folic acid deficiency in the diet and pancreatic disease may also lead to megaloblastic anemia. The elderly have the greatest risk for developing atrophic gastritis, which leads to decreased parietal cell function in the stomach. About 5% of people older than 65 years develop vitamin $B_{12}$ deficiency leading to anemia. In the United States, it is rare to see patients who have developed pernicious anemia because of dietary deficiency, although this occurs in extremely malnourished people, and pregnant women and alcoholics have a greater risk. Pernicious anemia is a disease in which an autoimmune process causes decreased vitamin $B_{12}$ absorption. There also is an increased familial risk for pernicious anemia. Pernicious anemia develops through a chronic autoimmune process in which autoantibodies form to both intrinsic factor and the parietal cell binding site for vitamin $B_{12}$. The autoimmune reaction causes complement fixation and inflammation of the parietal cells, and over years, the parietal cell mass atrophies. This then leads to both achlorhydria and lack of intrinsic factor in gastric juice. Intrinsic factor normally binds to dietary vitamin $B_{12}$; in its absence, vitamin $B_{12}$ is not adequately absorbed. Normally, intrinsic factors binds vitamin $B_{12}$ within the stomach, and then the complex is absorbed into the bloodstream through the brush border of the ileum. The binding with intrinsic factor alters the stereochemistry of the vitamin molecule, protecting it from attack by digestive enzymes. Without absorption of vitamin $B_{12}$ into the blood, neurologic symptoms occur, as well as a megaloblastic, reticulocytopenic anemia. The patient may seek care because of proprioceptive, cognitive, polyneuropathic, and balance problems and then is discovered to have pernicious anemia.

Deficiency of vitamin $B_{12}$ affects the final maturation of erythrocytes in the bone marrow. Both vitamin $B_{12}$ and folic acid are required for DNA synthesis, and decreased amounts of these substances results in an overproduction of RNA compared with DNA synthesis. This affects cells throughout the body, but the symptomatic effects are hematologic. Both white cells and erythrocytes show abnormalities, with multilobulated neutrophils commonly being observed. As red blood cells develop in the bone marrow, they go through the erythroblast stage before becoming reticulocytes. Maturation thus is halted at this stage, and the cells that form are large, oval, irregularly shaped, immature macrocytic cells. The membranes of these cells are osmotically fragile, and the cells do not stack readily because they are not biconcave discs. The hemoglobin in these cells can bind oxygen, but the cells lyse easily, so the patient develops anemia. Although vitamin $B_{12}$ is a water-soluble vitamin, the body does have large stores in the liver and kidney, and up to 5 years of deficient dietary absorption usually occur before the symptoms manifest themselves.

### Symptoms

Vitamin $B_{12}$ plays many roles in the body. It is necessary for myelin formation, gastrointestinal digestive and absorptive functions, fertility, and DNA and protein synthesis in all cells. The patient with pernicious anemia often presents first with

---

### *CLINICAL VIGNETTE 20.1*

Rose Howell is a 66-year-old widow who has come to the clinic with the chief complaint of fatigue. Her previous history includes peptic ulcer disease, mild osteoporosis, hypercholesterolemia, and hypertension. She has noticed increasing fatigue over the last month and reports becoming short of breath when she walks more than the length of a room or when going up stairs at her home. Her blood pressure and cholesterol levels are well controlled by medication. She has a good appetite and has not experienced weight loss or gain. She has noted that her stools are darker than normal. She has had some mild, intermittent abdominal pain, flatulence, and loose stools. Her skin and mucosa are pale, and she is tachycardic at 100, with a respiratory rate of 22. Her complete blood count is as follows: white blood cells, 5000; hemoglobin, 8 g/dL; hematocrit, 26%; and mean corpuscular volume, 78 fL

A stool for guiac is positive, and her stool is black. She is referred for colonoscopy, which shows colorectal carcinoma, Dukes stage C. Her microcytic anemia is iron deficiency anemia from gastrointestinal blood loss.

neurologic symptoms, since the anemia develops so slowly and the patient adjusts to the chronic hypoxia produced by this anemia. In addition, some patients with vitamin $B_{12}$ deficiency may have severe neuropsychiatric symptoms but are not anemic. The diagnosis is made based on the peripheral blood smear, which shows the typical macrocytic red blood cells and multilobulated neutrophils characteristic of this disease. The hemoglobin concentration is decreased, but the hematocrit may not show a proportional decrease because of the large oval cells, which occupy more space than biconcave discs. The mean corpuscular volume is increased markedly, and there is a reticulocytopenia because pernicious anemia is a maturation disease and the bone marrow is unable to produce normal reticulocytes. Early in the disease, the MCV may not be elevated because of the coexisting microcytic anemia. Red blood cell vitamin $B_{12}$ levels are low. The Schilling test is used to determine the cause of the vitamin $B_{12}$ deficiency. Radiolabeled vitamin $B_{12}$ absorption through the gastrointestinal tract can be determined with this test.

### Physiologic Basis of Treatment

Fortunately, pernicious anemia is a treatable illness in that vitamin $B_{12}$ can be given by intramuscular injection every 30 to 90 days. This needs to be done for the rest of the person's life. The clinician should be cautioned about administering folic acid to anemic patients without checking the vitamin $B_{12}$ levels, since folic acid can cause excessive utilization of vitamin $B_{12}$ stores. The vitamin $B_{12}$–deficient person can become seriously depleted and have severe neurologic effects when given additional folic acid.

## INFECTIOUS MONONUCLEOSIS

Infectious mononucleosis ("mono") is a common viral illness frequently diagnosed and managed by the primary care provider. Although first recognized in 1920, its etiology was not confirmed until 1968 (Hickey & Strasburger, 1997). The case frequency in the United States is about 45 to 50 cases per 100,000 population, with the highest frequency in the adolescent population. The two herpesviruses known to cause mono are the Epstein-Barr virus (EBV) and the cytomegalovirus (CMV). EBV causes most of the cases, and most persons have measurable antibodies to EBV by adulthood, indicating an infection at some point. Herpesviruses have the property of latency, so

once a person is infected, the virus remains latent and under surveillance by the immune system for the remainder of the person's life. The EBV is continuously replicated by the oral epithelial cells after the initial infection and by spreading the virus to B cells in the lymphoid tissues of the oropharynx. However, reactivation of EBV infection is rare unless a person becomes seriously immunosuppressed, as occurs in HIV disease. A recurrence of mono is not believed to be possible.

EBV infects several key cells, including cells of oropharyngeal epithelium, the cervix, and B lymphocytes. It is therefore found in high concentration in the saliva of an infected person, but many of its symptoms are largely related to the ensuing hematologic infection and the immune response that it evokes. The virus usually is spread through direct contact with infected saliva, so in popular parlance, mono has been called the "kissing disease." The person is infectious for a several days before symptoms appear and throughout the course of the infection. After exposure, the incubation period is 30 to 50 days.

### Pathogenesis

Once the EBV enters the oral cavity, it infects and replicates within the epithelial lining cells of the oropharynx and salivary ducts. From there, the virus spreads extensively through the lymphoreticular system because it specifically invades B lymphocytes (Fig. 20-2). EBV attaches to B lymphocytes at the CD21 marker and enters the cells, but does not result in excessive viral proliferation and cell killing in these cells as it does in the epithelial cells (Foerster, 1999). The B cells carry live virus throughout the lymphoid system and into the circulation. Once infected, B cells become activated plasma cells and secrete immunoglobulins to viral antigens and autoantibodies. The viral infection appears to "immortalize" these cells so that they are present for life. They also stimulate an extensive T-cell response, with proliferation of cytotoxic CD8 and natural killer cells. These cells are found in the blood of an infected person and are pleomorphic atypical lymphocytes, called Downy cells, which are characteristic of the disease. The presence of these cells is a positive sign because it is their function to hold the EBV cellular viral infection in check. These cells account for the widespread lymphadenopathy, splenomegaly, and hepatomegaly that occur in mono.

The disease is associated with a pattern of immune responses, which can be used as the basis for diagnosing the disease. The infected B cells initially secrete antibodies of the IgM class, but

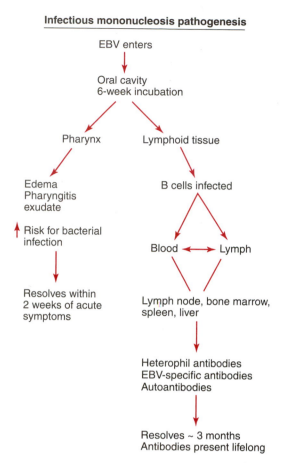

**Infectious mononucleosis pathogenesis**

**FIGURE 20.2**  •  Stages of infection in infectious mononucleosis.

nuclear antigen is confirmed. This antibody peaks 8 weeks after the onset of illness.

## Signs and Symptoms

There are three classifications of infectious mononucleosis (Hickey & Strasburger, 1997). *Anginose* mononucleosis is the most classic presentation in which the patient has the triad of fever, exudative tonsillopharyngitis with pharyngeal edema, and lymphadenopathy. *Typhoidal* mononucleosis is associated with prolonged high fever, little pharyngitis, and delayed onset of lymphadenopathy. *Glandular* mononucleosis is associated with a disproportionate enlargement of the lymph nodes compared with the degree of fever and pharyngitis. The major signs and symptoms of mono, which are present in most patients during the first week of infection, are a fever, pharyngitis, and lymphadenopathy. Many other signs and symptoms appear within a particular time course, such as fatigue, malaise, sweats, dysphagia, anorexia, nausea, headache, eyelid edema, palatal exanthema, hives, bradycardia, cough, liver or spleen enlargement and tenderness, and ocular muscle pain (Finch, 1969). The lymphadenopathy is seen early in the disease, peaking at 7 to 14 days, is bilateral, and involves both anterior and posterior bilateral chains, with occasional involvement of axillary and inguinal nodes. Hepatomegaly is present in half of the cases, with abnormal liver enzymes commonly seen. Splenomegaly is at highest incidence during the second and third week of illness, and splenic rupture is the most devastating complication of acute mononucleosis. The clinician should be cautioned about the danger of splenic palpation in these patients (Magnussen & Dolin, 1999). The spleen can enlarge tremendously and becomes friable and tender. Rupture of the spleen is rare (about 1.5/1000 cases) but can be fatal if not recognized. Another serious complication is upper airway obstruction from pharyngitis. Rarely, also, patients with mononucleosis can develop a hemolytic anemia.

The patient usually presents with a sore throat and adenopathy, and the results of streptococcal culture tests often are positive. The astute clinician should therefore understand that mononucleosis can coexist with streptococcal pharyngitis (Foerster, 1999). Laboratory tests show a leukocytosis, with an increase in the lymphocyte count to 60% of the differential. Ten percent or more of the peripheral lymphocytes are atypical. The diagnosis is made with antibody tests, most frequently, the heterophil antibody test. Heterophil antibodies are present in up to 70% of patients during the first

later switch to producing IgGs. Some of the antibodies are not specific to EBV. For example, the heterophil antibody, an early appearing IgM, agglutinates sheep erythrocytes, and its presence is tested by the mono "spot" test and by measuring blood titers. A titer of 1:256 or higher is diagnostic of acute infectious mononucleosis (Foerster, 1999). The heterophil antibody rises to its peak in the second to third week of the illness. The IgGs begin to appear around the time the heterophil is waning. Some of these are specific immunoglobulins to components of the EBV, whereas others are autoreactive antibodies against several different self-antigens. The polyclonal activation of B cells through EBV infection is believed to cause this nonspecific immune response, and these antibodies rarely cause pathophysiologic effects in infected patients. The patient with mononucleosis has a general increase in serum globulin levels. In some cases, the diagnosis of mono is not made until the presence of late-appearing IgGs to EBV

---

### CLINICAL VIGNETTE 20.2

Heather Brown is a 19-year-old college student who comes to the primary care provider because she has had a sore throat and swollen glands for about 10 days. She also complains of extreme fatigue, anorexia, and a constant headache. Her physical examination shows a temperature of 100°F, moderate anterior and posterior cervical lymphadenopathy, 3+ exudative tonsillitis, a slightly enlarged liver by palpation, and an enlarged spleen as determined by percussion. She reports exposure to mononucleosis, since her boyfriend was diagnosed about 6 weeks ago. Her throat culture is positive for β-hemolytic streptococcus. Her mononucleosis spot test is positive. She is treated with antibiotics, activity restriction, rest, and acetaminophen for fever and malaise. Note that many patients with mononucleosis develop a rash when given ampicillin, so other antibiotics are preferred.

---

week and in up to 90% after 3 months, and often stay positive for a year after the initial infection. Heterophil-negative cases of mononucleosis are related to other etiologic agents such as CMV. Other antibody titers may be measured in patients with mononucleosis and are related to early, late, or latent EBV antigens.

### Physiologic Basis of Treatment

The care of the patient with infectious mononucleosis is supportive and symptomatic. Controlling fever and pain, rest, good nutritional support, hydration, and preventing complications such as splenic rupture are the mainstay of care once the diagnosis is made. Some patients may require acyclovir or corticosteroid therapy if there is immi-

nent danger of airway obstruction (Hickey & Strasburger, 1997). Splenic rupture can be avoided by using laxatives and limiting activity. Controlling the spread of infection is another important aspect of care. Patients are infectious for several weeks after onset of symptoms and may be infectious for months, since the virus can be isolated from saliva for up to 1 year after infection.

Patients at risk for mono are students living in dormitories and young people in military service. Evidence shows that stress increases the risk of infection in those exposed, so recommending adequate rest and stress management are excellent approaches in this age group.

### REFERENCES

Bothwell, T.H. & Charlton, R.W. (1981). *Iron deficiency in women.* Washington, DC: The Nutrition Foundation.

Cavill, I. (1999). Iron status as measured by serum ferritin: The marker and its limitations. *American Journal of Kidney Diseases, 34* (4 Suppl 2), S12–S17.

Foerster, J. (1999). Infectious mononucleosis. In G.R. Lee, J. Foerster, J. Lukens, F. Paraskevas, J. Greer, & G. Rodgers (Eds.), *Wintrobes' clinical hematology.* Baltimore: Williams & Wilkins.

Hickey, S.M. & Strasburger, V.C. (1997). What every pediatrician should know about infectious mononucleosis in adolescents. *Pediatric Clinics of North America, 44* (6), 541–556.

Magnussen, C.R. & Dolin, R. (1999). Infectious mononucleosis and mononucleosis-like syndromes. In R. Reese, & R. Betts (Eds.), *A practical approach to infectious diseases.* In: *MAXX: Maximum access to diagnosis and therapy: The electronic library of medicine* [CD-ROM]. Philadelphia: Lippincott Williams & Wilkins.

Recommendations to Prevent and Control Iron Deficiency in the United States. (1998). *Morbidity and Mortality Weekly Report, Centers for Disease Control and Prevention, 47* (RR-3), 1–29.

Ungaro, P. (1999). Anemia. In L. Dornbrand, A. Hoole, & R. Fletcher (Eds.), *Manual of clinical problems in ambulatory care* (3rd ed.). In: *MAXX: Maximum access to diagnosis and therapy: The electronic library of medicine* [CD-ROM]. Philadelphia: Lippincott Williams and & Wilkins.

Walter, T. (1994). Effect of iron-deficiency anaemia on cognitive skills in infancy and childhood. *Baillieres Clinical Haematology, 7* (4), 815–827.

# HIV Disease

Kenneth D. Phillips

Marguerite L. Knox

Recent developments in the treatment of patients with HIV disease has led to the current recognition that AIDS is a chronic disease. Persons with AIDS are living both longer and higher quality lives. These individuals, nevertheless, require vigilant health care. This health care includes the specific regimens for treating HIV disease and primary care for prevention and treatment of other health problems. Most primary care practices have persons infected with the HIV virus among their patients. Primary care providers need an in-depth understanding of the pathophysiology of HIV disease to provide the best primary care for patients with this chronic disease. Usually, management of HIV disease is the purview of infectious disease specialists, but the primary care provider may manage these persons' common and ordinary health problems.

AIDS was first recognized in Los Angeles in 1981 among five young gay men who developed *Pneumocystis carinii* pneumonia, an opportunistic infection that does not ordinarily develop in people with healthy immune systems. Since the appearance of HIV disease almost 2 decades ago, remarkable scientific advances have been made regarding the genetics and molecular structure of HIV and the diagnosis and treatment of HIV disease. Yet, definitive treatments and vaccines for this life-threatening disease have not yet been found.

## EPIDEMIOLOGY

The World Health Organization estimates that more than 47 million people have been infected with HIV disease since it was first recognized. In 1998, 5.8 million new cases of HIV infection were diagnosed. Globally, there are 33.4 million people living with AIDS, and more than 95% of people living with HIV/AIDS reside in developing nations. Somewhere in the world, 11 people are infected with HIV every minute. Already, HIV/AIDS has taken the lives of nearly 14 million people, and most of the deaths have occurred in young adults in the most productive periods of their lives (UNAIDS Joint United Nations Programme on HIV/AIDS, 1998).

Since the beginning of the AIDS pandemic, a total of 688,200 persons with AIDS have been reported to the Centers for Disease Control and Prevention (CDC) in the United States (CDC, 1998). The continuing rapid spread of HIV disease is exemplified by the fact that during 1998 alone, 48,269 new cases of AIDS were reported in the United States. After several years of steady increase, the number of new cases (incidence) of AIDS declined by 6% in 1996 (CDC, 1997a). The changing demographics of the AIDS epidemic show that the greatest increases in the number of new cases of AIDS are among people of color, women, and heterosexuals (CDC, 1997a). African-American women comprise the group showing the greatest increases in new cases of AIDS (CDC, 1998). Decreased mortality; earlier diagnosis of HIV infection; better diagnosis, treatment, and prevention of opportunistic illnesses; and the use of highly active antiretroviral therapy (HAART) have led to an increase in the number of people living with HIV/AIDS (prevalence).

Most women with HIV disease are of reproductive age (16 to 44 years of age), resulting in a growing number of pediatric HIV/AIDS cases. Almost 90% of AIDS cases reported among children, and nearly all newly diagnosed cases of HIV infections among children, are attributed to perinatal transmission of HIV. Fewer than 10% of pediatric cases result from causes other than perinatal transmission, such as childhood sexual abuse and blood transfusions (CDC, 1998). By the year 2000, it is estimated that 10 million children worldwide will be HIV infected and 20 to 40 million children will have been orphaned by HIV/AIDS worldwide (UNAIDS Joint Union Nations Programme on HIV/AIDS, 1998).

## MODES OF TRANSMISSION

Three major ways by which HIV is transmitted are unprotected sexual intercourse, inoculation of infected blood, and perinatal exposure to HIV. The greatest risk of transmission is through unprotected sexual contact with infected semen or vaginal secretions (anal intercourse, vaginal intercourse). Although unprotected sexual intercourse holds the greatest risk for transmission of HIV, this virus is not easily transmitted in this way. Less than 15% of individuals exposed to HIV during unprotected sexual intercourse become infected (Bernard et al., 1999). The risk of infection from a single exposure is less than 0.3% (Peterman et al., 1988). However, some individuals have been infected after limited exposure to HIV (Staszewski et al., 1987), whereas others remain uninfected after multiple exposures (Alexander, 1990; Stratton et al., 1997). Unprotected anal, vaginal, or oral intercourse is considered to be risky sexual behavior. Unprotected anal intercourse carries the greatest risk, and the risk is greater for the receptive partner (Flemmig et al., 1997). Whereas unprotected vaginal intercourse is the behavior responsible for most cases of HIV infection in the world, vaginal intercourse is a less efficient vehicle for transmitting the virus than is anal intercourse. Transmission of HIV during vaginal intercourse is greater from male to female partner than from female to male partner (Alexander, 1990). Because saliva contains low amounts of HIV and has factors that may inactivate HIV, unprotected oral intercourse carries less risk than anal or vaginal sex for transmitting HIV (Moore et al., 1998). However, unprotected oral intercourse should not be considered safe, and protection should be used during every encounter. Examples of the relative risk of selected sexual activities are presented in Table 21-1.

## TABLE 21.1

### Relative Risk of Selected Sexual Activities

| Relative Risk | Sexual Activity |
| --- | --- |
| Very high risk | Receptive anal intercourse without a condom |
| | Receptive vaginal intercourse without a condom |
| High risk | Insertive anal intercourse without a condom |
| | Insertive vaginal intercourse without a condom |
| Medium risk | Receptive anal intercourse with a condom |
| | Receptive vaginal intercourse with a condom |
| | Receptive oral intercourse without a condom |
| Low risk | Insertive anal intercourse with a condom |
| | Insertive vaginal intercourse with a condom |
| | Insertive oral intercourse without a condom |
| Very low risk | Insertive or receptive oral intercourse with a condom |
| | Mutual masturbation |
| | Deep kissing |
| No risk | Sexual abstinence |
| | Hugging |
| | Massage |
| | Social kissing |

(Adapted from Flemmig, D. S. & Boyer, P. J. J. [1997]. Safer sex. In J. Fahey & D. S. Flemmig [Eds.], *AIDS/HIV reference guide for medical professionals* [pp. 378–389]. Baltimore: Williams & Wilkins.)

HIV is transmitted by inoculation of infected blood (sharing contaminated needles, tattooing, scarification, accidental needle sticks, or injury with other contaminated instruments and blood transfusions). As a result of better screening techniques, the risk of transmission of HIV through transfusion has been reduced dramatically. In the United States, the risk of transmitting HIV through transfusion is estimated to be 1 in 440,000 to 660,000 donations (Lackritz, 1998). Injecting drug use ranks second to sexual intercourse as the most common cause of HIV transmission. Transmission of HIV by drug injection carries a high risk when an individual uses the same equipment as an HIV-infected person has used. Transmission of HIV can be minimized by cleaning equipment with bleach between individuals and is eliminated only by using one's own equipment. Drug use may lower inhibition and cause an individual to participate in riskier sexual activities.

HIV may be transmitted in utero, during labor and delivery, or through breast feeding (Table 21-2). Several factors have been identified that influence the risk of transmission of HIV from a mother to her unborn child. The risk for transmitting HIV increases as the mother becomes more immunosuppressed (ie, greater viral load, lower CD4+ cell count) and during periods of rapid disease progression (European Collaborative Study, 1992). Malnutrition may contribute to the risk of HIV transmission. For instance, vitamin A deficiency is associated with a greater risk of transmission (Semba et al., 1994). Inflammation of the placenta, maternal co-infection (ie, syphilis), and prolonged rupture of the membranes may increase the risk of perinatal transmission (Sperling, 1997). Prematurity is associated with greater risk of vertical (mother-to-child) transmission (European Collaborative Study, 1992). Maternal HIV transmission rates have been reported to be as high as 40% among women living in developing countries (Ryder et al., 1989) and 25% to 30% in the United States (Goedert et al., 1989) in women not receiving antiretroviral therapy. In February 1994, the National Institutes of Health interrupted a clinical trial (ACTG076 Study) aimed at determining the efficacy of azidothymidine (AZT) administration during pregnancy. The study was interrupted for ethical reasons when it became evident that administration of AZT to pregnant women reduced vertical transmission from 32% to 8% (National Institute of Allergy and Infectious Diseases, 1994). Other antiretrovirals are being tested for their safety and efficacy in preventing vertical transmission. Recently, it has been shown that $4.00 worth of nevirapine may reduce the risk of vertical HIV

transmission. When a single dose of this drug is administered to the mother during labor and to the infant during the first 72 hours of extrauterine life, the risk of transmission may be reduced by as much as a half (Musoke et al., 1999). Several factors that increase the risk of perinatal transmission of HIV are summarized in Table 21-3.

## TABLE 21.2

### Percentage of Cases of HIV Infection Accounted for by Risk Factor

| Exposure Category | Percentage of Cases Worldwide |
|---|---|
| Vaginal intercourse | 70–85 |
| Anal intercourse | 10–15 |
| Intravenous drug abuse | 5–10 |
| Blood transfusion | 2–8 |
| Perinatal | 5–10 |
| Working as a health care worker | <0.01 |

(From Chernoff, D.N. [1995]. Human immunodeficiency virus disease and related opportunistic infections. In G.J. Lawlor, T.J. Fischer, & D.C. Adelman [Eds.], *Manual of allergy and immunology* [pp. 425–445]. Boston: Little, Brown & Company.)

## TABLE 21.3

### Factors Associated With Transmission of HIV From a Mother to Her Unborn Child

| Category | Factor |
|---|---|
| Maternal factors | Stage of illness |
| | Viral load |
| | Coinfections such as syphilis |
| | Malnutrition |
| Intrapartum factors | Chorioamnionitis |
| | Duration of rupture of membranes |
| | Mode of delivery |
| Fetal factors | Prematurity |
| | Genetic susceptibility |

(From Sperling R.S., [1997]. Perinatal transmission of HIV. In D. Cotton & D.H. Watts [Eds.], *The medical management of AIDS in women* [pp. 45–54]. New York: Wiley-Liss.)

## VIROLOGY OF HIV

HIV has been identified as the etiologic agent of AIDS. Currently, two strains of HIV are known to exist: HIV-1 and HIV-2. HIV-1 has a worldwide distribution and is the strain of HIV most often encountered in the United States. HIV-2 is seen primarily in West Africa.

HIV belongs to the Retroviridae family of viruses. Retroviridae are divided into three subfamilies: Oncovirinae, Spumavirinae, and Lentivirinae. Two Lentivirinae (HIV and simian immunodeficiency virus) cause disease in primates. Other Lentivirinae affect nonprimates: Visna virus, Maedi virus, Caprine arthritis virus, equine infectious anemia virus, and feline immunodeficiency virus. Retroviruses such as HIV contain their genetic material on strands of RNA rather than on DNA.

### Genetic Composition of HIV

HIV is a sphere (approximately 100 nm in diameter) that is comprised of an envelope and a core (Gallo, 1988) (Fig. 21-1). Seven genes provide the genetic structure of HIV. The genetic structure of HIV and the function of its proteins are presented in Table 21-4.

### Viral Structure

The envelope consists of glycoprotein 120 (gp120) and glycoprotein 41 (gp41). Glycoprotein 160 is the precursor of gp120 and gp41. The surface glycoprotein gp120 allows HIV to attach to the CD4+ receptor site of infected T-helper cells and other host cells that bear a CD4+ receptor site on their cell membranes. The transmembrane glycoprotein gp41 enables the viral envelope to fuse with the host cell membrane. The matrix is formed from p17 (Gallo, 1988; Phillips, 1996). The outer membrane of HIV's core, the capsid, is formed from p24. The core contains two strands of RNA and enzymes that are necessary for the replication of HIV (reverse transcriptase, RNAse, polymerase, integrase, and protease). The nucleocapsid protein

p9 lines the strands of RNA and directs these strands into newly forming viruses. The function of p6 is unknown. Reverse transcriptase (p65/p50) converts RNA to a single strand of viral DNA. RNAse (p15) removes the RNA template from the newly formed single strand of viral DNA. Polymerase produces an exact copy of the newly formed single strand of viral DNA and causes two strands of viral DNA to combine. Integrase (p31) inserts the newly formed double strand of viral DNA into the host's DNA. Protease (p10) cleaves long precursor proteins in the immature, noninfectious virions, allowing them to become mature, infectious viruses (Gallo, 1998; Phillips, 1996) (Fig. 21-2).

### Life Cycle of HIV-1

HIV replicates inside of host cells that bear a CD4+ cell marker. Replication takes place in eight well-defined stages:

*Stage I*—Glycoprotein 120 binds to the CD4+ marker on host cells.
*Stage II*—Glycoprotein 41 facilitates fusion of the viral coat with the CD4+ cell membrane.
*Stage III*—Inside the cell, HIV undergoes an uncoating process, and the two single strands of viral RNA are released into the cytoplasm of the host CD4+ cell.
*Stage IV*—A single strand of DNA is copied from the RNA by the enzyme reverse transcriptase. Reverse transcriptase is composed of two other enzymes: RNAse and polymerase. RNAse is necessary to remove the RNA from the DNA copy. Then, polymerase makes another exact copy of the viral DNA and causes the two strands of DNA to join.
*Stage V*—The newly formed, double strand of viral DNA moves into the nucleus of the host cell, where it is incorporated into the DNA of the host cell by the enzyme integrase. The host cell begins to make messenger RNA (mRNA). Then, mRNA moves from the host cell nucleus to the ribosomes, where it guides the production of viral proteins. Transfer RNA (tRNA) carries

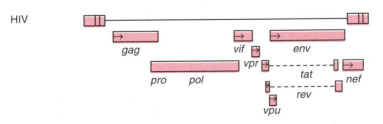

**FIGURE 21.1** ● Genes of the HIV retrovirus.

## TABLE 21.4

### Genetic Structure and Function of HIV

| HIV Protein | Functions |
| --- | --- |
| Gag | Codes for core proteins (p17, p24, p9, p6) |
| Env | Codes for envelope proteins (gp160, gp120, gp41) |
| Pol | Codes for reverse transcriptase (p65, p50), RNAse (p15), integrase (p31), and protease (p10) |
| Tat | Speeds transcription and viral replication in CD4+ cells |
| Rev | Allows unspliced and partially spliced HIV RNA to enter the cytoplasm |
| Nef | Allows high-titer growth of HIV in CD4+ cells by down regulating CD4+ cell function |
| Vif | Facilitates the release of viral particles from infected CD4+ cells |
| Vpr | Not required for in vitro HIV replication but may be required for in vivo HIV replication |
| Vif | Not required for in vitro HIV replication but is required for in vivo HIV replication. Facilitates the release of HIV from infected CD4+ cells |
| Vpu | Not required for in vitro HIV replication but may be required for in vivo replication. Facilitates the release of HIV from infected CD4+ cells. Prevents the gp120 from attaching to CD4+ receptor site in the endoplasmic reticulum of the host cell |

(From Ratner, L., Maseltine, W., Patarca, R., Livak, K.J., Starcich, B., Josephs, S.F., Doran, E.R., Rofalski, J.A., Whitehorn, E.A., Baumeister, K., Nomone, W.I., Petteway, S.R., Jr., Pearson, M.L., Lautzenberger, J.A., Papas, T.S., Ghrayeb, J., Chong, N.T., Gallor, R.C., Wong-Staal, F. [1985]. Complete nucleotide sequence of the AIDS virus, HTLV-III. *Nature, 313* [6000], 277–283.)

amino acids from the host cell cytoplasm to the ribosomes.

*Stage VI*—In the ribosomes, the amino acids are assembled into large, inactive precursor proteins.

*Stage VII*—During this stage, immature virions are released from the host cell through the process of budding. These virions, which are noninfectious, contain large precursor proteins that must be broken into smaller glycoproteins, proteins, and enzymes before they become infectious.

*Stage VIII*—By the action of protease, these large precursor proteins are split into a variety of

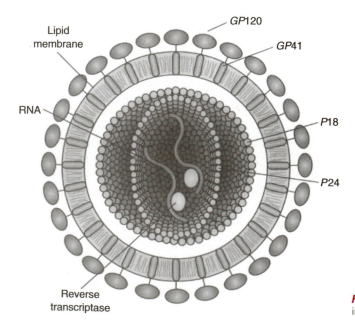

**FIGURE 21.2**  ●  The human immunodeficiency virus (HIV).

smaller glycoproteins and enzymes that are essential for the virus to become a mature, infectious retrovirus (Phillips, 1996)(Fig. 21-3).

Individuals who are HIV infected produce 100 million to 10 billion new virions per day (Robertson et al., 1996). As many as a billion CD4+ T-helper cells die and are replenished each day in the early stages of the illness (Pantaleo et al., 1993). When the immune system is no longer able to produce as many CD4+ cells as are lost, the CD4+ T-helper cell count begins to decline. CD4+ T-helper cells can die in the following ways: (1) binding of gp120 can lead to preprogrammed cell death known as apoptosis; (2) binding of gp120 can terminate cell division and protein synthesis by the CD4+ T-helper cells in a process known as anergy; (3) gp120 on the surface of virions budding form the surface of an infected CD4+ cell can bind to CD4+ receptors on other CD4+ cells, causing them to tear; (4) multiple CD4+ cells can join together in a process known as syncytium formation; (5) HIV may form superantigens that activate CD4+ cells in a nonspecific manner, allowing proliferation of numerous T-helper cells that could die in the absence of further activation; or (6) gp120 may inhibit early stages of T-helper cell activation (Peterson, 1995; Phillips, 1996).

## IMMUNOLOGIC CHANGES IN HIV DISEASE

### Cells

#### CD4+ T Lymphocytes

The CD4+ cells, or the T-helper cells, play an important part in initiating and orchestrating the cellular and the humoral immune response. There are two types of CD4+ cells, $T_H1$ and $T_H2$ (Clerici and Shearer, 1993). Clerici and Shearer (1993) proposed a mechanism in which the $T_H1$ subset (secretes gamma interferon [$\gamma$-IFN], interleukin [IL]-2, IL-12, and IL-15) switches to the $T_H2$ subset (secretes IL-4, IL-5, IL-10, and IL-13). The $T_H1$ subset primarily activates cellular immunity, whereas the $T_H2$ subset primarily activates humoral immunity. Switching from $T_H1$ to $T_H2$ subset favors progression to AIDS (Shearer et al., 1996).

One of the characteristics of HIV/AIDS is a progressive depletion of CD4+ lymphocytes, which begins at the time of HIV infection (Pantaleo et al., 1997). Destruction of CD4+ lymphocytes progresses at a rate of about 60 cells per year in untreated individuals until they are depleted (Anderson 1996). In acute HIV infection, the CD4+ cells decrease significantly during the first

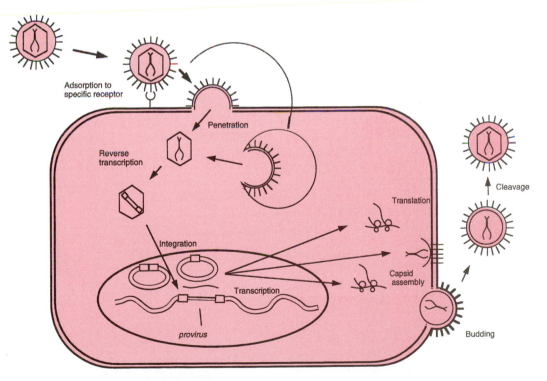

**FIGURE 21.3** ● Overview of retrovirus replication.

few weeks of infection but quickly return to near-normal levels. Over the next 12 to 18 months, during the asymptomatic period, the CD4+ cells drop rapidly (Saag et al, 1996), followed by a slowing of the rate of decline. The length of slowing of CD4+ cell destruction varies from individual to individual (Saag et al., 1996). About 2 years before AIDS becomes clinically evident, another period of accelerated decline in CD4+ cells occurs (Saag et al., 1996). In advanced stages of AIDS, the individual has almost no detectable CD4+ cells. The CD4+ cells lose their ability to respond to common antigens such as *Candida albicans*.

### CD8+ T lymphocytes

There are two types of CD8+ cells: cytotoxic T cells (directly kill virally infected or cancerous cells), and suppressor T cells (suppress the immune response created by the CD4+ cells when it is no longer needed). In healthy individuals, the number of CD8+ lymphocytes is approximately 500 cells/mm$^3$.

Approximately 33 days after HIV infection, the number of CD8+ lymphocytes increases (Cooper et al., 1999). In HIV disease, the number of CD8+ cells may increase to 1000 to 2000 cell/mm$^3$. CD8+ cells play a key role in the immune response to HIV during the primary response by killing cells that are HIV-infected (Zhu et al., 1993). CD8+ cells may secrete substances that suppress replication of HIV (Pantaleo et al., 1997). As HIV disease progresses, the CD8+ cells return to near-normal levels. The number of CD8+ cells bearing the marker CD8 are useful in predicting progression to AIDS.

### CD4+/CD8+ ratio

Normally, there are approximately twice as many CD4+ cells as CD8+ cells. In HIV disease, the decreasing CD4+ cells and the associated increasing CD8+ cells result in a reversed CD4+/CD8 ratio. In early HIV disease, the CD4+/CD8+ ratio falls to less than 1:0. During the later stages of HIV disease, the ratio becomes less than 0:2.

### Natural Killer Cells

A decrease in absolute NK cell number, both CD56+ and CD16+, is observed in HIV disease. The CD56+ and CD16+ NK cells have been shown to be severely decreased even in individuals with high levels of CD4+ cells (Hu et al., 1995). In early HIV infection, NK cells are cytotoxic for HIV-infected cells (Riviere et al., 1989). Natural killer cell activity (NKCA) becomes progressively depressed in HIV-infected individuals and severely depressed in persons with AIDS (Plaeger-Marshall et al., 1987). Decreased NKCA may be related to insufficiency of IL-2 production (Bonavida et al., 1986).

### B Lymphocytes

Activated T cells begin to secrete IL-2, IL-3, IL-4, IL-6, granulocyte-macrophage colony-stimulating factor (GM-CSF), macrophage colony-stimulating factor (M-CSF), and tumor necrosis factor-alpha (TNF-α). These cytokines enhance HIV replication by HIV-infected macrophages. TNF-α stimulates polyclonal expansion of the B cells, which results in hypergammaglobulinemia (Polk et al., 1987). Although the immunoglobulins are markedly increased, the antigen-specific response against HIV is weak. The TNF-α, TNF-β, and IL-1 factors produced by the activated T cells increase viral replication by HIV-infected CD4+ cells (Polk et al., 1987).

### Monocytes/Macrophages

Monocytes are macrophages that engulf and clear foreign substances that have formed complexes with antibodies. Monocytes participate in the immune response by processing and expressing an antigen of the class II major histocompatibility complex (MHC) on the macrophage's cell membrane and then presenting the antigen to the T cells. When antigen presentation has occurred, T cells become activated and secrete cytokines, which initiate the immune response.

Monocytes bear a CD4+ receptor and can be infected with HIV (Gartner et al., 1986). Monocytes replicate HIV at a slow rate, and unlike CD4+ T lymphocytes, monocytes do not die as a result of HIV infection and may serve as a reservoir for HIV (Pauza, 1988). Monocyte dysfunctions (decreased phagocytosis, defective intracellular killing, decreased cytotoxicity, and diminished class II MHC presentation) become progressively more pronounced in advanced stages of HIV disease (Braun et al., 1988).

## Cytokines

The primary functions of the cytokines are to stimulate the proliferation and differentiation of the cellular and humoral immune cells. Cytokines are integrally related to HIV replication. HIV directly infects CD4+ T lymphocytes and does not require presentation by antigen presenting cells such as the monocytes. HIV directly activates the CD4+ cells, thus initiating an immune response. Several interleukins and GM-CSFs and M-CSFs are positively related to increased HIV replication. In particular, increased levels of IL-1, IL-1β, IL-6, and TNF-α are positively associated with rapid progression of HIV disease (Fahey et al., 1990). Both TNF-α and TNF-β rapidly and powerfully enhance HIV replication (Poli et al., 1995) by inducing the production of cellular transcription nuclear factor, which increases the formation of mRNA from the proviral DNA found in the host cell chromosome (Rosenberg et al., 1991).

## STAGES OF HIV DISEASE

### Acute Infection

The CD4+ cell count in the acute stage of infection usually is greater than 750 cells/mm$^3$ (Mitsuyasu, 1997a). During this period, HIV replication proceeds at a rapid rate, and large quantities of HIV are detected in the blood. As high titers of HIV appear in the blood, there is a temporary and sometimes drastic decline in the CD4+ cell count that returns to near-normal levels (Tindall et al., 1991) of 589 to 1505 cells/mm$^3$ (Fischbach, 1996). For some individuals, the CD4+ cell count may precipitously drop as low as 100 cells/mm$^3$, placing the person at risk for opportunistic infection and even death (Flaskerud et al., 1999). In this period of rapid HIV replication, HIV disseminates to many other CD4+ cells, allowing mutations to occur with increased frequency. The acute infection stage may begin 1 to 3 weeks after infection with HIV and persists for 1 to 3 weeks (Parslow et al., 1996). If the person's blood is tested during the "window period" (6 to 12 weeks after infection), no antibodies are detected. The person may exhibit flu-like or mononucleosis-like symptoms that include headache, fever, lymphadenopathy, pharyngitis, rash, myalgia, arthralgia, diarrhea, headache, nausea and vomiting, oral ulcers, genital ulcers, thrombocytopenia, lymphopenia, elevated liver enzymes, thrush, altered mental status, dysasthesias, and Guillain-Barré syndrome (Katsufrakis et al., 1997).

### Asymptomatic Stage

In the asymptomatic stage, The CD4+ cell count usually is greater than 500 cells/mm$^3$ but may range from 200 to 750 cells/mm$^3$ (Mitsuyasu, 1997a). Seroconversion means that the person has developed enough antibodies to HIV to be detectable and signals advancement to this stage of HIV disease. Antibodies to HIV persist throughout the course of the disease. Viral replication continues at a high rate in lymphatic structures even though the person is asymptomatic (Pantaleo et al., 1993). Viral load in the blood declines (Flaskerud et al., 1999) during this phase, and CD4+ cells are progressively destroyed. Billions of CD4+ T-helper cells, which normally live for many years, die each day (Pantaleo et al., 1993). The immune system attempts to replenish the CD4+ cells that are destroyed by HIV. When the immune system can no longer keep up with the rate of destruction, the CD4+ cells decline. In the untreated person, the rate of CD4+ decline is about 60 cells per year (Anderson, 1996). Macrophages, on the other hand, survive for long periods, even though they are infected with HIV, and provide a site for HIV hidden away from the immune system and from drugs used to combat HIV (Meltzer et al., 1992). Although it is called the asymptomatic phase, most persons in this stage experience persistent, generalized lymphadenopathy and nonspecific constitutional symptoms. This stage lasts from 2 to 15 years or more.

### Early Symptomatic Stage

In the early symptomatic stage, the CD4+ cell count usually is greater than 200 cells/mm$^3$ (Mitsuyasu, 1997a), but it can range from 100 to 500 cells/mm$^3$ (Mitsuyasu, 1997a). This stage lasts from 1 to 5 years or more. Symptoms rarely appear until the the CD4+ cell count falls below 300 cells/mm$^3$. Persistent, generalized lymphadenopathy and constitutional symptoms (ie, persistent fever, diarrhea, or weight loss greater than 10% of normal body weight) are observed. Opportunistic organisms commonly seen in this stage are as follows: *Streptococcus pneumoniae*, *Haemophilus influenzae*, *Mycobacterium tuberculosis*, *C. albicans* and other *Candida* species, herpes simplex virus (HSV), varicella-zoster virus (VZV), Epstein-Barr virus (EBV), and *Coccidioides immitis* (Piemme, 1998).

### Late Symptomatic Stage

The CD4+ cell count in the late symptomatic stage ranges from 50 to 200 cells/mm$^3$ (Mitsuyasu, 1997a). This stage lasts from 1 to 4 years or more. A CD4+ cell count less than 200 cells/mm$^3$ indicates that the person has progressed to AIDS. Neurologic manifestations of immunodeficiency (ie, dementia, neuropathy, or myelopathy) may appear. When the T-helper cell count falls below 200 cells/mm$^3$, the person frequently is infected by a variety of opportunistic organisms, in particular *P.*

*carinii, Cryptosporidium parvum, Toxoplasma gondii*, microsporidia, *C. albicans* and other *Candida* species, *Cryptococcus neoformans*, *M. tuberculosis*, HSV, VZV, EBV, and *Histoplasma capsulatum* (Piemme, 1998).

### Advanced HIV Disease

The CD4+ cell count ranges from 0 to 50 cells/mm$^3$ in the advanced stage and may last from 0 to 2 years or more. Severe opportunistic infections and malignancies appear in this stage. In advanced HIV disease, the person becomes susceptible to *Mycobacterium avium-intracellulare*, cytomegalovirus (CMV), and Jakob-Creuzfeldt virus (Piemme, 1998). The CDC's revised classification system is presented in Table 21-5.

## DIAGNOSIS

### Enzyme-Linked Immunosorbent Assay

The enzyme-linked immunosorbent assay (ELISA) is the most common screening test for HIV infection. The ELISA has sensitivity and specificity greater than 99%. ELISA detects antibodies to HIV but does not directly detect HIV antigen. Because it takes 6 to 12 weeks for an individual to develop detectable antibodies to HIV, the diagnosis of HIV infection may be missed during this window period. The high sensitivity of this test results in very few false-negative results but in many false-positive findings. If the ELISA test is positive, it should be confirmed by the Western blot assay (WBA). A positive ELISA means that the individual may have been exposed to and developed antibodies to HIV; it does not mean that the person has AIDS (Saag, 1997b).

### Western Blot Assay

The Western blot assay (WBA) detects antibodies to specific proteins in HIV and is used to confirm the results of a ELISA. In the WBA, specific proteins of the HIV are separated by electrophoresis and blotted onto filter paper that is incubated with antibodies. Enzymes are used to change the colorless antigen-antibody complexes to a color. Specific regions on the filter paper correspond to the specific proteins that make up HIV. The WBA results may be positive, negative, or indeterminate. A positive WBA in conjunction with a positive ELISA test is accurate more than 99.9% of the time and is considered confirmatory for HIV infection.

### Polymerase Chain Reaction

Polymerase chain reaction (PCR) detects and quantifies HIV DNA or RNA in tissues. Unlike the ELISA and WBA, PCR does not detect antibodies to HIV but detects the virus itself. PCR amplifies specific segments of the viral RNA and is able to detect small quantities of HIV. During PCR, it is possible to make many copies of RNA or DNA from a single molecule. This makes PCR valuable in diagnosing HIV infection in persons with ambiguous antibody tests and in infants of HIV-infected mothers. Maternal antibodies to HIV persist for up to 6 months in infants who or may not be HIV-infected.

## ANTIRETROVIRAL THERAPY

### Nucleoside Reverse Transcriptase Inhibitors

Reverse transcriptase is an enzyme found within the core of retroviruses such as HIV that is necessary for viral replication. Reverse transcriptase inhibitors were the first major classification of antiretroviral drugs. Nucleoside reverse transcriptase inhibitors (NRTIs) work by substituting nucleoside analogues (ie, thymidine) for natural substrates necessary for the formation of viral DNA. Reverse transcriptase inhibitors inhibit RNA-directed DNA polymerase. The growing chains of viral DNA are prematurely terminated, resulting in the production of faulty HIV DNA, thus preventing viral replication (Phillips, 1996).

### Nonnucleoside Reverse Transcriptase Inhibitors

Nonnucleoside reverse transcriptase inhibitors directly combine with reverse transcriptase, causing this enzyme to be inactivated. This blocks the process by which the HIV RNA becomes HIV DNA.

### Protease Inhibitors

Proteases are enzymes that split the peptide bonds of larger proteins into smaller proteins. HIV protease is part of the gp160 molecule. In the viral replication process that occurs inside of the CD4+ cells, large precursor proteins are formed. HIV protease cleaves the large precursor proteins into the smaller, structurally essential proteins of HIV. Cleavage is necessary for immature, noninfectious viruses to become infectious (Phillips, 1996). Antiretroviral therapies are summarized in Table 21-6.

# TABLE 21.5

## Revised CDC Classification System for HIV Infection 1993

| CD4+ T-Cell Categories | (A) Asymptomatic, Acute (Primary) HIV or PGL | (B) Symptomatic, Not (A) or (C) Conditions | (C) AIDS-Indicator Conditions |
|---|---|---|---|
| (1) ≥ 500/mm³ | A1 | B1 | C1 |
| (2) 200–499/mm³ | A2 | B2 | C2 |
| (3) < 200/mm³ | A3 | B3 | C3 |

| Category | Defining Conditions |
|---|---|
| A | Asymptomatic HIV infection |
| | Persistent generalized lymphadenopathy |
| | Acute (primary) HIV infection with accompanying illness or history of acute HIV infection |
| B | Bacillary angiomatosis |
| | Candidiasis, oropharyngeal (thrush) |
| | Candidiasis, vulvovaginal; persists (> 1 mo duration), frequent or poorly responsive to therapy |
| | Cervical dysplasia (moderate or severe) or cervical carcinoma in situ |
| | Constitutional symptoms such as fever (38.5°C) or diarrhea lasting > 1 mo |
| | Hairy leukoplakia, oral |
| | Herpes zoster (shingles), involving at least two distinct episodes or more than one dermatome |
| | Idiopathic thrombocytopenic purpura |
| | Listeriosis |
| | Pelvic inflammatory disease, particularly if complicated by tuboovarian abscess |
| | Peripheral neuropathy |
| C | Candidiasis of bronchi, trachea, or lungs |
| | Candidiasis, esophageal |
| | Cervical cancer, invasive |
| | Coccidioidomycosis, disseminated or extrapulmonary |
| | Cryptococcosis, extrapulmonary |
| | Cryptosporidiosis, chronic intestinal (> 1 mo duration) |
| | Cytomegalovirus disease (other than the liver, spleen, or nodes) |
| | Cytomegalovirus retinitis (with loss of vision) |
| | Encephalopathy, HIV-related |
| | Herpes simplex, chronic ulcers (> 1 mo duration) |
| | Histoplasmosis, disseminated or extrapulmonary |
| | Isosporiasis, chronic intestinal (> 1 mo duration) |
| | Kaposi's sarcoma |
| | Lymphoma, Burkitt's |
| | Lymphoma, immunoblastic |
| | Lymphoma, primary, of brain |
| | *Mycobacterium avium* complex or *Mycobacterium kansasii,* disseminated or extrapulmonary |
| | *Mycobacterium tuberculosis,* any site (pulmonary or extrapulmonary) |
| | Mycobacteria, other species or unidentified species, disseminated or extrapulmonary |
| | *Pneumocystis carinii* pneumonia |
| | Pneumonia, recurrent |
| | Progressive multifocal leukoencephalopathy |
| | *Salmonella* septicemia, recurrent |
| | Toxoplasmosis of brain |
| | Wasting syndrome from HIV |

PGL, primary granulocytic lymphoma.
(Adapted from Centers for Disease Control and Prevention. [1992]. 1993 Revised classification system for HIV infection and expanded surveillance case definition for AIDS among adolescents and adults. *MMWR, 41,* 1–19.)

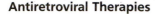

## TABLE 21.6

● ● ●

### Antiretroviral Therapies

| Classification | Generic Name | Trade Name | Abbreviations | Toxicities |
|---|---|---|---|---|
| Nucleoside RTIs | Zidovudine | Retrovir | AZT ZDV | Anemia Neutropenia |
| | Didanosine | Videx | DdI | Pancreatitis Peripheral neuropathy Elevated liver enzymes* |
| | Zalcitabine | HIVID | DdC | Peripheral neuropathy Stomatitis Pancreatitis |
| | Stavudine | Zerit | d4T | Peripheral neuropathy Pancreatitis Anemia Neutropenia Elevated liver enzymes* |
| | Lamivudine | Epivir | 3TC | None significant |
| Nonnucleoside RTIs | Delavirdine | Rescriptor | DLV | Neutropenia |
| | Nevirapine | Viramune | NVP | None significant |
| | Abacavir | Ziagen | ABC | None significant |
| | Efavirenz | | EFV | None significant |
| Protease inhibitors | Saquinavir | Invirase | SQV | Hyperglycemia Hypertriglyceridemia |
| | Ritonavir | Norvir | RTV | Hypertriglyceridemia Elevated liver enzymes* Hypertriglyceridemia |
| | Indinavir | Crixivan | IDV | Nephrolithiasis Hyperbilirubinemia Hypertriglyceridemia Hyperglycemia |
| | Nelfinavir | Viracept | NFV | Hypertriglycridemia Hyperglycemia Hypercholesterolemia |

RTIs, reverse transcriptase inhibitors.
*Rare.
(From Dolin, R., Masur, M., & Saag, M. [1999]. *AIDS therapy.* New York: Churchill Livingstone.)

## MONITORING DISEASE PROGRESSION AND THERAPEUTIC EFFECTIVENESS

### Viral Load

PCR is used to measure viral load. A new and more sensitive PCR makes it possible to measure viral loads lower than 50 copies/mL. Viral load increases as the CD4+ cell count decreases and as the disease progresses. In the early stages of HIV disease, the viral load or viral burden may be as low as 5000 copies/mL. When used as an indicator of the effectiveness of antiretroviral therapy, a decrease in viral load of 0.5 $\log_{10}$ indicates that the therapy is effective. If the viral load remains the same or does not drop 0.5 $\log_{10}$ after instituting a new therapy, the treatment regimen should be reevaluated and modified if necessary (Sax et al., 1996).

### CD4+ Cell Count

HIV targets and destroys CD4+ cells. As HIV disease progresses, the CD4+ cell count declines (Flaskerud & Ungvarski, 1999). Traditionally, antiretroviral therapy has been reserved for a

CD4+ cell count less than 500 cells/mm$^3$. Therapy should be initiated in patients who have a progressive decline of CD4+ cells to 500 cells/mm$^3$ or in those with a CD4+ cell count greater than 500 cells/mm$^3$ who have shown a rapid decline of CD4+ cells in a short time. Remember that CD4+ cell counts are labile and can rise in response to transient infections or can decline in response to other stimuli. CD4+ cells can vary by a much as 25 cells, more or fewer, on serial counts from a single sample (Fahey et al., 1997). A significant reduction in CD4+ cells indicates that the treatment plan needs to be reevaluated and possibly changed.

## β₂-Microglobulin

$\beta_2$-Microglobulin ($\beta_2$-M) is a part of class I MHC, which is present on all nucleated cells. $\beta_2$-Microglobulin is released into the blood when a cell dies. When cells (lymphocytes or otherwise) turn over rapidly, $\beta_2$-M levels increase (Fahey et al., 1990). As a result of the rapid turnover of lymphocytes in HIV disease, there is a significant correlation between $\beta_2$-M levels and disease progression. Levels of $\beta_2$-M greater than 3 mg/L are associated with more rapid progression to AIDS (Lazzarin, 1988).

## Serum Neopterin

Neopterin, a nonspecific marker of HIV disease progression, is a biologic molecule produced by macrophages in response to γ-IFN stimulation that can be detected in the blood. In asymptomatic seropositive patients, neopterin levels of 3 to 5 ng/mL are found, whereas levels greater than 15 ng/mL are found in persons who have progressed to AIDS (Reddy et al., 1989). Elevated levels of neopterin are associated with more rapid disease progression (Fahey et al., 1990).

## OPPORTUNISTIC INFECTIONS

### Fungal Infections

Fungi are prevalent opportunistic pathogens in HIV disease. As the CD4+ cells decrease during the progression of HIV disease, fungal infections surface. This section discusses the most common fungal opportunistic organisms: *P. carinii*, *C. albicans*, *C. neoformans*, *H. capsulatum*, and *C. immitis*.

### Pneumocystis Carinii

*Pneumocystis carinii* initially was thought to be a parasitic protozoan but has been identified as a fungus. *P. carinii* is found in nature in several mammals; however, transmission of *P. carinii* from one species to another is unlikely (Stansell et al., 1997). *P. carinii*, a nonpathogenic organism in a healthy adult that can become a lethal infection for an immunocompromised patient, most likely is transmitted from one person to another by inhalation. This fungus leads to hypoxic respiratory failure and has the highest mortality rate of any opportunistic infection (Stansell et al., 1997).

*P. carinii* attaches to type I alveoli membranes and sends branches into the alveoli, which may obtain needed nutrients. The alveoli fill with eosinophilic exudates containing *P. carinii*, cell membranes, surfactant, and host proteins. Surfactant production by type II alveoli is decreased, and a condition similar to the adult respiratory distress syndrome appears (Stansell et al., 1997). Early in the AIDS epidemic, *P. carinii* pneumonia (PCP) was the most common presenting opportunistic infection and the most common cause of death in persons with AIDS. Currently, PCP is much less common as a result of earlier diagnosis, HAART, and prophylaxis for PCP. There is a growing consensus that lifelong prophylaxis is no longer necessary since the advent of HAART (Furrer et al., 1999).

The primary site of *P. carinii* infection is lung tissue, but this organism also infects the spleen, lymphatic system, and blood (Stansell et al., 1997). Clinical manifestations of PCP are progressive dyspnea, acute tachypnea, cough, fever, hypoxemia, respiratory acidosis, and diffuse, bilateral pulmonary infiltrates (Stansell et al., 1997).

### Candida Albicans

*Candida* species are yeast-like fungi that are part of the normal flora of the skin, oropharynx, gastrointestinal (GI) tract, and vagina. *C. albicans* is the most common etiology of candidiasis in the person with HIV infection (Fichtenbaum, 1999). Immunosuppression allows *C. albicans*, an organism that normally is present in the human body, to flourish and produce infection. *C. albicans* infection most commonly involves the skin (intertrigo) but also can affect the oral mucosa (thrush), esophageal tract (esophageal candidiasis), and vagina (vaginal candidiasis). Common complaints associated with oral candidiasis include dry mouth and altered taste, whereas complaints related to esophageal candidiasis include dysphagia and odynophagia. Hallmark symptoms of esophageal candidiasis include fever and weight loss. Women with vaginal candidiasis present with purulent discharge, pruritus, frequent micturition, pain on urination, and redness and ulceration of mucous membranes. Often in vaginal candidiasis there is a red maculopapular rash of the intertriginous areas and inner thighs (Fichtenbaum, 1999).

### Cryptococcus Neoformans

*Cryptococcus neoformans* is the fungus that causes the most prevalent life-threatening infection found in AIDS patients (Powderly, 1999). This ubiquitous organism can be found in soil and bird droppings and is easily transmitted through inhalation. Cryptococcosis is more prevalent east of the Mississippi River (Powderly, 1999). Although the lungs are the portals of entry for this organism, the central nervous system (CNS) is the most common site of infection, frequently resulting in meningitis. Patients with cryptococcal meningitis may present with headache, fever, general malaise, stiff neck, and the inability to think clearly. Unfortunately, these classic symptoms of meningitis may wax and wane over time before diagnosis is certain.

Cryptococcal pneumonia is the second most common type of infection in immunosuppression, but it is believed that cryptococcal pneumonia is underdiagnosed and may not be recognized until extrapulmonary dissemination has taken place (Powderly, 1999). Cryptococcal pneumonia often manifests as dyspnea, pleuritic chest pain, a productive cough, and abnormal findings on chest x-rays.

### Coccidioides Immitis

*Coccidioides immitis* is a highly infectious organism that is endemic to the southwestern deserts of the United States in areas such as California, Arizona, New Mexico, and western Texas (Kirkland et al., 1996); it is transmitted by inhalation of the spores produced by this organism. Coccidiosis can present on a chest x-ray as focal or diffuse alveolar infiltrates or caseation mimicking the caseation seen in tuberculosis (TB) (Stephens, 1995). This virus can cause minimal disease (San Joaquin Valley fever) in immunocompetent persons to life-threatening pneumonitis or meningitis in persons with immunodeficiency. Manifestations of coccidioidal pneumonitis include fever, chills, weight loss, purulent cough, and dyspnea. Signs of coccidioidal meningitis include nuchal rigidity, headache, fever, and photosensitivity (Ampel, 1996).

### Histoplasma Capsulatum

*Histoplasma capsulatum*, a fungus that exists in the central and south central regions of the United States, is most prevalent along the Ohio and Mississippi River valleys. *H. capsulatum* is found in soil and in bird and bat droppings. The spores of this organism are transmitted through inhalation. In the warm environment of the human body, the spores enter the yeast phase. Infection with *H. capsulatum* can result in mild, asymptomatic, respiratory disease or can disseminate through the lymphatics, infecting the entire body. Fifty percent of patients presenting with mild disease have cough, dyspnea, and normal findings on chest x-rays, whereas disseminated histoplasmosis may present with fever, weight loss, lymphadenopathy, or hepatosplenomegaly. The most serious form of histoplasmosis affects approximately 10% of the patient population and presents with septic shock characterized by high fever, hypotension, and adult respiratory distress syndrome or disseminated coagulopathy (Saag, 1997a).

## Viral Infections

### Herpes Simplex Virus

Herpes simplex virus is another human pathogenic virus that is present throughout the world. Herpes simplex virus 1 (HSV-1) usually is present in oral secretions, whereas herpes simplex virus 2 (HSV-2) usually is present in the genital area. Both HSV-1 and HSV-2 can be transferred between the mouth and genitals through oral sex or touching. Although an active oral lesion can easily be transmitted to the genital area, HSV infection also can result from an inactive lesion (Hirsch, 1995). Also, HSV-2 can be transmitted during vaginal delivery from the mother to the infant. In AIDS patients, HSV can infect the prostate gland or the perianal region, resulting in symptoms of painful defecation, tenesmus, constipation, and impotence. Patients with HSV esophagitis often complain of odynophagia and dysphagia. Patients rarely develop HSV encephalitis, presenting with complaints of headache, fever, and altered mentation. The primary treatment for HSV infection is acyclovir (Casassus et al., 1997).

### Varicella-Zoster Virus

Varicella-zoster virus (herpes zoster) is a common virus among children spread by close, intimate contact through oropharyngeal secretions. Infection with VZV results in a characteristic rash of small, irregular, erythematous macules that become vesicular in 24 to 48 hours. Quickly, these lesions burst and crust over, resulting in contagious dissemination to others. As individuals grow and mature, this virus again can become harmful because of a secondary infection or the reactivation of dormant VZV in the sensory ganglia from previously acquired VZV infection. Patients usually complain of severe pain, pruritus, exquisite tenderness, and deep pain in an affected area before any skin lesions occur. Erythematous, vesicular lesions of thoracic dermatomes characterize shingles (HZV). HZV also can affect a single cervical, facial, lumbar, or sacral ganglion. The classic dermatomal pattern is diagnostic of HZV infection, based on clinical appearance. Involvement of the second or third cervical dermatome or involvement of the ophthalmic branch of the trigeminal ganglion may respectively result in facial paralysis or blindness (Katzenstein et al., 1994). The most common sequela of HZV infection is the persistent or intermittent pain that occurs for months to years, even after the resolution of acute HZV infection. In persons with HIV/AIDS, a HZV infection may be life threatening, leading to disseminated disease of the lung, pancreas, liver, or CNS. Acyclovir, famciclovir, valacyclovir, ganciclovir, and foscarnet are drugs used to treat HZV infection (McLigeyo, 1998).

## Cytomegalovirus

Cytomegalovirus, a herpesvirus, exists in most immunocompetent people throughout the world. Although 40% to 60% of the population within the United States have been exposed to this antigen, most do not have CMV disease (Piemme, 1998). Cytomegalovirus disease is common in HIV/AIDS and is more prevalent in men who have sex with men (Jones et al., 1999). Once the virus is reactivated, it can affect the following organ systems: retina, brain, lungs, liver, and mucosa of the GI tract (Staats et al., 1999). Cytomegalovirus produces polyradiculopathy, colitis, esophagitis, and pneumonia in an immunocompromised host (Arribas et al., 1996).

Retinitis, the most common presentation of CMV infection, leads to blindness if left untreated. Cytomegalovirus is responsible for more than 90% of HIV-related retinopathies. Retinitis from CMV infection most commonly appears when the CD4+ lymphocyte count has dropped below $50/mm^3$. Presenting signs and symptoms of CMV retinitis include decreased visual acuity, presence of floaters, visual loss, and the presence of yellowish white areas (cotton spots) and hemorrhages on the retina. CMV retinitis may progress to total blindness. The Food and Drug Administration has approved oral ganciclovir for the prevention of CMV retinitis.

Cytomegalovirus disease of the GI tract, the second most commonly affected organ system, produces esophageal ulcers, colitis, and even cholecystitis (Staats et al., 1999). When CMV infects the brain, it produces symptoms of encephalitis. Pulmonitis from CMV infection results in focal pneumonia manifested by the typical symptoms of fever, cough, dyspnea, and hypoxemia. Three drugs that have been approved for the treatment of CMV infection are ganciclovir, foscarnet, and cidofovir (Drew et al., 1997).

## Bacterial Infections

### Mycobacterium Tuberculosis

In the 1960s, public health officials believed they were well on their way to eradicating TB. Now, this highly infectious disease has resurged. At the recent pinnacle of this disease in 1993, there were 25,000 cases of active TB in the United States. It is estimated that there are 15 million people in the United States with inactive cases of TB that could become active (Ferri, 1999). One third of the world's population is estimated to be infected with *M. tuberculosis* (Basgoz et al., 1997). Tuberculosis is more prevalent in racial and ethnic minorities, the poor, and those living in crowded, enclosed spaces (Barnes et al., 1999; Classen et al., 1999; Piemme, 1998). Tuberculosis also is more prevalent among recent immigrants from countries with high TB prevalence rates, injection drug users, homeless people, prison inmates, inner city residents, residents of long-term care facilities, and HIV-infected persons (Ferri, 1999). Poor adherence to antitubercular regimens has resulted in multiple drug-resistant strains of *M. tuberculosis* (Sacks et al., 1998).

Diagnosis is made by administration of the purified protein derivative test (PPD) and chest x-ray. For individuals with healthy immune systems, an induration of 10 mm within 48 to 72 hours of the subcutaneous administration of PPD indicates that the individual has been exposed to *M. tuberculosis*. In immunocompromised individuals, an induration of only 5 mm indicates a positive exposure to *M. tuberculosis*. Notice that an immunocompromised person with an active case of TB may fail to develop an immune response because of anergy of the immune system. Generally, other common antigens such as mumps virus and *C. albicans* are placed subcutaneously near the PPD site. Failure to develop induration to any of these antigens may indicate anergy of the immune system. Chest x-ray generally shows caseous, cavitary lesions in the upper lobes of the lungs. Cavitary lesions may develop early in the course of HIV disease, when cellular immunity is near normal but may fail to develop in the later stages of the disease, when cellular immunity has decreased. The many other pulmonary infections of HIV disease may mask the diagnosis of pulmonary TB.

An obligate aerobe, *M. tuberculosis* is spread by inhalation of droplet nuclei that are produced when a person coughs or sneezes. The primary site of *M. tuberculosis* infection is the lungs. Normally, when a person inhales *M. tuberculosis*, the body initiates an inflammatory response. The organism is phagocytized by alveolar macrophages and carried to regional lymph nodes. From the lymph nodes, the infection enters the blood, where it is eliminated by cellular immunity (Basgoz et al., 1997). A caseous granuloma (tubercle) forms in the lungs to wall off the invading organism. When the body is unable to wall off the invading organism, active TB develops, and chronic inflammation leads to the formation of cavitary lesions. Tuberculosis may disseminate to other tissues including the spinal cord (Pott's disease), the CNS, the pericardium, the GI system, genitourinary tracts, bones, joints, and lymph nodes (Ferri, 1999). The symptoms of TB include productive cough, chest pain, hemoptysis, fever, chills, and night sweats. Pulmonary TB commonly occurs in the earlier stages of HIV disease and disseminates to other tissues in the later stages, when the CD4+ cell count has dropped below 200 cells/mm$^3$ (Piemme, 1998). In HIV disease, TB progresses more rapidly, disseminates more readily, and poses a greater threat to survival. Tuberculosis accelerates the acceleration rate of HIV disease.

### Mycobacterium avium-intracellulare

*Mycobacterium avium* and *Mycobacterium intracellulare* are two closely related species found in common surroundings such as water, soil, food, and animal sources. Together, these organisms are referred to as *Mycobacterium avium* complex (MAC). MAC invades through the GI tract or lungs, resulting in a systemic bacterial infection (French et al., 1997). Infection with MAC is likely to occur as macrophage dysfunction progresses in the disease process. Low levels of TNF, IFN-γ, and IL-2, contribute to the decreased host defense of an AIDS patient (Jacobson, 1997). Clinical manifestations of MAC infection are septicemia, fever, fatigue, weight loss, anorexia, nausea and vomiting, night sweats, diarrhea, abdominal pain, hepatosplenomegaly, and lymphadenopathy. Clinicians observe that CD4+ cell counts less than 50 cells/mm$^3$, a history of fever for fewer than 30 days, a hematocrit less than 30%, or a serum albumin level less than 3.0 g/dL are sensitive predictors of MAC bacteremia (Jacobson, 1997). Because MAC infection is a noncurable, chronic bacterial infection, the aim of treatment is clinical improvement with broad-spectrum antibiotics such as the macrolides. The CDC recommendations for the treatment of AIDS-related MAC infection include a macrolide in combination with one or more of the following drugs: ethambutol, rifabutin, ciprofloxacin, or amikacin (Havlir et al., 1996). Either azithromycin or rifabutin is used to prevent dissemination of MAC. Prophylaxis of AIDS-related MAC infection is recommended when the CD4+ count is less than 50 cells/mm$^3$ (CDC, 1997b; Desportes-Livage, 1996; Nightingale, 1997).

## Protozoal Infections

### Cryptosporidium Parvum

The most common cause of severe diarrhea in HIV/AIDS is infection with *Cryptosporidium parvum*. *Cryptosporidium parvum* infection produces diarrhea in humans (especially those who work in the meat processing industry) and in cattle. Cryptosporidiosis is transmitted by ingestion of contaminated food or water (even in the public water supply) and by person-to-person contact (Hayes et al., 1989). Persons with HIV/AIDS or another immunodeficiency should boil water before drinking it or drink bottled water. In immunocompetent individuals, cryptosporidiosis is self-limiting and lasts for about 10 to 14 days, but in persons with HIV/AIDS, it is chronic and difficult to treat. In advanced HIV/AIDS, cryptosporidiosis is manifested by profuse watery diarrhea, weight loss, abdominal pain, nausea, and vomiting. Fever is a rare manifestation in cryptosporidiosis. Cryptosporidiosis may result in the symptoms of cholangitis or cholecystitis. Pulmonary cryptosporidiosis sometimes occurs. The antibiotics most commonly used to treat cryptosporidiosis are paromomycin and azithromycin.

### Microsporidia

Two microsporidia cause diarrhea in HIV/AIDS, *Enterocytozoon bieneusi* and *Encephalitozoon intestinalis* (Asmuth et al., 1994). Microsporidiosis is more common in men who have sex with men. The mode of transmission and the reservoir of microsporidia have not been identified. Although the symptoms of microsporidiosis are the same as those of cryptosporidiosis, they are not as severe. Villus atrophy leads to malabsorption. Microsporidiosis is uncommon in persons with CD4+ cell counts greater than 50 cells/mm$^3$ (Heller, 1997). Albendazole is the most commonly prescribed drug for microsporidiosis (Lecuit et al., 1994).

### Isospora Belli

*Isospora belli* causes chronic diarrhea, abdominal cramping, malabsorption, and dehydration in persons with HIV/AIDS. This organism probably is spread by ingestion of contaminated food or water and less often by person-to-person contact. Infection with this organism can be prevented and treated with trimethoprim-sulfamethoxazole (Flanigan, 1999; Heller, 1997).

### Giardia Lamblia

Giardiasis has been called "the gay bowel syndrome"; however, the incidence of giardiasis is not any greater in persons with HIV/AIDS than in those who are seronegative for HIV. *Giardia* is transmitted by the fecal-oral route or by contaminated water or food sources. Giardiasis leads to flatulence, abdominal cramping, bowel hyperactivity, dyspepsia, diarrhea, and dehydration. The diagnosis is made by examination of a stool sample. The most common treatment for giardiasis is metronidazole (Wilcox et al., 1999). Treatments for the opportunistic infections are summarized in Table 21-7.

## TABLE 21.7

### Pharmacotherapeutic Interventions for Opportunistic Infections Related to HIV Disease

| Classification | Organism | Pharmacotherapeutic Intervention |
|---|---|---|
| Fungi | *Pneumocystis carinii* | Trimethoprim-sulfamethoxazole |
| | | Dapsone |
| | | Pyrimethamine |
| | | Pentamidine |
| | | Atovaquone |
| | | Clindamycin |
| | | Primaquine |
| | | Trimetrexate |
| | | Corticosteroids |
| | *Candida albicans* | Oropharngeal |
| | |    Clotrimazole troches |
| | |    Nystatin suspension |
| | |    Ketoconazole |
| | |    Itraconazole |
| | |    Fluconazole |
| | |    Amphotericin B |
| | | Esophageal |
| | |    Fluconazole |
| | |    Ketoconazole |
| | |    Itraconazole |
| | |    Amphotericin B |
| | | Vaginal |
| | |    Fluconazole |
| | |    Butaconazole |
| | |    Clotrimazole |
| | |    Miconazole |
| | |    Nystatin tablets |
| | |    Tioconazole |
| | |    Terconazole |

*(continued)*

**TABLE 21.7** (Continued)

| Classification | Organism | Pharmacotherapeutic Intervention |
|---|---|---|
| | *Cryptococcus neoformans* | Amphotericin B |
| | | Flucytosine |
| | | Fluconazole |
| | | Itraconazole |
| | *Coccidioides immitis* | Amphotericin B |
| | | Fluconazole |
| | | Itraconazole |
| | *Histoplasma capsulatum* | Amphotericin B |
| | | Itraconazole |
| | | Fluconazole |
| | | Ketoconazole |
| | *Blastomyces dermatitidis* | Amphotericin B |
| | | Itraconazole |
| Viruses | Herpes simplex | Acyclovir |
| | | Valacyclovir |
| | | Famciclovir |
| | | Foscarnet |
| | | Cidofovir |
| | Varicella-zoster | Acyclovir |
| | | Famciclovir |
| | | Valacyclovir |
| | | Foscarnet |
| | | Ganciclovir |
| | Cytomegalovirus | Ganciclovir |
| | | Foscarnet |
| | | Cidofovir |
| Bacteria | *Mycobacterium tuberculare* | Isoniazid |
| | | Rifampin |
| | | Pyrazinamide |
| | | Ethambutol |
| | | Streptomycin |
| | *Mycobacterium avium-intracellulare* | Clarithromycin |
| | | Azithromycin |
| | | Ethambutol |
| | | Rifabutin |
| | | Ciprofloxacin |
| | | Amikacin |
| | *Campylobacter* species | Erythromycin |
| | | Ciprofloxacin |
| | *Salmonella typhi* | Ciprofloxacin |
| | *Salmonella paratyphi* | |
| | *Listeria monocytogenes* | Ampicillin |
| | | Ampicillin + gentamycin |

*(continued)*

| TABLE 21.7 (Continued) | | ● ● ● |
|---|---|---|
| **Classification** | **Organism** | **Pharmacotherapeutic Intervention** |
| Protozoa | *Cryptosporidium parvum* | Paromomycin |
| | | Bovine colostrum |
| | | Letrazuril |
| | | Nitazoxanine |
| | Microsporidia | *Enterocytozoon intestinalis* |
| | |    Atovaquone |
| | |    Albendazole |
| | | *Enterocytozoon bieneusi* |
| | |    Atovaquone |
| | *Isospora belli* | Co-trimoxazole |
| | | Trimethoprim-sulfamethoxazole |
| | *Giardia lamblia* | Metronidazole |

(From Dolin R., Masur, H., & Saag, M. [1999]. *AIDS therapy.* New York: Churchill Livingstone.)

## OPPORTUNISTIC MALIGNANCIES

The HIV-mediated immunosuppressed state contributes to the high rate of opportunistic malignancies seen in AIDS. The opportunistic malignancies seen in HIV/AIDS include Kaposi's sarcoma (KS), non-Hodgkin's lymphoma (NHL), and invasive cervical cancer (Brown et al., 1996; CDC, 1992).

### Kaposi's Sarcoma

Epidemic KS identified in the AIDS patient can be distinguished from other forms of KS because of the uncontrolled, fulminant growth of spindle-shaped reticuloendothelial cells. Kaposi's sarcoma is the most common cancer seen in AIDS (Cooley et al., 1996). Kaposi's sarcoma results from a virus-related infection termed KS-associated herpesvirus and human herpesvirus (HHV)-8. KS lesions present as single, multinodular, red, macular patches that involve the torso, arms, head, or neck. Extracutaneous lesions can affect mucous membranes, GI tract, lung, spleen, adrenal gland, pancreas, and testes (Safai et al., 1994). The CDC's revised definition of AIDS in 1987 gives a presumptive diagnosis of KS based on the characteristic appearance of any erythematous or violaceous plaque-like lesion on skin or mucous membrane (Staats et al, 1999). Treatment is based on the extent and location of the lesions. Disseminated KS is treated with systemic therapy of specific, chemotherapeutic agents (Table 21-8) (Aboulafia, 1998).

### Non-Hodgkin's Lymphoma

Lymphomas are cancers of the immune system that originate with the development of abnormal cells, which eventually spread throughout the entire body (Staats et al., 1999). Non-Hodgkin's lymphoma is associated with multiple viruses (EBV, HIV-III, and HIV-I, and HHV-8) and with the cytokines induced by these infections. Non-Hodgkin's lymphoma originates either as a malignancy of the T or B lymphocytes (Staats et al., 1999), but most NHLs (95%) are of B cell origin. Non-Hodgkin's lymphoma is as much as 73 times higher in persons with HIV/AIDS than in the general population (Roth, 1998). Systemic NHL generally does not manifest until the CD4+ cell count is between 100 and 200 cells/mm$^3$, and primary CNS lymphomas generally do not manifest until the CD4+ cell count falls below 50 cells/mm$^3$. All lymphomas have a typical clinical presentation of uncontrolled, widespread lymphadenopathy. This uncontrolled proliferation of lymphatic tissues can spread from lymph nodes throughout the entire body to the heart, lung, oral cavity, GI tract, kidneys, abdomen, bone marrow, gonads, and genital tracts (Roth, 1998). Constitutional symptoms of advanced NHL include unexplained fever, night sweats, unintentional weight loss of greater than 10% of body weight, and diarrhea for more than 2 weeks (Safai et al., 1992). Non-Hodgkin's lymphoma is responsible for 15% to 20% of all AIDS-related deaths (Mitsayusa, 1997b).

## TABLE 21.8

**Treatments for Opportunistic Malignancies Associated With AIDS**

| Malignancy | Treatment |
|---|---|
| Kaposi's sarcoma | Local lesions |
| |     Liquid nitrogen cryotherapy |
| |     Intralesional injection of vinblastine |
| |     Intralesional injection of interferon-alfa |
| |     Intralesional injection of GM-CSF |
| |     Intralesional injection of recombinant platelet factor 4 |
| |     Intralesional injection of human chorionic gonadotropin |
| |     Intralesional injection of 9-*cis*-retinoic acid gel |
| |     Radiation therapy |
| | Chemotherapy |
| |     Recombinant interferon-$\alpha$2a |
| |     Recombinant interferon-$\alpha$2b |
| |     Etoposide |
| |     Teniposide |
| |     Vinblastine |
| |     Bleomycin |
| |     Doxorubicin |
| | Investigational |
| |     Synthetic retinoids |
| |     Thalidomide |
| |     Oral 9-cis-retinoic acid |
| |     Angiostatin |
| |     Endostatin |
| AIDS-related lymphoma | M-BACOD |
| |     Bleomycin |
| |     Doxorubicin |
| |     Cyclophosphamide |
| |     Vincristine sulfate |
| |     Dexamethasone |
| |     Methotrexate |
| |     Ara-C |
| |     Radiation therapy |
| |     Zidovudine |
| | m-BACOD |
| |     Methotrexate |
| |     Bleomycin |
| |     Doxorubicin |
| |     Cyclophosphamide |
| |     Vincristine |
| |     Dexamethasone |
| |     GM-CSF |
| |     Meningeal lymphoma prophylaxis |
| |     Pneumocystis prophylaxis |

*(continued)*

| Malignancy | Treatment |
|---|---|
| | CHOP |
| |   Cyclophosphamide |
| |   Doxorubicin |
| |   Vincristine |
| |   Prednisone |
| | Oral regimen |
| |   CCNU |
| |   Etoposide |
| |   Cyclophosphamide |
| |   Procarbazine |
| | Continuous infusion regimen |
| |   Cyclophosphamide |
| |   Doxorubicin |
| |   Etoposide |
| | ACVD dose-intensive chemotherapy regimen |
| |   Induction |
| |     Doxorubicin (Adriamycin) |
| |     Cyclophosphamide |
| |     Vindescine |
| |     Bleomycin |
| |     Prednisolone |
| |   Consolidation |
| |     Methotrexate |
| |     Folinic acid rescue |
| |     Ifosfamide |
| |     VP-16 |
| |     L-Asparaginase |
| |     Ara-C |
| | CNS prophylaxis |
| |   Methotrexate |
| | CNS treatment |
| |   Methotrexate |
| |   Radiation therapy |
| Cervical cancer | Cryotherapy |
| | Laser therapy |
| | Cone biopsy |
| | Loop excision |

Ara-C, cytosine arabinoside; CCNU, lomustine; CNS, central nervous system; GM-CSF, granulocyte-macrophage colony-stimulating factor; VP-16, vincristine, prednisone.

## Primary Central Nervous System Lymphoma

Primary central nervous system lymphoma (PCNSL) occurs in about 3% to 10% of AIDS cases (Roth, 1998) and is limited to the CNS. Most lesions are found in the cerebrum, but PCNSL may arise in the cerebellum, basal ganglia, and brainstem (Roth, 1998). Symptoms of PCNSL include headache, seizures, altered level of consciousness, focal neurologic abnormalities, weakness, confusion, lethargy, aphasia, and memory loss (Roth, 1998). Treatment for PCNSL includes radiation therapy and chemotherapy.

## Hodgkin's Lymphoma

Several large epidemiologic studies indicate that the risk for Hodgkin's lymphoma is significantly higher in persons with HIV/AIDS (Levine, 1996). Other studies report that there is no increased incidence of Hodgkin's lymphoma in HIV disease (Roth, 1998). The incidence of Hodgkin's lymphoma is higher in male intravenous drug users (Levine, 1996). Hodgkin's lymphoma occurs early in the course of HIV disease, when the CD4+ cell count is relatively high and other AIDS-defining illness have not appeared. Mediastinal involvement is less common in immunocompromised patients. B-cell symptoms such as generalized lymphadenopathy, fever, weight loss, and nocturnal sweats are frequent in HIV-infected patients. Histologic studies of immunocompromised patients reveal the predominance of type III mixed cellularity (presence of the EBV in Reed-Sternberg cells). Hodgkin's lymphoma often is widely disseminated to extranodal sites, and the bone marrow is involved in about 40% to 50% of patients (Levine, 1996; Roth, 1998). Immunodeficiency, antiretroviral treatments, and poor hematologic tolerance of chemotherapy often hampers disease management and may contribute to the development of other AIDS-related illnesses. Current therapeutic approaches often obtain complete remission; however, some deaths still are related to the disease progressing to AIDS (Costello et al., 1998).

## Cervical Cancer

Invasive cancer of the cervix is considered to be an AIDS-defining condition. HIV-mediated immunodeficiency predisposes individuals to both cervical intraepithelial neoplasia (CIN) and invasive cervical cancer. The risk of developing precancerous or cancerous cervical lesions is 7 to 10 times greater for an HIV-infected woman (Daley, 1998; Kuhn et al., 1999). Cervical cancer in women with AIDS progresses more rapidly and is less responsive to treatment than in HIV-negative women.

Human papillomavirus (HPV) is thought to be the viral carcinogen associated with both squamous cell neoplasia of the cervix and CIN (Maiman, 1997). More than 70 strains of HPV exist (Daley, 1998). Although HPV produces warts on the hands, feet, and knees, the most common form of HPV is genital warts (Daley, 1998). Human papillomavirus has a strong, causal relationship with cervical, penile, vulvar, anal, prostate, uterine, lung, esophageal, and laryngeal cancers (Daley, 1998). The most prevalent strain is HPV-16, which is associated with cervical cancer.

Risk factors for HPV infection and subsequent cervical cancer include early first intercourse, cigarette smoking, poor nutrition, multiple sex partners, and oral contraceptives (Daley, 1998). It has been estimated that 15% to 16% of women with genital warts will progress to cervical neoplasia within 9 years (Murthy et al., 1990; Syrjanen et al., 1990). The rate of progression is greater in HIV-infected women.

Cervical cancer often is diagnosed based on the morphologic features of the cells obtained from a cervical smear known as the Papanicolaou (Pap) smear. Cervical cancer occurs primarily in the transformational zone of the cervix. The transformational zone contains columnar epithelium and squamous epithelium. Cells in these tissues turnover rapidly, making them more susceptible to genetic mutations and carcinogenesis.

Unfortunately, the symptoms of cervical cancer do not become apparent to a woman until the later stages of the disease. Patients who complain of bleeding during or after intercourse, painful intercourse, watery discharge, foul-smelling discharge, or genital warts should be screened with a Pap smear. The stages of cervical cancer range from stage 0 (carcinoma in situ) to IVB (spread to distant organs) (Nelson et al., 1989). Recommended diagnosis and treatment for CIN in HIV-positive women include colposcopy, cone biopsy with laser cone, or loop electrosurgical excision procedure, as well as meticulous posttherapy surveillance with liberal repeat colposcopy and aggressive treatment for persistent or recurrent disease (Maiman, 1997). To cure cervical cancer, a simple or total abdominal or radical hysterectomy can be performed (Maiman, 1997).

# COMMON PROBLEMS IN HIV DISEASE

## Neurologic Problems

HIV directly infects microglial/macrophage cells in the CNS and produces HIV encephalitis in as many as 50% of AIDS cases. HIV can produce inflammatory changes, demyelinization, and axonal damage (Bell, 1998). The CNS is the site of several opportunistic infections and malignancies. Medications used to treat HIV disease and its complications can produce neurologic symptoms (Rachlis, 1998).

### AIDS Dementia Complex

AIDS dementia complex (ADC) refers to the cognitive, motor, and behavioral dysfunction seen in advanced HIV disease. ADC is believed to result from direct infection of nervous tissue by HIV (Price et al., 1988a). As ADC progresses, the symptoms advance from mild impairment of attention and memory to a nearly vegetative state (Price et al., 1988b). Symptoms of ADC include poor concentration, decreased memory, slower thinking, poor balance, incoordination, apathy, and irritability (Price, 1997). The most effective treatment for ADC is to suppress HIV replication by HAART (Filippi et al., 1998). Two other drugs that have been used experimentally to treat ADC are the calcium channel blocker, nimodipine, and the $N$-methyl-D-aspartate receptor inhibitor, memantine (Price, 1997).

## Progressive Multifocal Leukoencephalopathy

Progressive multifocal leukoencephalopathy (PML) is caused by a papovavirus, the JC virus. Sixty to eighty percent of adults throughout the world have been exposed to JC virus. Progressive multifocal leukoencephalopathy develops in about 3% to 4% of AIDS cases and results from reactivation of a latent JC virus infection. Characteristics of PML include focal neurologic changes such as dementia, aphasia, apraxia, visual deficits, and cranial nerve deficits. Magnetic resonance imaging is needed to detect the pathophysiologic changes of PML, which include demyelination from death of the oligodendrocytes (myelin-forming cells in the CNS) and loss of tissue (Price, 1999). No specific therapies for PML exist; however, improvement of symptoms has been reported after the initiation of HAART. Cytosine arabinoside, cidofovir, and topotecan have been tested for PML, but their effectiveness in treating PML has not been documented (Price, 1999).

## Peripheral Neuropathy

Peripheral neuropathy is the most common neurologic manifestation of HIV disease. Peripheral neuropathy manifests as paresthesia, numbness, or pain that usually begins in the toes and advances proximally. Peripheral neuropathy may result from direct HIV infection or may be a side effect of antiretroviral therapy. Tricyclic antidepressants, such as amitriptyline, have been used to relieve the symptoms of peripheral neuropathy.

## Myelopathy

Myelopathy refers to any pathologic condition of the spinal cord. Myelopathies are categorized as acute/subacute or as chronic/progressive. Three of the most common conditions that cause acute/subacute transverse myelopathy in HIV/AIDS are VZV infection, lymphoma, and toxoplasmosis.

Polyradiculopathy refers to any disorder of the spinal nerve roots or peripheral nerves. Cytomegalovirus infection may affect the spinal cord and produce polyradiculopathy. CMV polyradiculopathy is characterized by lower extremity weakness, spasticity, areflexia, urinary retention, and hypoesthesia (Drew et al., 1997). Vacuolar myelopathy, the most common type of chronic/progressive myelopathy, is characterized by cognitive dysfunction, upper extremity dysfunction, gait disturbance with ataxia and spasticity, and bowel and bladder dysfunction. Another type of chronic/progressive myelopathy is caused by coinfection with human T-cell lymphotropic virus type I (HTLV-I). Clinically, this type of myelopathy mimics vacuolar myelopathy. Coinfection with HTLV-I is seen primarily in intravenous drug users and their sexual partners.

## Meningitis

The most common cause of meningitis in HIV disease is *C. neoformans*. The person with cryptococcal meningitis may present with headache, photophobia, nausea, vomiting, and confusion (Price, 1997). The course of HIV meningitis ranges from a mild headache to hydrocephalus, cranial nerve palsies, or severe disability. Cryptococcal meningitis is treated with amphotericin B, flucytosine, fluconazole, and itraconazole. Other less common causes of meningitis include TB, syphilis, histoplasmosis, coccidioidomycosis, and lymphoma.

## Encephalitis

Inflammation of brain parenchymal cells may lead to either focal symptoms or diffuse symptoms of encephalitis. *T. gondii*, CMV, HSV-1 and HSV-2 are among the most common causes of encephalitis. Other less common conditions leading to encephalitis include TB, histoplasmosis, and coccidioidomycosis. Clinical manifestations of encephalitis include impaired cognition, decreased alertness, and changes in motor function from diffuse cerebral dysfunction. *T. gondii* usually produces focal neurologic symptoms from large abscesses but may present as encephalitis when numerous, smaller, more diffuse abscesses are present. Cytomegalovirus infection of brain is common in persons with AIDS; however, CMV is thought to be a minor contributor to neurologic dysfunction. In a few patients, CMV encephalitis results in decreased alertness, confusion, and seizures. Two drugs used to treat CMV infections are ganciclovir and foscarnet, but their efficacy has not been well established. Infection with HSV-1 and HSV-2 may result in focal encephalopathy or diffuse encephalopathy.

Other organisms that threaten vision are herpes simplex, VZV, *T. gondii*, *M. avium-intracellulare*, *Treponema pallidum*, *P. carinii,* and various fungi (Ah-Fat et al., 1997).

## Hematologic Problems

### Anemia

Anemia is characteristic of HIV/AIDS (Spivak et al., 1989), and it is more common in women with HIV disease (Means, 1997; Zon et al., 1988). As many as 66% to 85% of persons who have progressed to AIDS have some degree of anemia (Hambleton, 1996). As HIV disease progresses, the number of circulating erythrocytes decreases (Arevalo et al., 1997). HIV-related anemia is associated with decreased survival time (Moore et al., 1998).

The major etiology of anemia in HIV disease is impaired erythropoiesis (Coyle, 1997). Inappropriate secretion of IL-1$\beta$, TNF-$\alpha$, and the interferons may inhibit erythropoiesis. Opportunistic organisms (ie, B19 Parvovirus, *M. avium-intracellulare*, *M. tuberculare, H. capsulatum, C. neoformans, C. immitis*, CMV, and *P. carinii*) may infiltrate the bone marrow. Lymphomas can infiltrate the bone marrow (Viele, 1998) and suppress erythropoiesis (Mitsuyasu, 1999). Several drugs used to combat HIV and its complications may contribute to the anemia that is seen (Aboulafia, 1997). It has been demonstrated that iron metabolism is altered in HIV disease. Serum iron has been found to be lower and serum ferritin to be higher in an experimental group of HIV-infected subjects than in a healthy control group (Arevalo et al., 1997). Vitamin $B_{12}$ deficiency anemia sometimes is encountered in the care of the HIV-infected patient, and it responds well to the administration of vitamin $B_{12}$ (Aboulafia et al., 1991). Less commonly, folate deficiency anemia is seen in HIV disease (Kreuzer et al., 1997), which responds to oral administration of folic acid. Antibody-mediated hemolytic anemia is rare in HIV disease (Mitsuyasu, 1999). Anemia from blood loss may result from opportunistic infections and malignancies of the GI system (Mitsuyasu, 1999).

The typical anemia seen in HIV disease is the anemia of chronic illness. In the anemia of chronic illness and the anemia of HIV disease, there is an impaired erythropoietin response, but red blood cell production responds to administration of erythropoietin; erythrocyte progenitor cells are reduced; and iron metabolism is altered (Means, Jr., 1997).

Anemia in HIV disease typically is normocytic (mean corpuscular volume is normal) and normochromic (mean corpuscular hemoglobin and mean corpuscular hemoglobin concentration are normal). Reticulocytopenia is commonly observed (Kreuzer et al., 1997; Mitsuyasu, 1999). Low erythropoietin levels are found, and serum ferritin in HIV disease is even higher than that seen in the anemia of chronic illness (Arevalo et al., 1997; Kreuzer et al., 1997). Ideally, the hemoglobin should be kept greater than 10/dL. Transfusions are given when the hemoglobin falls below 8.0 g/dL (Viele, 1998); however, HIV disease progresses more rapidly after transfusion as a result of increased HIV expression or immunosuppression (Groopman, 1997).

### Thrombocytopenia

Thrombocytopenia is seen in 30% to 60% of HIV-infected patients (Abrams et al., 1986; Stricker, 1991). Thrombocytopenia results from bone marrow suppression, direct infection of megakaryocytes (Zauli et al., 1991), immune destruction of platelets (Dominguez et al., 1994), and nonimmune (ie, fever) destruction of platelets (Mitsuyasu, 1999). Immune destruction of platelets is the most common cause of thrombocytopenia in HIV disease. In HIV disease, platelets are coated with antibodies (Louache et al., 1991). Molecules of gp160/gp120 are similar to those on platelet membranes, and this may allow the host immune system to see platelets as foreign (Dominguez et al., 1994). HIV-associated thrombocytopenia is characterized by petechiae, ecchymosis, epistaxis, and occult blood in the stool. Significant hemorrhage is rare in HIV disease (Stricker, 1991). Zidovudine (Oksenhendler et al., 1989), corticosteroids (Stricker, 1991), immunoglobulin therapy (Yap et al., 1991), and splenectomy (Oksenhendler et al., 1993) are the most common modalities of treatment used successfully to treat the thrombocytopenia of HIV disease.

### Neutropenia

As many as 75% of people with advanced HIV infection exhibit neutropenia (Zon et al., 1988). The drugs used to treat HIV are the most common causes of neutropenia in HIV disease. Other causes for neutropenia are impaired myelopoiesis and deficient granulocyte colony stimulating factor (Mauss et al., 1997). Number and function of neutrophils decrease (Murphy et al., 1988). Neutropenia puts the patient with advanced HIV disease at even greater risk.

## Wasting Syndrome

Most people with advanced AIDS experience malnutrition (Bell et al., 1997). Malnutrition appears in the early stages of HIV disease before weight loss, when there is an increase in the ratio of extracellular mass to body cell mass. Malnutrition in AIDS is related to increased morbidity and mortality (Dobs et al., 1996).

Wasting is defined as an unintentional weight loss greater than 10%. In the wasting syndrome, the individual loses overall body weight (as much as 30%) and lean muscle mass (Elbein, 1992). Lean body mass is lost, while at the same time, the body preserves fat stores (Balog et al., 1998). In acute infections and chronic inflammation, skeletal muscle and connective tissue protein stores are mobilized, and the free amino acids are used for gluconeogenesis (Moldawer et al., 1998). During this same period, protein loss through the GI system increases. Resting energy expenditure increases an average of 10% for men and women alike in the early stages of HIV infection (Grinspoon et al., 1998; Melchior, 1997) and typically rises to approximately 25% in advanced HIV infection. Opportunistic infections and malignancies affect the entire GI system, creating five major conditions that affect nutritional intake: pain, nausea, vomiting, diarrhea, and malabsorption of proteins, fats, carbohydrates, and micronutrients (Table 21-9). Opportunistic infections may increase the resting energy expenditure to as much as 29% to 34% above normal (Moldawer et al., 1998). Compensatory mechanisms seen during chronic disease, severe burns, or starvation are activated in the HIV wasting syndrome. These compensatory mechanisms include the following: decreased conversion of thyroxine (most abundant thyroid hormone) to triiodothyronine (most active thyroid hormone), decreased synthesis of insulin-like growth factor I (a second messenger of growth hormone), and hypogonadism (decreased testosterone production) (Moldawer et al., 1998). Although these changes are intended to facilitate adaptation, they may worsen the catabolic state. Low levels of serum testosterone precede the wasting syndrome (Dobs et al., 1996). Because testosterone normally stimulates the production of growth hormone and the synthesis of insulin-like growth factor, hypogonadism leads to diminished levels of these anabolic molecules (Moldawer et al., 1998). Insulin-like growth factor is needed to increase the activity of gonadotropin and to promote the conversion of testosterone to its most active form, dihydrotestosterone. Cytokines that produce cachexia in the AIDS wasting syndrome include IL-1, IL-6, TNF-α, IFN-α, and IFN-γ (Von Roenn & Mulligan, 1999). Secretion of these cytokines is elevated in early HIV infection and progressively increases over the course of the infection (Poli et al., 1995). The mechanism by which these cytokines produce cachexia has not been fully elucidated. However, IL-1 and TNF-α suppress the appetite, stimulate the production of insulin-like growth factor, and activate the hypothalamic-pituitary axis, which results in increased production of glucocorticoids in the earlier stages of HIV (Moldawer et al., 1998). Profound cortisol deficiency can be seen in advanced HIV disease (Villette et al., 1990; Wilson et al., 1996). Hypercortisolemia is characteristic of HIV disease, producing muscle wasting and hyperglycemia (Coodley et al., 1994). Notice that hypocortisolemia complicates the later stages of AIDS (Abbott et al., 1995). Drugs used to treat the wasting syndrome include the following: HAART, anabolic steroids (testosterone, oxandrolone, oxymetholone, nandrolone, and recombinant growth hormone), appetite stimulants (megestrol acetate and dronabinol), and cytokine antagonists (thalidomide) (Von Roenn & Mulligan, 1999) (see Table 21-9).

## HIV DISEASE IN WOMEN

In many regards, women's experience of HIV/AIDS is the same as that of men. In many other ways, it is different. The incidence of AIDS is increasing the most in women and, in particular, among young women (CDC, 1998). Many women with HIV disease have long histories of physical, sexual, and emotional abuse and often need treatment for addiction. In addition to their battle with HIV disease, they often are the primary caretakers of their families.

In women, recurrent bacterial infections appear at higher CD4+ cell counts than in men and may provide the presenting symptoms for HIV infection. *S. pneumoniae* and *H. influenzae* are frequent etiologies of bacterial pneumonia in HIV-infected women.

Women infected with HIV are more prone to squamous intraepithelial lesions than HIV-seronegative women, and the lesions are more severe, more extensive, and more progressive. Pelvic inflammatory disease is more prevalent in HIV-infected women, and HIV-infected women

**TABLE 21.9**

## Conditions Associated With AIDS Wasting Syndrome

| Area of GI Tract | Condition | Effect on Nutrition |
|---|---|---|
| Mouth | Herpes simplex | Altered taste |
| | Cytomegalovirus | Pain and difficulty chewing |
| | *Candida albicans* | |
| | Kaposi's sarcoma | |
| Esophagus | *Candida albicans* infection | Dysphagia |
| | Kaposi's sarcoma | Odynophagia |
| Intestines | Bacteria | Diarrhea |
| |    *Campylobacter* | Abdominal pain |
| |    *Salmonella* | Malabsorption |
| |    *Shigella* | Steatorrhea |
| |    *Mycobacterium-avium intracellulare* | Hypermetabolism |
| |    *Escherichia coli* | Villus atrophy |
| | Viruses | |
| |    Cytomegalovirus | |
| |    HIV | |
| | Amebae | |
| |    *Entamoeba histolytica* | |
| | Flagellata | |
| |    *Giardia lamblia* | |
| | Coccidia | |
| |    *Isospora belli* | |
| |    *Cryptosporidium parvum* | |
| | Microsporidia | |
| |    *Enterocytozoon bieneusi* | |
| |    *Septata inestinalis* | |
| | Fungal | |
| |    *Histoplasma capsulatum* | |

GI, gastrointestinal.
(From Dolin, R., Masur, H., & Saag, M. [1999]. *AIDS therapy*. New York: Churchill Livingstone; Maiman, M. [1997]. Management of cervical neoplasia in HIV-positive women. In D. Cotton & D.H. Watts [Eds.], The medical management of AIDS in women [pp. 221–234]. New York: Wiley-Liss; and Saleh, M.N. & Scadden, D.T. [1999]. Non-Hodgkin lymphoma. In R. Dolin, H. Masur, & M. Saag [Eds.], *AIDS therapy* [pp. 592–603]. New York: Churchill Livingstone.)

● **Case Study 21.1**

The following case study exemplifies the pathophysiologic processes in the wasting syndrome associated with HIV/AIDS. It illustrates the importance of a holistic approach in assessing any individual with a chronic illness. This case study includes past medical history, a review of systems, and current clinical data.

David is a 38-year-old white, bisexual male, who works part time at a local AIDS support group. It has been 3 years since he first learned of his HIV infection. Since his last visit to the nurse practitioner 3 months ago, David has lost 18 lb. David's chief complaints are "difficulty swallowing" and "frequent diarrhea." He states that he has no appetite since he began a new regimen of antiretroviral therapy.

## History

### Past Medical History

| | |
|---|---|
| General state of health | Client states that although he has had AIDS for 3 years his health has been generally good except for the last 6 months |
| Allergies | No known drug allergies |
| Current medications | AZT, delavirdine, ritonavir, amitryptyline, Xanax |
| Surgeries | Tonsillectomy & adenoidectomy, age 6, no complications |
| Injury/Trauma | Fell from a tree at age 15 and fractured his right wrist |
| Childhood illnesses | Chickenpox, measles, unsure of immunization history, reports being healthy as a child; received tetanus in 1995, receives annual influenza vaccine |
| Adult illnesses | History of kidney stone at age 33; passed without surgical intervention |
| Psychiatric illnesses | None |

### Social History

| | |
|---|---|
| Marital status | Unmarried, partnered, continues to have unprotected receptive anal intercourse |
| Tobacco | 2 ppd × 17 years; denies marijuana use or dipping |
| Alcohol | Social drinker 1–2 beers on the weekend. Denies hard liquor |
| Social drugs | Admits to use of marijuana as a college student. States that he has not used any recreational drugs since that time |
| Exercise | Sedentary lifestyle due to chronic fatigue. Enjoys television and reading. Rises at 10 AM; retires 10–11 PM. No difficulty in getting to sleep or resting through the night. Requires a daily nap of 1–2 hours |
| Employment | Works 20 hours/week as a receptionist at the local AIDS support organization. States that he enjoys his relatively low-stress job |

*(Case study continued on page 436)*

*Family History*

| | |
|---|---|
| Father | Deceased, sudden death at age 58 |
| Mother | 60 years old, suffers from angina pectoris, history of MI at age 56 |
| Sister | Sister is in good health |

*24-Hour Recall*

| | |
|---|---|
| Breakfast | Coffee and 2 soft scrambled eggs |
| Lunch | Chocolate milkshake |
| Dinner | Mashed potatoes and green peas with ice cream for dessert |

## Review of Systems

| | |
|---|---|
| General | Weight has been relatively stable over his life, maximum weight 185 lb, minimum weight 132 lb; height 5'10"; normal ideal weight: 160 lb; current actual weight: 132 lb. Currently, he complains of difficulty swallowing, fatigue and diarrhea |
| Skin | Reports rashes on face chest and back |
| HEENT | Eyes: Wears contact lenses, annual eye examination 6 months ago, no report of redness or pain. Ears: No difficulty hearing, denies tinnitus, vertigo, or history of infections. Nose & sinuses: Denies nosebleeds, reports 1–2 sinus infections per year. Mouth & throat: Frequent sore throats about once every month. Reports redness and pain of the oral cavity and tongue. Dentitia is good. Receives bi-annual dental cleanings |
| Neck | "Swollen glands" in the neck, no pain or stiffness |
| Breasts | Denies lumps, pain, or nipple discharge |
| Lungs | Complains of shortness of breath upon exertion; history of *Pneumocystis carinii* pneumonia 3 months ago, antiretroviral therapy was started at that time and was treated with pentamadine during his hospital stay. He remains on maintenance TMP-SMX therapy. Denies cough, sputum, hemoptysis or wheezing at present. Is unaware of any exposure to TB. Last chest film: 02/99 |
| CV | Denies any heart trouble, HTN, rheumatic fever, heart murmers, chest pain, or palpitations. Has already reported dyspnea with increased activity. No orthopnea. Denies any lower extremity swelling |
| GI | Trouble swallowing × 1 month because of inflammation of oral cavity. His appetite has gradually decreased as his "stomach has shrunk." Complains of nausea or vomiting but reports increased amounts of watery brown stools about 2–3 times per day × 3 weeks. Denies any evidence of blood in his stool except for an occasional "bloody hemorrhoid aggravated by intercourse." No report of constipation, abdominal pain, or black tarry stools. No known history of jaundice, liver, or gallbladder trouble |

*(Case study continued on next page)*

| | |
|---|---|
| GU | Denies hernia, dysuria, urgency, or increase in frequency of urination. Has had "the clap," which he states cleared with medical treatment. Denies any discharge from or sores on the penis. Clearly describes his sexual preference to be "bisexual." No decrease in desire or satisfaction |
| PV | Denies any pain on walking, leg cramps, or varicosities |
| MS | Denies joint pain or swelling. No loss of range of motion from fracture of right arm. States right arm becomes stiff and painful in cold temperatures |
| Neurologic | Denies fainting, blackouts, seizures, paralysis or numbness. Admits to pain, weakness, and tingling of lower extremities |
| Hematologic | Iron deficiency anemia despite iron supplementation $\times$ 2 months. Denies bruising or bleeding. No report of past transfusions |
| Endocrine | No thyroid trouble, heat or cold intolerance, excessive sweating. States that he "stays thirsty." No excessive hunger, polyuria, or diabetes |
| Psychiatric | Has noticed that he continues to be irritable, nervous, and without energy. "The way I look makes me feel very depressed." No loss of short- or long-term memory |

## Physical Examination

| System | Findings |
|---|---|
| Vital signs | T-103.3°F P-102 R-20<br>BP-90/64<br>Height-5'10", Weight-132 lbs |
| General | Thin, relatively young, well-groomed man. Alert and oriented $\times$ 3 spheres. Appears anxious because of constant fidgeting and pacing. Does not appear in any distress |
| Skin | Skin is warm and dry with poor turgor. No lesions noted. Hair is coarse and dry but thick. No evidence of balding. Hands are diaphoretic with manicured nails |
| Head | Normocephalic, black, thick, coarse hair without balding. Face is clean and clear without evidence of acne |
| Eyes | Visual acuity is 20/20 with contact lenses. Normal visual fields. Normal sclera and conjuctivae. PERRLA. Funduscopic examination is normal without any evidence of vascular nicking, papilledema, or cotton wool spots |
| Ears | OD tempanic membrane obstructed with cerumen. OS tempanic membrane is intact. Rinne and Webber tests negative; hearing—normal |

*(Case study continued on page 438)*

| | |
|---|---|
| Nose & sinuses | Nasal bone structure is straight, nasal mucosa is pink, no deviation of the septum, no tenderness of frontal or maxillary sinuses |
| Mouth & pharynx | Oral pharynx is red and inflamed with cobblestone appearance. White patchy areas present on the buccal mucosa and tongue. Bluish brown lesions of the oral mucosa. Teeth and gums are well cared for without decay. Mucous membranes dry and sticky. Increased furrowing of tongue noted |
| Neck | Palpable preauricular cervical nodes. No carotid bruit. Neck size 16. Thyroid gland not palpable |
| Back | Spine with normal curvature. No costovertebral angle tenderness |
| Lungs | Clear to auscultation and percussion |
| Breasts | Breasts are flat without palpable masses or nodules. No signs of inflammation or discharge from either nipple. Axillary region is free of lymphadenopathy. No evidence of epitrochlear nodes |
| CV | Normal $S_1$, $S_2$. No rubs, clicks, or murmers. Apical pulse, 82 |
| Abdomen | Flat, scaphoid abdomen, no evidence of hernia. Hyperactive bowel sounds in all 4 quadrants. Soft, nontender, without any palpable masses. Normal liver span. Unable to palpate the spleen. No CVA tenderness |
| GU | Noncircumcised; no visible lesions, discharge. Testicles descended bilaterally without masses. Slight hypospadias. No inguinal hernias |
| Rectal | Anus reveals large external hemorrhoids. Normal sphincter tone with nonpalpable prostate gland. Occult blood sample is negative |
| Extremities | Palpable brachial, radial and ulnar pulses in upper extremities. Lower extremities reveal palpable femoral, popliteal, posterior tibial and pedal pulses. No evidence of varicosities or edema |
| MS | Normal curvature of spine, no loss of range motion in lower or upper extremities. Gait it is normal with correct alignment of legs and feet |
| Neurologic | Normal sensory is intact without evidence of pain. DTRs 5+ in upper and lower extremities. Romberg is negative |
| Mental status | Cognitive function is intact. Ability to subtract serial 7s is remarkable |

## Laboratory Studies

| Test |
|---|
| CBC |
| SMA-7 (serum electrolytes, glucose, BUN, creatinine) |
| CD4+ T-cell count |
| HIV-RNA viral load |

*(Case study continued on next page)*

Total serum protein
Serum albumin
Cholesterol
Triglycerides
Stool for *Clostridium difficile* toxin, culture, blood, ova and parasites
Stool for *Cryptosporidium muris*
D-Xylose absorption study
Endoscopy with biopsy

## Impression

Wasting syndrome:
   Diarrhea—rule out protozoal infection
   White patchy areas in oral cavity—rule out oral or systemic candidiasis
   Weight loss—rule out malnutrition

## Discussion

David has HIV-related wasting syndrome and is experiencing a constellation of symptoms that contribute to wasting: anorexia, oral and esophageal candidiasis, oral Kaposi's sarcoma, nausea, vomiting, diarrhea, fever, difficulty chewing, difficulty swallowing, and fatigue. These symptoms lead to decreased intake of nutrients, malabsorption, and increased metabolism. Because of his wasting, he is at risk for decreased cell-mediated immunity and increased incidence of opportunistic infections.

A full history and physical examination is imperative for this patient. A complete food history is required, including food preferences and intolerances, special dietary needs, use of nutritional supplements, and economic constraints. Anthropometric measurements should be taken.

Because of his wasting syndrome, antiretroviral therapy, and other factors, David is at risk for anemia. His hemoglobin and hematocrit should be assessed at least every 6 months. Other nutritional parameters are serum albumin, cholesterol, triglycerides, and total lymphocyte counts. Fecal fat and lactose intolerance should be measured to assess malabsorption.

David has oral and esophageal candidiasis and needs antifungal therapy. Intravenous amphotericin B will be administered in the acute phase. Then, he will be switched to oral diflucan.

David should receive 3000 to 3500 kilocalories per day with a high protein content and should take a daily multivitamin. Although oral nutrition is preferable, David is too weak to maintain oral nutrition; therefore, a nasogastric feeding tube needs to be placed. Because he is experiencing malabsorption, David will be given a liquid, high-protein supplement that contains free amino acids. David exhibits signs of hypertonic dehydration, which can be further assessed from his SMA-7. Rehydration with a hypotonic solution will be necessary. It is important to give him free water with his hypertonic enteral fluids.

When his condition improves, David will be switched to an oral, high-protein diet with frequent feedings and nutritional supplementation. Instructions will be given to help David increase protein and caloric intake. Food safety instructions will be given.

*(Case study continued on page 440)*

A variety of pharmacologic agents are available to improve David's nutritional status. These include appetite stimulants, anticytokines to inhibit the anorectic effects of TNF, IL-1, IL-6, interferons, metabolic inhibitors, antioxidants, growth hormone, and the androgens. Because antiretroviral therapy is strongly associated with hypercholesterolemia and hypertriglyceridemia, these parameters are being assessed. If they are elevated, a lipid-lowering drug will be initiated.

David's care is complex and requires intense intervention. David requires intervention in the physiologic, psychological, and social domains.

AZT, zidovudine; BP, blood pressure; BUN, blood urea nitrogen; CBC, complete blood count; CV, cardiovascular; CVA, costovertebral angle; DTRs, deep tendon reflexes; GI, gastrointestinal; GU genitourinary; HEENT, head, eyes, ears, nose, and throat; HTN, hypertension; IL, interleukin; MS, musculoskeletal; OD, right eye; OS, left eye; P, pulse; ppd, packs per day; PERRLA, pupils even, round, regular to light accommodation; PV, peripherovascular; R, respiration; T, temperature; TB, tuberculosis; TMP-SMZ, trimethoprim-sulfamethoxazole; TNF, tumor necrosis factor.

with pelvic inflammatory disease have greater incidence of endometritis, fever, pelvic masses, and abdominal tenderness. *Candida* vulvovaginitis is recognized as an AIDS-defining illness and is the most common presenting complaint (Carpenter et al., 1991). HPV causes a variety of skin and genital lesions, most notably genital warts (Vermund, 1997). A strong association between cervical (Schiffman, 1994) and anal cancer (Northfelt et al., 1996) and HPV has been demonstrated.

Survival has been demonstrated to be significantly shorter in HIV-infected women than in HIV-infected men. With the advent of HAART, gender differences in survival are not significantly different for those receiving combination antiretroviral therapy.

Pregnancy is a major concern in planning the treatment for an HIV-infected woman. Pregnancy does not accelerate the progression of HIV disease or adversely affect fetal development. Antiretroviral therapy is necessary to reduce the risk of transmission of HIV to the infant. Because HIV can be transmitted through breast milk, breast-feeding should be discouraged in women who have the resources to bottle feed the infant. In developing nations, malnutrition and diarrhea may pose greater risks to the infant's survival than breast-feeding.

## HIV DISEASE IN INFANTS AND CHILDREN

In children, HIV disease differs in several ways. Because maternal IgG persists in the newborn, all infants born to an HIV-infected mother are seropositive at birth, whether or not the infant is infected. Antibody tests such as the ELISA and WBA cannot be used to confirm HIV infection until the baby is 18 months of age. In children, every organ is affected by HIV infection. The signs and symptoms of HIV disease are different and include lymphadenopathy, hepatomegaly, splenomegaly, parotitis, recurrent diarrhea, failure to thrive, and recurrent fevers. Recurrent bacterial infections occur in early HIV disease in children as a result of humoral immune dysfunction. Later, opportunistic infections occur, related to cellular immune dysfunction (Grubman et al., 1998).

Lymphoid interstitial pneumonitis (LIP) is an AIDS-defining condition that occurs in more than 25% of children who are HIV infected. LIP may result from coinfection with HIV and EBV. In LIP, lymphocytes infiltrate the interstitium of lung tissue. This condition may lead to chronic bronchiectasis and hypoxemic respiratory failure. Treatment includes antimicrobial therapy and corticosteroids (Grubman et al., 1998).

### Bacterial Infections

Children experience recurrent bacterial infections of the skin, respiratory system, GI tract, and blood at a greater rate than do adults. Staphylococcal and streptococcal infections result in a high incidence of cellulitis, abscess, otitis media, chronic sinusitis, and pneumonia. In children, *M. avium-intracellulare* most commonly affects the GI tract.

### Fungal Infections

*Coccidioides immitis* and *H. capsulatum* are fungi that rarely cause infection in children. *P. carinii* pneumonia has a more virulent onset and more rapid progression in HIV-infected children than is seen in HIV-infected adults. Candidiasis generally is localized but may disseminate in some instances. Symptoms of oral and esophageal candidiasis such as dysphagia, odynophagia, and altered taste may result in malnutrition and dehydration. *C. neoformans* infection is seen less frequently in HIV-infected children than HIV-infected adults but may produce a life-threatening meningoencephalitis.

## Viral Infections

In adults, CMV disease results from reactivation of a latent CMV infection. children infected with HIV are more likely to get CMV disease by primary infection. CMV disease may cause retinitis, enteritis, pneumonia, or hepatitis in HIV-infected children. In HIV-infected children, HSV-1 infection most commonly causes gingivostomatitis, esophagitis, encephalitis, or pneumonia.

## Protozoal Infections

*Toxoplasma gondii* and *Cryptosporidium muris* are two protozoa that are particularly problematic for HIV-infected children. *Toxoplasma gondii* may be transmitted congenitally or horizontally (from ingestion of undercooked meat or contact with cats). Toxoplasmosis generally results from reactivation of a latent infection in an immunocompromised host. The most common presentation of toxoplasmosis is encephalitis. Signs and symptoms of toxoplasmosis encephalitis are fever, altered level of consciousness, focal neurologic abnormalities, cranial nerve palsies, and sensory deficits. *C. muris* infection most commonly produces a profuse, watery diarrhea.

## Opportunistic Malignancies

Opportunistic malignancies are not as frequent in HIV-infected children as they are in adults. Kaposi's sarcoma is rarely seen. The most common types of malignancies are NHL, Burkitt's lymphoma, and smooth muscle tumors. Lymphomas in children are manifested by lymphadenopathy, fever, night sweats, weight loss, hepatomegaly, splenomegaly, and pain. Primary CNS lymphoma is characterized by changes in level of consciousness, seizures, and focal neurologic deficits.

Diarrhea and vomiting are symptoms requiring urgent care in HIV-infected infants and children. Organisms such as CMV, *C. muris*, *M. avium-intracellulare*, and *G. lamblia* are frequent etiologies of diarrhea and vomiting in children with HIV/AIDS.

## VACCINES FOR THE PREVENTION AND TREATMENT OF HIV INFECTION

Many variants exist for each of the two strains of HIV, HIV-1 and HIV-2. For HIV-1, six genetic groups (clades) have been identified based on genetic sequences of its envelope genes. Considerable genetic variation is evident in each of the six clades. Billions of new viruses may be formed each day in HIV-infected persons during certain periods of the disease progression. During rapid replication, the virus mutates at an accelerated rate. Serum from HIV-infected persons in one community may not be effective against HIV in another community. Preventive and therapeutic vaccines have been approved and are in stage III clinical trials. There is a theoretical basis for at least four types of vaccines.

### Active Acquired Immunity

In active acquired immunity, an individual is exposed to an antigen (live, attenuated, dead, or portions of the antigen), or to molecules produced by the antigen, and subsequently develops antibodies to the antigen. The goal of this type of vaccination is to prevent HIV infection or disease (Lambert, 1997).

### Immunotherapy

Immunotherapy refers to interventions that produce or enhance immunity. The goals of this type of therapy are to reduce viral burden, to lessen infectivity, and to slow disease progression (Lambert, 1997).

### Perinatal Immunization

A therapeutic vaccine (passive) given to the mother at the time of delivery is not only therapeutic for the mother but may decrease the risk of HIV transmission from the mother to the infant. The goals of this type of vaccine are to reduce viral burden, lessen infectivity, slow disease progression, and to prevent transmission of HIV from the mother to the infant (Lambert, 1997).

### Passive Acquired Immunity

In passive acquired immunity, antibodies against a specific antigen are given. The goals of this type of immunity are to reduce viral burden, lessen infectivity, slow disease progression, and prevent transmission of HIV from the mother to the infant (Lambert, 1997).

The ideal HIV vaccine would be one that could be given to an HIV-seronegative person and that would completely eradicate the virus on exposure. A less ideal vaccine would be one that reduces HIV viral replication and destroys virally infected cells. The host must be able to mount a cellular and a humoral immune response to the antigen. The HIV-specific antibodies will need to develop. Several possibilities exist for the ways these antibodies may function. The antibodies may bind the antigen, activate complement mediated lysis, neutralize the antigen, prevent syncytium formation, or block HIV from binding to the gp120 receptor (Lambert, 1997).

Four major types of vaccines have been developed. Recombinant subunit vaccines have been developed using HIV's envelope proteins (gp160, gp120) (Gorse et al., 1999; Ratto-Kim et al., 1999) and other HIV proteins (p17, p24) (Anthony et al., 1999; Benson et al., 1999; Sarin et al., 1999). It is hoped that recombinant subunit vaccines, by imitating a complete virus, will induce an immune response that includes antibody production and proliferation and differentiation of cytotoxic T lymphocytes (Gonzalo et al., 1999; Hanke et al., 1999). A second type is recombinant live vaccine. In this type of vaccine, microorganisms are used to produce live subunits of HIV. These types of vaccines are hoped to induce the proliferation and differentiation of cytotoxic T lymphocytes (Dyer et al., 1999; Hanke et al., 1999). Whole, killed viruses have induced an immune response against simian immunodeficiency virus (Hayami et al., 1999). Whole, killed viruses pose a problem in humans in that there is the concern that all of the viruses have not been completely killed. Certain peptide sequences in the proteins of HIV have been demonstrated to be immunogenic (Howie et al., 1999; Sitz et al., 1999). It would be relatively inexpensive to combine a number of peptide sequences from various protein regions of HIV, from each of the six clades, and from a wide geographic area (Wagner et al., 1999). Another possibility is that by using recombinant technology, a live attenuated virus could be formed that lacks one of its structurally essential proteins. The danger exists that a noninfectious virus could mutate to a virulent one (Berkhout et al., 1999; Lambert, 1997). Many clinical trials for the safety and efficacy of preventive vaccines are under way. At this point, there are no vaccines to prevent or treat HIV infection.

## REFERENCES

Abbott, M., Khoo, S.H., Hammer, M.R., & Wilkins, E.G. (1995). Prevalence of cortisol deficiency in late HIV disease. *Journal of Infection, 31*, 1–4.

Aboulafia, D.M. (1997). Use of hematopoietic hormones for bone marrow defects in AIDS. *Oncology, 11* (12), 1827–1834, 1839, 1843–1844.

Aboulafia, D.M. (1998). Regression of acquired immunodeficiency syndrome-related pulmonary Kaposi's sarcoma after highly active antiretroviral therapy. *Mayo Clinic Proceedings, 73*(5), 439–443.

Aboulafia, D.M. & Mitsuyasu, R.T. (1991). Hematologic abnormalities in AIDS. *Oncology Clinics of North America, 5* (2), 195–214.

Abrams, D.I., Kiprov, D.D., Goedert, J.J., Samgadharan, M.G., Gallo, R.C., & Volberding, P.A. (1986). Antibodies to human T-lymphotropic virus type III and development of the acquired immunodeficiency syndrome in homosexual men presenting with immune thrombocytopenia. *Annals of Internal Medicine, 104* (1), 47–50.

Ah-Fat, F.G. & Batterbury, M. (1997). Ophthalmic complications of HIV/AIDS. *Postgraduate Medical Journal, 72* (854), 725–730.

Alexander, N.J. (1990). Sexual transmission of human immunodeficiency virus: Virus entry into the male and female genital tract. World Health Organization: Global Programme on Acquired Immune Deficiency Syndrome. *Fertility and Sterility, 54* (1), 1–18.

Ampel, N.M. (1996). Emerging disease issues and fungal pathogens associated with HIV infection. *Emerging Infectious Diseases, 2* (2), 109–116.

Anderson, R.M. (1996). The spread of HIV and sexual mixing patterns. In J. Mann & D. Tarantola (Eds.), *AIDS in the world: II* (pp. 71–86). New York: Oxford University Press.

Anthony, L.S., Wu, H., Sweet, H., Turnnir, C., Boux, L.J., & Mizzen, L.A. (1999). Priming of CD8+ CTL effector cells in mice by immunization with a stress protein–influenza virus nucleoprotein fusion molecule. *Vaccine, 17* (4), 373–383.

Arevalo, V.A., Mateo, R.F., Sanchez, P.M., Alonso, C., Perez, A.J., & Fuertes, M.A. (1997). Iron metabolism in patient infected by human immunodeficiency virus type 1. *Sangre, 42* (5), 345–349.

Arribas, J.R., Storch, G.A., Clifford, D.B., & Tselis, A.C. (1996). Cytomegalovirus encephalitis. *Annals of Internal Medicine, 125* (7), 577–587.

Asmuth, D.M., DeGirolami, P.C., Federman, M., Ezratty, C.R., Pleskow, D.K., Desai, G., & Wanke, C.A. (1994). Clinical features of microsporidiosis in patients with AIDS. *Clinical Infectious Diseases, 18*, 819–825.

Balog, D.L., Epstein, M.E., & Amodio-Groton, M.I. (1998). HIV wasting syndrome: Treatment update. *Annals of Pharmacotherapy, 32* (4), 446–458.

Barnes, P.F., Yang, Z., Pogoda, J.M., Preston-Martin, S., Jones, B.E., Otaya, M., Knowles, L., Harvey, S., Eisenach, K.D., & Cave, M.D. (1999). Foci of tuberculosis transmission in central Los Angeles. *American Journal of Respiratory & Critical Care Medicine, 159* (4 Pt 1), 1081–1086.

Basgoz, N., & Schecter, G. (1997). *Mycobacterium tuberculosis* infection in HIV. In D. Cotton & D.H. Watts (Eds.), *The medical management of AIDS in women* (pp. 253–267). New York: Wiley-Liss.

Bell, J.E. (1998). The neuropathology of adult HIV infection. *Revue Neurologique, 154* (12), 816–829.

Bell, S.J., Bistrian, B.R., Connolly, C.A., & Forse, R.A. (1997). Body composition changes in patients with human immunodeficiency virus infection. *Nutrition, 13* (7-8), 629–632.

Benson, E.M., Clarkson, J., Law, M., Marshall, P., Kelleher, A.D., Smith, D.E., Patou, G., Stewart, G.J., Cooper, D.A., & French, R.A. (1999). Therapeutic vaccination with p24-VLP and zidovudine augments HIV-specific cytotoxic T lymphocyte activity in asymptomatic HIV-infected individuals. *AIDS Research and Human Retroviruses, 15* (2), 105–113.

Berkhout, B., Verhoef, K., van Wamel, J.L., & Back, N.K. (1999). Genetic instability of live, attenuated human immunodeficiency virus type 1 vaccine strains. *Journal of Virology, 73* (2), 1138–1145.

Bernard, N.F., Yannakis, C.M., Lee, J.S., & Tsoukas, C.M. (1999). Human immunodeficiency virus (HIV)-specific cytotoxic T lymphocyte activity in HIV-exposed seronegative persons. *Journal of Infectious Diseases, 179* (3), 538–547.

Bonavida, B., Katz, J.D., & Gottlieb, M.S. (1986). Mechanism of defective NK cell activity in patients with acquired immunodeficiency syndrome (AIDS) and AIDS-related complex: I. Defective trigger on NK cells for NKCF production by target cells and partial restoration by IL-2. *Journal of Immunology, 137* (4), 1157–1163.

Braun, P., Kessler, H., Falk, L., Paul, D., Harris, J., Blaauw, B., & Landay, A. (1988). Monocyte functional studies in asymptomatic human immunodeficiency disease virus (HIV)–infected individuals. *Journal of Clinical Immunology, 8* (6), 486–494.

Carpenter, C.J.C., Mayer, K.H., Stein, M.D., Leibman, B.D., Fisher, A., & Fiore, T.C. (1991). Human immunodeficiency virus infection in North American women: Experience with 200 cases and a review of the literature. *Medicine, 70* (5), 307–325.

Casassus, P., Padrazzi, B., Lhote, F., & Jarrousse, B. (1997). Prevention of opportunistic infections in HIV seropositive patients: Prevention of bacterial infections. *Presse Medicale, 26* (7), 340–343.

Centers for Disease Control and Prevention. (1992). 1993 Revised classification system for HIV infection and expanded surveillance case definition for AIDS among adolescents and adults. *Morbidity and Mortality Week Report, 41* (RR-17), 1–19.

Centers for Disease Control. (1997a). Update: Trends in AIDS incidence—United States, 1996. *Morbidity and Mortality Weekly Report, 46* (37), 861–866.

Centers for Disease Control and Prevention. (1997b). 1997 USPHS/IDSA guidelines for the prevention of opportunistic infections in persons infected with human immunodeficiency virus. *Morbidity and Mortality Weekly Report, 46* (RR-12), 1–46.

Centers for Disease Control and Prevention. (1998). *HIV/AIDS surveillance report*. Atlanta: Centers for Disease Control and Prevention.

Chernoff, D.N. (1995). Human immunodeficiency virus disease and related opportunistic infections. In G.J. Lawlor, T.J. Fischer, & D.C. Adelman (Eds.), *Manual of allergy and immunology* (pp. 425–445). Boston: Little, Brown & Company.

Classen, C.N., Warren, R., Richardson, M., Hauman, J.H., Gie, R.P., Ellis, J.H., van, Helden, P.D., & Beyers, N. (1999). Impact of social interactions in the community on the transmission of tuberculosis in a high incidence area. *Thorax, 54* (2), 136–140.

Clerici, M. & Shearer, G.M. (1993). A $T_H1–T_H2$ switch is a critical step in the etiology of HIV infection. *Immunology Today, 14* (3), 107–111.

Coodley, G.O., Loveless, M.O., Nelson, H.D., & Coodley, M.K. (1994). Endocrine function in the HIV wasting syndrome. *Journal of Acquired Immune Deficiency Syndrome, 7*, 46–51.

Cooley, T.P., Hirschhorn, L.R., & O'Keane, J.C. (1996). Kaposi's sarcoma in women with AIDS. *AIDS, 10* (11), 1221–1225.

Cooper, D.A., Tindall, B., Wilson, E.J., Imrie, A.A., & Penny, R. (1999). Characterization of T lymphocyte responses during primary infection due to human immunodeficiency virus. *Journal of Infectious Diseases, 157* (5), 889–896.

Costello, R., Heuberger, L., Petit, N., Olive, D., & Gastaut, J.A. (1998). Hodgkin's disease in patients infected with the human immunodeficiency virus. *Revue de Medecine Interne, 19* (8), 558–564.

Coyle, T.E. (1997). Hematologic complications of human immunodeficiency virus infection and the acquired immunodeficiency syndrome. *Medical Clinics of North America, 81* (2), 449–470.

Daley, E.M. (1998). Clinical update on the role of HPV and cervical cancer. *Cancer Research, 21* (1), 31–35.

Dobs, A.S., Few, W.L., Blackman, M.R., Harman, S.M., Hoover, D.R., & Graham, N.M. (1996). Serum hormones in men with human immunodeficiency virus–associated wasting. *Journal of Clinical Endocrinology & Metabolism, 81* (11), 4108–4112.

Dolin, R., Masur, H., & Saag, M. (1999). *AIDS therapy*. New York: Churchill Livingstone.

Dominguez, A., Gamallo, G., Garcia, R., Lopez-Pastor, A., Pena, J.M., & Vazquez, J.J. (1994). Pathophysiology of HIV related thrombocytopenia: An analysis of 41 patients. *Journal of Clinical Pathology, 47*, 999–1003.

Drew, W.L., Stempien, M.J., & Erlich, K.S. (1997). Management of Herpesvirus infections (CMV, HSV, VZV). In M. Sande & P.A. Volberding (Eds.), *The medical management of AIDS* (pp. 381–398). Philadelphia: W.B. Saunders.

Dyer, W.B., Ogg, G.S., Demoitie, M.A., Jin, X., Geczy, A.F., Rowland-Jones, S.L., McMichael, A.J., Nixon, D.F., & Sullivan, J.S. (1999). Strong human immunodeficiency virus (HIV)–specific cytotoxic T-lymphocyte activity in Sydney Blood Bank Cohort patients infected with nef-defective HIV type 1. *Journal of Virology, 73* (1), 436–443.

Elbein, R.C. (1992). Nutritional assessment and management. In M.L. Galantino (Ed.), *Clinical assessment and treatment of HIV: Rehabilitation of a chronic illness* (pp. 43–63). Thorofare, NJ: SLACK.

European Collaborative Study. (1992). Risk factors for mother-to-child transmission of HIV-1. *Lancet, 339* (8800), 1007–1012.

Fahey, J., Taylor, J., Detels, R., Hofmann, B., Melmed, R., Nishanian, P., & Giorgi, J. (1990). The prognostic value of cellular and serologic markers in infection with human immunodeficiency virus type 1. *New England Journal of Medicine, 322*, 166–172.

Fahey, J.L. & Nishanian, P. (1997). Laboratory diagnosis and evaluation of HIV infection. In J.L. Fahey & D.S. Flemmig (Eds.), *AIDS/HIV reference guide for medical professionals* (pp. 75–95). Baltimore: Williams & Wilkins.

Ferri, R.S. (1999). HIV-related conditions: Focus on tuberculosis. *HIV Frontline* (37), 6

Fichtenbaum, C.J. (1999). Candidiasis. In R. Dolin, H. Masur, & M. Saag (Eds.), *AIDS therapy* (pp. 432–443). New York: Churchhill Livingstone.

Filippi, C.G., Sze, G., Farber, S.J., Shahmanesh, M., & Selwyn, P.A. (1998). Regression of HIV encephalopathy and basal ganglia signal intensity abnormality at MR imaging in patients with AIDS after the initiation of protease inhibitor therapy. *Radiology, 206* (2), 491–498.

Fischbach, F. (1996). *A manual of laboratory & diagnostic tests* (5th ed.). Philadelphia: J.B. Lippincott.

Flanigan, T.P. (1999). *Cryptosporidium, Isospora,* and *Cyclospora* infections. In R. Dolin, H. Masur, & M. Saag (Eds.), *AIDS therapy* (pp. 328–335). New York: Churchill Livingstone.

Flaskerud, J. & Ungvarski, P.J. (1999). Overview and update of HIV disease. In P.J. Ungvarski & J. Flaskerud (Eds.), *HIV/AIDS: A guide to primary care management* (pp. 1–25). Philadelphia: W.B. Saunders.

Flemmig, D.S. & Boyer, P.J.J. (1997). Safer sex. In J. Fahey & D.S. Flemmig (Eds.), *AIDS/HIV reference guide for medical professionals* (pp. 378–389). Baltimore: Williams & Wilkins.

French, A.L., Benator, D.A., & Gordon, F.M. (1997). Nontuberculosis *Mycobacterium* infections. *Medical Clinics of North America, 81* (2), 361–379.

Furrer, H., Egger, M., Opravil, M., Bernasconi, E., Hirschel, B., Battegay, M., Telenti, A., Vernazza, P.L., Rickenbach, M., Flepp, M., & Malinverni, R. (1999). Discontinuation of primary prophylaxis against *Pneumocystis carinii* pneumonia in HIV-1–infected adults treated with combination antiretroviral therapy: Swiss HIV Cohort Study. *New England Journal of Medicine, 340* (17), 1301–1306.

Gallo, R. (1988). HIV, the cause of AIDS: An overview on its biology, mechanisms of disease induction, and our attempts to control it. *Journal of Acquired Immune Deficiency Syndromes, 1* (6), 521–535.

Gartner, S., Markovits, P., Markovitz, D., Kaplan, M., Gallo, R., & Popovic, M. (1986). The role of mononuclear phagocytes in HTLV-III/LAV infection. *Science, 233* (4760), 215–218.

Goedert, J.J., Mendez, H., Drummond, J.E., Robert-Guroff, M., Minkoff, H.L., Holman, S., Stevens, R., Rubenstein, A., Blattner, W.A., & Willoughby, A. (1989). Mother-to-infant transmission of human immunodeficiency virus type 1: Association with prematurity or low anti-gp120. *Lancet, II,* 1351–1354.

Gonzalo, R.M., Rodriguez, D., Garcia-Sastre, A., Rodriguez, J.R., Palese, P., & Esteban, M. (1999). Enhanced CD8+ T cell response to HIV-1 env by combined immunization with influenza and vaccinia virus recombinants. *Vaccine, 17* (7-8), 887–892.

Gorse, G.J., Corey, L., Patel, G.B., Mandava, M., Hsieh, R.H., Matthews, T.J., Walker, M.C., McElrath, M.J., Berman, P.W., Eibl, M.M., & Belshe, R.B. (1999). HIV-1MN recombinant glycoprotein 160 vaccine–induced cellular and humoral immunity boosted by HIV-1MN recombinant glycoprotein 120 vaccine: National Institute of Allergy and Infectious Diseases AIDS Vaccine Evaluation Group. *AIDS Research and Human Retroviruses, 15* (2), 115–132.

Grinspoon, S., Corcoran, C., Miller, K., Wang, E., Hubbard, J., Schoenfeld, D., Anderson, E., Basgoz, N., & Klibanski, A. (1998). Determinants of increased energy expenditure in HIV-infected women. *American Journal of Clinical Nutrition, 68* (3), 720–725.

Groopman, J.E. (1997). Impact of transfusion on viral load in human immunodeficiency virus infection. *Seminars in Hematology, 34* (3 Suppl. 2), 27–33.

Grubman, S. & Oleske, J. (1998). HIV infection in infants, children, and adolescents. In G.P. Wormser (Ed.), *AIDS and other manifestations of HIV infection* (pp. 349–371). Philadelphia: Lippincott Williams & Wilkins.

Hambleton, J. (1996). Hematologic complications of HIV infection. *Oncology, 10* (5), 671–680.

Hanke, T., Neumann, V.C., Blanchard, T.J., Sweeney, P., Hill, A.V., Smith, G.L., & McMichael, A. (1999). Effective induction of HIV-specific CTL by multi-epitope using gene gun in a combined vaccination regime. *Vaccine, 17* (6), 589–596.

Havlir, D.V., Dube, M.P., & Sattler, F.R. (1996). Prophylaxis against disseminated *Mycobacterium avium* complex with weekly azithromycin, daily rifabutin, or both. *New England Journal of Medicine, 335* (6), 392–398.

Hayami, M., Igarashi, T., Kuwata, T., Ui, M., Haga, T., Ami, Y., Shinohara, K., & Honda, M. (1999). Gene-mutated HIV-1/SIV chimeric viruses as AIDS live attenuated vaccines for potential human use. *Leukemia, 13* (Suppl. 1), S42–S47.

Hayes, E.B., Matte, T.D., O'Brien, T.R., McKinley, T.W., Logsdon, G.S., Rose, J.B., Ungar, B.L., Word, D.M., Pinsky, P.F., Cummings, M.L., Wilson, M.A., Long, E.G., Hurwitz, E.S., & Juranek, D.D. (1989). Large community outbreak of cryptosporidiosis due to contamination of a filtered public water supply. *New England Journal of Medicine, 320* (21), 1372–1376.

Heller, H.M. (1997). Management of enteric protozoan infections. In D. Cotton & D.H. Watts (Eds.), *The medical management of AIDS in women* (pp. 367–377). New York: Wiley-Liss.

Hirsch, M.S. (1995). Herpes simplex virus. In G.L. Mandell, J.E. Bennett, & R. Dolin (Eds.), *Principles and practice of infectious diseases* (pp. 1336–1345). New York: Churchill Livingstone.

Howie, S.E., Fernandes, M.L., Heslop, I., Hewson, T.J., Cotton, G.J., Moore, M.J., Innes, D., Ramage, R., & Harrison, D.J. (1999). A functional, discontinuous HIV-1 gp120 C3/C4 domain–derived, branched, synthetic peptide that binds to CD4 and inhibits MIP-1alpha chemokine binding. *FASEB Journal, 13* (3), 503–511.

Hu, P.F., Hultin, L.E., Hultin, P., Hausner, M.A., Hirji, K., Jewett, A., Bonavida, B., Detels, R., & Giorgi, J.V. (1995). Natural killer cell immunodeficiency in HIV disease is manifest by profoundly decreased numbers of CD16+CD56+ cells and expansion of a population of CD16$^{\text{dim}}$ CD56− NK cells with low lytic activity. *Journal of Acquired Immune Deficiency Syndrome, 10* (3), 331–340.

Jacobson, M.A. (1997). Disseminated *Mycobacterium avium* complex and other bacterial infections. In M. Sande & P.A. Volberding (Eds.), *The medical management of AIDS* (pp. 301–310). Philadelphia: W.B. Saunders.

Jones, J.L., Hanson, D.L., Dworkin, M.S., Alderton, D.L., Fleming, P.L., Kaplan, J.E., & Ward, J. (1999). Surveillance for AIDS-defining opportunistic illnesses, 1992–1997. *Morbidity and Mortality Weekly Report, 48* (SS-2), 1–22.

Katsufrakis, P.J., & Daar, E.S. (1997). HIV/AIDS assessment, testing, and natural history. *Primary Care: Clinics in Office Practice, 24* (3), 479–496.

Katzenstein, D.A. & Jordan, M.C. (1994). Herpes virus infection (Herpes simplex virus, varicella zoster virus, cytomegalovirus, Epstein-Barr virus). In J.H. Stein, J.J. Hutton, P. Kohler, R.A. O'Rourke, H.Y. Reynolds, M.A. Samuels, M.A. Sande, J.S. Trier, & N.J. Zvaifler (Eds.), *Internal medicine* (pp. 2035–2045). St. Louis: Mosby.

Kirkland, T.N. & Fierer, J. (1996). Coccidiodomycosis: A reemerging infectious disease. *Emerging Infectious Diseases, 2* (3), 192–199.

Kreuzer, K.A. & Rockstroh, J.K. (1997). Pathogenesis and pathophysiology of anemia in HIV infection. *Annals of Hematology, 75* (5-6), 179–187.

Kuhn, L., Sun, X.W., & Wright, T.C., Jr. (1999). Human immunodeficiency virus infection and female lower genital tract malignancy. *Current Opinion in Obstetrics and Gynecology, 11* (1), 35–39.

Lackritz, E.M. (1998). Prevention of HIV transmission by blood transfusion in the developing world: Achievements and continuing challenges. *AIDS, 12* (Suppl. A), S81–S86.

Lambert, J.S. (1997). Preventive and therapeutic HIV-1 vaccines. In D. Cotton & D.H. Watts (Eds.), *The medical management of AIDS in women* (pp. 415–436). New York: Wiley-Liss.

Lazzarin, A. (1988). Raised serum $\beta_2$-microglobulin levels in different stages of human immunodeficiency virus infection. *Journal of Clinical Laboratory Immunology, 27,* 133–137.

Lecuit, M., Oksenhelder, E., & Sarfati, C. (1994). Use of albendazole for disseminated microsporidian infection in a patient with AIDS. *Clinical Infectious Diseases, 19,* 332–333.

Levine, A.M. (1996). HIV-associated Hodgkin's disease: Biologic and clinical aspects. *Hematology-Oncology Clinics of North America, 10* (5), 1135–1148.

Louache, F., Bettaieb, A., Henri, A., Oksenhenler, E., Farcet, J.P., Bierling, P., Seligmann, M., & Vainchenker, W. (1991). Infection of megakaryocytes by human immunodeficiency virus in seropositive patients with immune thrombocytopenic purpura. *Blood, 78,* 1697–1705.

Maiman, M. (1997). Management of cervical neoplasia in HIV-positive women. In D. Cotton & D.H. Watts (Eds.), *The medical management of AIDS in women* (pp. 221–234). New York: Wiley-Liss.

Mauss, S., Steinmetz, H.T., Willers, R., Manegold, C., Kochaner, M., Haussinger, D., & Jablonowski, H. (1997). Induction of granulocyte colony-stimulating factor by acute febrile infection but not by neutropenia in HIV-seropositive individuals. *Journal of Acquired Immune Deficiency Syndromes and Human Retrovirology, 14* (5), 430–434.

McLigeyo, S.O. (1998). Herpes zoster in HIV/AIDS: A little recognised opportunistic infection with important clinical and cost implications. *East African Medical Journal, 75* (7), 377–378.

Means, R.T., Jr. (1997). Cytokines and anaemia in human immunodeficiency virus infection. *Cytokines, Cellular and Molecular Therapy, 3* (3), 179–186.

Melchior, J.C. (1997). Metabolic aspects of HIV: Associated wasting. *Biomedicine and Pharmacotherapy, 51* (10), 455–460.

Mitsuyasu, R.T. (1997a). Neoplastic aspects. In J.L. Fahey & D.S. Flemmig (Eds.), *AIDS/HIV reference guide for medical professionals* (pp. 149–161). Baltimore: Williams & Wilkins.

Mitsuyasu, R.T. (1997b). Spectrum of illness, disease staging, and natural history. In J.L. Fahey & D.S. Flemmig (Eds.), *AIDS/HIV reference guide for medical professionals* (pp. 100–115). Baltimore: Williams & Wilkins.

Mitsuyasu, R.T. (1999). Hematologic disease. In R. Dolin, H. Masur, & M. Saag (Eds.), *AIDS therapy* (pp. 666–679). New York: Churchill Livingstone.

Moldawer, L.L. & Sattler, F.R. (1998). Human immunodeficiency virus-associated wasting and mechanisms of cachexia associated with inflammation. *Seminars in Oncology, 25* (1 Suppl. 1), 73–81.

Moore, R.D., Keruly, J.C., & Chaisson, R.E. (1998). Anemia and survival in HIV infection. *Journal of Acquired Immune Deficiency Syndromes and Human Retrovirology, 19* (1), 29–33.

Murphy, P.M., Lane, N.C., Fauci, A.S., & Gallin, J.I. (1988). Impairment of neutrophil bactericidal capacity in patients with AIDS. *Journal of Infectious Diseases, 158* (3), 627–630.

Murthy, N., Seghal, A., Satyanarayana, L., Das, D., Singh, V., Das, B., Gupta, M., Mitra, A., & Luthra, U. (1990). Risk factors related to biological behavior or precancerous lesions of the uterine cervix. *British Journal of Cancer, 61,* 732–736.

Musoke, P., Guay, L.A., Bagenda, D., Mirochnick, M., Nakabiito, C., Fleming, T., Elliott, T., Horton, S., Dransfield, K., Pav, J.W., Murarka, A., Allen, M., Fowler, M.G., Mofenson, L., Hom, D., Mmiro, F., & Jackson, J.B. (1999). A phase I/II study of the safety and pharmacokinetics of nevirapine in HIV-1–infected pregnant Ugandan women and their neonates (HIVNET 006). *AIDS, 13* (4), 479–486.

National Institute of Allergy and Infectious Diseases. (1994). *Executive summary: Abstract ACTG076. A phase III randomized, placebo controlledtrial to evaluate the efficacy, safety, and tolerance of zidovudine (ZDV) for the prevention of maternal-fetal transmission.* Washington, DC: Government Printing Office.

Nelson, J., Averett, H., & Richart, R. (1989). Cervical intraepithelial neoplasia (dysplasia and carcinoma in situ) and early invasive cervical carcinoma. *Ca: Cancer Journal for Clinicians, 39,* 159.

Northfelt, D.W., Swift, P.S., & Palefsky, J.M. (1996). Anal neoplasia: Pathogenesis, diagnosis, and management. *Hematology-Oncology Clinics of North America, 10* (5), 1177–1187.

Oksenhendler, E., Bierling, P., Chevret, S., Delfraissy, J.F., Laurian, Y., Clauvel, J.P., & Seligmann, M. (1993). Splenectomy is safe and effective in HIV-related immune thrombocytopenia. *Blood, 82* (1), 29–32.

Oksenhendler, E., Bierling, P., Ferchal, F., Clauvel, J.P., & Seligmann, M. (1989). Zidovudine for thrombocytopenia purpura related to human immunodeficiency virus infection. *Annals of Internal Medicine, 110* (5), 365–368.

Ortona, L. & Fantoni, M. (1998). Tuberculin skin test and chemoprophylaxis of tuberculosis. *Rays, 23* (1), 218–224.

Pantaleo, G., Cohen, O., Graziosi, C., et al. (1997). Immunopathogenesis of human immunodeficiency virus infection. In V.T. Devita, S. Hellman, & S.A. Rosenberg (Eds.), *AIDS: Biology, diagnosis, treatment and prevention* (pp. 75–88). Philadelphia: Lippicott-Raven.

Pantaleo, G., Graziosi, E., Demarest, J.F., Butini, L., Mantroni, M., Fox, C.H., Orenstein, J.M., Kotler, D.P., & Fauci, A.S. (1993). HIV-1 infection is active and progressive in lymphoid tissue during the clinically latent stage of the illness. *Nature, 362* (6418), 355–358.

Parslow, T.G. & Elder, M.E. (1996). Pathobiology of immunodeficiency disorders. In A.E. Sirica (Ed.), *Cellular and molecular pathogenesis* (pp. 199–217). Philadelphia: Lippincott-Raven.

Pauza, C. (1988). HIV persistence in monocytes leads to pathogenesis and AIDS. *Cellular Immunology, 112* (2), 414–424.

Peterman, T.A., Stoneburner, R.L., Allen, J.R., Jaffe, H.W., & Curran, J.W. (1988). Risk of human immunodeficiency virus transmission from heterosexual adults with transfusion-associated infection. *JAMA, 259* (1), 55–58.

Phillips, K.D. (1996). Protease inhibitors: A new weapon and a new strategy against HIV. *Journal of the Association of Nurses in AIDS Care, 7* (5), 57–71.

Piemme, J.A. (1998). Opportunistic infections. In M.E. Ropka & A.B. Williams (Eds.), *HIV nursing and symptom management* (pp. 110–142). Boston: Jones and Bartlett Publishers.

Plaeger-Marshall, S., Spina, C.A., Giorgi, J.V., Mitsuyasu, R.T., Worlfe, P., Gottlieb, M.S., & Beall, G. (1987). Alterations in cytotoxic and phenotypic subsets of natural killer cells in acquired immunodeficiency syndrome (AIDS). *Journal of Clinical Immunology, 7* (1), 16–23.

Poli, G. & Fauci, A.S. (1995). Role of cytokines in the pathogenesis of human immunodeficiency virus infection. In B. Aggarwal & R.K. Puri (Eds.), *Human cytokines: Their role in disease and therapy.* (pp. 421–449). Cambridge, MA: Blackwell Science.

Polk, B., Fox, R., Brookmeyer, R., Kanchanaraksa, S., Kaslow, R., Visscher, B., Rinaldo, C., & Phair, J. (1987). Predictors of the acquired immunodeficiency syndrome developing in a cohort of seropositive homosexual men. *New England Journal of Medicine, 316* (2), 61–66.

Powderly, W.G. (1999). Cryptococcosis. In R. Dolin, H. Masur, & M. Saag (Eds.), *AIDS therapy* (pp. 400–411). New York: Churchill Livingstone.

Price, R. (1997). Management of the neurologic complications of HIV-1 infection and AIDS. In M. Sande & P.A. Volberding (Eds.), *The medical management of AIDS* (pp. 197–216). Philadelphia: W.B.Saunders.

Price, R. & Brew, B. .(1988) The AIDS dementia complex. *Journal of Infectious Diseases, 158* (5), 1079–1083.

Price, R., Brew, B., Sidtis, J., Rosenblum, M., Scheck, A.C., & Cleary, P. (1988). The brain in AIDS: Central nervous system HIV-1 infection and AIDS dementia complex. *Science, 239* (4840), 586–592.

Price, R.W. (1999). Neurological disease. In R. Dolin, H. Masur, & M. Saag (Eds.), *AIDS therapy* (pp. 620–638). New York: Churchill Livingstone.

Rachlis, A.R. (1998). Neurologic manifestations of HIV infection. Using imaging studies and antiviral therapy effectively. *Postgraduate Medicine, 103* (3), 147–150.

Ratner, L., Haseltine, W., Patarca, R., Livak, K.J., Starcich, B., Josephs, S.F., Doran, E.R., Rofalski, J.A., Whitehorn, E.A., Baumeister, K., Nomone, W.I., Petteway, S.R., Jr., Pearson, M.L., Lautzenberger, J.A., Papas, T.S., Ghrayeb, J., Chong, N.T., Gallo, R.C., & Wong-Staal, F. (1985). Complete nucleotide sequence of the AIDS virus, HTLV-III. *Nature, 313* (6000), 277–283.

Ratto-Kim, S., Sitz, K.V., Garner, R.P., Kim, J.H., Davis, C., Aronson, N., Ruiz, N., Tencer, K., Redfield, R.R., & Birx, D.L. (1999). Repeated immunization with recombinant gp160 human immunodeficiency virus (HIV) envelope protein in early HIV-1 infection: Evaluation of the T cell proliferative response. *Journal of Infectious Diseases, 179* (2), 337–344.

Reddy, M.M. & Grieco, M.H. (1989). Neopterin and alpha and beta interleukin 1 levels in sera of patients with human immunodeficiency virus infection. *Journal of Clinical Microbiology, 27* (9), 1919–1923.

Riviere, P., Tanneau-Salvadori, F., Regnault, A., Lopez, O., Sansonetti, P., Guy, B., Kieny, M.P., Fournel, J.J., & Montagnier, L. (1989). Human immunodeficiency virus–specific cytotoxic responses of seropositive indiviudals: Distinct types of effector cells mediate killing of targets expressing gag and env proteins. *Journal of Virology, 63* (5), 2270–2277.

Robertson, M.N. & Emerman, M. (1996). Pathogenesis. In D.H. Spach & T.M. Hooton (Eds.), *The HIV manual: A guide to diagnosis and treatment* (pp. 3–13). New York: Oxford University Press.

Rosenberg, Z. & Fauci, A.S. (1991). Immunopathogenesis of HIV infection. *FASEB J, 5*, 2382–2390.

Roth, E.L. (1998). Acquired immunodeficiency syndrome–related lymphoma. *Seminars in Oncology Nursing, 14* (4), 284–292.

Ryder, R.W., Nsa, W., Hassig, S.E., Behets, F., Rayfield, M., Ekungola, B., Nelson, A.M., Mulenda, U., & Francis, H. (1989). Perinatal transmission of the human immunodeficiency virus type 1 to infants of seropositive women in Zaire. *New England Journal of Medicine, 320*, 1637–1642.

Saag, M.S. (1997a). Cryptocococcosis and other fungal infections (histoplasmosis, coccidioidmycosis). In M. Sande & P.A. Volberding (Eds.), *The medical management of AIDS* (pp. 327–342). Philadelphia: W.B. Saunders.

Saag, M.S. (1997b). Quantitation of HIV viral load: A tool for clinical practice? In M. Sande & P.A. Volberding (Eds.), *The medical management of AIDS* (pp. 57–74). Philadelphia: W.B. Saunders.

Saag, M.S., Holodniy, M., Kuritzkes, D.R., O'Brien, W.A., Coombs, R., Poscher, M.E., Jacobsen, D.M., Shaw, G.M., Richman, D.D., & Volberding, P.A. (1996). HIV viral load markers in clinical practice. *Nature Medicine, 2* (6), 625–629.

Sacks, L.V. & Pendle, S. (1998). Factors related to in-hospital deaths in patients with tuberculosis. *Archives of Internal Medicine, 158* (17), 1916–1922.

Safai, B. & Dias, B.M. (1994). Kaposi's sarcoma and cloagenic carcinoma associated with AIDS. In S. Broder, T.C. Merigan, & D. Bolognesi (Eds.), *Textbook of AIDS medicine* (pp. 401–415). Baltimore: Williams & Wilkins.

Safai, B., Dias, B.M., & Schwartz, J. (1992). Malignant neoplasms associated with human immunodeficiency virus infection. *Ca: Cancer Journal for Clinicians, 42* (2), 74–95.

Saleh, M.N. & Scadden, D.T. (1999). Non-Hodgkin lymphoma. In R. Dolin, H. Masur, & M. Saag (Eds.), *AIDS therapy* (pp. 592–603). New York: Churchill Livingstone.

Sarin, P.S., Talmadge, J.E., Heseltine, P., Murcar, N., Gendelman, H.E., Coleman, Kelsey, L., Beckner, S., Winship, D., & Kahn, J. (1999). Booster immunization of HIV-1 negative volunteers with HGP-30 vaccine induces protection against HIV-1 virus challenge in SCID mice. *Vaccine, 17* (1), 64–71.

Sax, P. & Flory, J. (1996). Information for patients: Viral load testing. *AIDS Clinical Care, 8*, 31.

Schiffman, M. (1994). Epidemiology of cervical human papillomavirus infections. *Current Topics in Microbiology and Immunology, 186*, 55–81.

Semba, R.D., Miotti, P.F., Chiphangwi, J.D., Saah, A.J., Canner, J.K., Dallabetta, G.A., & Hoover, D.R. (1994). Maternal vitamin A deficiency and mother-to-child transmission of HIV-1. *Nature, 323*, 1593–1597.

Shearer, G.M. & Clerici, M. (1996). Type 1 and type 2 responses in HIV infection and exposure. In S. Gupta (Ed.), *Immunology of HIV infection* (pp. 229–241). New York: Plenum.

Singer, E.J. (1997). Neurologic aspects. In J.L. Fahey & D.S. Flemmig (Eds.), *AIDS/HIV reference guide for medical professionals* (pp. 161–174). Baltimore: Williams & Wilkins.

Sitz, K.V., Ratto-Kim, S., Hodgkins, A.S., Robb, M.L., & Birx, D.L. (1999). Proliferative responses to human immunodeficiency virus type 1 (HIV-1) gp120 peptides in HIV-1-infected individuals immunized with HIV-1 rgp120 or rgp160 compared with nonimmunized and uninfected controls. *Journal of Infectious Diseases, 179* (4), 817–824.

Sperling, R.S. (1997). Perinatal transmission of HIV. In D. Cotton & D.H. Watts (Eds.), *The medical management of AIDS in women* (pp. 45–54). New York: Wiley-Liss.

Spivak, J., Barnes, D.C., Fuchs, E., & Quinn, T.C. (1989). Serum immunoreactive erythropoietin in HIV-infected patients. *JAMA, 261*, 3104–3107.

Staats, J.A., Sheran, M., & Herr, R. (1999). Adolescents and adults: Care management of AIDS-indicator diseases. In P.J. Ungvarski & J. Flaskerud (Eds.), *HIV/AIDS: A guide to primary care management.* (pp. 194–254). Philadelphia: W.B. Saunders.

Stansell, J.D., & Huang, L. (1997). *Pneumocystis carinii* pneumonia. In M. Sande & P.A. Volberding (Eds.), *The medical management of AIDS* (pp. 275–300). Philadelphia: W.B. Saunders.

Staszewski, S., Schieck, E., Rehmet, S., Helm, E.B., & Stille, W. (1987). HIV transmission from a male after only two sexual contacts. *Lancet, II*, 628.

Stephens, D.A. (1995). Coccidioides immitis. In G.L. Mandell, J.E. Bennet, & R. Dolin (Eds.), *Principles and practices of infectious diseases* (pp. 2365–2374). New York: Churchill Livingstone.

Stratton, P. & Alexander, N.J. (1997). Heterosexual spread of HIV infection. In D. Cotton & D.H. Watts (Eds.), *The medical management of AIDS in women* (pp. 15–43). New York: Wiley-Liss.

Stricker, R.B. (1991). Hemostatic abnormalities in HIV disease. *Hematology - Oncology Clinics of North America, 5*, 249.

Syrjanen, K., Hakama, M., Saorikoski, S., Vayrynen, M., Yliskioski, M., Syrjanen, S., Katajaca, V., & Castren, O. (1990). Prevalence, incidence, and estimated life-time risk of cervical human papillomavirus infections in a non-selected Finnish female population. *Sexually Transmitted Diseases, 17*, 15–19.

Tindall, B. & Cooper, D.A. (1991). Primary infection: Host responses and intervention strategies. *AIDS, 5* (1), 1–14.

UNAIDS Joint United Nations Programme on HIV/AIDS. (1998, December). *AIDS epidemic update.* Geneva: World Health Organization.

Vermund, S. (1997). Genital human papillomavirus infection. In D. Cotton & D.H. Watts (Eds.), *The medical management of AIDS in women* (pp. 125–159). New York: Wiley-Liss.

Viele, C.S. (1998). Hematologic abnormalities. In M.E. Ropka & A.B. Williams (Eds.), *HIV nursing and symptom management* (pp. 387–399). Boston: Jones and Bartlett Publishers.

Villette, J.M., Bourin, P., Doinel, C., Mansour, I., Fiet, J., Boudou, P., Dreux, C., Roue, R., Debord, M., & Levi, F. (1990). Circadian variations in plasma levels of hypophyseal, adrenocortical, and testicular hormones in men infected with human immunodeficiency virus. *Journal of Clinical Endocrinology and Metabolism, 70* (3), 572–577.

Von Roenn, J.H., & Mulligan, K. (1999). Wasting syndrome. In R. Dolin, H. Masur, & M. Saag (Eds.), *AIDS therapy* (pp. 607–619). New York: Churchill Livingstone.

Wagner, R., Shao, Y., & Wolf, H. (1999). Correlates of protection, antigen delivery and molecular epidemiology: Basics for designing an HIV vaccine. *Vaccine, 17* (13-14), 1706–1710.

Wilcox, C.M. & Mönkemüller, K.E. (1999). Gastrointestinal disease. In R. Dolin, H. Masur, & M. Saag (Eds.), *AIDS therapy* (pp. 752–765). New York: Churchill Livingstone.

Wilson, L.D., Truong, M.P., Barber, A.R., & Aoki, T.T. (1996). Anterior pituitary and pituitary-dependent target organ function in men infected with the human immunodeficency virus. *Metabolism, 45*, 738–746.

Yap, P.L., Todd, A.A., William, P.E., Hague, R.A., Mok, J., Burns, S.M., & Brettle, R.P. (1991). Use of intravenous immunoglobulin in acquired immune deficiency syndrome. *Cancer, 68* (Suppl. 6), 1440–1450.

Zauli, G., Re, M.C., Gulgiotta, L., Visani, G., Vianelli, Furlini, & LaPlaca, M. (1991). Lack of compensatory megakaryocytopoiesis in HIV-1–seropositive thrombocytopenic individuals compared with immune thrombocytopenic purpura patients. *AIDS, 5* (11), 1845–1850.

Zhu, T., Mo, H., Wang, N., Nam, D.S., Cao, Y., Koup, R.A. & Ho, D.D. (1993). Genotypic and phenotypic characterization of HIV-1 patients with primary infection. *Science, 261* (5125), 1179–1181.

Zon, L.I. & Groopman, J.E. (1988). Hematologic manifestations of the human immune deficiency virus. *Seminars in Hematology, 25* (3), 208–218.

# Alzheimer's Disease

Maureen Groer

Four million Americans have the progressive, degenerative, debilitating disease known as Alzheimer's disease (AD). Since most people with AD are older than 65 years, the incidence of this disease is expected to increase as the proportion of elderly in the population rises. In a growing segment of the elderly, the "old old," AD is a significant cause of death, with about 20% of those older than 80 years expected to develop AD. The risk for AD doubles in each decade after the age of 65 (McNeil, 1999). The cost of the disease stands at $100 billion dollars annually. Primary care providers are facing an epidemic of AD. Many clients and their families will deal with this devastating disease if a cure or new treatments are not discovered.

## EPIDEMIOLOGY

Alzheimer's disease is the most common cause of dementia, affecting men slightly more frequently than women. As the fourth to fifth leading cause of death in adults in the United States, AD causes 100,000 deaths per annum, with most patients dying from respiratory infection and respiratory failure. The risk for AD is associated with familial incidence, particularly for the early-onset form (younger than 60 years of age), which accounts for about 5% of cases. For late-onset AD, genetic factors have been discovered, but it may be the interaction of environmental exposure and genetic susceptibilities that ultimately produce AD in this population. Environmental factors undergoing research include viral infection (particularly herpes), metal exposure (zinc), electromagnetic fields, and head injuries. There also is evidence of an association of AD with cerebrovascular disease.

Ethnic differences in risk occur, with African Americans having four times the risk, and Hispan-

ics having two times the risk, of whites. The incidence is lower in Native-American and Asian-American populations (NOAH, 1999).

## GENETICS OF ALZHEIMER'S DISEASE

Familial AD has been associated with an autosomal dominant mode of transmission in which genetic mechanisms produce increased amounts of the protein, β-amyloid. A candidate location for a suspect gene is chromosome 21, since persons with Down syndrome have a trisomy of chromosome 21 and a nearly a 100% possibility of developing AD during early middle age. Mutations of a gene on chromosome 21, as well as genes on chromosome 1 and 14, are implicated. Through several genetic linkage analyses of kindred with early-onset AD, a gene on chromosome 21 that codes for an amyloid precursor protein (APP) has been identified. Amyloid precursor protein is continuously synthesized in neurons and then makes its way to the cell membrane, where it spans the membrane and protrudes. Proteases in the membrane cleave the APP, producing the 42–amino acid protein, β-amyloid. In early-onset AD, the defect may be the production of excessive amounts of APP, which then forms β-amyloid. Amyloid accumulates in the brain, and deposits of amyloid lead to neuritic plaques. However, amyloid deposition occur in normal-aged brains and in other diseases, and the presence of amyloid is not enough, in itself, to account for the dementia and degeneration of AD. It is uncertain whether amyloid is involved directly in pathogenesis or is secondary to the disease process, being merely a marker. Amyloid could be directly toxic to neurons or may generate free radicals, which then cause damage. Another idea is that amyloid disrupts neuronal electrolyte permeability, such as calcium channels (McNeil, 1999).

The form that amyloid takes in plaques is Aβ1-42, which is a sticky, insoluble protein that precipitates into fibrillar structures. Aβ1-42 forms from APP, which is coded for on chromosome 21, and may be overexpressed in early-onset AD. Amyloid deposition in the brain, then, might begin early in life, ultimately leading to neurologic damage and degeneration. A target for amyloid's neurotoxic effects is the intracellular protein ERAB, which appears to be involved in fatty acid metabolism. Amyloid binds with ERAB, and this interaction increases its intracellular toxicity.

Research has discovered another potential genetic mechanism for late-onset AD—the more common form of the disease. This link also is thought to be associated with early-onset AD. The suspect gene is ApoE (chromosome 19), which codes for apolipoprotein E. It is found in 40% of patients with late-onset AD (St. George-Hyslop, 1994). This lipoprotein and its role in atherosclerosis are described in Chapter 14. A normal function of apolipoproteins is cholesterol transport, but the specific role of ApoE in the brain is unknown.

Particular alleles of the ApoE gene both increase risk and lower the age at which symptoms appear. An allele associated with greatest risk is known as ApoE ∈4, and its presence is associated with amyloid deposition. The ApoE ∈4 protein binds with amyloid, causing amyloid to become insoluble and, thus, more likely to be deposited in the brain. Another mechanism for the association may be related to abnormal fragility in the microtubules in the nerve cells of the brain. If a person has two alleles, one from each parent, the risk of AD is between 50% and 90%. However, an individual with only one copy, which normally confers about a 25% to 60% risk, has a 10-fold increase in risk for AD after experiencing major head trauma. This suggests that environmental insults may play a role in the pathogenesis of AD.

Other genes speculated to be involved in AD include mitochondrial DNA mutations, which are passed to progeny only through maternal inheritance. A prominent theory of AD involves oxidative damage to neurons, implicating mitochondrial oxidative phosphorylation mechanisms, which could increase the rate of apoptosis in neuronal cells or decrease the production of acetyl coenzyme A, which then results in decreased acetylcholine formation (Meier-Ruge & Bertoni-Freddari, 1999).

The genes for the proteins presenilin 1 (chromosome 14) and 2 (chromosome 1) also are speculated to be involved in the etiology of AD, particularly the early-onset form. The role of these proteins is not completely understood, although they may divert amyloid metabolism toward increased expression of Apoβ1-42 (Tanzi et al., 1996). Overexpression of presenilin 2 also may result in an increased rate of apoptosis in the brain. This type of programmed cell suicide leading to death of neurons in critical areas of the cortex, hippocampus, and midbrain provides another explanation of AD pathogenesis.

The tau protein is another target of investigation into genetic mechanisms involved in AD. The tau protein normally is involved in microtubular integrity within neuronal axons. The microtubules are important in transporting materials from the cell body of the neuron down to its dendritic endings. In AD, the microtubules become tangled because the tau proteins twist into structures termed paired helical filaments. These are the basic components of the intracellular neurofibrillary tangles (NFTs) associated with AD (McNeil, 1999). Elevated levels of tau protein can be found in the cerebrospinal fluid of AD patients early in the course of the disease (Galasko et al., 1997).

The ongoing revolution in molecular biology and genetics has led to important understandings regarding the etiology of AD in the last few years. It is anticipated that several new pharmaceutical approaches will be generated from the knowledge gained through these explorations.

## NONGENETIC INFLUENCES

Although genetic factors are important, they are not the only factor involved in pathogenesis. People who carry the mutations described earlier have a certain increase in risk, but environmental influences also are likely to play a major role in pathogenesis.

### Metals

#### Aluminum

Many different environmental agents have been implicated as etiologic in AD. The most well known is aluminum because of the similarity of aluminum neurotoxicity seen in dialysis patients with the symptoms of AD. However, the evidence for aluminum as a cause of AD has been outweighed by the evidence against it. Studies on occupational exposure, drinking water, food, antiperspirant use, and cooking utensils do not provide a strong argument for aluminum's role in AD. Whereas aluminum can accumulate in the brains of patients with AD, so can other metal ions.

However, although controversial, research suggests that aluminum is found in NFTs, a hallmark of AD. Aluminum's highly reactive properties could stabilize the tangled protein structures of the NFTs (Perl & Good, 1992).

### Zinc

Zinc is another metal more recently implicated in AD. Abnormalities in zinc metabolism have been observed in patients with AD, and some studies have found higher levels of zinc in the AD brain. Zinc can accelerate the aggregation of amyloid and can promote oxidative damage. It also is involved in apoptosis, a mechanism that may be accelerated in AD.

### Mercury

Mercury has been speculated to be involved in AD pathogenesis, and dental amalgam is known to give off mercury vapors. However, a study of autopsy data of 68 subjects with AD and 33 controls showed no difference in brain mercury levels, nor was there any association of dental amalgam and restorations with brain mercury levels (Saxe et al., 1999).

## Viruses

The neurodegenerative processes seen in AD are similar to those found in slow viral infections of the brain such as kuru and scrapie. The fact that herpesviruses reside in latent states in neurologic tissue suggests a possible relation between AD and herpesvirus infection. Individuals who carry the apoE $\epsilon$4 allele have a higher risk for AD when herpes simplex virus type 1 (HSV-1) is present in their brain tissues (Dobson & Itzhaki, 1999). Therefore, some interaction is speculated between the ApoE $\epsilon$4 lipoprotein and HSV-1 that increases the risk of AD. The HSV-1 is found in the brain of elderly people, but it is found in higher amounts in patients with AD. The presence of the virus alone probably is not sufficient, but when combined with the allele, there is a significantly greater risk of developing AD.

## Electromagnetic Fields

Some epidemiologic evidence associates neurodegenerative diseases, including AD, with exposure to electromagnetic fields (Sobel et al., 1996). Other studies refute this connection (Graves et al., 1999). Occupational exposure is highest among electrical utility workers and power plant operators. Electromagnetic fields may alter nervous system physiology by altering calcium homeostasis or inappropriately activating immune system cells such as microglial cells.

## Head Injury

Individuals who repeatedly experience head trauma may develop a dementia that in many ways mimics AD. Dementia pugilistica is found in boxers, head bangers, and football player. The brains of these persons show NFTs, indicating that after physical injury to the brain, a mechanism develops that also is seen in AD, perhaps of a vascular nature (Geddes et al., 1999). A history of a previous head injury with loss of consciousness increases the ultimate risk of developing AD (O'Meara et al., 1997). Several studies show that this risk is greatest for individuals carrying the ApoE $\epsilon$4 lipoprotein allele. It is speculated that ApoE $\epsilon$4 may detrimentally affect neuronal branching and viability, and this, in combination with head injury, perpetuates neuronal degenerative disease. Another phenomenon may be that head injury causes the upregulation of the presenilin 1 gene, perhaps inducing apoptosis.

## Other Factors

Several studies suggest interesting relationships between AD and educational level, cognitive ability, social factors, and mood. For example, a greater risk for AD exists in the never-married individual (Helmer et al., 1999). A history of preceding depression also is a possible risk factor, and depression may be the presenting symptom in many early stage AD patients. It is not known if depression increases the risk of AD or is an early manifestation of the disease (Devanand et al., 1996).

Linguistic ability, which is related to cognitive function, is an additional factor that may be related to AD. Snowdon has been conducting the well-known Nun's Study, a longitudinal study in which writing samples from 678 Catholic nuns were analyzed on their entry into the convent and were related to their later cognitive function, including risk of AD (Snowdon, 1996). This group is unique in that their living conditions, diet, and other lifestyle and environmental influences are similar or the same throughout their lives. A direct relationship seems to exist between linguistic abilities early in life and cognitive abilities in old age. Of the nuns who died, AD was present in all who wrote in simple prose ("low idea density") on entry into the convent, but in only one who wrote in a complex prose style ("high idea density"). This nun died at 101 years and did not show signs of dementia while alive, but had NFTs and senile plaques at death. This evidence has led to the idea that greater intellectualism (the "use it or lose it" argument) decreases the risk of AD.

## PATHOPHYSIOLOGY

Several nonspecific findings regularly occur in the AD brain, but these findings also occur in the normal-aged brain. No pathognomonic finding specific for AD has been discovered. However, hallmarks of the disease include neuronal cell loss, NFTs, and senile plaques—all present to a greater degree in the AD brain than in the normal-aged brain.

### Cerebral Atrophy

A characteristic feature of AD is loss of neurons, loss of synapses, and generalized atrophy and widespread loss of cells throughout the neocortex. Loss of cells also occurs within subcortical structures such as the nucleus basalis, locus caeruleus, dorsal raphe nucleus, and ventral tegmentum. The degree of atrophy does not, however, coincide directly with the degree of dementia. The causes of cell death are controversial. Apoptosis may be the mechanism, in which case, cells die by a programmed noninflammatory process in which intracellular enzymes digest the cell. Another possibility is that excessive calcium enters through calcium channels and ultimately accumulates, killing the cell.

### Senile Plaques

Senile, or neuritic, plaques occur throughout the cortex in AD. They appear earliest in the entorhinal cortex, which is close to the hippocampus. Figure 22-1 depicts the appearance of such a plaque. The plaque is filled with a core of insoluble amyloid, thought to be mostly Aβ1-42, which is surrounded by rings of distended neurites and proliferating microglial cells. The plaques occur throughout the cortex and often are found in association with blood vessels. Amyloid deposition in the brain is thought to be the initiating event in plaque formation. Amyloid is neurotoxic, possibly causing neuronal degeneration through the production of dystrophic neurites, as well as an amyloid angiopathy (Caselli & Boeve, 1999). The dystrophic neurites have abnormal sprouting of dendritic endings so that synaptic connections with other neurons are diminished. This absence of innervation may lead to degeneration (Masliah et al., 1991).

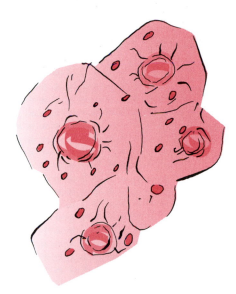

**FIGURE 22.1** ● Neuritic plaques seen in Alzheimer's disease.

### Neurofibrillary Tangles

Another feature of AD is the presence of NFTs, which are intracellular accumulations of microtubular debris made of insoluble, paired helical fragments of tau protein. The presence of this filamentous microarchitectural disturbance in the neuron's cytoskeleton causes impairment in synaptic transmission and intracellular communications. Neurofibrillary tangles are found in cells in the entorhinal cortex, the limbic cortex, amygdala, and the association cortex of the frontal, temporal, and parietal lobes, and the basal forebrain cholinergic systems (Pearson et al., 1985). A correlation exists between the number of NFTs and the degree of dementia, whereas plaque density and dementia are not highly correlated. Neurofibrillary tangles develop in the neuronal cell body and then extend into the dendrites. Figure 22-2 shows the structural changes in the neuron as NFTs accumulate. The filaments cause flame-shaped tangles in the cells, with remnant "ghost" tangles left behind once the affected neuron has degenerated. β-Amyloid is found within NFTs, although it is not known if the amyloid deposits first or is secondary to the formation of NFTs.

The distribution of NFTs in the brain occurs in a particular sequence, suggesting that AD spreads through the brain initially from damaged cortical neurons to subcortical neurons. Cells in the cortical association areas send projections into the hippocampus and amygdala, which in turn become damaged. The hippocampus is the part of the brain

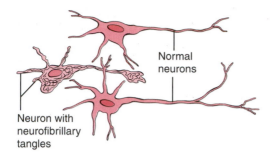

**FIGURE 22.2** ● Neuron with neurofibrillary tangles.

involved in memory, whereas the amygdala is involved in emotions. The effect is to disconnect memory, mood, cognitive, and intellectual functions from the higher centers of the brain.

## Energy Metabolism

Glucose utilization is drastically reduced in AD, but it is not clear if this is a primary problem or is related to neuronal degeneration. The ability of the brain to use glucose can be visualized using positron emission tomography scans. When brain function and activity diminish with time in AD, the uptake and utilization of glucose in different parts of the brain drops. Glucose uptake into the cerebral cortex may be decreased because of decrease in the GLUT1 and GLUT3 transporters (McNeil, 1999). When neurons receive less than adequate amounts of glucose, they are unable to synthesize and transport neurotransmitters. Acetylcholine deficits are known to occur in AD, in part because of inadequacies of glucose and energy metabolic pathways. The abnormalities in glucose metabolism may precede memory loss.

## Neurotransmitters

Abnormalities in several neurotransmitter systems have been found in AD, but decreased amounts of acetylcholine are the most dramatic. The loss of acetylcholine occurs first in the nucleus basalis, which has many cholinergic projections to other parts of the brain. Because acetylcholine is a critical neurotransmitter in both the cerebral cortex and hippocampus, deficits may be associated with the typical memory losses of AD. Not only is there evidence for a decreased amount of acetylcholine produced in the brain, but also for decreased or abnormal acetylcholine receptors. The loss of cholinergic neurons in the nucleus basalis eventually can reach a level of 90% loss.

## CLINICAL FEATURES

An older term for AD was senile dementia. Several diseases have features of dementia, particularly memory loss. The term dementia implies a decline in intellectual function severe enough to interfere with activities of daily living and social relationships. With AD, there is progressive, irreversible memory loss; decreased ability to perform normal tasks; disorientation to time and space; impaired language and communication abilities; impaired judgment; decreased abstract thinking; and a decreased ability to calculate. Usually, a significant change in the personality also occurs (McNeil, 1999). The diagnosis of AD is definitive only after death, but most clinicians are accurate in ruling out other causes of dementia (encephalopathies, multi-infarction dementia, severe depression, substance abuse, brain tumors, Creutzfeldt-Jakob disease, Parkinson's disease, Pick's disease) before making the diagnosis. The diagnostic criteria for AD are indicated in Table 22-1.

## Stages of the Disease

Generally, AD occurs in early, middle, and late stages. The early stage lasts about 2 to 4 years and often ends with the diagnosis. The first sign of AD is memory loss, a problem that occurs to some degree in all elderly persons. However, the memory loss in AD is more severe and clearly progressive. The loss is most striking for short-term memory, reflecting degeneration of the hippocampal neurons. The symptoms develop slowly and may not be noticeable at first by casual contacts. The memory loss of AD often is associated with confusion, a phenomenon not seen in the well elderly person who may have some problems with short-term memory. With memory loss in AD, there is aphasia (impaired ability to communicate through language or writing), apraxia (impaired ability to carry out purposeful activity), and agnosia (impaired ability to recognize objects). Thus, these individuals begin to exhibit difficulty in managing their lives. The symptoms may become particularly noticeable if the patient is stressed or taken out of the familiar environment. Many patients in the early stage of AD experience significant clinical depression. Their depression may be manifested by weight loss, quietness, sadness, excessive sleeping, and anhedonia. However, vegetative symptoms and depression rarely persist through the course of the disease. Psychotic symptoms such as delusions and hallucinations show moderate persistence, whereas behavioral disturbances,

# TABLE 22.1

## NINCDS-ADRDA Criteria for Diagnosis of Alzheimer's Disease

*I. Clinical Diagnosis of Probable Alzheimer's Disease*
1. Dementia established by clinical examination and mental status testing and confirmed by neuropsychologic testing
2. Deficits in at least two cognitive domains
3. Progressive cognitive decline, including memory
4. Normal level of consciousness
5. Onset between ages 40 and 90 (most common after 65) y
6. No other possible medical or neurologic explanation

*II. Probable Alzheimer's Disease Diagnosis Supported by*
1. Progressive aphasia, apraxia, and agnosia
2. Impaired activities of daily living
3. Family history of similar disorder
4. Brain atrophy on CT/MRI, especially if progressive
5. Normal CSF, EEG (or nonspecific abnormal)

*III. Other Clinical Features Consistent With Probable Alzheimer's Disease*
1. Plateau in course
2. Associated symptoms: depression; insomnia; incontinence; illusions; hallucinations; catastrophic verbal, emotional, or physical outbursts; sexual disorders; weight loss; during more advanced stage, increased muscle tone, myoclonus, and abnormal gait
3. Seizures in advanced disease
4. CT normal for age

*IV. Features That Make Alzheimer's Disease Uncertain or Unlikely*
1. Acute onset
2. Focal sensorimotor signs
3. Seizures or gait disorders early in course

*V. Clinical Diagnosis of Possible Alzheimer's Disease*
1. Dementia with atypical onset or course in the absence of another medical/neuropsychiatric explanation
2. Dementia with another disease not believed otherwise to be the cause of dementia
3. For research purposes, a progressive focal cognitive deficit

*VI. Definite Alzheimer's Disease*
1. Meets clinical criteria for probable Alzheimer's disease
2. Tissue confirmation (autopsy or brain biopsy)

*VII. Research Classification of Alzheimer's Disease Should Specify*
1. Familial?
2. Early onset (before age 65)?
3. Down's syndrome (trisomy 21)?
4. Coexistent with other neurodegenerative disease (eg, Parkinson's disease)?

CSF, cerebral spinal fluid; CT, computed tomography; EEG, electroencephalogram; MRI, magnetic resonance imaging; NINCDS-ADRDA, National Institute of Neurological and Communicative Disorders and Stroke and the Alzheimer's Disease and Related Disorders Associations.
(From McKhann, G., Drachman, D., Folstein, M., Katzman, R., Price, D., Stadlam, E. [1984]. Clinical diagnosis of Alzheimer's disease: Report of the NINCDS-ADRDA Work Group under the auspices of the Department of Health and Human Services Task Force on Alzheimer's Disease. *Neurology, 34,* 939–944.)

particularly agitation, persist through the course of the disease (Devanand et al., 1997). When considering AD as a diagnosis, notice that AD is not associated with level of consciousness.

The length of the middle stage varies, depending on the length of the disease, which normally averages between 4 and 8 years. The middle stage is characterized by more significant symptoms of memory loss, and patients often are unable to recognize their loved ones, need assistance for basic activities of daily living, and are easily stressed. They also lose much of their communication abilities and become reliant on others for their care. They often have significant emotional outbursts and expressions of anger. During this stage, the patients' circadian rhythms become confused, and they do not have normal sleep patterns. They often are awake during the night and are subject to restlessness and periods of aimless wandering. They need close supervision at all times by their caretakers, which places an enormous burden and stress on caregivers of patients with AD. Caregiver stress clearly has been identified as significant, immunosuppressive, and harmful to the health of the caregiver.

The late stage typically lasts 1 to 3 years. During this terminal phase, patients have progressively less affect and become more withdrawn, delusional, and disabled. They may become bedridden and incontinent of bowel and bladder. Eventually, they may lapse into a comatose-like stage, and the cause of death typically is pneumonia.

Diagnosis of AD usually requires either a computed tomography (CT) scan or magnetic resonance imaging of the brain, complete cognitive assessment, a complete physical examination including thyroid function tests and vitamin $B_{12}$ levels, testing for syphilis, chest x-ray and electrocardiogram, blood chemistries including liver and kidney chemistries, and an erythrocyte sedimentation rate. Many of these tests merely rule out another cause for the dementia (Caselli & Boeve, 1999), so that AD becomes a diagnosis of exclusion.

## Physiologic Basis of Treatment

### Cholinergic Approaches

Because acetylcholine deficit is so marked in the AD brain, pharmacologic approaches to increase acetylcholine have been used. The drug type used with greatest success is a cholinesterase inhibitor such as tacrine (Cognex) and donepezil (Aricept). The use of these drugs is problematic if patients have cholinergic side effects, but several studies demonstrate a small but significant clinical improvement in patients, particularly in early and middle stages of AD (Farlow, 1999).

### Hormone Replacement Therapy

Several studies have found that using estrogen replacement therapy either prevents or slows AD progression. Six or more months of estrogen therapy at menopause was associated with a 50% reduction in incidence of AD in an epidemiologic study in Rochester, Minnesota (Waring et al., 1999). Cholinergic neurons have estrogen receptors, and estrogen appears to increase the level of nerve growth factor. Estrogen also seems to have its major biologic effects in the hippocampus and cerebral cortex. Estrogen may prevent cholinergic neuron degeneration, thus protecting against AD (McNeil, 1999). The evidence is strong enough to prompt use of estrogen in early stage AD patients and to encourage perimenopausal women to consider the protective effects of estrogen for AD as well as osteoporosis and heart disease.

### Antioxidants

One of the major theories about AD implicates oxidative stress causing damage through the production of free radicals. Aging is a major risk factor associated with AD, and an abundance of evidence indicates that oxidative damage accumulates in aging. This "free radical theory of aging" suggests that reactive oxygen species (ROS) are produced and enzyme systems that defend against ROS are reduced in aging (Smith & Perry, 1999). These ROS are oxygen free radicals produced by oxidases and in oxidative phosphorylation. They have an unpaired electron in their outer shell and thus are highly reactive, short-lived species. Molecules to which ROS readily attach include lipids and nucleic acid. Lipids become peroxidated in this way, and nucleic acid can become mutated through the action of free radicals. Although the body has several powerful enzyme systems that remove free radicals before they can damage biologic molecules (catalase, superoxide dismutase), with aging these enzymes systems may be less effective and can become overwhelmed by free radical production. Evidence indicates that oxidative damage occurs in both normal aging and in AD. In AD, the senile plaques and NFTs contain oxidatively damaged molecules (Smith & Perry, 1999). Inflammatory processes in the brain may be provoked by oxidative damage in AD. ApoE and β-amyloid require oxygen for their interaction. DNA fragmentation, a sign of oxidative damage, is widespread throughout affected neurons in AD. The ROS may mutate the APP gene. Evidence for oxidative damage playing a role in AD is sufficient to warrant clinical trials of various agents that protect against free radical generation. The most well-known and acceptable agent is vitamin E. Evidence for slight delay in disease progression was noted in one study of vitamin E supplementation in AD patients (*www.noah.cuny.edu/wellconn/alzheimers.html*).

## Anti-Inflammatory Drugs

Some studies suggest that people who take nonsteroidal anti-inflammatory drugs such as aspirin and ibuprofen have a reduced risk for AD. Because there is evidence of inflammatory reactions to amyloid plaques and nerve cell death with release of cell-damaging cytokines, suppression of inflammation theoretically might oppose the disease processes.

## Treatment of Symptoms

Caregivers of AD patients must deal with a range of patient management issues such as basic hygiene and nutrition, as well as behavioral, psychotic, and sleep disturbance symptoms. It is appropriate to use medications for depression, antipsychotic medications, and sleep medications to keep patients at home and out of institutions. Most patients with AD eventually require institutionalization during the latter stages of illness. As mentioned previously, caregiver burden and stress is enormous in this disease, and the provider must treat both the patient and the caregiver to achieve the best outcome for both.

## Conclusions

Primary care providers can keep current on the research on AD pathogenesis and pathophysiology through several web sites. Current research and information about clinical trials is updated on *http://www.alzforum.org*. Many management issues concerning providers and AD patients are discussed at *http://www.alzheimers.org*. The primary AD organization web site, which provides information about local chapters, resources, and advice, is found at *http://www.alz.org*.

---

● **Case Study 22.1**

Gladys Washburn is a 75-year-old patient in the primary care clinic who is brought in by her 77-year-old husband because she has been "acting strangely." Her husband reports that she has become increasing forgetful and confused. Today, he found her turning on the microwave oven so that she could watch her favorite television show. Mr. Washburn is concerned and nervous and asks the provider, "It isn't Alzheimer's disease, is it?"

Mrs. Washburn appears to be a pleasant, well-groomed lady. She is a retired librarian and has been active within her retirement community. Lately, she has been less interested in playing bridge or social activities. Her demeanor is flat and she appears sad. On questioning, she voices great fear that she is "losing her mind."

### *History*

#### *Past Medical History*

| | |
|---|---|
| Allergies | NKDA |
| Current medications | Takes atenolol and chlorthiazide for HTN for last 6 years |
| Surgeries | Caesarean childbirth 45 years previously |
| Injury Trauma | MVA 20 years ago; sustained head injury with LOC. MVA 6 months ago; concussion without LOC |

*(Case study continued on page 456)*

| | |
|---|---|
| Childhood illnesses | Had the usual illnesses as child (measles, rubella, mumps, chickenpox). Had nonparalytic polio in 1953 with no known sequelae |

### Social History

| | |
|---|---|
| Marital status | Has not been sexually active in about 10 years. States she and her husband "just lost interest" |
| Alcohol | Uses moderately, mostly wine at dinner |
| Tobacco | Does not smoke |
| Social drugs | Does not use other drugs |
| Exercise | None except for occasional game of golf |
| Employment | Retired for 5 years. Lives in a retirement community and is involved in social activities, bridge club, golf |

### Family History

| | |
|---|---|
| Mother | Died from stroke |
| Father | Died from AD |
| Children | Has three adult children who live in different states. Sees them only at Christmas. Feels closest to eldest daughter, who lives about 500 miles away |

### 24-Hour Dietary Recall

| | |
|---|---|
| | Can't remember what she ate yesterday. Thinks she had meals that her husband prepared. Husband states that she can't remember her recipes and gets confused while cooking. States that her appetite is poor and that she has lost weight |

### Review of Systems

| | |
|---|---|
| General | Withdrawn, pale, sad |
| Skin | Skin is dry and she has noted hair loss over last few months |
| HEENT | Wears glasses. Slight hearing loss. No headaches, nosebleeds, dizziness, ear aches, sore throats |
| Lungs | No SOB, asthma, bronchitis, pneumonia |
| CV | No chest pains, palpitations. Prior ECG indicated slight LVH |
| GI | No nausea, vomiting, diarrhea. Poor appetite. Frequent bouts of constipation |
| GU | No UTIs, dysuria, frequency. Sees gynecologist yearly for Pap smear and examination. Has yearly mammograms, which have always been normal |
| MS | Has mild arthritis in hands and knees. Denies joint swelling. Feels "weak" and tired lately, with no energy for activities |
| Neurologic | Denies numbness, tingling, weakness, fainting, seizures. Gets easily confused; is forgetful; cries easily; appears nervous and depressed. Sleeps more than usual |

*(Case study continued on next page)*

## Physical Examination

| System | Findings |
| --- | --- |
| Vital signs | T-97.8°F P-56 R-14<br>BP-110/62<br>Height-5'3", Weight-124 lb |
| General | Thin, withdrawn, quiet women who sits with head down, noncommunicative. Appears pale, skin cool to touch |
| HEENT | Normocephalic, cranial nerves intact. Rinne and Weber indicate mild conductive hearing loss, bilateral, but patient had difficulty understanding directions. TMs clear.<br>Nasal mucosa pale. No lymphadenopathy. Throat clear. Vision without glasses 20:60 OD; 20:50 OS. Conjunctiva slightly injected (patient crying)<br>Funduscopic examination WNL.<br>Thyroid examination suggests moderate bilateral enlargement. No carotid bruits |
| Lungs | Clear to auscultation and percussion bilaterally |
| CV | HR regular; no murmurs, thrills. Slight cardiomegaly by percussion |
| Abdomen | Soft, nontender to palpation. BS heard in all 4 quadrants. Liver, spleen not palpable. No CVA tenderness |
| GU/rectal | Deferred |
| Extremities | Cool to touch. All pulses 2+. Capillary refill 5 seconds. Grip strength poor. Gait somewhat ataxic |
| Neurologic | General cognitive assessment: unable to state name of President; uncertain about month and day of week; unable to count backwards from 10. Failed memory test of sequence of numbers. Unable to perform simple multiplications. Unable to understand how to perform heel-shin, finger to hand and nose<br>Sensations intact. Romberg negative. DTRs 2+ in upper and lower extremities |

## Impression

Dementia of unknown origin, possibly AD
Rule out multi-infarct dementia, depression, postconcussive syndrome, hypothyroidism, vitamin $B_{12}$ deficiency

## Discussion

Mrs. Washburn has many of the early signs and symptoms of dementia such as confusion, forgetfulness, balance problems, depression, memory loss, and disorientation. She also has a positive family history for AD. However, she has some indications of hypothyroidism (enlarged thyroid, dry skin, slow pulse, fatigue, hair loss, anorexia, constipation), so this should be ruled out. In addition, her age, pallor, fatigue, cool skin, and decreased reflexes suggest vitamin $B_{12}$

*(Case study continued on page 458)*

deficiency, although it is rare for this degree of dementia to result entirely from vitamin B$_{12}$ deficiency. Because she has HTN with LVH, she is at risk for cerebral infarction. She has had two significant, previous head injuries, which increases her risk for AD or for brain injury from the previous concussion. Finally, it is important to determine if her depression is the primary problem, although her symptoms are more consistent with AD than with depression.

Her workup needs to include more extensive neuropsychiatric testing with standardized instruments used with dementia patients, CT scan, spinal tap, blood chemistries, thyroid scan, CBC, vitamin B$_{12}$ levels, and, possibly, genetic testing for ApoE g-4.

AD, Alzheimer's disease; ApoE g-4, apolipoprotein E g-4; BP, blood pressure; BS, bowel sounds; CBC, complete blood count; CT, computed tomography; CV, cardiovascular; CVA, costovertebral angle; DTRs, deep tendon reflexes; ECG, electrocardiogram; GI, gastrointestinal; GU, genitourinary; HEENT, head, eyes, ears, nose, and throat; HR, heart rate; HTN, hypertension; LOC, loss of consciousness; LVH, left ventricular hypertrophy; MS, musculoskeletal; MVA, motor vehicle accident; NKDA, no known drug allergies; P, pulse; R, respiration; SOB, shortness of breath; T, temperature; TMs, typanic membranes; UTIs, urinary tract infections; WNL, within normal limits.

## REFERENCES

Caselli, R. & Boeve, B. (1999). The degenerative dementias. In C. Goetz & E. Pappert (Eds.), *Textbook of clinical neurology* (1st ed.). Philadelphia: W.B. Saunders.

Devanand, D.P., Sano, M., Tang, M.X., Taylor, S., Gurland, B.J., Wilder, D., Stern, Y., & Mayeux, R. (1996). Depressed mood and the incidence of Alzheimer's disease in the elderly living in the community. *Archives of General Psychiatry, 53* (2), 175–182.

Devanand, D.P., Jacobs, D.M., Tang, M.X., Del Castillo-Castaneda, C., Sano, M., Marder, K., Bell, K., Bylsma, F.W., Brandt, J., Albert, M., & Stern, Y. (1997). The course of psychopathologic features in mild to moderate alzheimer disease. *Archives of General Psychiatry, 54,* 257–263.

Dobson, C.B. & Itzhaki, R.F. (1999). Herpes simplex virus type 1 and Alzheimer's disease. *Neurobiology of Aging, 20* (4), 457–465.

Farlow, M.R. (1999). Therapeutic advances for Alzheimer's disease and other dementias. Available at: http://www. medscape.com.

Galasko, D., Clark, C., Chang, L., Miller, B., Green, R.C., Motter, R., & Seubert, P. (1997). Assessment of CSF Levels of tau protein in mildly demented patients with Alzheimer's disease. *Neurology, 48,* 632–635.

Geddes, J.F., Vowles, G.H., Nicoll, J.A., & Revesz, T. (1999). Neuronal cytoskeletal changes are an early consequence of repetitive head injury. *Acta Neuropathologica, 98* (2), 171–178.

Graves, A.B., Rosner, D., Echeverria, D., Yost, M., & Larson, E.B. (1999). Occupational exposure to electromagnetic fields and Alzheimer disease. *Alzheimer Disease Association Disorders, 13* (3), 165–170.

Helmer, C., Damon, D., Letenneur, L., Fabrigoule, C., Barberger-Gateau, P., Lafont, S., Fuhrer, R., Antonucci, T., Commenges, D., Orgogozo, J.M., & Dartigues, J.F. (1999). Marital status and risk of Alzheimer's disease: A French population-based cohort study. *Neurology, 53* (9), 1953–1958.

Masliah, E., Mallory, M., Hansen, L., Alford, M., Albright, T., DeTeresa, R. Terry, R., Boudier, J., & Saiton, T. (1991).

Patterns of aberrant sprouting in Alzheimer's disease. *Neuron, 6,* 729–739.

McKhann, G., Drachman, D., Folstein, M., et al. (1984). Clinical diagnosis of Alzheimer's disease: Report of the NMINCDA-ADRDA Work Group under the auspices of the Department of Health and Human Services Task Force on Alzheimer's Disease. *Neurology, 34,* 939–944.

McNeil, C. (1999). Alzheimers disease: Unraveling the mystery. http://www.alzheimers.org/unravel.html.

Meier-Ruge, W.A. & Bertoni-Freddari, C. (1999). Mitochondrial genome lesions in the pathogenesis of sporadic Alzheimer's disease. *Gerontology, 45* (5), 289–297.

New York Access to Online Health (NOAH) (1999). Alzheimer's disease: Well connected [NIDUS information services]. Available at: http://www.noah.cuny.edu/well-conn/alzheimers.html.

O'Meara, E.S., Kukull, W.A., Sheppard, L., Bowen, J.D., McCormick, W.C., Teri, L., Pfanschmidt, M., Thompson, J.D., Schellenberg, G.D., & Larson, E.B. (1997). Head injury and risk of Alzheimer's disease by apolipoprotein E genotype. *American Journal of Epidemiology, 146* (5), 373–384.

Pearson, R.C., Esiri, M., Hiorns, R., Wilcock, G., & Powell. T.P. (1985). Anatomical correlates of the distribution of the pathological changes in the neocortex in Alzheimer's disease. *Proceedings of the National Academy of Sciences, 82,* 4531–4534.

Perl, D.P. & Good, P.F. (1992). Auminium and the neurofibrillary tangle: Results of tissue microprobe studies. *Ciba Foundation Symposium, 169,* 217–236.

Saxe, S.R., Wekstein, M.W., Kryscio, R.J., Henry, R.G, Cornett, C.R., Snowdon, D.A., Grant, F.T., Schmitt, F.A., Donegan, S.J., Wekstein, D.R., Ehmann, W.D., & Markesbery, W.R. (1999). Alzheimer's disease, dental amalgam and mercury. *Journal of the American Dental Association, 130* (2), 191–199.

Smith, M.A. & Perry, G. (1999). Oxidative stress is central to the pathogenesis of Alzheimer's disease [On-line forums]. Available at: http://www.alzforum.org/members/forums/hypotheses/index.html.

Snowdon, D.A. (1996). Linguistic ability in early life and cognitive function and Alzheimer's disease in late life:

Findings from the Nun Study. *Journal of the American Medical Association, 275,* 528–532

Sobel, E., Dunn, M., Davanipour, Z., Qian, Z., & Chui, H.C. (1996). Elevated risk of Alzheimer's disease among workers with likely electromagnetic field exposure. *Neurology, 47* (6), 1477–1481.

St. George-Hyslop, P.H. (1994). The molecular genetics of Alzheimer's disease. In R.D. Terry, R. Katzman, & K.L. Bick (Eds.), *Alzheimer's disease.* New York: Raven Press.

Tanzi, R.E., Kovacs, D.M., Kim, T., Moir, A., Guenette, S., & Wasco, W. (1996). The presenilin genes and their role in early-onset familial Alzheimer's disease. *Alzheimer's Disease Reviews, 1,* 96–98.

Waring S., Rocca, W., Petersen, R., O'Brien, P., Tangalos, E., & Kokmen, E. (1999). Postmenopausal estrogen replacement therapy and risk of AD: A population-based study. *Neurology, 52,* 965–970.

# INDEX

NOTE: A *t* following a page number indicates tabular material, an *f* following a page number indicates a figure, and a *v* following a page number indicates a clinical vignette. Insofar as possible, drugs are listed under their generic names. When a drug trade name is listed, the reader is referred to the generic name.